Updates in Clinical Dermatology

Series Editors

John Berth-Jones, University Hospitals Coventry & Warwickshire,
NHS Trust, Coventry, UK

Chee Leok Goh, National Skin Centre, Singapore, Singapore

Howard I. Maibach, Department of Dermatology
University of California San Francisco Department of Dermatology
ALAMEDA, CA, USA

Shari R. Lipner, Dermatology, Weill Cornell Medicine
New York, NY, USA

Updates in Clinical Dermatology aims to promote the rapid and efficient transfer of medical research into clinical practice. It is published in four volumes per year. Covering new developments and innovations in all fields of clinical dermatology, it provides the clinician with a review and summary of recent research and its implications for clinical practice. Each volume is focused on a clinically relevant topic and explains how research results impact diagnostics, treatment options and procedures as well as patient management. The reader-friendly volumes are highly structured with core messages, summaries, tables, diagrams and illustrations and are written by internationally well-known experts in the field. A volume editor supervises the authors in his/her field of expertise in order to ensure that each volume provides cutting-edge information most relevant and useful for clinical dermatologists. Contributions to the series are peer reviewed by an editorial board.

Wanda Robles

Editor

Skin Disease in Travelers

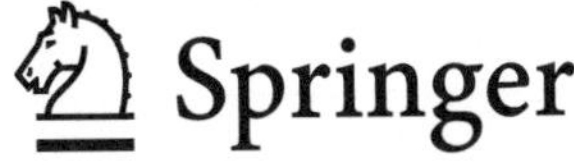 Springer

Editor
Wanda Robles
Royal Free Hospitals NHS Trust
London, UK

ISSN 2523-8884   ISSN 2523-8892   (electronic)
Updates in Clinical Dermatology

ISBN 978-3-031-57838-0   ISBN 978-3-031-57836-6   (eBook)
https://doi.org/10.1007/978-3-031-57836-6

This Springer imprint is published by the registered company Springer Nature Switzerland AG
The registered company address is: Gewerbestrasse 11, 6330 Cham, Switzerland

If disposing of this product, please recycle the paper.

Dedicated to my husband Ken and to my children Daniel, Otto and James

Foreword

One of the major features of our changing world is the regular movement of individuals and groups from one region to another. In some cases, this reflects the ease of travel leading, in turn, to large numbers of tourists leaving their home environment to visit different regions and people. There has also been an increase of movement for a different reason, in that wars, civil unrest and natural disasters have led to large numbers of people fleeing their homes and seeking refuge in other countries; in other cases, the motivation for travel is to escape from a cycle of poverty and deprivation. Whatever the reasons the consequences are that the full range of human disease follows these trends leading to people presenting with illnesses in another country where health workers are often unfamiliar with disease common or endemic in a different part of the world. This is not simply restricted to encounters with infectious diseases; it also extends to physical reactions to different climates, hot and cold, as well as the different elements that make up those climatic zones from jungles to mountains to seas and lakes. All these environments are associated with the need to address different and unfamiliar diseases, presentations and treatments.

The skin, being the largest organ of the human body and the site exposed to the natural environment, is often the first place where these diseases are seen. They range from infections, which are normally confined to specific regions now presenting in outside their normal endemic area to the consequences of overcrowding and deprivation amongst large mobile populations which also lead to dermatological diseases such as scabies and leishmaniasis.

This book addresses all these issues. Written by subject experts in the different areas, it draws a comprehensive picture of a range of infections presenting in the skin caused by bacteria, virus, fungi and parasites as well as the skin signs that develop as a consequence of encounters with different climates; these include cold injury as well as infections and trauma associated with swimming in unfamiliar seas. It addresses the pathology, the clinical manifestations and treatment of these imported diseases and, as such, will be useful for both dermatologists and non-dermatologists; it addresses the full range of conditions experienced by travellers and migrants. This book is a welcome addition to more conventional works on skin disease, while helping to inform those encountering the new and less familiar manifestations of skin disease that result from travel.

Professor (Emeritus) of Cutaneous Infection Roderick Hay
King's College,
London, UK

Preface

With the increased ability of people to travel around the world, a great number of skin diseases, mainly infectious, can be acquired by travellers. These may represent a challenge not just to the medical community but particularly to dermatologists. Signs and symptoms may be nonspecific. Furthermore, many infections by different organisms may share a similar set of signs and symptoms making definitive diagnosis even more difficult. Whenever possible, this is achieved only in isolation or demonstration of the causative organism. However, this can be very difficult if the diagnosis is not considered, on clinical suspicion by the physician. Though infectious skin diseases should be high in the differential diagnosis at presentation of any traveller with skin disease, there are also some conditions produced by physical agents, for example, exposure to extreme temperatures: heat or cold.

The aim of this book is to raise awareness in the medical world in order to consider a potential infectious cause for many of the skin rashes in travellers, as well as over exposure to different climatic conditions. It also aims to give advice on potential ways of prevention but foremost to acquaint the physician with the different signs and symptoms of skin diseases in travellers, as well as the best available treatments. I very much believe this book will be a valuable contribution to all medical communities including young and experienced physicians as well as junior and senior dermatologists.

Contributors are from 14 different countries, all of whom have a special interest and outstanding expertise in their particular field or disease, confirming that this book in the series is an international effort. I am very grateful to my mentor Professor Rod Hay and my colleague John Berth-Jones for encouraging me to take on this task.

London, UK   Wanda Robles

Contents

Influence of the New Environment on the Skin

Environmental Related Skin Disorders in Immigrants and Tourists

A. L. Nguyen and S. Badeloe

Key Points

- A new environment can induce a wide variety of skin disorders in people travelling between different global climates (tropical, arid, temperate, cold, and polar).
- Skin disorders can occur in travellers due to interaction between genetic and biological traits of the individual, on the one hand, and changes in environmental factors (i.e. physical factors, biological and immunological factors, social and cultural factors), on the other hand.
- Physical environmental factors in a climate include low humidity and dry environment, hot and humid environment, sunlight/ultraviolet radiation, cold environment, and water hardness.
- Changes in biological and immunological environmental factors can induce new infectious skin disorders in travellers, such as varicella zoster virus infection and strongyloidiasis.
- Social and cultural factors may lead to skin problems in the new environment; this includes habits such as sunbathing and skin bleaching.
- Climate change causes global warming, leading to higher average temperatures, changes in humidity and precipitation. This can lead to increased cutaneous infectious diseases, marine dermatoses, pollution-induced or aggravated skin disorders, and skin cancer.

Introduction

Worldwide travel has increased enormously; according to the United Nations World Tourism Organization, the estimated tourist arrivals were 25 million in 1950, which has increased 56-fold to 1.4 billion international arrivals per year in 2018. Europe is the most important touristic region and accounts for about half of the international travel, followed by Asia & Pacific (24.5%), America (15.5%), Africa (4.8%), and Middle East (4.6%) [1]. Not only tourists but also business travellers, researchers, volunteers, immigrants, refugees etcetera contribute to the worldwide travel, which can occur between different climatic zones across the globe.

The term 'climate' encompasses the composite or generally prevailing weather conditions in an area over a long time such as temperature, air pressure, humidity, precipitation, sunshine, cloudiness, and wind [2]. Global climates can be

A. L. Nguyen (✉) · S. Badeloe
Department of Dermatology, Leiden University Medical Center, ZA, Leiden, The Netherlands
e-mail: a.l.nguyen@lumc.nl; s.badeloe@lumc.nl

© The Editor(s) (if applicable) and The Author(s), under exclusive license to Springer Nature Switzerland AG 2024
W. Robles (ed.), *Skin Disease in Travelers*, Updates in Clinical Dermatology,
https://doi.org/10.1007/978-3-031-57836-6_1

divided into five types according to the Köppen-Geiger climate classification system: tropical (A), arid (B), temperate (C), cold (D), and polar (E) (Fig. 1). In tropical climate, the mean temperature of all months exceeds 18 °C (64.4 ° F) combined with significant amount of precipitation. An arid climate is hot (mean annual temperature ≥ 18 °C) or cold (mean annual temperature < 18 °C) with little precipitation. A temperate climate has a temperature between 0 °C (32 ° F) and 18 °C in the coldest month and a temperature of >10 °C (50 °F) in the hottest month and with a variable amount of precipitation determining the dryness of a season. A temperate climate can be subdivided into several subclimates such as Mediterranean climate with dry summers, humid subtropical climates with hot humid summers and mild winters, and oceanic climates without a dry season. Cold climate has a temperature of >10 °C in the hottest month and ≤ 0 °C in the coldest month, which can be further subdivided in numerous subclimates without dry season, with dry summers, and dry

winters. In polar climate, the temperature in the hottest month is ≤10 °C. Figure 1 illustrates different type of climates for all countries across the world according to the Köppen-Geiger climate classification [3].

All types of travellers including immigrants, refugees, tourists can travel across the world between countries with different climatic zones, for instance they can travel from a (sub)tropical climatic zone to a temperate, cold or polar climatic zone, and vice versa. Travelling between these five climatic zones can induce numerous infectious and non-infectious skin disorders due to several environmental factors, which can be subdivided in:

1. Physical factors, e.g. ambient temperature (heat, cold), degree of humidity (dryness, moistness), amount of precipitation, sunlight, ultraviolet (UV) radiation, and water hardness.
2. Biological and immunological factors, e.g. micro-organisms.

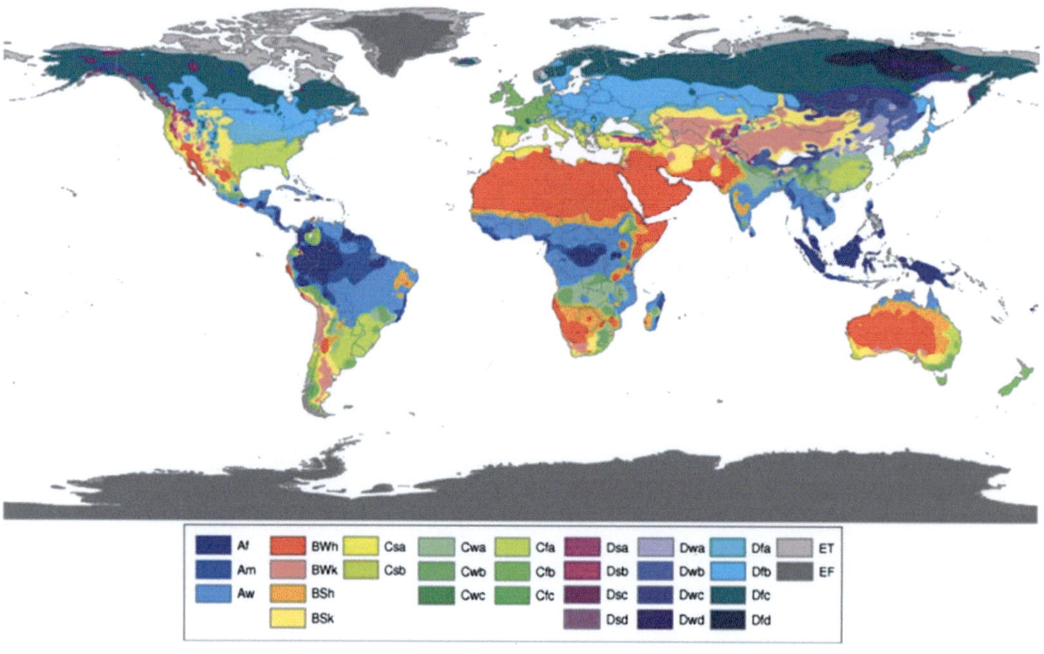

Fig. 1 Köppen-Geiger climate classification (1980–2016). Main climates: (**a**) (tropical): f (rainforest), m (monsoon), w (savannah) (**b**) (arid): W (desert), S (steppe); temperature h (hot) or k (cold) (**c**) (temperate) and (**d**) (cold): s (dry summer), w (dry winter), f (without dry season); temperature a (hot summer), b (warm summer), c (cool summer), d (very cold winter) (**e**) (polar): f (frost), T (tundra). Figure was adopted from *Peel* et al [3]

3. Social and cultural factors, e.g. cultural habits such as bathing habits and skin bleaching.

Other non-environmental factors determining the development of skin diseases are the structure and function of the skin, genetic constitution, and psychological factors, including behaviour. The interaction between factors present in a certain climatic zone, on the one hand, and biological traits and behaviour of the individual, on the other hand, can induce 'new' skin disorders in individuals that originated from different climatic zones.

This chapter discusses skin disorders induced by change in environment and climatic zone or to be more precise: the lack of adaptation to the new environment. We will also discuss specific skin disorders physicians should be aware of when treating immigrants and refugees, as they will experience a long-term and possibly a permanent change in climatic environment. In this chapter, we will discuss few disorders as an example of this topic. Tropical infectious disorders that can occur in (returning) travellers will be discussed in chapter "Cellulitis and Erysipelas".

Skin Function and Racial Differences

The skin primarily serves as a barrier against the external environment. The epidermis is the outer layer of the skin, which mainly consists of keratinocytes. It undergoes a continuous process of regeneration, proliferation, and desquamation. The skin barrier is maintained by formation of tight junctions and desmosomes between the keratinocytes. The stratum corneum is the outer layer of the epidermis and consists of corneocytes, lipids, and proteins. The tight lipid barrier and desmosomes between the corneocytes protect the skin, like a brick wall, to prevent trans epidermal water loss (TEWL) and penetration by micro-organisms (e.g. bacteria, viruses, fungi), allergens, toxins, and irritants. The corneocytes also contain a natural moisturising factor (a mixture of hygroscopic amino acids resulting from filaggrin breakdown), which is essential for skin hydration, water retention within the stratum corneum, and plasticity of the skin. An impaired skin barrier function is associated with increased TEWL and low corneum water content, which leads to dry skin. Another main function of the skin is thermoregulation. Skin blood flow plays an important factor in thermoregulation; vasodilatation and vasoconstriction of the cutaneous vasculature help regulate heat loss. Evaporation of water through skin and respiratory tract reduces excess heat from the body. However, in hot and humid conditions evaporation can become ineffective in releasing heat into the environment.

Structure and function of the skin in people originating from tropical countries are in some aspects different compared to people from a temperate, less sunny climate. Skin colour is a complex adaptive trait facilitated by a particular environment: natural selection influences genetic and phenotypic diversity in humans. In a wide range of geographical populations, several genetic differences associated with skin colour variation have been identified [4]. Skin colour is highly correlated with geographical latitude and ultimately UV radiation, therefore people living closer to the equator (0° latitude) tend to have darker pigmented skin [4, 5]. Darker skin contains larger and more numerous melanosomes, which are more evenly distributed throughout the epidermis, and also has a higher eumelanin to pheomelanin ratio. Eumelanin absorbs lights, prevents the formation of free radical species, protects against UV light, and lowers the risk of UV induced carcinogenesis [6]. Lighter skin has a lower melanin content, smaller melanosomes mostly located (supra)basal in the epidermis, higher pheomelanin content, and higher penetration of UV light to the upper dermis. People living at higher latitudes, north or south of the equator, tend to have paler skin to ensure adequate absorption of UV rays to maximize vitamin D synthesis in the basal layer of the epidermis, however they are also more prone to phototoxic reactions and UV-induced carcinogenesis [4–6]. In addition to skin colour variation in humans across the world, other anatomical differences related to skin type have been identified. For instance, the TEWL appears to be greater in black skin compared to white skin and the desquamation rate is 2.5 times higher compared to Caucasians and Asians [7]. Also the stratum corneum of black people appeared to be more compact than that of white people, reflecting a stronger intercellular cohesion [5]. This may be responsible for the fact that continuous scratching in black people often leads to lichenification. Black skin also contains larger mast cell granules compared to white skin, which could account for differences in pruritus sensation between these groups [7]. The skin surface pH is lower in black people, and they appear to have larger apocrine sweat glands and in greater numbers compared to white people [5, 7]. Racial differences with regard to other skin properties such as water content, corneocyte variability, blood vessel variability, elastic recovery, lipid content, and surface microflora are inconclusive and often contradictory [7].

Skin Disorders Due to Physical Environmental Factors

A seasonal variation is often seen in a variety of skin disorders such as atopic dermatitis, psoriasis, acne, miliaria, polymorphic light eruption, lupus erythematosus, fungal dermatitis, and perniosis [2]. The conditions of a certain climate such as temperature and humidity influence skin disorders by affecting the skin barrier function. Several studies have reported that low humidity causes a decrease in skin hydration, initial increase in TEWL, decreased elasticity of the skin, increased dryness of skin and complaints such as pruritus and irritation [8]. Eventually, the TEWL will decrease under dry conditions and declining temperatures [9]. Furthermore, studies have shown that skin symptoms improve with increasing absolute and relative humidity. A low temperature decreases skin hydration, which leads to dry skin and increased sensation of itchiness [8]. Also short- and long-term effects of change in climate for, respectively, tourists and immigrants can influence symptoms of atopic dermatitis, for instance flares of atopic dermatitis

occur more frequently under cold and dry weather conditions. A higher prevalence of paediatric eczema was seen in American states with low humidity, low UV exposure, low outdoor temperature, indoor heating, and increased precipitation. The combination of high UV exposure and high outdoor temperature with low indoor heating demonstrated a protective effect against eczema, whilst combined high humidity and precipitation with low UV exposure were associated with increased eczema prevalence [10].

In this paragraph, we focus on skin disorders that can develop in all types of travellers (including immigrants, refugees and tourists) due to a change in climatic zone, for instance from a cold climate to a (sub)tropical climate and vice versa. We shall discuss a few examples of skin disorders that can develop due to different physical environmental factors in a certain climate, such as low humidity and dry environment, a hot and humid environment, sunlight / UV radiation, cold environment, and water hardness (Table 1).

Low Humidity and Dry Environment

Dry Skin and Asteatotic Eczema

Dry skin or xerosis is one of the most common skin disorders in immigrants originally from a (sub)tropical climate migrating to a temperate climatic zone. Dry skin and subsequently asteatotic eczema (eczéma craquelé) can develop very soon after arrival, especially during wintertime due to low environmental humidity caused by cold, dry weather, and central heating. Dry skin can also develop or worsen due to prolonged and excessive showering and bathing, especially with hot water and excessive use of soap. Racial differences in skin properties of immigrants can also explain certain differences in susceptibility to the development of dry skin or asteatotic eczema. The increased TEWL in black skin could explain the increased frequency of xerosis cutis in individuals with black skin [7].

The signs of the dry skin syndrome range from mild to severe: dry scaly skin, ichthyosiform skin (Fig. 2), and asteatotic eczema (mildly infiltrated erythematous scaling plaques with

Table 1 Skin disorders related to physical environmental factors

Low humidity and dry environment	Hot and humid environment	Sunlight/ultraviolet radiation	Cold environment
Itch Dry skin Ichthyosiform skin Asteatotic eczema	Miliaria Bacterial infections Viral infections Fungal infections Yeast infections Parasitic infections Mycobacterial infections	*Idiopathic, probably immunologically mediated photodermatoses* – Polymorphic light eruption. – Juvenile spring time eruption. – Solar urticaria. – Chronic actinic dermatitis. – Actinic prurigo. – Hydroa vacciniforme. *Photodermatoses caused by exogenous sensitizers* – Phototoxicity including phytophotodermatitis. – Photo-allergy contact dermatitis. *Photoaggravated dermatoses*	Raynaud phenomenon Livedo reticularis Acrocyanosis Erythrocyanosis Perniones (chilblains) Cold erythema Cold urticaria Cold agglutinins Cold panniculitis Cryoglobulinaemia

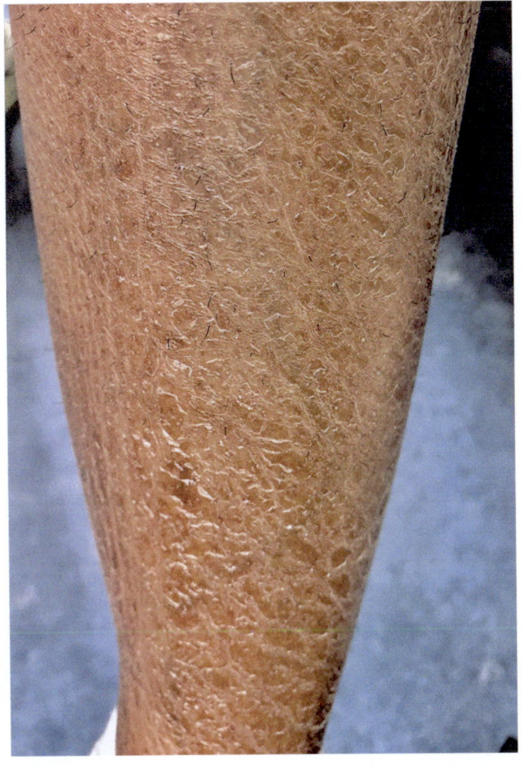

Fig. 2 Ichthyosiform skin

characteristic polygonal cracks and superficial fissuring). If the skin is dark, the erythema cannot be identified. Symptoms are a 'dry feeling', pruritus (sometimes severe and even causing sleep disturbances), and sometimes pain. The disorder most commonly involves upper and lower extremities, but can be localized anywhere on the body including the face, especially the lips. This diagnosis can be easily made on clinical grounds. However, it should be differentiated from other types of eczema, e.g. contact and atopic dermatitis, as other forms of eczema can be worsened by dry skin. A secondary infection can occur as a complication of the eczema.

Management of dry skin consists of humidifying the environment and adjusting bathing habits. Patients should decrease the frequency and duration of showering, use lukewarm (not hot) water, use oily-based products instead of soap, gently dry the skin with a towel; patting is better than rubbing and use of a hydrating ointment after drying the skin. Emollient ointments, with or without urea, should be used abundant and multiple times a day and continued as maintenance therapy to prevent recurrences. The eczema needs intermittent treatment with a topical corticosteroid ointment (class 2 or 3).

Hot and Humid Environment

We will discuss miliaria as an example of skin disorder that can occur in travellers in a hot and humid environment. A hot and humid environment can also induce skin disorders caused by bacteria (e.g. pyoderma, impetigo, erysipelas/cellulitis), fungi and yeast infections (e.g. pityriasis versicolor, mycoses), these will be discussed in chapter "Ecthyma".

Miliaria

Miliaria (prickly heat) is a disorder caused by blockage of the eccrine sweat duct. Miliaria is a common disorder in tourists visiting a hot and humid climate. It can develop within a few days after arrival. Three subtypes of miliaria can be distinguished dependent on the level of obstruction:

1. Miliaria crystallina: sweat duct blockage is located in the stratum corneum. It presents with thin-walled superficial, clear vesicles of 1–2 mm, that easily rupture. There is no inflammation or erythema. The lesions are asymptomatic.
2. Miliaria rubra: sweat duct blockage is located in the epidermis. This the most common type, which is characterized by itchy or stinging non-follicular papules or papulovesicles, on erythematous background. Miliaria pustulosa is a variant in which pustules form. A secondary bacterial infection, usually caused by staphylococci, can occur and may lead to sweat gland abscesses.
3. Miliaria profunda: sweat duct blockage is located at the dermo-epidermal junction, causing leakage of sweat in surrounding tissues. This presents as erythematous to skin-coloured non-follicular firm papules of 1–4 mm. Due to deep obstruction of the sweat ducts little to no sweating occurs at affected sites.

The lesions are most commonly localized in friction areas with clothing or occluded sites such as flexural areas, head-neck region, and upper trunk. Sweating is the most important means of heat regulation in a hot environment and blockage of sweating can cause hyperthermia, heat exhaustion and eventually heatstroke with malaise, nausea and vomiting, tachycardia, dyspnoea, and ultimately cardiovascular collapse. Miliaria is generally easily diagnosed; however, it must be differentiated from folliculitis, herpes simplex virus, varicella, acne, or insect bites.

Management of miliaria is primarily aimed at minimizing sweating and obstruction of sweat ducts by means of a cooler (air-conditioned) environment, cool baths, or showers combined with daily gentle exfoliation and wearing breathable non-occlusive clothing. Miliaria rubra can be treated with topical corticosteroids to decrease the pruritus and inflammation. Topical or oral antibiotics can be needed in case of a secondary bacterial infection. These disorders normally disappear within a few days after arrival in a cooler climate.

Sunlight/UV Radiation

Solar radiation is composed of three components of the electromagnetic spectrum: UV radiation, visible light, and infrared radiation. UV radiation can be subdivided based on wavelength into UVA (400–320 nm), UVB (320–290 nm), and UVC (290–200 nm). A higher wavelength can penetrate deeper into the skin. During a holiday in a (sub)tropical climate, short-term effects of UV radiation can cause sunburn (UVB > UVA) and tanning (immediate tanning: mostly UVA; delayed tanning: UVB). UVB exposure induces epidermal hyperplasia, which relatively protects the skin from UV radiation. Furthermore, UV radiation also leads to vitamin D synthesis, pro-inflammatory responses, and immunosuppression. UVC is filtered by the atmosphere and very little reaches the earth's surface. Photodermatoses can develop due to exposure to specific wavelengths of electromagnetic radiation. Skin disorders caused by solar radiation in tourists, and other travellers can be categorized in three main groups: idiopathic or immunologically mediated photodermatoses, photodermatoses caused by exogenous sensitizers, and photoaggravated dermatoses.

Idiopathic, Probably Immunologically Mediated Photodermatoses

The group of idiopathic, probably immunologically mediated photodermatoses comprises of the following more common disorders such as polymorphous light eruption, solar urticaria, chronic actinic dermatitis and actinic prurigo. As an example, we will discuss the occurrence of polymorphous light eruption in travellers.

Polymorphous Light Eruption

Polymorphous light eruption is a recurrent delayed-type hypersensitivity response to sunlight. It usually occurs in the spring and early summer in temperate climates, but it can also occur after sudden intense sun exposure during a holiday in a (sub)tropical climate. The occurrence is more frequent at higher latitudes. In the United States, blacks more frequently have polymorphous light eruption than Caucasians [11–13]. Symptoms present as symmetric pruritic skin-coloured to red papules, papulovesicles, and plaques on sun-exposed skin. In darker skin types, 1–2 mm pinpoint papules a more frequently seen, which constitute a morphologic pinpoint variant of polymorphous light eruption. In case of initial sunlight exposure, these symptoms can develop after 30 min up to 2–3 days, whilst after repeated sun exposure it can already present as soon as after 10 min up to several hours. After avoidance of sunlight, the skin eruption usually resolves in a few days to 2 weeks. The differential diagnosis consists of solar urticaria, cutaneous lupus, and photoallergic contact dermatitis.

The treatment for polymorphous light eruption consists of sun avoidance and adequate photoprotection (e.g. broad spectrum photoprotection, hats, clothing). It can also be preventively treated through photohardening of the skin, preferably with narrow-band UVB in early spring. A mild to moderate eruption can be treated with topical corticosteroids, whilst a severe eruption may require short courses of oral corticosteroids, antimalarial agents (i.e. hydroxychloroquine), or in rare cases azathioprine or ciclosporin.

Photodermatoses Caused by Exogenous Sensitizers

Travellers visiting a (sub)tropical climatic zone are exposed to a greater amount of UV radiation, which could lead to photosensitivity due to exogenous drugs and chemicals that can present as phototoxicity or a photoallergy.

Phototoxicity develops after exposure to UV radiation (UVA > UVB) and a photosensitive agent that has been ingested or applied to the skin, which causes direct tissue and cellular damage to the skin through a non-immunological mechanism. These reactions present as exaggerated sunburn, usually appear within minutes to hours after sun exposure. In severe cases, vesicles and bullae may develop. A phytophotodermatitis is a form of phototoxicity caused by contact with photosensitizing substances in plants. It is mainly caused by furocoumarin-containing plants such as (giant) hogweed, parsnip, dill, fennel, parsley, celery, lime, lemon, and fig. This can induce a reaction consisting of pruritic, burning or painful erythema, oedema, vesicles, and bullae in linear streaky configurations on sun-exposed skin, healing with post-inflammatory hyperpigmentation.

Photoallergy is a delayed-type hypersensitivity reaction to a photoallergen on sun-exposed skin. This type develops after 24–48 h of sun exposure and usually presents as a pruritic eczematous eruption on sun-exposed areas.

The extensive list of photosensitive drugs includes tetracyclines (especially doxycycline), diuretics, nonsteroidal anti-inflammatory drugs, sulphonamides, metformin, amiodarone, hydroxychloroquine, psoralens, retinoids, and azathioprine. Examples of topical photosensitizing agents are sunscreens, fragrances, nonsteroidal anti-inflammatory drugs, dyes, and psoralens. Phototests and photopatch test can be performed in order to identify the offending agent. These photosensitivity reactions should be differentiated from chronic actinic dermatitis, porphyria cutanea tarda, lupus erythematosus, or solar urticaria.

Management consists of cessation or avoidance of the offending drug or chemical, sun avoidance and adequate sun protection with broad-spectrum sunscreens and (UV-)protective clothing. Symptomatic treatment with emollients and topical corticosteroids may be needed to reduce pruritus and the inflammatory response.

Photoaggravated Dermatoses

Photoaggravated dermatoses are skin disorders that can be exacerbated by UV radiation or visible light. A change in climate to a (sub)tropical or sunny temperate climatic zone can cause exacerbation of existing skin disorders due to a greater exposure to sunlight. The list of photoaggravated dermatoses is extensive and includes acne, atopic dermatitis, bullous pemphigoid, disseminated superficial actinic porokeratosis, erythema multiforme, Hailey-Hailey disease, Darier disease, dermatomyositis, Grover's disease, herpes simplex infection, lichen planus, lupus erythematosus, melasma, pemphigus, pityriasis rubra pilaris, and rosacea. Some skin disorders such as atopic dermatitis generally improve with sun exposure and also respond to treatment with phototherapy; however, a minority of patients with atopic dermatitis can experience aggravation due to sun exposure.

Management of these photodermatoses consists of adequate photoprotection and treatment of the underlying skin disorder.

Lack of Exposure to Sunlight and UV Radiation

Lack of exposure to sunlight and subsequent UVB radiation can lead to a vitamin D deficiency, which is common in Europe and the Middle East [14]. Non-western immigrants or refugees usually have darker skin, which requires more UVB to produce vitamin D. A higher latitude, winter season, and shorter duration and exposure to sunlight negatively influence the amount of vitamin D that can be produced in the skin [15]. A poor vitamin D status was observed in non-Western immigrants, therefore it has been advocated that vitamin D supplements should be considered in order to prevent the consequences of vitamin D deficiency such as rickets in children and osteomalacia in adults [14]. It is well known that sunlight exposure can reduce disease severity in several skin disorders such as atopic dermatitis, psoriasis, and vitiligo, whilst the lack thereof can lead to exacerbations [16].

Psoriasis

Psoriasis is a common chronic relapsing inflammatory skin disorder with a genetic component. Worldwide prevalence is estimated at approximately 1–3%; however, the prevalence is quite variable depending on ethnicity and geographic areas. The prevalence rate appears to be higher in whites compared with non-white ethnic groups.

It has been noted that psoriasis is more common in people from South Asian descent than people from African descent. Also, within Africa, a wide variation has been reported with higher prevalence in Eastern Africa (1.9–3.5%) compared to western Africa (0.025–0.9%) [17]. Overall, psoriasis is more common in the colder northern climates than in tropical climates [18]. The clinical course of psoriasis in immigrants could be negatively influenced by environmental triggers in the new environment such as cold weather, low humidity, less exposure to sunlight and UV radiation, and psychological stress related to life in a new environment. Immigrants from (sub)tropical countries can also have their first episode of psoriasis after arriving in a temperate climate.

Chronic plaque psoriasis, the most common form of psoriasis, is characterized by sharply demarcated indurated erythematous plaques with a coarse silvery scale. The typical localizations are the scalp, extensor sides of elbows, knees, and sacral region, but lesions can appear on virtually any part of the body. In 30% of patients, the lesions are not or slightly itchy. In black patients, psoriasis lesions are less erythematous, more violaceous, or hyperpigmented, plaques appear to be thicker with more scaling and affected body surface area tend to be more extensive. In dark skin, active lesions more frequently resolve with hyper- or hypopigmentation, which can make it difficult to distinguish active lesions from postinflammatory dyspigmentation [17]. The clinical characteristics are usually sufficient to diagnose psoriasis. However, darker skin can make it challenging to determine the right diagnosis; postinflammatory hyperpigmentation, nummular eczema, neurodermatitis circumscripta, dermatophytosis, lichen planus, and parapsoriasis should be considered. Histopathological investigation can sometimes be helpful.

Treatment for psoriasis is diverse and consists of topical therapies (corticosteroids, vitamin D analogues, combination corticosteroid-vitamin D analogues, calcineurin inhibitors), phototherapy, systemic medications, and biological therapies. Physicians should be aware of the country of origin and travel history of immigrants and refugees as they should be adequately screened for various endemic infectious diseases such as tuberculosis, human immunodeficiency virus, hepatitis B and C before starting immunosuppressive therapies.

Cold Environment

A cold, damp, and non-freezing environment with a shortage or lack of sunlight (visible and UV-radiation) can induce new skin disorders or worsen existing skin disorders in immigrants from (sub)tropical countries moving to a temperate climatic zone.

Cold-induced disorders consists of acrocyanosis, perniosis (chilblains), Raynaud's phenomenon, livedo reticularis, cold urticaria, cold panniculitis, and cryoglobulinemia. As an example, we will discuss perniosis in travellers. Other cold-induced skin disorders will be discussed in chapter "Cold Injuries".

Perniosis

Perniosis presents as cold-induced erythrocyanotic lesions on skin vulnerable to cold exposure. It is caused by an abnormal vascular reaction to cold in probably genetically predisposed persons. Immigrants or refugees from (sub)tropical countries, not using gloves and wearing inadequate footwear in cold seasons are prone to developing perniosis.

It is a common disorder that occurs during the cold months of the year. The clinical signs are erythematous to blue-violet macules, papules, plaques, or nodules on the hands or feet. It can also affect the nose, ears, calves, thighs, or buttocks. Sometimes blisters and ulceration can occur. The symptoms are pruritus, burning, and pain. It must be differentiated from other cold-induced disorders with similar symptoms, like acrocyanosis, chilblain lupus erythematosus, and lupus pernio (a variant of sarcoidosis). It typically resolves in 1 to 3 weeks.

The management of perniosis is primarily targeted at avoiding exposure to cold by wearing adequate and warm gloves, clothes, and footwear. In recalcitrant cases, treatment with nifedipine, a calcium antagonist with vasodilatory properties, can be effective in terms of accelerated clearance of existing skin lesions and prevention of new perniosis lesions [19].

Water Hardness

Hard water contains a high mineral content, typically calcium and magnesium ions. It has been hypothesized that exposure to hard water aggravates atopic dermatitis, as high concentrations of calcium and magnesium act as chemical irritants which can cause irritation and dryness of the skin [20]. Travellers moving to another country can be exposed (short or long term) to domestic water with a higher degree of water hardness. Several studies have demonstrated that higher water hardness is associated with an increase in atopic dermatitis during childhood [20–22]. Two studies have demonstrated that children exposed to hard water have an increased risk at atopic dermatitis when they have a positive atopic status or a filaggrin mutation [23, 24]. However, an observer-blinded randomized controlled trial of 12 weeks conducted amongst 336 children with moderate to severe atopic dermatitis supplied by hard water demonstrated no additional benefit of an ion-exchange water softener, regardless of filaggrin mutation [25]. Further prospective studies regarding this topic are needed.

Skin Disorders Related to Biological and Immunological Factors

The immune system, including the so-called skin immune system, plays a major role in defending the body against microbial intruders [26]. In a new environment with micro-organisms in the ecosystem which are immunologically unknown to the traveller, infectious diseases including skin infections can develop, which otherwise would not appear in the old environment. The so-called hygiene theory hypothesizes that exposure to pollutants or infectious diseases in poorer less developed nations would protect against atopy [27]. According to this theory, epidemiological and laboratory studies have implied that the environment during early childhood is important for the risk of developing atopic disorders [28].

Skin disorders related to immunological and changed biological environment such as the occurrence of varicella zoster virus infection and strongyloidiasis in travellers such as immigrants and refugees will be discussed.

Varicella Zoster Virus (VZV) Infection

A primary VZV infection results in varicella (chickenpox) and is a highly contagious disease. In temperate, industrialized countries, it is a very common and self-limiting disease amongst healthy children [29, 30]. It has been reported that about 90% of primary VZV infections occur in children under the age of 10 years. It is more common in cooler winter and spring months. The incidence of varicella amongst children is lower in tropical climates compared to temperate climates. In the tropics, it more often develops in adolescents and adults. About 30% of individuals from tropical regions are susceptible to varicella at 20 years of age and 5–10% remain susceptible at 30 years of age [29]. Varicella outbreaks have been reported in immigrant populations in temperate climates. In a group of Tamil refugees in Denmark, 38% of the adults and 68% of the children developed varicella in the first few months after arrival due to lack of immunity [30]. Varicella is more severe in adults than in children and is associated with significant morbidity (e.g. secondary bacterial infection, pneumonitis, hepatitis, encephalitis) and mortality. Non-immune female immigrants or refugees are also at risk of acquiring varicella during pregnancy, with potential complications for mother and baby. Congenital varicella syndrome may develop during the first 20 weeks of pregnancy and neonatal varicella during 5–7 days before delivery to 2 days after, with a reported mortality of 30%. Therefore, serological screening of immigrants and refugees without a self-reported history of varicella and subsequent vaccination of seronegative immigrants and refugees has been advocated [29].

Varicella is spread by droplet-airborne transmission or by direct contact of skin and mucosa with the contents of blisters. The incubation period ranges between 10 and 21 days. After a prodromal phase of 2–3 days with fever, malaise and flu-like symptoms, the skin eruption appears. It is characterized by erythematous macules, papules, vesicles, pustules, and crusts, which present in different stages of development. It occurs mainly on scalp and face, which can progress to trunk, extremities, oral mucosa, and occasionally on other mucous membranes such as conjunctiva and genitalia. Total healing takes about 2–3 weeks. The eruption can be extremely itchy. On a dark skin, the initial erythematous macules are obscure, and after healing 'polka dot', hyperpigmented scars can be present for many months and sometimes even years.

In immigrants and refugees, with an unknown varicella history or serologic status, a varicella infection should be distinguished from a disseminated herpes zoster or herpes simplex infection. Herpes zoster infection (shingles) is caused by reactivation of latent VZV in sensory ganglia and most frequent occurs in older adults and immunocompromised individuals. Typically, this presents as an intense painful unilateral progressing erythematous macules, papules, and vesiculopustular eruption following a dermatomal distribution. In case of a disseminated herpes zoster infection, several dermatomes are involved or lesions can develop at distance from the primary affected dermatome. Early herpes zoster can occur in infants who have been exposed to VZV in utero or postnatally. A definite diagnosis can be made by performing polymerase chain reaction of vesicle fluid or by serological antibody assessment.

Non-immune adolescent or adult immigrants and refugees with uncomplicated varicella should be treated with oral antiviral therapy (e.g. acyclovir, valacyclovir) to reduce the severity of symptoms and risk of complications. Pregnant women, newborns, and immunocompromised individuals should be treated with intravenous acyclovir. In healthy children ≤12 years, varicella is typically self-limited old and therefore generally does not require antiviral treatment [31].

Strongyloidiasis

Strongyloidiasis is caused by an infection with the parasite *Strongyloides stercoralis*. About 30–100 million are estimated to be infected worldwide, however, this might be an underestimation. Strongyloidiasis occurs in warm, especially damp, climates and is endemic in (sub) tropical areas such as South-East Asia, sub-Saharan Africa, Latin America, mainly in the rural areas. Sporadically this also occurs in temperate areas such as North America, Southern Europe, Japan, and Australia. In the United states, the infection rates are high amongst those who resided in endemic areas (including immigrants, refugees, travellers, and military personnel) [32]. High risk of exposure to *S. stercoralis* is considered in immigrants from endemic areas, adopted children who have been living ≥1 year in a highly endemic area, and expatriates living >1 year in endemic countries and visiting rural areas [33].

Transmission of this infection occurs via skin contact with contaminated soil, faecal-oral transmission, and from person-to-person transmission through faecal contaminated fomites. More than half of cases can be asymptomatic or are associated with nonspecific symptoms. In an acute or chronic infection gastrointestinal symptoms, respiratory symptoms and dermatologic manifestations can occur. Thirty percent of patients have urticarial wheals and flares of migrating subcutaneous larvae anywhere between nipples and knees, particularly around anus and buttocks. The erythematous urticarial tracks can disappear within a day. Eosinophilia can occur up to two-thirds of a chronic infection. Chronic asymptomatic infection can sustain for decades due to the autoinfection cycle of the *S. stercoralis* in skin, lungs, and gastrointestinal tract within the human host. Immunosuppressed patients are at risk for developing a *S. stercolaris* hyperinfection (accelerated autoinfection within organs normally involved in autoinfection cycle) or disseminated infection (hyperinfection with spread of larvae to organs and tissues outside autoinfection cycle). Serologic screening of asymptomatic individuals is warranted in immigrants and refugees from endemic areas, immunosuppressed patients, or candidates for immunosuppressive therapies with a high-intermediate risk to strongyloidiasis, epidemiologic exposure in military personnel [32, 33]. In patients with gastrointestinal symptoms additional stool testing (polymerase chain reaction or agar plate culture) can be performed, however, due to intermittent larval excretion the sensitivity is relatively low [32].

Treatment of strongyloidiasis consists of ivermectin 200 microgram/kg daily for 2 days, repeated at 2 weeks for immunocompromised patients or those who require immunosuppression. Amongst patients with hyperinfection or a disseminated infection, the mortality rate is 70–100% [18, 32].

Skin Disorders Related to Social and Cultural Factors

Different social and cultural factors related to an old environment can cause skin disorders in travellers moving between different climatic zones. For instance, sunbathing habits of tourists in (sub)tropical climates could lead to massive sunburn and subsequent complications. Whilst, veiled female immigrants or refugees wearing covering clothes often suffer from vitamin D deficiency in Western countries. We report on adverse reactions to skin bleaching as a common practice amongst travellers such as immigrants and refugees with skin of colour.

Adverse Reactions to Skin Bleaching

Worldwide, in several communities with dark-skinned inhabitants, a clear and light skin has been viewed as a cultural beauty ideal and deemed to represent a superior socio-economic status. Skin bleaching has been practiced in order to achieve this beauty ideal. Skin bleaching is therefore a common phenomenon in countries such as sub-Saharan Africa, Middle East, Asia (i.e. India, Philippines, Hong Kong), Southern, and Central America [34]. The skin bleaching practices are frequently continued as an "imported phenomenon" amongst immigrant populations in North America and Europe [35]. There are indications that due to "psychosocial pressure" the skin bleaching practise is intensified in the new environment by some individuals in certain groups of immigrants. Mostly adult woman practice skin bleaching. The most common compounds that are used are hydroquinone (in several concentrations) and 0.05% clobetasol proprionate. In this cosmetic context, these skin bleaching products can be obtained without a doctor's prescription from their country of origin, tropical convenience stores in immigrant countries, or online via the internet. The active ingredients may be indicated on the packages of the skin bleaching products, however, it can also be inaccurate or undocumented [34]. Inadequate use of skin bleaching products can lead to various adverse reactions.

Misuse of hydroquinone can lead to periorbital hyperpigmentation, irritant, and/or allergic contact dermatitis with subsequent post-inflammatory dyspigmentation and exogenous ochronosis. Exogenous ochronosis can develop due to long-term or excessive use of hydroquinone. It represents as reticulated and ripple-like sooty or blue-black pigmented macules, papules, and plaques on sun-exposed skin, also pigmented colloid milia can be seen. It must be differentiated from post-inflammatory hyperpigmentation and melasma. The histological picture is pathognomonic, with a dermal infiltrate and yellow-brown banana-shaped fibers in papillary dermis in the haematoxylin eosinophilic staining. Unfortunately, there is no effective treatment known for this disease.

Misuse of topical corticosteroids can induce local complications such as striae, skin atrophy, acne, folliculitis, purpura, persistent erythema, tinea corporis. Prolonged and excessive application of topical corticosteroids, especially on large body surface areas, can lead to systemic complications like hyperglycaemia, hypothalamic-pituitary-adrenal axis suppression, Cushing's syndrome an hypertension [35].

Awareness and adequate recognition by physicians of cosmetic skin bleaching practices amongst immigrants is important in order to prevent potential permanent local and systemic complications. Physicians should educate immigrants and refugees about the cutaneous and systemic complications including paradoxical hyperpigmentation of prolonged, extensive, and incorrect use of skin bleaching products. The use of these products should be immediately discontinued [35].

Climate Change and Skin Disorders

The global climate is changing. Skin disorders aren't only influenced by a change in environment due to travelling to another climatic zone, but they can also be affected by the overall change in the global climate and environment. Climate change describes the regional or global variation in climate over time in terms of temperature, humidity, precipitation, atmospheric pressure, cloud cover, and wind. Climate change has been considered to be the cause of global warming, leading to higher average temperatures, changes in humidity and precipitation. The average surface temperature has increased by 0.6 °C over the past 100 years and will probably increase by 2 °C by the end of 2100 [2]. Warming oceans, melting of arctic ice cap and rising sea levels contribute to more severe hurricanes and storms. Climate change overall also leads to a global rise in extreme climatic events such as floods, droughts, and wildfires [36]. These conditions are associated with increased cutaneous infectious diseases and expanding geographic range of vector-borne diseases (e.g. Lyme disease, malaria, leishmaniasis, dengue) [34], which will be discussed in chapters. "Ecthyma", "Boils or Furunculosis", and "Cellulitis and Erysipelas". Water-associated climate changes such as increasing ocean temperatures also cause increases in marine dermatoses such as jellyfish stings, seabather eruption, and Swimmer's itch [37], which will be further discussed in chapter "Marine Dermatoses". Environmental pollutants from fossil fuel emissions and wildfires can also negatively affect inflammatory disorders such as atopic dermatitis [36]. Ozone depletion increases UV radiation on earth, which leads to skin aging and increases the risk at skin cancer. It has been estimated that each 1% reduction in thickness of the ozone layer increases the incidence of melanoma by 1–2% and the risk for squamous cell carcinoma by

3–4.6% and for basal cell carcinoma by 1.7–2.7% [38]. Dermatologists should be aware that climate change could cause changing patterns in skin disorders.

References

1. Roser M. Tourism [Internet]. 2020 [cited 21-07-2020]. Available from: https://ourworldindata.org/tourism.
2. Andersen LK, Hercogova J, Wollina U, Davis MD. Climate change and skin disease: a review of the English-language literature. Int J Dermatol. 2012;51(6):656–61. quiz 9, 61
3. Peel MC, Finlayson BL, McMahon TA. Updated world map of the Koppen-Geiger climate classification. Hydrol Earth Syst Sci. 2007;11:1633–44.
4. Deng L, Xu S. Adaptation of human skin color in various populations. Hereditas. 2018;155:1.
5. Taylor SC. Skin of color: biology, structure, function, and implications for dermatologic disease. J Am Acad Dermatol. 2002;46(2 Suppl Understanding):S41–62.
6. Sharma VK, Sahni K. Photodermatoses in the pigmented skin. Adv Exp Med Biol. 2017;996:111–22.
7. Wesley NO, Maibach HI. Racial (ethnic) differences in skin properties: the objective data. Am J Clin Dermatol. 2003;4(12):843–60.
8. Engebretsen KA, Johansen JD, Kezic S, Linneberg A, Thyssen JP. The effect of environmental humidity and temperature on skin barrier function and dermatitis. J Eur Acad Dermatol Venereol. 2016;30(2):223–49.
9. Singh B, Maibach H. Climate and skin function: an overview. Skin Res Technol. 2013;19(3):207–12.
10. Silverberg JI, Hanifin J, Simpson EL. Climatic factors are associated with childhood eczema prevalence in the United States. J Invest Dermatol. 2013;133(7):1752–9.
11. Gutierrez D, Gaulding JV, Motta Beltran AF, Lim HW, Pritchett EN. Photodermatoses in skin of colour. J Eur Acad Dermatol Venereol. 2018;32(11):1879–86.
12. Kerr HA, Lim HW. Photodermatoses in African Americans: a retrospective analysis of 135 patients over a 7-year period. J Am Acad Dermatol. 2007;57(4):638–43.
13. Nakamura M, Henderson M, Jacobsen G, Lim HW. Comparison of photodermatoses in African-Americans and Caucasians: a follow-up study. Photodermatol Photoimmunol Photomed. 2014;30(5):231–6.
14. Lips P, Cashman KD, Lamberg-Allardt C, Bischoff-Ferrari HA, Obermayer-Pietsch B, Bianchi ML, et al. Current vitamin D status in European and Middle East countries and strategies to prevent vitamin D deficiency: a position statement of the European calcified tissue society. Eur J Endocrinol. 2019;180(4):P23–54.
15. van der Meer IM, Middelkoop BJ, Boeke AJ, Lips P. Prevalence of vitamin D deficiency among Turkish, Moroccan, Indian and sub-Sahara African populations in Europe and their countries of origin: an overview. Osteoporos Int. 2011;22(4):1009–21.
16. Kechichian E, Ezzedine K. Vitamin D and the skin: an update for dermatologists. Am J Clin Dermatol. 2018;19(2):223–35.
17. Kaufman BP, Alexis AF. Psoriasis in skin of color: insights into the epidemiology, clinical presentation, genetics, quality-of-life impact, and treatment of psoriasis in non-white racial/ethnic groups. Am J Clin Dermatol. 2018;19(3):405–23.
18. Chandran V, Raychaudhuri SP. Geoepidemiology and environmental factors of psoriasis and psoriatic arthritis. J Autoimmun. 2010;34(3):J314–21.
19. Rustin MH, Newton JA, Smith NP, Dowd PM. The treatment of chilblains with nifedipine: the results of a pilot study, a double-blind placebo-controlled randomized study and a long-term open trial. Br J Dermatol. 1989;120(2):267–75.
20. Miyake Y, Yokoyama T, Yura A, Iki M, Shimizu T. Ecological association of water hardness with prevalence of childhood atopic dermatitis in a Japanese urban area. Environ Res. 2004;94(1):33–7.
21. McNally NJ, Williams HC, Phillips DR, Smallman-Raynor M, Lewis S, Venn A, et al. Atopic eczema and domestic water hardness. Lancet. 1998;352(9127):527–31.
22. Perkin MR, Craven J, Logan K, Strachan D, Marrs T, Radulovic S, et al. Association between domestic water hardness, chlorine, and atopic dermatitis risk in early life: a population-based cross-sectional study. J Allergy Clin Immunol. 2016;138(2):509–16.
23. Chaumont A, Voisin C, Sardella A, Bernard A. Interactions between domestic water hardness, infant swimming and atopy in the development of childhood eczema. Environ Res. 2012;116:52–7.
24. Jabbar-Lopez ZK, Craven J, Logan K, Greenblatt D, Marrs T, Radulovic S, et al. Longitudinal analysis of the effect of water hardness on atopic eczema: evidence for gene-environment interaction. Br J Dermatol. 2020;183(2):285–93.
25. Thomas KS, Dean T, O'Leary C, Sach TH, Koller K, Frost A, et al. A randomised controlled trial of ion-exchange water softeners for the treatment of eczema in children. PLoS Med. 2011;8(2):e1000395.
26. Salmon JK, Armstrong CA, Ansel JC. The skin as an immune organ. West J Med. 1994;160(2):146–52.
27. English JS, Dawe RS, Ferguson J. Environmental effects and skin disease. Br Med Bull. 2003;68:129–42.
28. Hjern A, Rasmussen F, Hedlin G. Age at adoption, ethnicity and atopic disorder: a study of internationally adopted young men in Sweden. Pediatr Allergy Immunol. 1999;10(2):101–6.
29. Merrett P, Schwartzman K, Rivest P, Greenaway C. Strategies to prevent varicella among newly arrived adult immigrants and refugees: a cost-effectiveness analysis. Clin Infect Dis. 2007;44(8):1040–8.
30. Kjersem H, Jepsen S. Varicella among immigrants from the tropics, a health problem. Scand J Soc Med. 1990;18(3):171–4.

31. Treatment of varicella (chickenpox) infection [Internet]. UpToDate. 2020 [cited 21-07-2020]. Available from: https://www.uptodate.com/contents/treatment-of-varicella-chickenpox-infection?search=varicella.

32. Strongyloidiasis [Internet]. UpToDate. 2020 [cited 21-07-2020]. Available from: https://www.uptodate.com/contents/strongyloidiasis.

33. Requena-Méndez A, Buonfrate D, Gomez-Junyent J, Zammarchi L, Bisoffi Z, Muñoz J. Evidence-based guidelines for screening and Management of Strongyloidiasis in non-endemic countries. Am J Trop Med Hyg. 2017;97(3):645–52.

34. Mahe A. The practice of skin-bleaching for a cosmetic purpose in immigrant communities. J Travel Med. 2014;21(4):282–7.

35. Topical skin-lightening agents: complications associated with misuse [Internet]. 2020 [cited 21-07-2020]. Available from: https://www.uptodate.com/contents/topical-skin-lightening-agents-complications-associated-with-misuse.

36. Coates SJ, McCalmont TH, Williams ML. Adapting to the effects of climate change in the practice of dermatology-a call to action. JAMA Dermatol. 2019;155(4):415–6.

37. Kaffenberger BH, Shetlar D, Norton SA, Rosenbach M. The effect of climate change on skin disease in North America. J Am Acad Dermatol. 2017;76(1):140–7.

38. Balato N, Megna M, Ayala F, Balato A, Napolitano M, Patruno C. Effects of climate changes on skin diseases. Expert Rev Anti-Infect Ther. 2014;12(2):171–81.

Part I

Dermatoses Caused by Infection: Bacterial Infections

Impetigo

Patricia Chang
and Monica Vanessa Vasquez Acajabon

Key Points
- Impetigo is the most common bacterial skin infection.
- Non-bullous impetigo and bullous impetigo.
- Primary and secondary impetigo.
- *Staphylococcus aureus* or *Streptococcus pyogenes.*
- Treatment: topical antibiotics such as mupirocin, retapamulin, and fusidic acid.
- For limited impetigo.

Impetigo, written for the first time in 1864 by Tilbury Fox [1], is an acute bacterial-origin dermatosis caused by *Staphylococcus aureus or Streptococcus pyogenes* that affects the superficial layers of the epidermis [2, 3]. It is also called impetigo contagious, impetigo bullosa, or impetigo of Tilbury fox [4].

It is highly contagious and self-inoculable [4, 5], and a linear distribution secondary to scratching is frequently observed [6].

Impetigo is among the first five causes of dermatological consultation in children [2, 4, 5]. A higher prevalence is observed in malnourished and immunocompromised patients, but the main risk factor is the alteration of the integrity of the skin due to trauma, bites or insect bites, preexisting dermatoses, pyogenic infections, and poor hygiene [2, 4, 7, 8], as well as diseases that affect the host's immune status, such as diabetes mellitus, HIV, autoimmune, hematological diseases, chemotherapy, steroid and biological treatments.

As for the ethiopathogenesis, it can be caused by S. aureus and S. pyogenes or beta hemolytic group A, or both. In immunocompetent patients, 60% of impetigo is due to staphylococcus, 20% to streptococcus, and 20% to both [4].

Streptococcal infections are more prevalent in the summer and in tropical or humid climates [4, 6]. Staphylococcal impetigo primarily affects newborns and school children [2]. In the case of infants, the highest frequency is explained by the lack of specific antibodies to neutralize the staphylococcal exfoliative toxin that acts against desmoglein (DSG) [4], which causes blisters due to epidermal separation. If it is very severe, it causes staphylococcal scalded skin syndrome (Ritter's disease) [4, 7, 8]. 60% of healthy people are staphylococcus carriers in nostrils, armpits, groins, and perineum, so their frequent participation as a primary site of infection is observed [8]. In addition, staphylococci of phage type 71 may reduce the population of group A streptococci [4].

P. Chang (✉)
Dermatologist at Paseo Plaza Clinic Center,
Guatemala City, Guatemala

M. V. V. Acajabon
Private Practice Dermatologist in Antigua,
Antigua, Guatemala

W. Robles (ed.), *Skin Disease in Travelers*, Updates in Clinical Dermatology,
https://doi.org/10.1007/978-3-031-57836-6_2

There are two main types of impetigo: the non-bullos which occurs in 70% of cases and is also called contagious impetigo, and the bulloso, which occurs in 30% of cases [9].

Non-bullous impetigo can also be classified as primary or secondary, which is the most common one [5, 6]. It is generally caused by S. aureus, but S. pyogenes may also be involved, especially in warm, humid climates (Table 1).

It is clinically characterized by blisters and pustules, which erode and subsequently dry out quickly and are covered by meliceric scabs. They are classified as primary and secondary impetigo, and according to their cause and morphology, in blister or staphylococcal, and crusty or streptococcal [3, 4].

Primary impetigo occurs by direct bacterial invasion of previously normal skin [6] and is mainly located on the face, around the natural holes: mouth, nostrils, ear pavilions, and eyes (Figs. 1, 2, 3, and 4) [2, 4], although in infants it predominates in the perineum, in the periumbilical region or in disseminated form [4, 8]. Vesiculopustular lesions predominate in the lower extremities, face, and can be extended by self-inoculation (Figs. 5, 6, 7, and 8) [4, 5, 7].

The secondary form, also called impetiginization, is preceded by an underlying pruritic dermatosis that alters the skin barrier [4, 6] (Figs. 9, 10, 11, and 12). It can appear on any part of the body. The lesions are erythema, blisters, pustules, and meliceric scabs [4]. The secondary form, also called impetiginization, is preceded by a pruritic dermatosis that alters the underlying skin barrier [4, 6]. Usually S. aureus is associated in secondary forms [6].

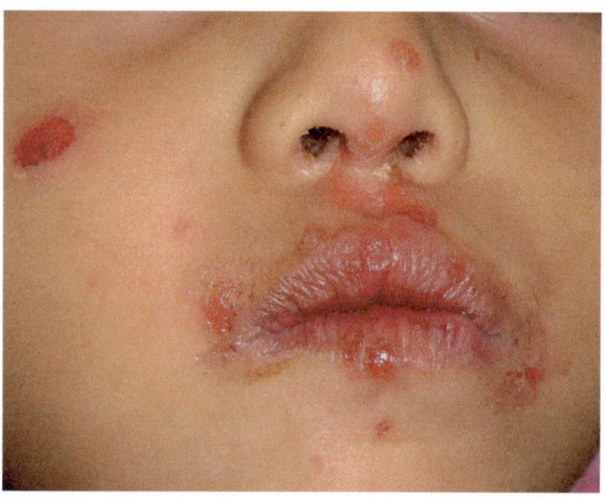

Fig. 1 Primary impetigo around natural holes

Table 1 Main types of impetigo

Bullous impétigo	Non-Bullous impetigo
Caused only by *S. Aureus*	*S. Aureus S. pyogenes*
Large, fragile, flaccid bullae that can rupture and ooze yellow fluid	Primary or secondary (more common form)
The pathognomonic collarette of scales on its periphery develops after the bullae rupture, leaving a thin, brown crust on the remaining erosions	Primary impetigo is a direct bacterial invasion of intact healthy skin
Exfoliative toxins produced by *S. Aureus* strains that cause loss of cell adhesion in the superficial epidermis That form the bullaes	Secondary impetigo is a bacterial infection of disrupted skin caused by trauma, eczema, insect bites, scabies, or herpetic outbreaks and other diseases. Diabetes or other underlying systemic conditions also increase susceptibility.
Trunk, axilla, and extremities, and in intertriginous (diaper) areas	Maculopapular lesions that transition into thin-walled vesicles that rapidly rupture, leaving superficial, sometimes pruritic or painful erosions covered by the classic honey-colored crusts
It is the most common cause of ulcerative rash on the buttocks of infants	Exposed skin of the face (nares, perioral region) and the extremities are the most affected sites
Systemic symptoms are uncommon but can include fever, diarrhea, and weakness	Systemic symptoms are unlikely
Topical antibiotics: Mupirocin, retapamulin, and fusidic acid	Topical antibiotics: Mupirocin, retapamulin, and fusidic acid
Resolve within 2 to 3 weeks without scarring	Resolve within 2 to 3 weeks without scarring

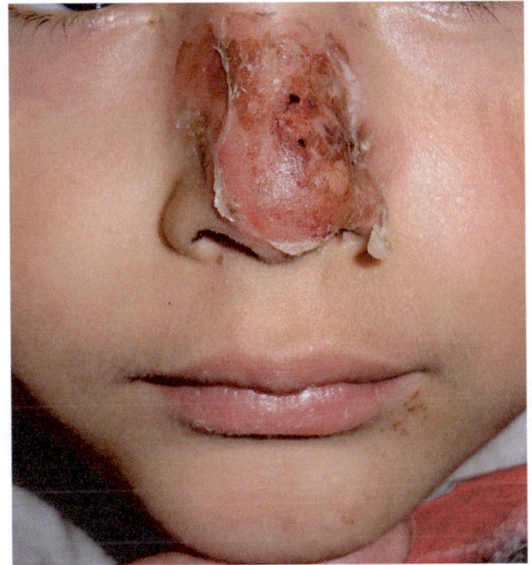

Fig. 2 Bullous impetigo on nose

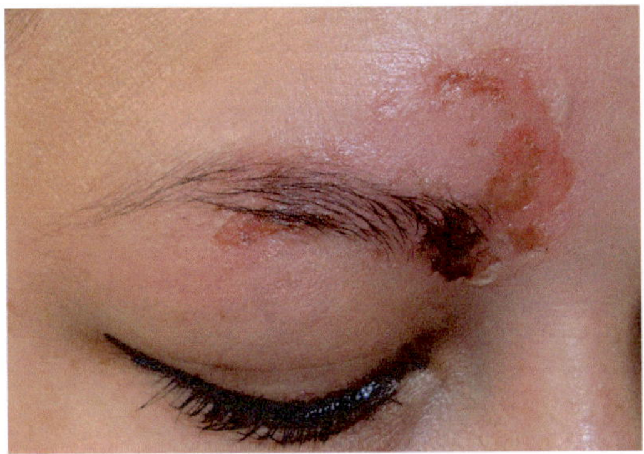

Fig. 3 Erosive pustular lesions on the right eyebrow

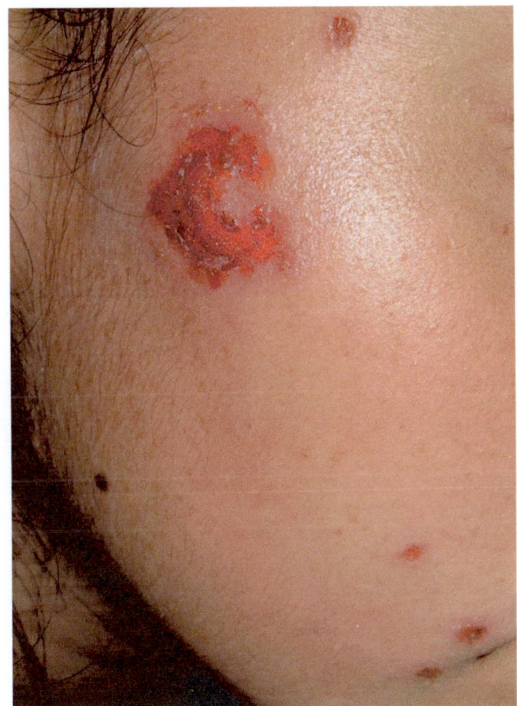

Fig. 4 Crusty lesions on cheek

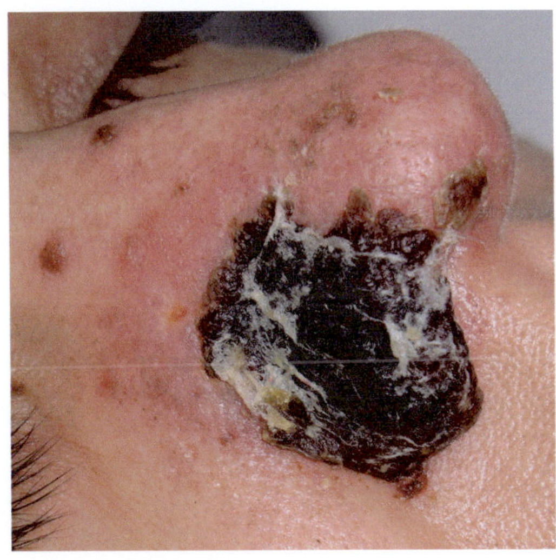

Fig. 5 Lesions with meliceric blood crust in a patient with sytemic lupus

Some authors classify this entity as true blister or staphylococcal impetigo, which usually affects the face, buttocks, trunk, and perineum [1], and contagious impetigo of Tilbury Fox or non-bullous (the most common) [1, 4, 6, 7], the latter caused mostly by S. aureus and less frequently by S. pyogenes [8]. Other less frequent forms have been described, such as layer impetigo of the scalp, where there are scabs that agglutinate the hair; impetigo of the mucous membranes, consisting of erosive plaques on the lips and oral mucosa, and which, if affecting the corners, produces angular cheilitis and may be accompanied by phlyctenas keratitis; Circinated or geographical impetigo where squamous circles form; miliary impetigo in which micro vesicles and pyogenic intertrigos are observed [4].

The evolution is acute and tends to a spontaneous resolution in 2 to 3 weeks. It leaves an eroded skin that subsequently evolves to a pinkish spot,

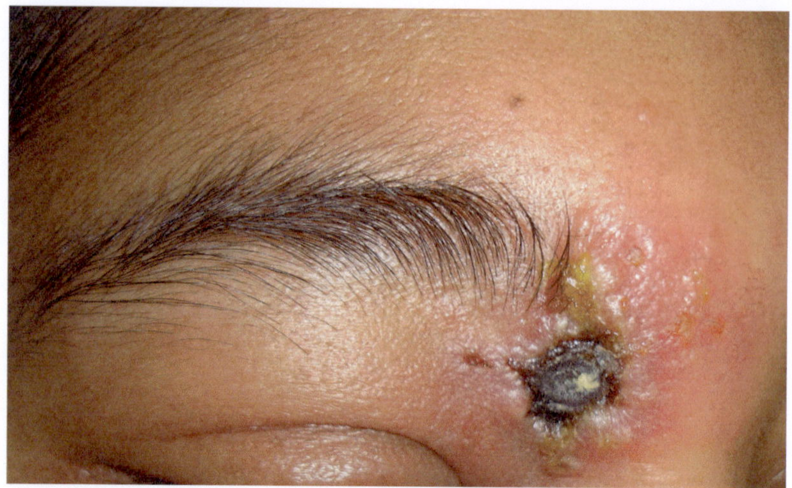

Fig. 6 Melicerous crusts surrounded by erythema on eyebrow

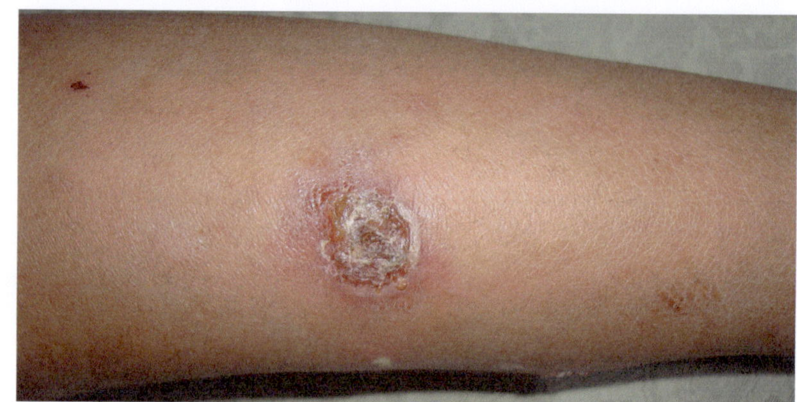

Fig. 7 Meliceric crust on leg

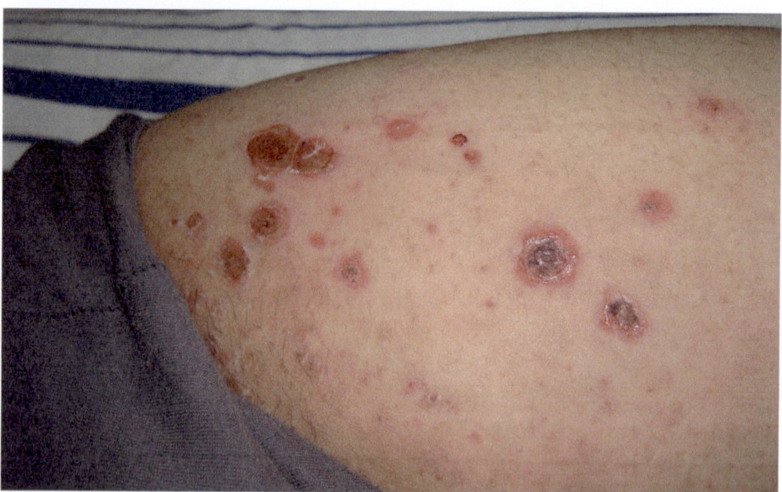

Fig. 8 Crusty lesions on leg

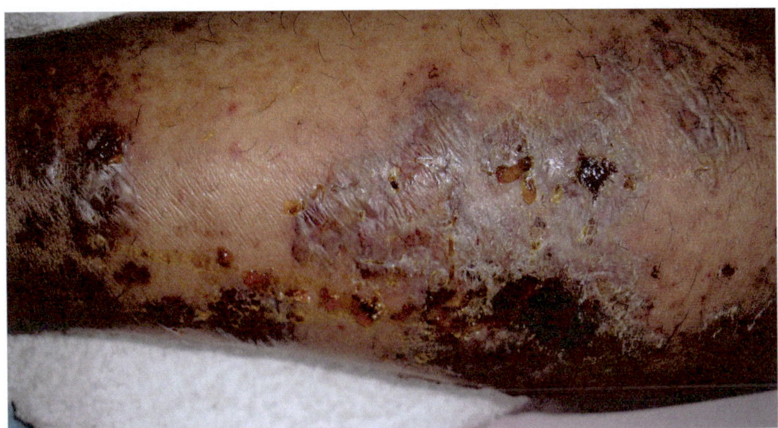

Fig. 9 Secondary impetigo on leg with meliceric crust

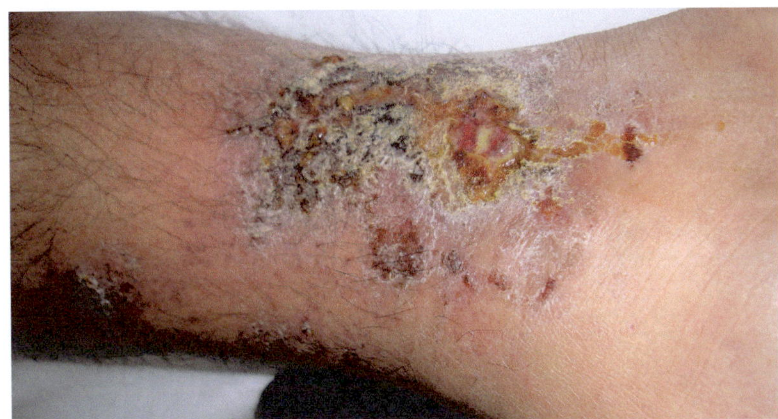

Fig. 10 Melicerous crusts in venous insufficiency

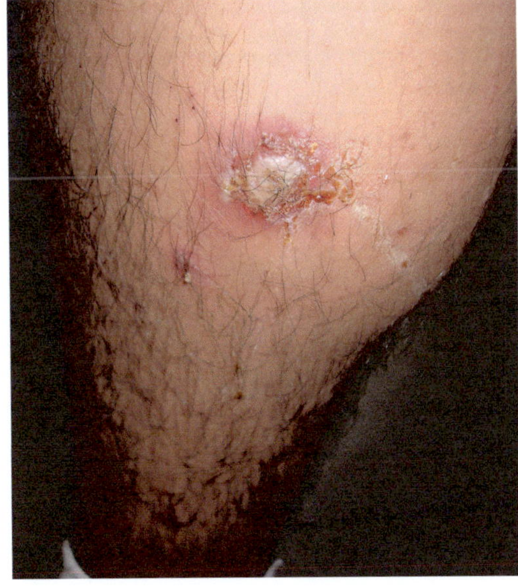

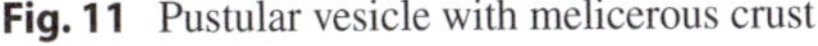

Fig. 11 Pustular vesicle with melicerous crust

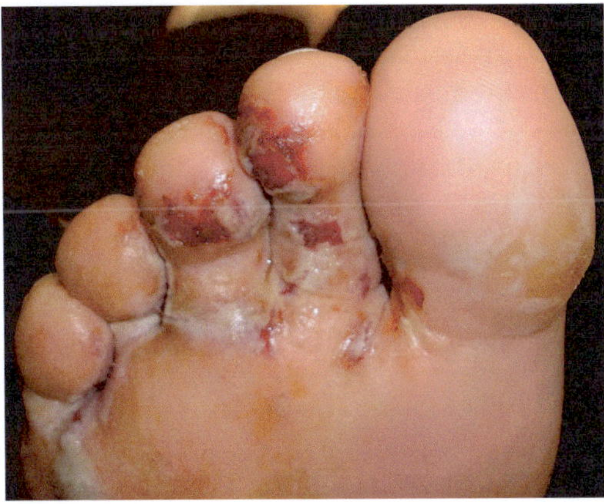

Fig. 12 Impetiginized ringworm of the feet

with the epidermis regenerating without scarring [4–6]. There are usually no systemic symptoms, but it can be accompanied by fever, malaise, and regional adenopathy [4, 6]. In rare cases, it can complicate to deep infections such as cellulite, or spread and cause lymphangitis or septicemia. The evolution is sharp and tends to spontaneous resolution in 2 to 3 weeks. Non-infectious complications of S. pyogenes have been described, including psoriasis gutata, scarlet fever [4] and, in very large cases, glomerulonephritis in 1% to 5% of cases, so it is vital to eradicate streptococcus by systemic treatment [2, 4, 5].

The diagnosis is clinical and can be confirmed by gram-staining bacterial culture [5] and does not require biopsy. There may be diagnostic confusion with entities such as herpes simplex, acute contact dermatitis, papulocostrosal syphilis, inflammatory ringworm, pemphigus, pemphigoid and herpetiformis dermatitis, eczema among others [4, 6].

The treatment varies depending on the extent and severity of the disease. The nature of localized impetigo is to resolve spontaneously, and washing with soap and water, mechanical removal of scabs, and local application of weak antiseptic in baths or baths [2–4, 7] is recommended. The use of alibour solution (copper sulfate + zinc sulfate) or chlorhexidine gluconate solution has been described. Cream with 0.5–3% yodoclorhydroxyquinoline, fusidic acid or 2% mupirocin can be used twice a day for 7 days [2, 4, 5, 7]. Other options are topical bacitracin, polymyxin, gentamicin, rifampin, and erythromycin. In resistant cases, 1% nadifloxacin cream or ratapamulin ointment may be alternatives [4, 5].

In patients with highly disseminated lesions, particularly pediatric patients, the use of systemic antibiotics is warranted. Specific treatments against streptococci or staphylococci are recommended, although resistance has been observed [4]. In impetigo caused by staphylococcus the treatment is based on dicloxacillin 50–100 mg/kg/day, divided into four doses, and in adults 500 mg every 6 h for 7 to 10 days [2–4].pediatric patients, justify the use of systemic in streptococcal infections in general just a dose of benzathine penicillin of 1,200,000 or in patients 6 years or more (27 kg or more) and 600.000 or in patients under the age of 6 years [2]. In case of allergies, use erythromycin 40 mg/kg/day in four doses for 7 to 10 days, or other macrolides such as azithromycin or clarithromycin. Other options are cephalosporins, cloxacillin, clindamycin, and ampicillin plus clavulanic acid or sulbactam [2, 4, 7].

No Conflict of Interest No financial support.

References

1. Ajay G, Rubin G. A systematic review and meta-analysis of treatments for impetigo. Br J Gen Pract. 2003;53(491):480–7.
2. Diez de Medina J. Piodermitis: Impetigo, folliculitis, boils, Ectimas anthrax. In: Antibiotics in dermatology. 1st ed. Venezuela: Editorial pentagráfica. p. 151–4.
3. Brown J, Shriner D, Schwartz R, Janniger C. Impetigo: an update. Int J Dermatol. 2003;42:251–5.
4. Arenas R. Impetigo Vulgaris. In: Arenas R, editor. Atlas dermatology, diagnosis and treatment. 5th ed. Mexico: Mc Graw-Hill; 2019.: Inter-american. p. 391–6.
5. Cole C, Gazewood J. Diagnosis and treatment of impetigo. Am Fam Physician. 2007;75(6):859–64.
6. Koning S, van der Sande R, Verhagen AP, van Suijlekom-Smit LWA, Morris AD, Butler CC, Berger M, van der Wouden JC. Interventions for impetigo. Cochrane Database Syst Rev. 2012;1:CD003261. https://doi.org/10.1002/14651858.CD003261.pub3.
7. Baptista L. Impetigo–review magazine. An Bras Dermatol. 2014;89(2):293–9.
8. Craft N. Superficial skin infections and Piodermas. In: Fitzpatrick dermatology in general medicine. 8th ed. Spain: Editorial Médica Panamericana; 2012. p. 2128–34.
9. Banvard Hartman-Adams HC, Juckett G. Impetigo: diagnosis and treatment. Am Fam Physician. 2014;90(4):229–35.

Ecthyma

Jose Dario Martinez, Jesus Alberto Cardenas-de la Garza, and Kenneth J. Tomecki

Abbreviations

EG   Ecthyma gangrenosum
CL   Cutaneous leishmaniasis

Key Points

- Ecthyma is a cutaneous infection caused by *S pyogenes* or *S aureus*.
- Travelers returning from tropical climates are most often affected.
- Ecthyma is characterized by small ulcers with central necrosis and crust.
- Differential diagnosis is broad and endemic infections should be considered.
- Treatment consists of systemic antibiotics.

J. D. Martinez (✉)
Department of Internal Medicine, University Hospital "Dr. José E. González" Universidad Autónoma de Nuevo León, Monterrey, Mexico

J. A. Cardenas-de la Garza
Department of Rheumatology, University Hospital "Dr. José E. González" Universidad Autónoma de Nuevo León, Monterrey, Mexico

K. J. Tomecki
Department of Dermatology, Cleveland Clinic Foundation, Cleveland, OH, USA
e-mail: tomeckk@ccf.org

Introduction

Ecthyma (from Greek meaning "to break out") is a cutaneous infection with deep dermal involvement caused by the Gram-positive cocci *Streptococcus pyogenes* and *Staphylococcus aureus* [1, 2]. People living in or traveling to tropical climates are most often affected. Infection is often secondary to trauma or scratching due to arthropod bites. Predisposing factors include malnutrition, immunosuppression, homelessness, and poor hygiene [1–3].

Ecthyma should not be confused with ecthyma gangrenosum or ecthyma contagiosum, two infectious diseases that sound and look similar. Ecthyma gangrenosum (EG) is an uncommon disseminated infection that usually affects immunocompromised individuals. It is classically associated with *Pseudomonas aeruginosa* bacteremia and occasionally other pathogens including *Escherichia coli* and *S. aureus* can cause it [4]. Ecthyma contagiosum (Orf) or Orf nodule is a viral infection caused by a parapoxvirus. It predominantly affects shepherds, veterinarians, and farmers who handle sheep, goats, or deer. It may affect travelers who have had direct contact with such animals in petting-zoos, hunting, or during religious rituals [5, 6].

© The Editor(s) (if applicable) and The Author(s), under exclusive license to Springer Nature Switzerland AG 2024
W. Robles (ed.), *Skin Disease in Travelers*, Updates in Clinical Dermatology,
https://doi.org/10.1007/978-3-031-57836-6_3

Epidemiology

Skin diseases are a common cause of illness in international travelers. Only gastrointestinal disorders and fever are more common. Cutaneous larva migrans, pyodermas, and insect bites are the most common dermatologic diagnosis in travelers returning from tropical countries [7–9]. The most frequent pyodermas are impetigo, erysipelas, ecthyma, and abscesses [9].

Clinical Characteristics

Ecthyma begins as a vesicle or pustule that progresses to a 2–3 cm punched-out ulcer with necrotic base, green-yellow crust, and purulent discharge (Figs. 1 and 2). The borders are erythematous and slightly elevated. The most common sites are the legs, thighs, buttocks, or feet [1, 2, 10]. Insect bites, scabies, or impetigo lesions may occur with ecthyma. Systemic symptoms like fever rarely occur. Resolution may leave atrophic scarring. Occasionally, ecthyma may be a prelude to poststreptococcal glomerulonephritis, toxic shock syndrome, cellulitis, necrotizing fasciitis, or sepsis [3].

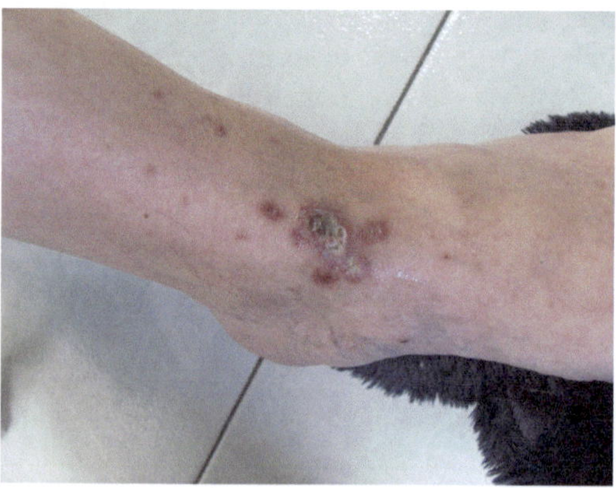

Fig. 1 Ecthyma with multiple, small ulcers with yellow crust. Insect bites are also present

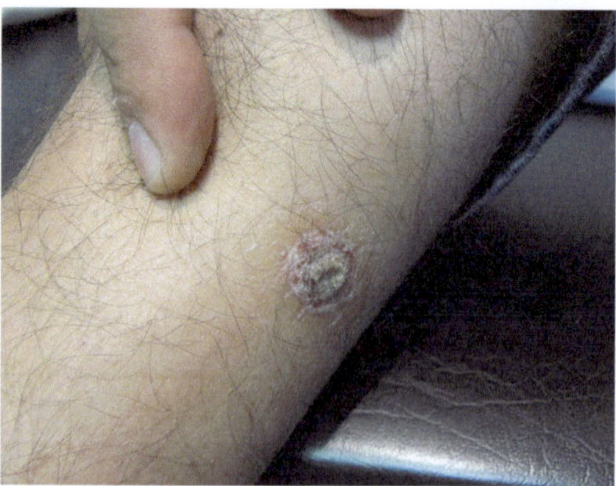

Fig. 2 Ecthyma as a single ulcer with thick, yellow crust surrounded by an erythematous raised border

Diagnosis

Diagnosis can be established by presence of characteristic skin disease. Gram stain and culture from exudate or pus help to identify the causative organism and the antibiotic susceptibility [11, 12]. Recent travel history is critical for consideration of differential diagnoses that may share a similar clinical picture, including some zoonoses.

Skin biopsy is advisable for any atypical clinical presentation, if the diagnosis is uncertain, or to exclude other conditions. In these cases, samples should be obtained for culture (for fungi, mycobacteria, and bacteria) and histopathology. Hematoxylin and eosin staining typically shows an ulcer with a sharp border, covered by a crust, with a central neutrophilic infiltrate in the superficial dermis. Bacterial colonies can be identified with tissue Gram stains.

Differential Diagnosis

The differential diagnosis of ecthyma is broad and includes other infections, insect or spider bites, pyoderma gangrenosum, vasculitis, zoonoses, and vasculopathies. Travel history is critical to identify causes of endemic tropical infections. Table 1 summarizes differential diagnosis of ecthyma in travelers.

Ecthyma gangrenosum (EG) is a rare infection classically associated with *P. aeruginosa* septicemia. In recent years, many other etiological agents have been associated with EG and controversy exists if these clinical presentations should be labeled as ecthyma gangrenosum or as ecthyma gangrenosum-like skin disease [13–15].

Table 1 Differential diagnosis of ecthyma in travelers

Ecthyma gangrenosum
Rickettsial infections
Cutaneous anthrax
Cutaneous diphtheria
Tularemia
Buruli ulcer
Atypical mycobacteriosis
Tuberculids
Sexually transmitted diseases, e.g. syphilis
Other pyogenic infections
Cutaneous leishmaniasis
Sporotrichosis
Orf or milker's nodule
Insect or spider bites
Scabies
Pyoderma gangrenosum
Vasculitis and vasculopathy

EG begins as a macule or vesicle with erythematous border which rapidly progresses into an ulcer with a black central eschar. Ulcers may be single or multiple. The most frequently affected site is the pelvis followed by the extremities [14]. Multiple ulcers at different locations should raise the suspicion of hematogenous spread. Characteristically, EG has scant or absent suppuration [16, 17]. Systematic symptoms and multiple ulcers in immunocompromised travelers (particularly those with neutropenia or HIV disease) should raise the suspicion of ecthyma gangrenosum as a diagnosis. Wound cultures are necessary to identify the etiological agent. Early treatment with parenteral antibiotics is warranted [17].

Several rickettsioses may produce skin disease that initially resembles ecthyma. Some rickettsia infections from the spotted fever group initially produce one or more small ulcers with a necrotic scab with an erythematous border at the inoculation site, known as *tache noir* (black spot in French) [18–20]. Mediterranean spotted fever (Boutonneuse fever) is a tick-transmitted infection caused by *Rickettsia conorii*, endemic in regions around the Mediterranean Sea and the Black Sea and some African countries [19, 21]. Clinical features include an eschar, maculopapular rash, fever, lymphadenopathy, arthralgia, and myalgia. Diagnosis is confirmed with PCR or serology, the treatment of choice is doxycycline [19–21]. African tick bite fever is a tick-borne infection due to *Rickettsia africae*, which has a clinical presentation similar to Mediterranean spotted fever but exhibits multiple eschars more frequently. African thick bite fever should be suspected in travelers to African countries especially if they engaged in outdoor activities like safaris or hunting. Diagnosis and treatment are similar to Mediterranean spotted fever. Other rickettsial diseases that with eschars include ricketssialpox by *R. akarii*, scrub typhus by *Orientia tsutsugamushi*, and *Rickettsia parkeri* rickettsiosis [20, 22].

Other rare bacterial infection are a possibility depending on travel, country of origin, contact with animals, and clinical presentation, e.g. cutaneous anthrax, cutaneous diphtheria, and tularemia [10]. Buruli ulcer and other mycobacteriosis may occasionally resemble ecthyma.

Cutaneous leishmaniasis (CL) is an endemic infection in specific areas of Central and South America, Asia, and Africa. It is a vector-borne disease transmitted by sandflies and caused by more than 20 different species of parasites from the genus *Leishmania*. Clinical manifestations vary depending on the species involved. CL may initially develop as a nodule that evolves to a non-painful ulcer [23, 24]. It should always be part of the differential diagnosis in chronic cutaneous ulcers in travelers, military, or refugees from endemic countries.

Treatment

The treatment of ecthyma includes wound care and systemic antibiotics. Initially, empiric treatment with of an antibiotic that covers both *S. aureus* and *S. pyogenes,* e.g., dicloxacillin or cephalexin should be started. If *S. pyogenes* is the primary isolate, treatment is penicillin. When methicillin-resistant *S. aureus* is isolated or suspected, treatment should be doxycycline, trimethoprim/sulfamethoxazole, or clindamycin. Treatment should last from 7 to 10 days [11, 12]. Dosage information is shown in Table 2.

Table 2 Oral antibiotics for ecthyma in adults

Empirical treatment (*S. pyogenes* and/or methicillin-susceptible *S. aureus*)	Dosage
Dicloxacillin	250–500 mg every 6 h
Cephalexin	250–500 mg every 6 h
S. pyogenes	
Penicillin V	250–500 mg every 6 h
Methicillin-resistant *S. aureus*	
Doxycycline	100 mg every 12 h
Trimethoprim/sulfamethoxazole double strength	160–800 mg every 12 h
Clindamycin	300–450 mg every 6 h

Prognosis

Complete resolution without complications happens in most cases. Atrophic scarring may occur specially with deep ulcers. Other complications are infrequent. Lack of resolution should prompt consideration of other maladies coupled with additional diagnostic tests including cultures and biopsy.

Conclusions

Ecthyma is a cutaneous infection caused by *S. pyogenes* or *S. aureus* that exhibits as punched-out ulcers with a crust and erythematous borders. The differential diagnosis is broad and endemic infections, especially zoonoses, should be considered in returned travelers. Treatment consists of wound care and systemic antibiotics.

References

1. Matz H, Orion E, Wolf R. Bacterial infections: uncommon presentations. Clin Dermatol. 2005;23(5):503–8.
2. Empinotti JC, Uyeda H, Ruaro RT, Galhardo AP, Bonatto DC. Pyodermitis. An Bras Dermatol. 2012;87(2):277–84.
3. Wasserzug O, Valinsky L, Klement E, Bar-Zeev Y, Davidovitch N, Orr N, et al. A cluster of ecthyma outbreaks caused by a single clone of invasive and highly infective streptococcus pyogenes. Clin Infect Dis. 2009;48(9):1213–9.
4. Martinez-Longoria CA, Rosales-Solis GM, Ocampo-Garza J, Guerrero-Gonzalez GA, Ocampo-Candiani J. Ecthyma gangrenosum: a report of eight cases. An Bras Dermatol. 2017;92(5):698–700.
5. Caravaglio JV, Khachemoune A. Orf virus infection in humans: a review with a focus on advances in diagnosis and treatment. J Drugs Dermatol. 2017;16(7):684–9.
6. Veraldi S, Esposito L, Pontini P, Vaira F, Nazzaro G. Feast of sacrifice and Orf, Milan, Italy, 2015-2018. Emerg Infect Dis. 2019;25(8):1585–6.
7. Sanford CA, Fung C. Illness in the returned international traveler. Med Clin North Am. 2016;100(2):393–409.
8. Lederman ER, Weld LH, Elyazar IR, von Sonnenburg F, Loutan L, Schwartz E, et al. Dermatologic conditions of the ill returned traveler: an analysis from the GeoSentinel surveillance network. Int J Infect Dis. 2008;12(6):593–602.
9. Hochedez P, Canestri A, Lecso M, Valin N, Bricaire F, Caumes E. Skin and soft tissue infections in returning travelers. Am J Trop Med Hyg. 2009;80(3):431–4.
10. Orbuch DE, Kim RH, Cohen DE. Ecthyma: a potential mimicker of zoonotic infections in a returning traveler. Int J Infect Dis. 2014;29:178–80.
11. Stevens DL, Bisno AL, Chambers HF, Dellinger EP, Goldstein EJ, Gorbach SL, et al. Practice guidelines for the diagnosis and management of skin and soft tissue infections: 2014 update by the infectious diseases society of America. Clin Infect Dis. 2014;59(2):147–59.
12. Kwak YG, Choi SH, Kim T, Park SY, Seo SH, Kim MB, et al. Clinical guidelines for the antibiotic treatment for community-acquired skin and soft tissue infection. Infect Chemother. 2017;49(4):301–25.
13. Vaiman M, Lasarovitch T, Heller L, Lotan G. Ecthyma gangrenosum versus ecthyma-like lesions: should we separate these conditions? Acta Dermatovenerol Alp Pannonica Adriat. 2015;24(4):69–72.
14. Vaiman M, Lazarovitch T, Heller L, Lotan G. Ecthyma gangrenosum and ecthyma-like lesions: review article. Eur J Clin Microbiol Infect Dis. 2015;34(4):633–9.
15. Jiang Y, Al-Hatmi AM, Xiang Y, Cao Y, van den Ende AH, Curfs-Breuker I, et al. The concept of Ecthyma Gangrenosum illustrated by a fusarium oxysporum infection in an immunocompetent individual. Mycopathologia. 2016;181(9–10):759–63.
16. Wuyts L, Wojciechowski M, Maes P, Matthieu L, Lambert J, Aerts O. Juvenile ecthyma gangreno-

sum caused by Pseudomonas aeruginosa revealing an underlying neutropenia: case report and review of the literature. J Eur Acad Dermatol Venereol. 2019;33(4):781–5.

17. Karimi K, Odhav A, Kollipara R, Fike J, Stanford C, Hall JC. Acute cutaneous necrosis: a guide to early diagnosis and treatment. J Cutan Med Surg. 2017;21(5):425–37.

18. Haemel AK, Bearden A, Longley BJ, Crnich C. Black spots in the returning traveler. Dermatol Online J. 2013;19(11):20393.

19. Oaks JB, Lasam G, LaCapra G. Mediterranean spotted fever: a rare non-endemic disease in the USA. Cureus. 2017;9(1):e974.

20. Fischer M. Rickettsioses: cutaneous findings frequently lead to diagnosis–a review. J Dtsch Dermatol Ges. 2018;16(12):1459–76.

21. Rovery C, Raoult D. Mediterranean spotted fever. Infect Dis Clin N Am. 2008;22(3):515–30. ix

22. Blanton LS. The rickettsioses: a practical update. Infect Dis Clin N Am. 2019;33(1):213–29.

23. Vasievich MP, Villarreal JD, Tomecki KJ. Got the travel bug? A review of common infections, infestations, bites, and stings among returning travelers. Am J Clin Dermatol. 2016;17(5):451–62.

24. Burza S, Croft SL, Boelaert M. Leishmaniasis. Lancet. 2018;392(10151):951–70.

Boils or Furunculosis

Guadalupe E. Estrada-Chávez

Key Points
- Furunculosis main causal agent is *Staphylococcus aureus.*
- Clinical features are abscesses with a central pustule in main folds.
- Imunosupresion, obesity, and external factors as humidity are related.
- Treatments include fusidic acid, mupirocine, or dicloxaciline.
- Treat according to the severity of the infection and age of patient.

Bacterial diseases among travelers is one of the main complications especially in tropical or subtropical areas, either during the visit or after returning to their hometown, as high environmental humidity and temperature are some of the main triggering factors for superficial or even deep infectious skin diseases. Together with the former, there are multiple other associated external causes that can aggravate initial mild skin problem, evolving to severe health conditions [1]. There are also multiple predisposing factors but not exclusive, as triggering or aggravators for the disease which include immunodeficiency or health issues such as diabetes, obesity, malnutrition, alcoholism, hyperhidrosis, anemia, etc. [2]

The term "boils" has been known since antiquity, having references as the sixth Egyptian plague in the Book of Exodus (the second book of the Pentateuch or Torah) and was related to dust and how polluted environment can cause health issues [3].

Boils is also known as furunculosis and, is caused by *Staphylococcus aureus* which is the most frequent causal agent of skin and soft tissues infections (SSTI) in tropical environments, it is in most cases preceded by folliculitis. It can affect all ages, and the complexity of the clinical manifestations are related to the host immune response, both innate and acquired immunity; together with the inherent pathogenicity of the causal agent [4] and co-morbidities, in most cases, diabetes and obesity determine the severity of each case. Much has been told regarding the relevance of identifying causal agents as well as cultures to provide sensitivity information, which will allow an adequate future comparison, based on solid ground. *S. aureus* methicillin-resistant strains (MRSA) have caused great concern especially whenever acquired at the community as it can cause from 8 to 50% in mortality rate bacteremia [2]. Community-associated MRSA epidemic clones are Panton-Valentine leukocidine (PVL) genes carriers, with multiple reports regarding the severity of infections in immuno-

Community Dermatology Mexico

G. E. Estrada-Chávez (✉)
Faculta de Medicina, Universidad Autonoma de Guerrero Mexico, Acapulco, Mexico

© The Editor(s) (if applicable) and The Author(s), under exclusive license to Springer Nature Switzerland AG 2024

W. Robles (ed.), *Skin Disease in Travelers*, Updates in Clinical Dermatology, https://doi.org/10.1007/978-3-031-57836-6_4

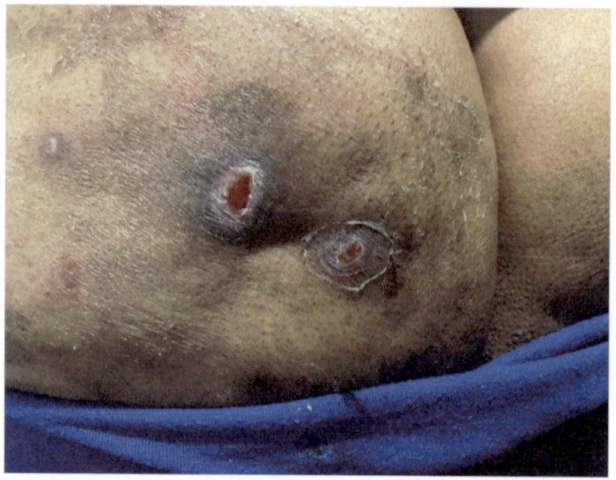

Fig. 1 Furunculosis with residual hyperpigmentation and desquamation

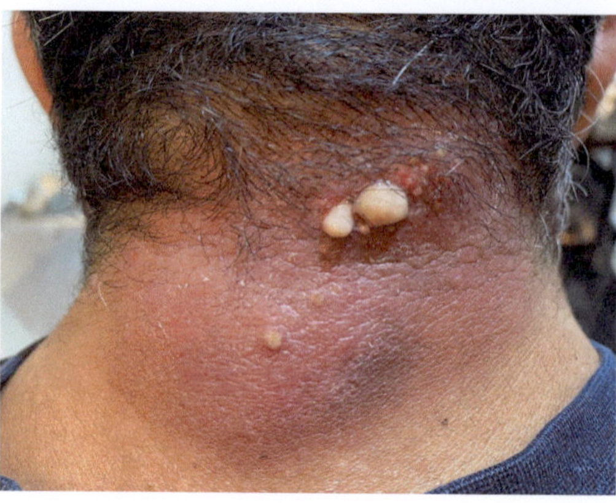

Fig. 2 Carbuncle on the neck with intense erythema and draining fistulae with thick yellowish pus

competent, young, healthy people, with furunculosis, necrotizing pneumonia, and osteomyelitis [5]. Unfortunately, the trend of MRSA and multi-resistant *S. aureus* bacterial infections is on the increase [6, 7]. It has become more relevant as one of the main agents responsible for pulmonary and cardiac complications evolving to severe health threat.

As Furunculosis is a deep follicular infection, with necrosis and perifollicular inflammation, the main clinical features observed include, erythema, edema, or local swelling of a nodular-like lesion or abscesses, which contains purulent collections and can be centered by a superficial pustule. Lesions are usually very painful and can be single or multiple. Malaise, fever, and fatigue are not uncommon. The affected areas are mostly in main folds, as neck, axillae, inguinal, and buttocks (Fig. 1), especially if obesity is present, as humidity and maceration of the superficial skin increases the risk of bacterial proliferation.

Areas where hair follicles are abundant are also frequently affected. Furuncules can converge and can cause a larger affected area with abundant pus-discharging openings which is considered as Carbuncle (Fig. 2) [2, 8], with clear modification of the aspect of the skin; hair follicles can be displaced or lost due to purulent exudate and local necrosis.

Even though furunculosis affects any age group, children from early infancy and school age frequently have evident lesions at the anterior

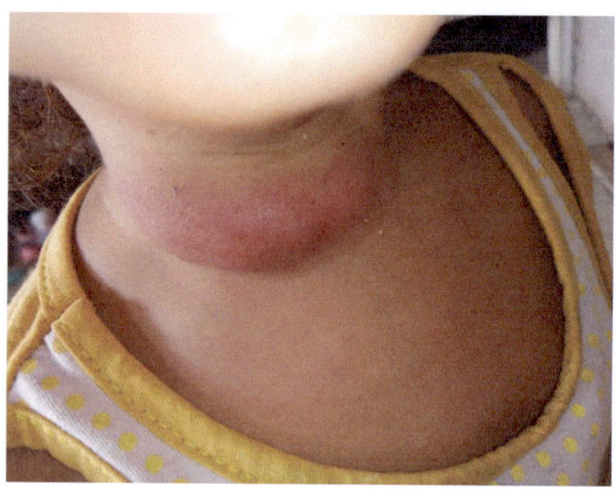

Fig. 3 Neck boils in a 4 y-o child, with characteristic erythema and oedema of the affected area

neck fold (Fig. 3), especially as sweat and dust, and food debris are commonly accumulated in soft and redundant fat tissue (dewlap). Due to the nature of this bacterial infection and its numerous variables and triggering factors, it is worth mentioning some of the most frequent factors to which travelers are exposed. These include sand or abrasive surfaces, synthetic fabric clothing, use of oil-based sun block, prolonged contact with the latter and even prolonged exposure to, either environmental humidity, sweating or brackish/sea water together with all of the above mentioned in infants rapidly evolve into severely painful lesions that cause parental distress and seek for prompt medical attention. Some of these are consistent with seasonal variants of pediatric skin problems which are more frequent during rainy season and summer [9].

There are several aspects that have to be taken into account whenever a skin problem is identified in a patient with a recent travel history. These include age, other health problems such as diabetes or immunosuppressive treatments, which, associated with environmental factors e.g., high humidity weather, sweating, use of synthetic clothing, prolonged contact with water and/or wet clothing may trigger the condition. Occlusion is a well-known element that will play a role in the pathogenicity of *S. aureus* to produce deeper or more severe lesions on the skin [10] Swimming pool water contains highly chlorinated water and acid, among other chemicals, in order to maintain water clearness. Salted sea water, due to salinity can cause, as well, skin barrier alteration, cutaneous dehydration, scaling and microabrations related to activities on sand or harsh surfaces, especially on the folds, can change pH and microflora. Similar cases have been reported in active military members who, due to their work activities, together with environmental factors, can spend prolonged time with the gear and exposed to environmental factors that favor bacterial infections becoming prone to develop SSTIs [11] which can cause a prolonged treatment or inability to promptly return to their daily activities. There are other groups that, related to humidity conditions, have developed similar lesions, as in athletes from different disciplines, as abrasions due to equipment, clothing or objects over wet, macerated skin provide a favorable environment for bacterial proliferation [12]. Small epidemics have been reported in athletes especially swimmers, both fresh and saltwater, as most athletes interact with environmental-related factors that can cause cutaneous infectious diseases [13], which may resemble the conditions that travelers are exposed to.

Therefore, medical chart and direct medical interrogatory is essential in order to obtain valuable information that allows us to identify causal agents or triggering factors that could have influenced the skin problem. We propose a series of questions that could allow identifying possible cutaneous triggers for boils, besides the basic medical interrogatory including concomitant diseases.

Seven days before the onset of any visible skin lesions specify:

- Visited countries.
- Climate at the visited countries or regions.
- Frequency of aquatic activities.
- Type of water exposure (treated, pool, brackish (sea water or cave water), lagoon, river, muddy, etc.)
- Time of permanency of wet, humid or sweaty clothing on the skin per day, either continuously or discontinuously.
- Type of fabric clothing most frequently used.
- Hygienic habits daily during travelers stay (shower or bath with soap and water).

Recurrences of furunculosis can be in some cases a severe inconvenience, it has been proposed that transient immune change influences in the recalcitrant boils, especially in returning travelers from tropical regions, and can occur up to 8.4 months after with over four recurrences in average [14].

Differential diagnosis of boils in early stages can include several superficial cutaneous infections, like folliculitis, *hydradenitis suppurativa*, acneiform dermatitis, etc. And depending on the topography other diseases should be considered, as osteomyelitis, atypical mycobacteriosis, and even tumoral lesions such as angiosarcoma. One of the most frequently reported in literature are myasis mimicking furunculosis [15], especially as clinical aspect can be very similar, and particularly as it is a frequent skin problem in tropical and subtropical environments. Whenever a clinical furunculosis has recidivant lesions or is resistant to treatment with a recent history of travel, myasis (*Diptera* larvae) should be kept in mind, which is usually endemic and presents and has been reported as "vacation" disease, most of the reported cases are in young adults with lesions in the abdomen and chest and with antibiotic-resistant furunculosis [16, 17].

Treatment: Due to the nature of boils and the notorious lesions, together with intense symptomatology, treatment can be challenging, whenever travelers are suffering from this disease. Bacterial infections can initiate as apparently simple mildly symptomatic cutaneous lesions. Nevertheless, consider that travelers are often without the means to receive adequate or specific treatment, and in some cases, can be reluctant to receive therapy whenever are not in an accessible or "trustful" medical area, allowing skin infections to evolve into more severe health problems.

Every case should be treated according to the severity of the infection, and age of the patient, always considering co-morbidities. Though there are multiples reports regarding treatment options, both topical and systemic, early diagnosis and treatment in essential in order to avoid future complication such as cellulitis or lymphadenitis. Initial hygienic measures are essential together with local antiseptics; allowing a reduction on local bacterial colonization. In hot weather environments, usage of talcum and Zinc oxide powder over clean and dry skin can provide a partial reduction on the humidity and secondary maceration on folds. Topical antibiotics include bacitracin, mupirocin, fusidic acid, eritromycin and retapamulin, depending on the availability of each country, is usually recommended for 1 week but can be extended depending individual cases. Systemic antibiotic treatment, as with most of antibiotic treatments, needs to be indicated depending on the severity of infection, as well as sensitivity; these include dicloxacilin, oxacillin, ryfampicyn, eritromycin, ciprofloxacin, or azytromycin among others [18] always with a previous interrogation regarding allergic reactions related to antibiotics. There has been multiple analysis to compare the efficacy of antibiotics, but evidence suggests that regarding treating boils, there is no significant difference between them [19]. Treatment options will need to be reviewed in each country, Nevertheless, dicloxaciline 500 mg four times a day for 1 week is a regular dosage especially in acute episodes, with a general world-wide availability, clindamycin 300 mg every 8 h for 1 week or ciprofloxacine 500 mg every 12 h for 1 week are effective and usually well tolerated. Azithromycine 500 mg daily for 3 days has shown a positive response

and can be used to prevent relapse in chronic furunculosis [20]. In diabetics or immunosuppressed patients, a double scheme can be considered in order to avoid complications or deep tissue infections. Generally, antibiotic sensitivity is not particularly considered, but whenever possible, culture should be performed. Depending on the elected antibiotic and related to individual patients' conditions, anti-inflammatory medication can be added. Drainage of a furuncule is an option whenever an abscess is well delimited, and with a fluctuant center, always should be performed with all hygienic measures as complications related to self-performed or in-house lancing of the lesions is not uncommon, but can lead to complications [21]. MRSA infections can be treated systemically with Vancomycin or Rifampicin.

References

1. Marques SA, Abbade LPF. Severe bacterial skin infections. An Bras Dermatol. 2020;95(4):407–17. https://doi.org/10.1016/j.abd.2020.04.003. Epub 2020 May 16
2. Venkatesan R, Baskaran R, Asirvatham AR, Mahadevan S. Carbuncle in diabetes': a problem even today! BMJ Case Rep. 2017;2017:bcr-2017220628.
3. Mazokopakis EE, Karagiannis CG. Environmental and medical aspects related to the sixth plague of Egypt. Maedica (Bucur). 2019 Sep;14(3):310–3. https://doi.org/10.26574/maedica.2019.14.3.310.
4. Nowicka D, Grywalska E. Staphylococcus aureus and host immunity in recurrent Furunculosis. Dermatology. 2019;235(4):295–305. https://doi.org/10.1159/000499184. Epub 2019 Apr 17
5. Nimmo GR, Coombs GW. Community-associated methicillin-resistant Staphylococcus aureus (MRSA) in Australia. Int J Antimicrob Agents. 2008;31(5):401–10. https://doi.org/10.1016/j.ijantimicag.2007.08.011. Epub 2008 Mar 14
6. Zetola N, Francis JS, Nuermberger EL, Bishai WR. Community-acquired meticillin-resistant Staphylococcus aureus: an emerging threat. Lancet Infect Dis. 2005 May;5(5):275–86. https://doi.org/10.1016/S1473-3099(05)70112-2.
7. Macmorran H, Harch S, Athan E, Lane S, Tong S, Crawford L. The rise of methicillin resistant *Staphylococcus aureus*: now the dominant cause of skin and soft tissue infection in Central Australia. Epidemiol Infect. 2017;145:2817–26.
8. Craft N. Chapter 176 Fitzpatrick's dermatology in general medicine. 2012.

9. Banerjee S, Gangopadhyay DN, Jana S, Chanda M. Indian J Dermatol. 2010;55(1):44–6.

10. Firsowicz M, Boyd M, Jacks SK. Follicular occlusion disorders in down syndrome patients. Pediatr Dermatol. 2020;37(1):219–21. https://doi.org/10.1111/pde.14012. Epub 2019 Oct 18

11. Stahlman S, Williams VF, Oh GT, Tribble DR, Millar EV. Skin and soft tissue infections, active component, U.S. armed forces, January 2016-September 2020. MSMR. 2021 Apr;28(4):27–38.

12. Levy JA. Common bacterial dermatoses: protecting competitive athletes. Phys Sportsmed. 2004 Jun;32(6):33–9. https://doi.org/10.3810/psm.2004.06.380.

13. Adams BB. Dermatologic disorders of the athlete. Sports Med. 2002;32(5):309–21. https://doi.org/10.2165/00007256-200232050-00003.

14. Artzi O, Sinai M, Solomon M, Schwartz E. Recurrent furunculosis in returning travelers: newly defined entity. J Travel Med. 2015;22(1):21–5. https://doi.org/10.1111/jtm.12151. Epub 2014 Aug 25

15. Rodríguez-Cerdeira C, Gregorio MC, Guzman RA. Dermatobia Hominis infestation misdiagnosed as abscesses in a traveler to Spain. Acta Dermatovenerol Croat. 2018 Oct;26(3):267–9.

16. Pathania V, Kashif AW, Aggarwal RN. Cutaneous myiasis: think beyond furunculosis. Med J Armed Forces India. 2018;74(3):268–72. https://doi.org/10.1016/j.mjafi.2017.03.005. Epub 2017 Apr 7

17. Ajili F, Abid R, Bousseta N, Mrabet A, Karoui G, Louzir B, Battikh R, Othmani S. Des furoncles résistants aux antibiotiques: penser à la myiase !! [Antibiotic resistant furuncles: think myiasis]. Pan Afr Med J, 2013 Jun 4. 15:41. https://doi.org/10.11604/pamj.2013.15.41.2621.

18. Daum RS, Miller LG, Immergluck L, Fritz S, Creech CB, Young D. A placebo-controlled trial of antibiotics for smaller skin abscesses. N Engl J Med. 2017;376:2545–55.

19. Lin HS, Lin PT, Tsai YS, Wang SH, Chi CC. Interventions for bacterial folliculitis and boils (furuncles and carbuncles). Cochrane Database Syst Rev. 2021 Feb 26;2(2):CD013099. https://doi.org/10.1002/14651858.CD013099.pub2.

20. Aminzadeh A, Demircay Z, Ocak K, Soyletir G. Prevention of chronic furunculosis with low-dose azithromycin. J Dermatolog Treat. 2007;18(2):105–8. https://doi.org/10.1080/09546630601165125.

21. Medows M, Sharma A. Lancing of a boil leading to severe invasive methicillin-sensitive Staphylococcus aureus infection in an adolescent. BMJ Case Rep. 2013 Dec 11;2013:bcr2013200651. https://doi.org/10.1136/bcr-2013-200651.

Cellulitis and Erysipelas

Paola De Mozzi

Key Points

- Cellulitis and erysipelas are common dermatoses in travelers.
- Pathophysiology and microbiology: the most common pathogens responsible for cellulitis and erysipelas are Streptococci and Staphylococcus Aureus. Unusual and atypical pathogens may be implicated in travelers, depending on travel itinerary and environmental exposures.
- Treatment is based on antimicrobial agents directed to the responsible microorganism. The vast majority of cases resolve without sequelae with appropriate treatment. In severe cases, especially in the presence of underlying systemic disorders or immunosuppression, the course of the disease may be severe.
- Preventative measures in travelers are recommended.

Epidemiology

Bacterial skin and soft tissue infections are one of the leading causes of cutaneous problems in travelers [1–4], however there is no validated data on the real prevalence of cellulitis and erysipelas in this group [5].

P. De Mozzi (✉)
Royal Free Hospital NHS Foundation Trust,
London, UK
e-mail: paolademozzi@nhs.net

The challenge in assessing epidemiologic data on cellulitis and erysipelas in travelers is due not only to the limited number of studies available and their small sample size but also to the large variability of demographics and travel characteristics. Travel characteristics are numerous and heterogeneous, for example: region of travel, purpose of travel (i.e., tourism, business, education, volunteering), travel duration, timing to healthcare provider visit, point of assessment (primary care, specialised centres in secondary care). Another compounding factor is that cellulitis and erysipelas are not reportable infectious diseases.

Indeed, travelers should be considered at higher risk than the general population to acquire cellulitis and erysipelas, especially in the context of activities exposing them to environments and circumstances leading to these presentations.

The largest retrospective series of returned travelers presenting with dermatologic conditions reported in the literature to date [1] found cellulitis to be more common in geriatric patients.

Pathophysiology and Microbiology

Cellulitis and erysipelas are caused by inoculation of normal skin flora and other bacteria through a breakdown in the skin barrier. The

W. Robles (ed.), *Skin Disease in Travelers*, Updates in Clinical Dermatology,
https://doi.org/10.1007/978-3-031-57836-6_5

introduction of these bacteria leads to an acute superficial infection which affects the upper dermis in erysipelas and the deep dermis and subcutaneous fat in cellulitis.

The microorganism involved in the vast majority of classic erysipelas and cellulitis is beta-haemolytic Streptococcus, usually group A organisms (i.e. Streptococcus pyogenes), although other groups may be involved (especially G but also C and B) in both conditions, followed by methicillin-sensitive Staphylococcus Aureus [6].

A wider spectrum of pathogenetic microorganisms should be considered in travelers in the context of their travel characteristics, especially when travel destinations or activities may expose them to unusual or more aggressive pathogens, for example in the case of marine activities or animal bites.

Here, we analyse some types of common and uncommon cellulitis and erysipelas in travellers and associated pathogens, although this is not exhaustive of the entire spectrum of potential pathogens or travel scenarios.

Cellulitis and Erysipelas Caused by Insect Bites

Insect bites are a common cause of cellulitis or erysipelas in the traveler (for example mosquitoes, bedbugs, fleas, midges, spiders, mites, ticks, bees, ants). Insect bites and superinfected insect bites is one of the most common skin-related diagnosis in returning travelers [1].

Increased susceptibility to insect bites in travelers is often linked to destinations with hot and humid climates, where insect bites are ubiquitous, and the skin surface area covered by clothes is reduced, or to low level of accommodation in non-urban areas.

Following a local inflammatory allergic reaction, cellulitis and erysipelas may develop as a secondary phenomenon, due to inoculation of pre-existing bacteria on the surface of the skin into the wound or as a result of exogenous pathogenic bacteria inoculated into the wound from an insect that served either as a reservoir or vector

for them [7]. Cellulitis and erysipelas may also be caused by excoriations (breach in the skin barrier) secondary to itch associated with insect bites and subsequent inoculation of bacteria.

It can often be challenging to clinically distinguish between a local reaction to insect bites and cellulitis or erysipelas caused by insect bites. Factors which may indicate cellulitis or erysipelas include. The presence of systemic upset, worsening reactions with spreading erythema after expected time to improvement, the presence of purulent discharge, or lymphangitis.

Cellulitis and Erysipelas Caused by Animal Bites

Cellulitis and erysipelas may present following animal bites in travelers. This may occur in the context of rural or remote destinations and activities where animal exposure is more likely. If travel purpose is tourism, then this may also be favoured by a relaxed attitude towards safety, when domestic or wild animals are at reaching distance. Children are at greatest risk, as they are often unaware of the dangers and are more likely to approach animals.

Human-infected wounds caused by animal bites are usually polymicrobial. The organisms involved tend to originate from the oral cavity of the offending biter, as well as the environment where the injury occurred.

The most commonly reported animal bites in travellers are from dogs, followed by cats and monkeys, although any mammalian could be implicated.

Pathogens in cat and dog bites include Pasteurella multocida, Capnocytophaga canimorsus, Streptococcus, Staphylococcus, Neisseria, Corynebacterium, Moraxella, Fusobacterium, Porphyromonas, Prevotella, Bacteroides, Propionibacterium [8]. The severity of infection can range from localised cellulitis to systemic dissemination, leading to severe disease, hence prompt diagnosis and antimicrobial treatment of severe infections are paramount, as well as any appropriate post-exposure prophylaxis or immunization [8, 9] (i.e., rabies, tetanus, other viral infections).

Pasteurella multocida is the most common pathogen in dog and cat bites. It is an anaerobic, gram-negative coccobacillus. Pasteurella wound infection typically presents with early onset of local intense cellulitis associated with purulent discharge, and lymphangitis, usually within 12–24 h after the injury. If untreated, this infection can lead to sepsis and multiple organ failure [10]. In monkey bites, the increased risk from rabies and simian herpes B virus should be considered as well as post exposure prophylaxis or immunisation as appropriate [8].

Prompt and adequate wound cleaning is the first step in the management of animal bites and may prevent development of cellulitis.

Cellulitis and Erysipelas Caused by Aquatic Environment

The aquatic environment includes seawater, freshwater (i.e. lakes, ponds, rivers), swimming pools and spas.

Travelers engaging in aquatic activities, (sport or recreational) such as swimming, snorkelling, diving, or fishing, may be susceptible to injuries, for example skin abrasions, aquatic animal bites, stings, and other minor traumas, leading to cellulitis or erysipelas.

Wounds sustained in the aquatic environment or pre-existing the aquatic activity are exposed to a milieu of bacteria rarely encountered in the more common settings of land-based trauma.

Although Staphylococcus and Streptococcus species that colonise the skin remain the most common etiologic agents associated with salt-water and freshwater skin and soft tissue infections, other significant pathogens should be considered in the aquatic environment, including Vibrio spp., Aeromonas spp., Shewanella spp., Edwardsiella spp., Chromobacterium violaceum, Erysipelothrix rhusiopathiae, Pseudomonas aeruginosa, Mycobacterium marinum and other Mycobacterium spp., Streptococcus Iniae, Plesiomonas, Clostridium, [11] although this listing is not all-inclusive.

The spectrum of manifestations with aquatic pathogens varies from cases of mild cellulitis to severe life-threatening necrotizing fasciitis, sepsis, and death. The most severe presentations are especially seen with Vibrio, Aeromonas, and Shewanella spp. infections. Travelers at greater risk of severe infection include those with pre-existing open wounds, individuals with suppressed immune systems, liver disease, alcoholism, hemochromatosis, haematological disease, diabetes, chronic renal disease, acquired immunodeficiency syndrome, and cancer. Early detection and appropriate management with antibiotic therapy in severe cases is paramount as it can significantly decrease morbidity and mortality [12].

Methicillin-Resistant Staphylococcus Aureus (MRSA)

The increasing international travel, except for the slowdown associated with the COVID-19 pandemic, has facilitated the transmission of multidrug-resistant bacteria across continents, including Methicillin-Resistant Staphylococcus Aureus (MRSA), resulting in a global concern. MRSA burden has a great geographical variation, ranging from low prevalence in Scandinavia to the highest prevalence in parts of America and Asia [13].

MRSA may be acquired by travelers via recreational travelling (community-acquired) or overseas healthcare exposure (hospital-acquired) and medical tourism, resulting in either asymptomatic colonisation or clinically significant MRSA disease.

MRSA cellulitis and erysipelas are uncommon, but they should be considered in the appropriate context. They may be associated with a more severe or purulent clinical picture and lack of response to conventional antibiotics.

Risk Factors

Risk factors for the first episode of cellulitis and erysipelas in travelers can be divided into two main groups: general and travel-specific.

General Risk Factors

General risk factors for cellulitis and erysipelas are the same as in the general population [14] and can be classified in local and systemic.

Local Risk Factors

1. Trauma to skin barrier (i.e. cut, abrasion, laceration, excoriation, burn).
2. Pre-existing skin ulcer (i.e. leg ulcer).
3. Tinea pedis.
4. Excoriated underlying inflammatory dermatosis (i.e. eczema, psoriasis).
5. Oedema from any cause.
6. Venous insufficiency or other venous compromise (i.e. saphenous harvest for bypass).
7. Lymphoedema or other lymphatic compromise (i.e. previous lymph node dissection).

Systemic Risk Factors

1. Diabetes mellitus.
2. Obesity.
3. Immunosuppression.
4. Peripheral vascular disease.
5. Intravenous drug abuse.
6. Chronic kidney disease.
7. Liver disease.
8. Malignancy.

Travel-Specific Risk Factors

Travel-related risk factors include travel destination (i.e., insect bites acquired in hot and humid climates), type of itinerary, duration of travel, level of accommodation, activities undertaken during travel, environmental exposures (i.e., animal, plants, aquatic setting), adherence to prescribed and over-the-counter preventative medications and measures.

Clinical Presentation

Cellulitis and erysipelas present with expanding erythema, warmth, tenderness, and swelling.

Cellulitis typically affects the deep dermis and subcutaneous tissues. It has ill-defined borders and is slower to develop. Erysipelas affects the more superficial layers of the skin (upper dermis) and has a characteristic well-demarcated and raised oedematous edge and faster development. Both conditions can be associated with blistering, bullae, which may be haemorrhagic in nature.

When extending to the superficial cutaneous lymphatics, lymphatic involvement (i.e., ascending lymphangitis, and regional lymph node involvement) may be present, which is a common finding in erysipelas.

Systemic symptoms (i.e. fever, malaise, chills, and nausea) may be present and in classic erysipelas they can be more prominent. These may be associated with raised white cell count and inflammatory markers [15].

In many instances, it may be challenging to clinically distinguish between erysipelas and cellulitis, as cellulitis may extend superficially and erysipelas deeply. When this is the case, then erysipelas can be regarded as a superficial form of cellulitis rather than a distinct entity.

Cellulitis and erysipelas can affect any part of the body, however they both most commonly occur in the legs. In the traveler, when cellulitis is secondary to a new traumatic wound or insect bites, any anatomical site exposed to the external environment can be affected. Both conditions share similar risk factors and management principles.

In most severe cases, cellulitis and erysipelas can progress to dermal necrosis, abscess, necrotising fasciitis, myositis or osteomyelitis, and septicaemia.

Diagnosis and Differential Diagnosis

Accurate history and thorough clinical examination are essential steps to make a correct diagnosis of erysipelas or cellulitis in the traveler.

In the history, key questions include timing of symptoms and/or signs, history of skin trauma or injuries, type of activity engaged with during travel (i.e., exposure to sea or freshwater, to swimming pools, exposure to animals, fish, etc.), history of insect bites, the presence of local and/or systemic symptoms (such as fever, malaise, etc.), pattern, and speed of progression. Additionally, a complete past medical history and drug history should be conducted to evaluate underlying chronic medical conditions or immunosuppression, any known pre-existing predisposing factors such as venous stasis, lymphoedema, peripheral vascular disease and chronic tinea pedis, and the presence of inflammatory dermatosis (i.e., psoriasis, eczema, or other pruritic dermatoses leading to excoriations).

A careful clinical examination is paramount, as the diagnosis of cellulitis and erysipelas is mainly clinical. Furthermore, this may also reveal a portal of entry (such for example an injury, insect bites, eczema, or cutaneous mycosis).

While in mild cellulitis and erysipelas no diagnostic tests are usually required, some important considerations should apply to travelers, as follows [16, 17]:

- In the presence of an open wound, penetrating injury, drainage, or an obvious portal for microbial entry, or if there is history of exposure to water-borne organisms, a swab or sample for culture should be taken, as it may yield relevant organisms.
- Surface swabs from intact skin are not routinely recommended, as they are unlikely to be helpful. In the case of facial infections, the pathogen should be sought in nose, throat, conjunctive, and sinuses.
- Imaging is not necessary in uncomplicated cellulitis. It can be considered if suspecting cellulitis with an underlying abscess and when this proves clinically challenging to differentiate from non-purulent cellulitis; if suspecting a drainable fluid collection, or when clinical examination is equivocal, for example with ultrasonography. Magnetic resonance imaging (MRI) may be helpful for distinguishing cellulitis from osteomyelitis, when the latter is suspected but cannot be ruled out clinically. Radiographic examination with X-ray, CT scan, and MRI may be performed when suspecting necrotising fasciitis, although if there is clinical suspicion, this should not delay surgical intervention.

- A skin biopsy can be considered only where there is doubt about the diagnosis and to help identifying any unusual pathogens in subjects who are unresponsive to initial treatment.
- White blood cell count, erythrocyte sedimentation rate (ESR), and C-reactive protein (CRP), although non-specific and not routinely performed, may support the diagnosis, when this is challenging to make, by detecting acute inflammation through elevated levels, or in severe presentations.
- When there is a history of recurrent cellulitis, serologic testing for beta-haemolytic streptococci may be a useful diagnostic tool. Various assays are available, for example anti-streptolysin-O (ASO) reaction, anti-deoxyribonuclease B test (anti-DNAse B), anti-hyaluronidase test (AHT), or Streptozyme antibody assay.
- Blood cultures are warranted in the traveler, in the following circumstances:
  - Severe and extensive infection.
  - Systemic signs of infection (e.g., fever).
  - Aquatic injuries and animal bites.
  - Failure of initial antibiotic therapy.
  - Presence of underlying comorbidities (lymphedema, malignancy, neutropenia, immunodeficiency, splenectomy, diabetes, etc.).

The differential diagnosis of cellulitis and erysipelas, includes other soft tissue infections, (such as erysipeloid and necrotising fasciitis). When localised to the lower limbs, differential diagnosis includes deep vein thrombosis, stasis dermatitis (varicose eczema), superficial thrombophlebitis, and panniculitis (i.e., erythema nodosum, lipodermatosclerosis), chronic inflammation secondary to lymphoedema/chronic oedema. Other differential diagnoses include inflammatory causes of 'pseudocellulitis' such as allergic contact dermatitis, exaggerated insect bite reactions, erythema migrans, fixed drug eruptions, Sweet's syndrome, inflammatory granuloma annulare, Well's syndrome, inflammatory morphoea, interstitial granulomatous dermatitis [6].

Treatment

In uncomplicated cellulitis and erysipelas in travelers, for example when caused by superficial or minor injuries or by insect bites, the same general principles as in the general population apply. Outlining treatment guidelines is beyond the scope of this chapter, as these may vary at a national and local level, with substantial practice variation, and they also depend on the source or body of recommendations [18–21].

As a general rule, the antibiotic of choice should be one that is active against Gram-positive pathogens, especially streptococci (i.e. penicillins, first- or second-generation oral cephalosporins, macrolides, or clindamycin).

If there are exposure histories suggesting infection with an unusual pathogen, empiric regimens should include coverage targeting the organisms suggested by the exposure history. In these instances, the aid of microbiology data (i.e., wound, tissue or blood cultures) will guide on targeted treatment. In immunocompromised travelers, a wide variety of organisms may be implicated as cause of cellulitis or erysipelas, and broader antimicrobial coverage should be considered for fungal, viral, and parasitic organisms as appropriate, in addition to bacteria.

Specific guidelines on treatment of patients with soft tissue infections following water exposure are available [22], and may be applicable to travelers who develop cellulitis or erysipelas following exposure to the aquatic environment. In this scenario, clinical concern of unusual gram-negative organisms should be raised and an initial empirical treatment should cover for these. Obtaining specimens (i.e., wound, exudate, tissue, blood cultures) for microbiologic examination and to guide on antibiotic therapy when possible, is recommended. Suitable antimicrobial agents include first-generation cephalosporin or clindamycin or linezolide if penicillin allergic, plus a fluoroquinolone plus doxycycline, if seawater exposure, for coverage of Vibrio species.

In animal bites, antimicrobial treatment should be directed against the typical pathogens associated with the oral flora of the biting animal and the skin of the victim. Guidelines on the treatment of animal bites are available, and in non-severe cases they include initial empiric treatment with co-amoxiclav in adults and children or doxycycline with metronidazole [23] in the outpatient setting. Appropriate treatment and wound care are important in animal bites, to prevent them from progressing to cellulitis or a more severe clinical picture.

MRSA coverage may be required in travelers whose cellulitis is associated with purulent drainage, penetrating trauma, evidence of MRSA infection elsewhere or nasal colonisation with MRSA, if there is a history of intravenous drug use or in the presence of severe infection not responding to conventional treatment [19]. MRSA colonisation or infection should be also considered when there is history of exposure to healthcare facilities during travel or if the purpose of travel is medical tourism.

Anti-MRSA agents include trimethoprim-sulfamethoxazole, doxycycline, clindamycin, linezolid, glycopeptides and newer antimicrobials and treatment should be chosen based on local susceptibility profiles and local MRSA treatment protocols [24, 25].

The recommended duration of antibiotic therapy for cellulitis and erysipelas in the outpatient setting is 7 days, but treatment should be extended if the infection has not improved within this time period.

Hospitalisation and intravenous antimicrobial treatment may be required in the following circumstances [26]:

1. When uncommon pathogens are suspected, for example, after a penetrating injury or exposure to water-borne organisms.
2. If the traveller is severely unwell.
3. When the infection occurs near the eyes or nose (including periorbital cellulitis), because of risk of a serious intracranial complication.
4. If the infection is rapidly progressing and is not responding to oral antibiotics or if there is concern for a deeper or necrotising infection.
5. In a severely immunocompromised traveler.

Following hospitalisation, review of clinical response is recommended every 24 to 72 hours and treatment regimen should be adjusted, as appropriate.

Prognosis and Complications

Erysipelas and cellulitis have, in the vast majority of cases, a benign course, as they can be treated successfully with antimicrobial agents and do not result in permanent sequelae.

Rarely, they may progress to serious illness by a more aggressive contiguous spread via the lymphatic or circulatory systems, manifesting with lymphangitis, abscess formation, and rarely, myositis, gangrenous cellulitis, septic arthritis, osteomyelitis, or necrotizing fasciitis [27].

Toxins produced by certain bacterial species, such as group A beta-hemolytic Streptococcus and Staphylococcus aureus, or the exposure to unusual and more virulent bacterial pathogens (i.e., certain marine injuries or animal bites), may mediate a more severe systemic infection, especially in travelers who are elderly or have underlying medical conditions, and can lead to septic shock and death in the worse scenario.

Cellulitis and erysipelas in the traveler, as in the general population, is associated with a risk of recurrence. Each episode increases the likelihood of subsequent recurrence and also of length of hospitalisation [28]. Persistent leg ulceration and lymphoedema (caused by lymphatic inflammation and subsequent permanent damage to lymphatic vessels) are potential chronic complications of cellulitis and erysipelas [29].

Prevention

As rupture of the cutaneous barrier, whatever is its cause, is a common factor in cellulitis, travelers should avoid skin injuries as much as possible, maintain good skin hygiene, increase their self-protection against insect bites, and avoid contact with wild or domestic animals.

Travel essentials (travel kits) and travel recommendations to minimise the risk of cellulitis and erysipelas [30] include:

1. Insect repellent (such as DEET or picaridin) to protect against insect bites.
2. Wearing clothing that covers the limbs, especially in the early evening, and tucking trousers into socks to reduce insect bites exposure.
3. Products to counteract skin irritation and itch from insect bites or stings (i.e. oral or topical antihistamines and low dose topical corticosteroids).
4. A broad-spectrum sunscreen with appropriate SPF to avoid getting sunburnt.
5. Emollient to prevent and treat any skin dryness.
6. Anti-fungal products (from over-the-counter or on prescription) in the presence of fungal infection or athlete's foot.
7. Good wound care and hygiene practice in the presence of a wound (cleaning the wound with soap and water, using clean dry bandages where necessary, using a topical antiseptic, avoiding aquatic activities).
8. Wearing shoes to protect the feet on the beach and in the sea and using appropriate shoe wearing when accessing remote destinations.
9. Staying at sensible distance from animals to avoid being bitten or scratched.
10. Prescription of oral, as well as topical antibiotics against staphylococcal/streptococcal infections should be considered in selected cases, for example for remote and/or prolonged itineraries where self-treatment may be necessary.

Paediatric travelers require parental supervision to ensure that preventative measures are properly employed, especially with regards to contact with water, animals, sand, and soil.

In the presence of pre-existing host-related local or general factors which may predispose to cellulitis and erysipelas, preventative measures are recommended.These also recommended when an episode of cellulitis or erysipelas has already occurred, since recurrence of cellulitis is common after the first episode.

Examples of pre-existing factors and actions recommended include:

1. Oedema and venous insufficiency: compression therapy after resolution of cellulitis. This has been shown to be effective in reducing recurrent cellulitis [31].
2. Tinea pedis (fissuring or maceration of the interdigital spaces on the feet): foot hygiene and early treatment, especially in elderly people, can significantly reduce the incidence of cellulitis and erysipelas [32].
3. Obesity: weight management.
4. Diabetes: optimisation of diabetic control.
5. Pre-existing inflammatory dermatosis associated with dryness and itch causing scratching and subsequent areas of skin breakdown (i.e. eczema, psoriasis) or ulceration: appropriate treatment of underlying inflammatory dermatosis prior to travelling.

References

1. Lederman ER, Weld LH, Elyazar IR, von Sonnenburg F, Loutan L, Schwartz E, Keystone JS. Dermatologic conditions of the ill returned traveler: an analysis from the GeoSentinel surveillance network. Int J Infect Dis. 2008;12:593–602.
2. Lucchina LC, Wilson ME, Drake LA. Dermatology and the recently returned traveler: infectious diseases with dermatologic manifestations. Int J Dermatol. 1997;36:167–81.
3. Hill DR. Health problems in a large cohort of Americans traveling to developing countries. J Travel Med. 2000;7:259–66.
4. Lockwood DN, Keystone JS. Skin problems in returning travelers. Med Clin North Am. 1992;76: 1393–411.
5. Caumes E, Carriere J, Guermonprez G, et al. Dermatoses associated with travel to tropical countries: a prospective study of the diagnosis and management of 269 patients presenting to a tropical disease unit. Clin Infect Dis. 1995;20:542–8.
6. Bolognia JL, Lorizzo JL, Rapini RP. Dermatology. 2nd ed. Mosby Elsevier; 2008.
7. Darlet RW, Richards JR. Cellulitis from insect bites: a case series. Cal J Emerg Med. 2003;4:27–30.
8. Thomas N, Brook I. Animal bite-associated infections: microbiology and treatment. Expert Rev Anti-Infect Ther. 2011;9:215–26.
9. Boillat N, Frochaux V. Animal bites and infection. Rev Med Suisse. 2008;4(2149–52):2154–5.
10. Evgeniou E, Markeson D, Iyer S, et al. The management of animal bites in the United Kingdom. Eplasty. 2013;13:e27.
11. Finkelstein R, Oren I. Soft tissue infections caused by marine bacterial pathogens: epidemiology, diagnosis, and management. Curr Infect Dis Rep. 2011;13:470–7.
12. Diaz JH. Skin and soft tissue infections following marine injuries and exposures in travelers. J Travel Med. 2014;21:207–1.
13. Lee AS, de Lencastre H, Garau J, et al. Methicillin-resistant Staphylococcus aureus. Nat Rev Dis Primers. 2018;4:18033.
14. Bjornsdottir S, Gottfredsson M, Thorisdottir AS, et al. Risk factors for acute cellulitis of the lower limb: a prospective case-control study. Clin Infect Dis. 2005;41:1416–22.
15. Rook. Rook's textbook of dermatology. 8th ed. Wiley-Blackwell; 2010.
16. Stevens DL, Bisno AL, Chambers HF, et al. Practice guidelines for the diagnosis and management of skin and soft tissue infections: 2014 update by the infectious diseases society of America. Clin Infect Dis. 2014;59(2):e10–52.
17. Spelman D, Baddour LM. Cellulitis and skin abscess: epidemiology, microbiology, clinical manifestations, and diagnosis 2021. https://www.uptodate.com/contents/cellulitis-and-skin-abscess-epidemiology-microbiology-clinical-manifestations-and-diagnosis#H3993200902.
18. Herchline TE. Cellulitis treatment and management. 2021. https://emedicine.medscape.com/article/214222-treatment
19. National Institute for health and care excellence. Cellulitis and erysipelas: antimicrobial prescribing. NICE guideline. 2019. https://www.nice.org.uk/guidance/ng141/chapter/Recommendations#treatment
20. Stevens DL, Bisno AL, Chambers HF, et al. Infectious Diseases Society of America. Practice guidelines for the diagnosis and management of skin and soft tissue infections: 2014 update by the Infectious Diseases Society of America. Clin Infect Dis. 2014;59:e10–52.
21. Johns Hopkins Guides. Cellulitis. http://www.hopkinsguides.com/hopkins/view/Johns_Hopkins_ABX_Guide/540106/all/Cellulitis.
22. Baddour LM. Soft tissue infections following water exposure. 2021. https://www.uptodate.com/contents/soft-tissue-infections-following-water-exposure.
23. NICE. Human and animal bites: antimicrobial prescribing. 2020. https://www.nice.org.uk/guidance/ng184/chapter/recommendations#choice-of-antibiotic
24. Bystritsky RJ. Cellulitis. Inf Dis Clin North Am. 2021;35:49–60.
25. Sartelli M, Guirao X, Hardcastle TC, et al. WSES/SIS-E consensus conference: recommendations for the management of skin and soft-tissue infections. World J Emerg Surg. 2018;13:58.
26. Gunderson CG, Cherry BM, Fisher A. Do patients with cellulitis need to be hospitalized? A systematic review and meta-analysis of mortality rates of inpatients with cellulitis. J Gen Intern Med. 2018;33:1553–60.
27. Herchline TE. What is the prognosis of cellulitis? 2019. https://www.medscape.com/answers/214222-3111/what-is-the-prognosis-of-cellulitis

28. Cannon J, Dyer J, Carapetis J, et al. Epidemiology and risk factors for recurrent severe lower limb cellulitis: a longitudinal cohort study. Clin Microbiol Infect. 2018;24:1084–8.

29. Dalal A, Eskin-Schwartz M, Mimouni D, et al. Interventions for the prevention of recurrent erysipelas and cellulitis (Cochrane review/Cochrane intervention protocol), vol. 6. John Wiley & Sons, Ltd; 2017.

30. Wilcock J, Etherington C, Hawthorne K, et al. Insect bites. BMJ. 2020;370:m2856.

31. Webb E, Neeman T, Bowden FJ, et al. Compression therapy to prevent recurrent cellulitis of the leg. N Engl J Med. 2020;383:630.

32. Korecka K, Mikiel D, Banaszak A, et al. Fungal infections of the feet in patients with erysipelas of the lower limb: is it a significant clinical problem? Infection. 2021;49:671–6.

Dengue, Chikungunya and Zika

Omar Lupi

Key Points

- Arthropod or mosquito-borne viral diseases are a major public health problem.
- Ecological changes may be responsible for increased susceptibility of populations in endemic areas.
- Urbanisation, globalisation and lack of effective mosquito control are also responsible for increased incidence and development of epidemics.
- Non-specific skin rashes and co-infection can make the diagnosis very difficult.
- Treatment is supportive.

Dengue

Introduction

Dengue is a major international public health concern, and the number of outbreaks has escalated greatly. Human migration and international trade and travel are constantly introducing new vectors and pathogens into novel geographic areas [1].

Dengue is a mosquito-borne endemo-epidemic viral disease, caused by any one of the four serotypes, designated dengue virus (DENV-1, DENV-2, DENV-3 and DENV-4), belonging to the *Flavivirus* genus in the family *Flaviviridae*, can cause dengue fever (DF), an acute viral infection characterised by fever, rash, headache, muscle and joint pain, and nausea, as well as more severe forms of the disease. A possible fifth (DENV-5) serotype has recently been detected, but its global significance remains to be seen [2].

The Flavivirus genus comprises more than 68 arthropod-transmitted viruses, of which 30 are known to cause human disease. 1 The flaviviral infections include dengue, yellow fever, as well as Japanese encephalitis, and tick-borne encephalitis [3, 4]. The clinical picture of dengue was described by Benjamin Rush during an epidemic that occurred in Philadelphia in 1778. Later, during the nineteenth century, several outbreaks were reported in tropical regions around the world.

It is believed that the global dengue pandemic began in the Asian and Pacific regions during and after World War II. Ecological changes occurring at that time probably favoured the geographic expansion of the vector and its increase in den-

O. Lupi (✉)
Dermatology—Federal University of the State of Rio de Janeiro (UNIRIO), Rio de Janeiro, Brazil

Postgraduate Course in Internal Medicine at the Federal University of Rio de Janeiro (UFRJ), Rio de Janeiro, Brazil

Immunology Service—HUCFF/UFRJ, Rio de Janeiro, Brazil

Dermatology Department—Policlínica Geral do Rio de Janeiro (PGRJ), Rio de Janeiro, Brazil

W. Robles (ed.), *Skin Disease in Travelers*, Updates in Clinical Dermatology,
https://doi.org/10.1007/978-3-031-57836-6_6

sity. The high number of susceptible individuals (local populations, soldiers) and their movement due to the war probably created the conditions for the dissemination of the virus [5].

In the second half of the last century, a severe disease, Dengue haemorrhagic fever/Dengue shock syndrome (DHF/DSS), was recognised as a clinical syndrome of dengue infection, and the first cases were described by Hammon in Manila and Bangkok during the 1950s [6]. Since then, the number of cases has steadily increased worldwide and DHF/DSS emerged in new areas of the world, such as the American region, where the first devastating epidemic was reported in 1981. Currently, dengue is the most important arthropod-borne viral disease in terms of morbidity and mortality worldwide [7].

The pathophysiology of dengue was largely inferred from vaccine studies in rhesus monkeys using the attenuated vaccines [3]. After inoculation in rhesus monkeys, the virus replicated initially in local lymph nodes, followed by blood-borne spread and subsequent replication, mostly occurring in regional lymph tissue, spleen, and bone marrow, followed by the liver, lung and adrenal glands [5].

Epidemiology

Dengue transmission has increased geographically during the past few decades [8]. Tropical countries have undergone uncontrolled dengue epidemics, which may expand beyond the supposed climatic and geopolitical boundaries. A combination of urbanisation, globalisation and lack of effective mosquito control has promoted the rapid spread of dengue [9]. Epidemics have been reported in tropical and subtropical regions of Asia and Africa and more recently in the American region. Successive introduction of new serotypes into the Caribbean, Central and South America has occurred since 1977. [8, 10, 11] Dengue diffusion is due to a complex process involving the spread of Aedes mosquitoes and their adaptation to urban environments, population mobility that facilitates the circulation of the virus, and changes in climate that accelerate the

transmission cycle. This is especially marked in cities where, due to urban heat island effects, ambient temperatures are warmer than in surrounding rural areas and rainfall regime alterations may favour the maintenance of mosquito breeding sites [12].

A DHF epidemic was first reported in Cuba in 1981 and was followed 8 years later by the second DHF epidemic in Venezuela. Since then, epidemics have occurred in many other Latin American countries [7, 8]. Currently, more than 3.5 billion people are at risk of DENV infection. It has recently been estimated that there are 390 million DENV infections every year, of which up to 96 million are symptomatic [13]. Previous estimates indicated that there were 50–100 million cases of DENV infection and 250,000–500,000 cases of DHF/DSS each year, placing over 2.5 billion people at risk [14].

Complex and different factors play a causative role in the emergence and re-emergence of this disease, in particular population growth and unscheduled urbanisation, resulting in substandard housing and inadequate water supply, sewage and waste management systems. This is worsened by air travel, migration and deteriorated health programmes. However, poverty and health inequities are behind almost all of these factors [15, 16].

The transmission dynamics of dengue viruses are determined by the interaction of the environment, the agent, the host population and the vector [17].

The macro-determinants of transmission include environmental factors such as latitude (35°N to 35°S), elevation (<2200 m), ambient temperature range (15–40 °C), relative humidity (moderate to high) and the social factors mentioned above (population density, settlement patterns, unscheduled urbanisation, inadequate water supply and waste management) and insufficient knowledge about the disease. The microdeterminants of dengue transmission include host factors (gender, age, immune status, occupation), dengue virulence factors (serotype, level of viremia) and vector factors (abundance and types of mosquito production sites, density of adult females, age of females, host preference, frequency of feeding, etc.) [17, 18].

Aedes aegypti is the main vector although Aedes albopictus has been described as an important vector in some epidemics in Southeast Asia. Aedes aegypti is a domestic mosquito, which lives in the human environment, mainly anthropophilic, bites during daylight and usually breeds in clean water. Once the vector bites a person during the viraemic phase, the virus multiplies within the mosquito (extrinsic incubation period) and within a few days, usually 7–11, it can transmit the virus to another person. After 3–7 days (intrinsic incubation period), the infected individual begins to show symptoms of the disease. Aedes aegypti transmits dengue (horizontal transmission) and can also pass the virus via infected eggs to its offspring (vertical transmission) [3, 19]. Therefore, the mosquito is the true reservoir and the vector for dengue disease. This vector, flourishing in urban and suburban environments, has disseminated the disease to many parts of the world. Furthermore, an Asian tiger mosquito called *A. albopictus* is the major vector to transmit the virus of DENV in Europe, although the most important vector world-wide, *A. aegypti*, was identified in Madeira Island, Portugal, in October 2005. A major epidemic occurred in Madeira in 2012 [20]. Autochthonous transmission of DENV in the United States has also been reported intermittently over the past decade in Texas, Hawaii and Florida [21].

Pathogenesis

Secondary infection by a different dengue serotype has been recognised as a major DHF/DSS risk factor since the 1950s. Severe disease was observed mainly in children experiencing secondary dengue virus and infants born to dengue-immune mothers who experienced their first infection. Seroepidemiologic studies first performed in Thailand and later in Cuba suggested that the presence of heterotypic antibodies from primary dengue infection is a risk factor for developing DHF/DSS [22–24].

It is accepted that the infection with one dengue serotype produces lifelong immunity to reinfection with the same serotype, but only temporal and partial protection to the other serotypes. One of the most important questions with regard to dengue pathogenesis is the identity of the cells that play a crucial antiviral role during the innate immune response to DENV at the earliest stages of infection [25]. Recently, Gandini et al. have shown that DENV2 efficiently activated IFN-α production by plasmacytoid dendritic cells (pDCs), which produced up to 1000-fold more IFN-α than other cell types in response to virus exposure. Elevated IFN-α plasmatic levels are observed shortly after onset of symptoms in children and adult DENV-infected patients. [26]

Neutralising antibodies could attenuate the severity of the disease: the presence of low amounts of heterotypic neutralising antibodies could prevent severe disease; in contrast, non-neutralising, cross-reactive antibodies can augment dengue virus infection of Fcg receptor-positive cells such as monocytes and macrophages. This phenomenon termed antibody-dependent enhancement (ADE) of infection has been hypothesised to occur in vivo during secondary infections [27].

It has been demonstrated that following primary infection, the dengue virus-specific memory T lymphocyte population is composed predominantly of serotype cross-reactive T lymphocyte clones. This observation has led to a new integrated hypothesis arguing that during secondary infection, non-neutralising antibodies can increase the number of dengue-infected monocytes via ADE. In addition, serotype cross-reactive CD8+ and CD4+ T lymphocytes are activated and produce high levels of lymphokines. Marked T cell and monocyte activation results in the production of higher levels of cytokines and chemical mediators that consequently induce malfunction of vascular endothelial cells and derangement of blood coagulation with the final outcome of plasma leakage, shock and haemorrhagic manifestations [28, 29]. Massive complement activation is also present [30]. Recently, it has been suggested that an inappropriate "T cell" response could contribute to immunopathology while doing little to clear the virus. T cells with relatively low affinity for the serotype of the secondary infection and high affinity for those that produced the primary infection have been demonstrated [30].

Besides secondary infection, other factors depending on the host, the virus and the epidemiological/ecological conditions contribute to the development of DHF, both in individuals and in epidemics [31]. Age (children have a higher risk of developing DHF/DSS), chronic diseases such as intrinsic asthma, diabetes mellitus, sickle cell anaemia, ethnicity (higher risk in Whites than Blacks) and the genetic background of the individual represent host factors for severe disease. [31–33] Four viruses have been associated with DHF/DSS epidemics. However, serotypes 2 and 3 and some particular genotypes are the most frequently reported. Several mutations that are associated with changes in virulence have been identified in the genome of Dengue 2 virus belonging to the Asian genotype; a decreased ability to replicate in human monocyte-derived macrophages of American strains has also been observed [34, 35].

Clinical Features

The spectrum of the disease is broad. Most of the infections are asymptomatic or very mild, characterised by undifferentiated fever with or without rash mainly in infants and young children. Studies performed in Cuba provide evidence that for each clinically reported case at least 10 sub-clinical or asymptomatic infections may occur [7]. Given limited access to medical services in many countries, it is conceivable that this relation could be higher.

Classic dengue fever is a febrile viral syndrome of sudden onset, characterised by fever for 2–5 days, severe headache, intense myalgia, arthralgia, retroorbital pain and, sometimes, a diffuse morbilliform rash that may be pruritic and heals with desquamation [3]. Skin haemorrhage and petechiae are frequently observed. Leukopenia and thrombocytopenia may be observed. Recovery is slow, characterised by massive fatigue and severe depression, especially in adults. In some epidemics, unusual bleeding has been described [3, 17].

DHF is characterised by high fever, haemorrhagic phenomena [10, 17, 36, 37]—often with enlargement of the liver—and circulatory failure. Thrombocytopenia (below 100,000/mm3) and haemoconcentration (haematocrit > = 20% or associated signs of plasma leakage such as pleural effusion, ascites, hypoproteinaemia) are regularly present. Plasma leakage is the major pathophysiological alteration that determines the severity of the disease in DHF and differentiates it from dengue fever.

DHF is more likely to develop if an individual previously infected with one serotype is later infected with a different viral serotype [22]. It is primarily recognised in children less than 15 years and has a more severe course, including vomiting, facial flushing and circumoral cyanosis, and weakness [1]. Minor bleeding phenomena such as epistaxis, petechiae and gingival bleeding may occur at any time but major bleeding phenomena such as menorrhagia and gastrointestinal haemorrhage are poor prognostic indicators.

Diffuse capillary leakage of plasma is responsible for the haemoconcentration. In the presence of haemoconcentration and thrombocytopenia, the patient is considered to have DHF as classified according to the World Health Organisation (Table 1). [17] DHF is a potentially deadly complication that is characterised by high fever, haemorrhagic phenomena—often with enlargement of the liver—and, in severe cases, circula-

Table 1 World Health Organisation (WHO) classification of dengue hemorrhagic fever

	Signs and symptoms
Grade I	Thrombocytopenia + hemoconcentration. Absence of spontaneous bleeding
Grade II	Thrombocytopenia + hemoconcentration. Presence of spontaneous bleeding
Grade III	Thrombocytopenia + hemoconcentration. Hemodynamic instability: Filiform pulse, narrowing of the pulse pressure (< 20 mmHg), cold extremities, and mental confusion
Grade IV	Thrombocytopenia + hemoconcentration. Declared shock, patient pulseless and with arterial blood pressure = 0 mmHg (dengue shock syndrome: DSS)

tory failure [17]. The illness commonly begins with a sudden rise in temperature accompanied by facial flush and other non-specific constitutional symptoms of dengue fever. The fever usually continues for 2–7 days and can be as high as 40–41 °C, possibly with febrile convulsions and haemorrhagic phenomena [17]. In moderate DHF cases, all signs and symptoms abate after the fever subsides (grades I and II). In severe cases, the patient's condition may suddenly deteriorate after a few days of fever; the temperature drops, followed by signs of circulatory failure, and the patient may rapidly go into a critical state of shock and die within 12–24 h (dengue shock syndrome: DSS) [17]. The case-fatality of DHF/DSS is 10% or higher if untreated. With supportive treatment, fewer than 1% of such cases succumb.

Warning signs are valuable as early predictors of DHF/DSS. Intensive and on-going abdominal pain, intense vomiting, sudden decrease of temperature, irritability, depression lethargy or ultrasound evidence of plasma leakage indicate that a rapid and appropriate treatment must be administered [17, 37].

Diagnosis and Differential Diagnosis

The differential diagnosis in the early phase of dengue is difficult. Meningococcaemia, leptospirosis, malaria, typhus, yellow fever, other haemorrhagic viral fevers, influenza, rubella and other diseases producing rash must be considered [3, 8, 37].

Confirmation of the suspected diagnosis can be done by serological studies and by virus detection. Dengue IgM detection is routinely used as a serological marker of recent infection. 5–6 days after the onset of fever, dengue IgM can be detected by IgM ELISA. This assay is 95% sensitive and is widely employed. The determination of IgG antibodies in paired sera provides serological confirmation. A fourfold increase in anti-dengue IgG titer is confirmatory. Viral isolation mainly in mosquito cell lines followed by identification using immunofluorescence techniques with specific dengue antibodies and genome

detection using the polymerase chain reaction (PCR) represent methods for virus detection. The virus can be recovered from acute serum samples collected in the first days after onset of fever and in tissues (liver, spleen, lymph nodes and others) in fatal cases [38, 39].

Serotype determination should be done by PCR and virus isolation. At present, the neutralisation test is the only serological assay for serotype determination.

Treatment

Treatment of dengue is non-specific and supportive. For patients with severe bleeding and shock syndrome, measures to correct hypovolemia, hypoxia and shock can reduce complications and death. The use of high doses of corticosteroids has not been shown to alter mortality rates in this situation [3, 10]. Specific chemotherapies under investigation include interferon and ribavirin [40]. When interferon is administered to monkeys within 8 h of infection, mortality is reduced; however, interferon is ineffective when given at 24 h [40]. The use of interferon in combination with other immune-enhancing drugs is continuing to be researched. Ribavirin, although effective in vitro, has not been proven effective in vivo because of an inability to achieve sufficient concentrations in the blood [40].

An effective vaccine against dengue is a difficult task since the different serotypes of the dengue virus are present in most countries, and a future infection with other serotypes can predispose to DHF [10].

Prophylaxis

Prevention and control of the arthropod vector rely on insecticides, barrier measures, protective clothing, bed netting and insect repellents [3, 11]. In Asia and the Americas, Aedes aegypti breeds primarily in artificial containers like earthenware jars, metal drums and concrete cisterns used for domestic water storage, as well as discarded plastic food containers, used automobile tires, and other items that collect rainwater. In Africa, it also breeds extensively in natural habitats such as tree holes and leaf axils. In recent years, A. albopictus, a secondary dengue vector in Asia, has become established in the United States, several Latin American and Caribbean countries, and in parts of Europe [11].The rapid geographic spread of this species has been largely attributed to the international trade in used tires [11].

Vector control is implemented using environmental management and chemical methods. Proper solid waste disposal and improved water storage practices, including covering containers to prevent access by egg-laying female mosquitoes, are amongst the methods that are encouraged through community-based programmes [11, 17]. The application of appropriate insecticides to larval habitats, particularly those that are considered useful by householders, e.g. water storage vessels, prevent mosquito breeding for several weeks but must be reapplied periodically [11, 17]. Biocontrol efforts include the use of predatory fish to reduce larvae populations. These methods are interesting option for the long-term control of the infection in endemic areas [11].

A dengue vaccine must confer long-lasting protective immunity against the four dengue serotypes in order to avoid the ADE phenomenon and sensitisation to future dengue infections and consequently DHF/DSS [41].. Although an effective DENV vaccine has not yet reached the market, there are several candidates currently in clinical trial and it is likely that at least one or more of these vaccine platforms will provide protective immunity against this important, yet previously neglected disease. Although the current frontrunner, CYD-TDV, has yet to demonstrate effective protection in Phase IIb field trials, there is still hope that the Phase III trials will be successful [42].

Four principles are crucial for dengue control: political will (financial support, human resources); improvement of public health infrastructure and vector control programmes, as well as intersectoral coordination (partnerships amongst donors, the public sector, civil society, non-government organisations and private, as well as commercial sectors); active community participation; and reinforcement of health legislation [43]. Currently, new initiatives for dengue management are being conducted by international organisations in order to supply endemic countries with affordable tools for dengue control. Integrated dengue monitoring and control, insecticide-treated curtains, improved formulations of larvicides, the implementation of the dengue/Net, a global system for standardised epidemiological and virological surveillance and the COMBI approach (Communication for Behavioural Impact) will assist planners in developing sustained community action plans for dengue prevention and control [44].

Zika Fever

Zika virus (ZIKV) is a mosquito-borne flavivirus related to yellow fever virus, dengue virus and West Nile virus (WNV). It is a single-stranded positive RNA virus that is transmitted by many *Aedes* spp. mosquitoes, including Ae. aegypti. The virus was identified in rhesus monkeys during sylvatic yellow fever surveillance in the Zika Forest in Uganda in 1947 and was reported in humans in 1952 [45]. In 2007, an outbreak of ZIKV was reported in Yap Island, Federated States of Micronesia [46]. ZIKV also caused a major epidemic in the French Polynesia in 2013–2014 [45], and New Caledonia reported imported cases from French Polynesia in 2013 and reported an outbreak in 2014 [45]. A new challenge has arisen in Brazil with the emergence of ZIKV and co-circulation with others arboviruses (i.e. dengue and chikungunya virus [CHIKV]) [45], but also in Thailand and the Philippines (Buathong). During the Brazilian outbreak in 2015, Zika fever was correlated for the first time to increased cases of microcephaly that forced the country to declare a health emergency after more than 1500 new cases observed in a few months after the arrival of ZIKV to the country [45]. In addition, pregnant women should follow specific recommendations about protection from mosquito bites, such as keeping doors and windows closed or screened, wearing trousers and long-sleeved shirts and using repellents authorised during pregnancy [45]. Considering the geographic spread of the disease and the fact that the vector is the same one closely related to dengue is probably just a matter of time to see the first cases of Zika fever in the United States.

Clinical manifestations can be difficult to differentiate from dengue and chikungunya infections. In addition, co-infection with dengue has also been recently reported [47]. In humans, ZIKV infection is characterised by mild fever (37.8 °C–38.5 °C); arthralgia, notably of small joints of hands and feet; myalgia, headache; retroorbital pain; conjunctivitis; and cutaneous maculopapular rash. ZIKV infection is believed to be asymptomatic or mildly symptomatic in most cases [48]. Thus, Zika can be misdiagnosed during the acute (viraemic) phase because of nonspecific influenza-like signs and symptoms. Haemorrhagic signs have not been reported in ZIKV-infected patients [48, 49]. However neurologic complications, including Guillain-Barré syndrome, have been observed [48, 49].

The most common symptoms of Zika infection are maculopapular skin rash that starts on the face or trunk and becomes more diffuse, headaches, low-grade fever, arthralgias, myalgia and conjunctivitis. For ZIKV infection, date of onset of illness is difficult to establish because of sporadic and frequently mild fever. Although rash has been reported 3–5 days after the febrile phase [48], most patients present light asthenia and mild fever 2–3 days before the rash was observed; these symptoms are considered indicative of disease onset. Therefore, at the time the rash is observed, viremia was probably decreasing, which makes detection of virus in serum samples extremely challenging. It is important to observe that ZIKV can also be detected in urine and semen [48]. This observation supports the suitability of urine samples for diagnosis of ZIKV infection by showing that ZIKV RNA is detectable in urine at a higher load and with a longer duration than in serum. However, it also supports the possibility of the transmission of ZIKV as a possible sexually transmitted disease.

There is no specific treatment against ZIKV, so it is critical to control the vector. The impact the use of community peer educators in promoting reduction of mosquito habitats for mosquitoes, especially *Ae. Albopictus* and *Ae. aegyptii*, important vectors of dengue, chikungunya, and Zika viruses can be critical to control these arboviral infections. Since Culex vectors of WNV also utilise container habitats, there is an added benefit for the control of these important species as well. Studies have shown that the most effective education campaigns are those where the community has ownership of the programme [50]. Although public health educational campaigns do not always have an immediate effect on the population of mosquitoes, community participation can help reduce mosquito habitats of important vectors, while developing long-term, low-cost, sustainable programmes [50]. In the event of a public health emergency, such as an outbreak of a vector-borne disease, community peer educators can both help in the reduction of vector habitats, as well as provide reassurance back to the community regarding mosquito control programmes in the area.

Chikungunya Infection

Chikungunya fever (CF) is an arboviral acute febrile illness transmitted by the bite of infected Aedes mosquitoes. A human–mosquito–human cycle is responsible for the maintenance of the virus in the South-East Asia region in contrast to the sylvatic transmission cycle occurring in the African continent [51]. The recrudescence of CF worldwide has been attributed to a multitude of factors including mutation of the virus, absence of herd immunity, lack of efficient vector control activities, and globalisation and emergence of another vector, *A. albopictus*, in addition to *A. aegypti*, as an efficient transmitter of Chikungunya virus. CF presents a risk for importation now that *A. aegypti* populations have become established in central and southern California as the vector preferences are the same as dengue; recent modelling approaches forecasting the spread of chikungunya identified Los Angeles as a high-risk area for the importation of chikungunya cases but a low-risk area for local transmission [52]. In agreement with these predictions, a single case of CF was identified in Los Angeles in a traveller returning from a visit to Haiti in 2013. By the end of 2014, a total of 46 imported cases of chikungunya in California were reported to and confirmed by CDC [52]. The risks here appear real: A single chikungunya outbreak occurred in temperate northern Italy in 2007 that was transmitted by A. albopictus and sparked by the return of a single infected traveller from India [52, 53]. As of 2014, cases of locally acquired CF have been identified in Florida [52]. As Aedes populations spread across California and continue to successfully overwinter, the possibility of local transmission of both dengue and CHKV will surely increase [53].

A large variety of skin and mucous membrane lesions have been documented to occur in association with CF. The dermatological manifestations of the disease may occur in about 40–50% of all cases [54]. Morbilliform eruption is the most common pattern of cutaneous lesions found. It usually appears 3–5 days after the appearance of fever and subsides within 3–4 days usually without any sequelae. The rash is asymptomatic in about 80% of the patients, and the remainder may complain of mild pruritus [51]. The eruption most frequently appears on the first 2 days of onset of fever, but may appear simultaneously with the fever or after defervescence [54]. The first site of appearance of the skin lesions are most frequently the upper limbs, followed by the face and trunk. The skin rash in CF commonly affects the extremities, trunk, neck and ear lobes. Although the face is said to be relatively spared, facial involvement in up to 77% of the cases have been documented. Recurrent episodes have also been observed.

Hypermelanosis of the skin may develop soon after the rash has resolved. The hypermelanosis appears to be postinflammatory in nature and may develop rapidly [54]. The hyperpigmentation may be of different types including centrofacial and freckle-like, diffuse pigmentation of face, pinna, and extremities, flagellate pigmentation and pigmentation of existing acne lesions. Predominant affection of the exposed skin raises the possibility of the role of ultraviolet exposure in the distribution pattern of the pigmentary anomaly [55]. Xerosis of skin and associated scaling is also commonly seen. Desquamation of palms was also noted in some patients. Excoriated papules due to itching are often present. Generalised urticarial lesions have also been reported to be associated with CF. Generalised macular erythema, usually found within 24–48 h of appearance of fever, is another important finding of this infection [51, 54].

Acute intertrigo-like lesions and peno-scrotal or perianal ulceration are other distinctive manifestations of CF and may be hard to differentiate from genital herpes, chancroid and even Behçet's disease [55]. The patients usually develop these ulcers about 2–5 weeks after the onset of fever. The ulcerations are usually punched-out, deep-seated with undermined edges showing healthy granulation tissue in the floor and erythema and thickening in the surrounding skin.54 The size of the ulcers varies from 0.5 to 2 cm in diameter and their shape is round to be oval or asymmetrical. Multiple aphthous-like ulcers may also be found on axillae, tongue, palate and other areas of oral mucosa [54, 55]. Lymphedema, mainly in acral distribution, may also appear 2–3 weeks after the appearance of fever. Flaccid vesiculobullous lesions in infants have also been reported. These lesions were of sudden-onset and often multiple and healed without scarring or pigmentary changes. Vesiculobullous lesions appeared around the fourth day of fever over the lower limb and spread to involve the perineum, abdomen, chest and upper limb [54]. Generalised erythema, maculopapular rash and peripheral cyanosis were amongst the other dermatological findings in the infants [56].

Vasculitic lesions and erythema nodosum like lesions have also been reported to occur in CF. Targetoid lesions over the extremities and trunk simulating erythema multiforme was seen in some patients [54, 55]. Although the acute febrile illness caused by the Chikungunya virus remits spontaneously without any sequelae in most patients, the joint manifestations may linger for a prolonged period of time. Persistent joint affection has been described to occur in about 12% of patients in the forms of residual stiffness without pain and persistent painful restriction of joint movements [54, 55].

The vast majority of cases are diagnosed on clinical and epidemiological grounds. A positive virus culture supplemented with neutralisation provides a definitive proof for the presence of Chikungunya vírus [54, 55]. A RT-PCR test can also provide proof of infection. Demonstration of a fourfold increase in specific IgG antibody titer against the virus between the acute and convalescent phase sera, or the demonstration of IgM antibodies specific for Chikungunya virus in acute-phase sera, offers serological confirmation of the disease.

There is no specific antiviral therapy available for CF. The disease is generally self-limiting and the goal of the therapy is symptomatic relief of complaints like fever and joint pain with paracetamol or NSAIDs. Since no vaccines are commercially available for inducing active immunity against the disease, the mainstays of prevention remain the vector control measures at the household and community levels and the avoidance of mosquito bites by appropriate measures [51, 55].

References

1. Lambrechts L, Scott TW, Gubler DJ. Consequences of the expanding global distribution of *Aedes albopictus* for dengue virus transmission. PLoS Negl Trop Dis. 2010;4:64–6.
2. Normile D, Tropical medicine. Surprising new dengue virus throws a spanner in disease control efforts. Science. 2013;342:41–5.
3. Halstead SB. Dengue. Curr Opin Infect Dis. 2002;15:471–6.
4. Mahe A, Lamaury I, Strobel M. Mucocutaneous manifestations of dengue. Presse Med. 1998;27:1909–13.
5. Gubler DJ. In: Gubler DJ, Kuno G, editors. Dengue and dengue hemorrhagic fever: its history and resurgence as a global public health problem, vol. 8. New York: Cab International; 1997. p. 1–22.
6. Hammon WM, Rudnick A, Sather G, et al. New hemorrhagic fevers of children in The Philippines and Thailand. Trans Assoc Am Phys. 1960;73:140–55.
7. Kouri GP, Guzman MG, Bravo JR, et al. Dengue haemorrhagic fever/dengue shock syndrome: lessons from the Cuban epidemic, 1981. Bull World Health Organ. 1989;67:375–80.
8. Isturiz RE, Gubler DJ, Brea del Castillo J. Dengue and dengue hemorrhagic fever in Latin America and Caribbean. Infect Dis Clin N Am. 2000;14: 121–40.
9. Gubler DJ. Dengue, urbanization and globalization: the unholy trinity of the 21(st) century. Trop Med Health. 2011;39(4):3–11.
10. Guzman MG, Kouri G. Dengue: an update. Lancet Infect Dis. 2002;2:33–42.
11. Guzman MG, Kouri G. Dengue and dengue hemorrhagic fever in the Americas: lessons and challenges. J Clin Virol. 2003;27:1–13.
12. Jetten TH, Focks DA. Potential changes in the distribution of dengue transmission under climate warming. Am J Trop Med Hyg. 1997;57:285–97.
13. Bhatt S, Gething P, Brady O, Messina J, Farlow A, Moyes C, et al. The global distribution and burden of dengue. Nature. 2013;496:504–7.
14. World Health Organisation (WHO). Dengue and Dengue Haemorrhagic Fever. Fact sheet. 2014. No. 117. Geneva.
15. Farmer P. Social inequalities and emerging infectious diseases. Emerg Infect Dis. 1996;2:259–69.
16. Gubler DJ. The changing epidemiology of yellow fever and dengue, 1900 to 2003: full circle? Comp Immunol Microbiol Infect Dis. 2004;27:319–30.
17. Pan American Health Organization. Dengue and dengue hemorrhagic fever in the Americas: guidelines for prevention and control. Scientific Publication. No. 548; 1994.
18. Kuno G. In: Gubler DJ, Kuno G, editors. Factors influencing the transmission of dengue viruses. New York: Cab International; 1997. p. 61–88.
19. Lindback H, Lindback J, Tegnell A, et al. Dengue fever in travelers to the tropics, 1998 and 1999. Emerg Infect Dis. 2003;9:438–42.
20. Alves MJ, Fernandes PL, Amaro F, Osório H, Luz T, Parreira P, et al. Clinical presentation and laboratory findings for the first autochthonous cases of dengue fever in Madeira island, Portugal, October 2012. Euro Surveill. 2013, 18:203–8.
21. Murray KO, Rodriguez LF, Herrington E, Kharat V, Vasilakis N, Walker C, et al. Identification of dengue fever cases in Houston, Texas, with evidence of autochthonous transmission between 2003 and 2005. Vector Borne Zoonotic Dis. 2013;13:835–45.
22. Halstead SB. The Alexander D. Langmuir Lecture. The pathogenesis of dengue. Molecular epidemiology in infectious disease. Am J Epidemiol. 1981;114:632–48.
23. Sangkawibha N, Rojanasuphot S, Ahandrik S, et al. Risk factors in dengue shock syndrome: a prospective epidemiologic study in Rayong, Thailand. I. The 1980 outbreak. Am J Epidemiol. 1984;120:653–69.
24. Guzman MG, Kouri G, Valdes L, et al. Epidemiologic studies on dengue in Santiago de Cuba, 1997. Am J Epidemiol. 2000;152:793–9. discussion 804
25. Schmidt AC. Response to dengue fever—the good, the bad, and the ugly? N Engl J Med. 2010;363:484–7.
26. Gandini M, Gras C, Azeredo EL, Pinto LM, Smith N, Despres P, et al. Dengue virus activates membrane TRAIL relocalization and IFN-alpha production by human plasmacytoid dendritic cells in vitro and in vivo. PLoS Negl Trop Dis. 2013;7(6):1–14.

27. Halstead SB. Antibody, macrophages, dengue virus infection, shock, and hemorrhage: a pathogenetic cascade. Rev Infect Dis. 1989;11(Suppl 4):S830–9.
28. Kurane I, Takasaki T. Dengue fever and dengue haemorrhagic fever: challenges of controlling an enemy still at large. Rev Med Virol. 2001;11:301–11.
29. Rothman AL. Dengue: defining protective versus pathologic immunity. J Clin Invest. 2004;113:946–51.
30. Mongkolsapaya J, Dejnirattisai W, Xu XN, et al. Original antigenic sin and apoptosis in the pathogenesis of dengue hemorrhagic fever. Nat Med. 2003;9:921–7.
31. Kouri GP, Guzman MG, Bravo JR. Why dengue haemorrhagic fever in Cuba? 2. An integral analysis. Trans R Soc Trop Med Hyg. 1987;81:821–3.
32. Bravo JR, Guzman MG, Kouri GP. Why dengue haemorrhagic fever in Cuba? 1. Individual risk factors for dengue haemorrhagic fever/dengue shock syndrome (DHF/DSS). Trans R Soc Trop Med Hyg. 1987;81:816–20.
33. Guzman MG, Kouri GP, Bravo J, et al. Effect of age on outcome of secondary dengue 2 infections. Int J Infect Dis. 2002;6:118–24.
34. Leitmeyer KC, Vaughn DW, Watts DM, et al. Dengue virus structural differences that correlate with pathogenesis. J Virol. 1999;73:4738–47.
35. Cologna R, Rico-Hesse R. American genotype structures decrease dengue virus output from human monocytes and dendritic cells. J Virol. 2003;77:3929–38.
36. John TJ. Dengue fever and dengue hemorrhagic fever. Lancet. 2003;361:181–2.
37. Martinez E. Dengue hemorrágico en criancas. La Habana: Editorial Jose Marti; 1992. p. 1–180.
38. Guzman MG, Kouri G. Dengue diagnosis, advances and challenges. Int J Infect Dis. 2004;8:69–80.
39. Guzman MG, Kouri G. Advances in dengue diagnosis. Clin Diagn Lab Immunol. 1996;3:621–7.
40. Crance JM, Scaramozzino N, Jouan A, et al. Interferon, ribavirin, 6-azauridine and glycyrrhizin: antiviral compounds active against pathogenic flaviviruses. Antivir Res. 2003;58:73–9.
41. Jacobs M, Young P. Dengue vaccines: preparing to roll back dengue. Curr Opin Investig Drugs. 2003;4:168–71.
42. Slifka MK. Vaccine-mediated immunity against dengue and the potential for long-term protection against disease. Front Immunol. 2014;6(5):195.
43. Kroeger A, Nathan M, Hombach J, et al. Dengue. Nat Rev Microbiol. 2004;2:360–1.
44. Guzman MG, Kouri G, Diaz M, et al. Dengue, one of the great emerging health challenges of the 21st century. Expert Rev Vaccines. 2004;3:511–20.
45. Musso D. Zika virus transmission from French Polynesia to Brazil. Emerg Infect Dis. 2015;21(10):1887.
46. Duffy MR, Chen T-H, Hancock WT, Powers AM. Zika virus outbreak on Yap Island, Federated States of Micronesia. N Engl J Med. 2009;360:2536–43.
47. Rodriguez-Morales AJ. Zika: the new arbovirus threat for Latin America. J Infect Dev Ctries. 2015 Jul 4;9(6):684–5.
48. Gourinat AC, O'Connor O, Calvez E, Goarant C, Dupont-Rouzeyrol M. Detection of Zika vírus in urine. Emerg Infect Dis. 2015 Jan;21(1):84–6.
49. Buathong R, Hermann L, Thaisomboonsuk B, Rutvisuttinunt W, Klungthong C, Chinnawirotpisan P, Manasatienkij W, Nisalak A, Fernandez S, Yoon IK, Akrasewi P, Plipat T. Detection of Zika virus infection in Thailand, 2012-2014. Am J Trop Med Hyg. 2015 Aug 5;93(2):380–3.
50. Healy K, Hamilton G, Crepeau T, Healy S, Unlu I, Farajollahi A, Fonseca DM. Integrating the public in mosquito management: active education by community peers can lead to significant reduction in peridomestic container mosquito habitats. PLoS One. 2014 Sep 25;9(9):e108504.
51. Inamadar AC, Palit A, Sampagavi VV, Raghunath S, Deshmukh NS. Cutaneous manifestations of chikungunya fever: observations made during a recent outbreak in South India. Int J Dermatol. 2008;47:154–9.
52. Vega-Rúa A, Lourenço-de-Oliveira R, Mousson L, Vazeille M, Fuchs S, Yébakima A, Gustave J, Girod R, Dusfour I, Leparc-Goffart I, Vanlandingham DL, Huang YJ, Lounibos LP, Mohamed Ali S, Nougairede A, de Lamballerie X, Failloux AB. Chikungunya virus transmission potential by local Aedes mosquitoes in the Americas and Europe. PLoS Negl Trop Dis. 2015 May 20;9(5):e0003780.
53. Fredericks AC, Fernandez-Sesma A. The burden of dengue and chikungunya worldwide: implications for the southern United States and California. Ann glob. Health. 2014 Nov-Dec;80(6):466–75.
54. Bandyopadhyay D, Ghosh SK. Mucocutaneous manifestations oc chikungunya fever. Indian J Dermatol. 2010 Jan-Mar;55(1):64–7.
55. Prashant S, Kumar AS, Mohammed Basheeruddin DD, Chowdhary TN, Madhu B. Cutaneous manifestations in patients suspected of chikungunya disease. Indian J Dermatol. 2009;54:128–31.
56. Valamparampil JJ, Chirakkarot S, Letha S, Jayakumar C, Gopinathan KM. Clinical profile of chikungunya in infants. Indian J Pediatr. 2009;76:151–5.

Coronavirus

Veronique Bataille

Key Points
- Covid pandemic in early 2020 was responsible for lockdown almost worldwide.
- Clinical symptoms were predominantly of respiratory disease with often the need for hospital admissions.
- Skin manifestations with different types of rashes were soon evident.
- The commonest skin manifestation was an erythemato-papular rash followed by urticaria and rash on acral sites.
- Collaboration through social media with phone apps enabled collection of clinical data.

On the 11th of March 2020, the WHO declared the spread of the SARS-COV2 virus across the globe as a pandemic. Reports of atypical flu infections had already been reported in China and other parts of the world since the autumn of 2019 [1]. The most common COVID symptoms, at that time, were fever and chronic cough with severe lung complications leading to hospital admissions. For dermatologists, establishing a link between COVID infection and skin manifestations took a little longer. Early case reports in 2020 reported skin changes in severe hospitalized cases of COVID often from ITU [2, 3]. These were more likely to be showing cutaneous vasculitis but patients were on many drugs and may have suffered from organ failure. More subtle community base dermatology presentations were slowly emerging afterwards as dermatologists started to report cases on multi-media [4]. Later many published case reports and larger series of different COVID skin presentations appeared [5–8]. COVID digits or pseudo-perniosis was the most intriguing skin presentation and many dermatologists, at first, were not convinced of a connection with COVID. The weather was very warm in Europe in the spring of 2020 and the high incidence of these pseudo-perniosis was very atypical. These acral eruptions were also seen in patients who had no previous history of vascular disorders. It then became clear that this was the most specific cutaneous sign of exposure to SARS-COV2 [6, 9, 10]. Another common presentation was an erythemato-papular rash (sometime vesicular) but, this again, was often missed or thought not to be relevant, as this type of eruption often occurred well after the acute phase of infection with negative PCR [5, 6]. These rashes were also more likely to occur in young individuals in the community, and this may have been why series on hospital based patients did not reflect on the full breadth of skin manifestations of COVID in early publications. Cases of urti-

V. Bataille (✉)
Department of Twin Research and Genetic Epidemiology, Kings College, London, UK

Dermatology Department, West Herts NHS Trust, Hertfordshire, UK
e-mail: bataille@doctors.org.uk

W. Robles (ed.), *Skin Disease in Travelers*, Updates in Clinical Dermatology,
https://doi.org/10.1007/978-3-031-57836-6_7

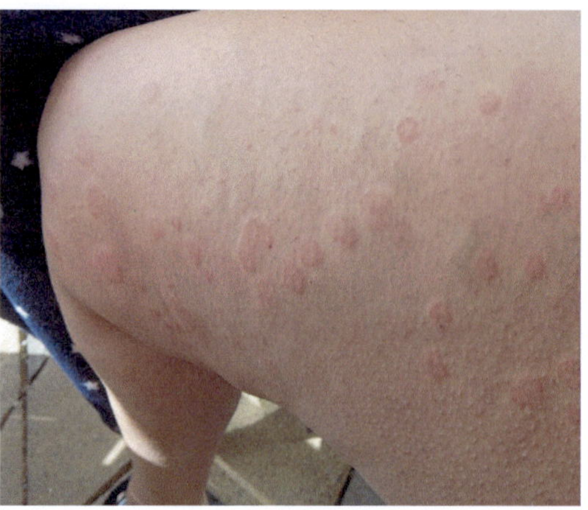

Fig. 1 Urticaria with short-lived erythematous wheals on the limbs

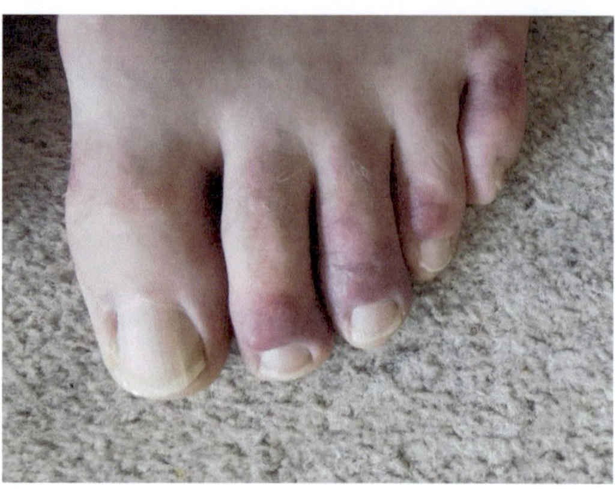

Fig. 2 COVID toes with erythematous and purplish lesions on the toes often affecting the nail bed and dorsum of the toes

caria were also becoming much more common and it was clear that these cases were also virally induced at a time when COVID was very much prevalent [6, 11] (Fig. 1).

In late March 2020, the COVID symptom study app (The Zoe symptom COVID app) was launched in the United Kingdom and later on in the United States [12]. The app could be downloaded on iphones or android handsets and was not a COVID tracker like the NHS app. Instead, it widened significantly the number of potential symptoms of COVID which were reported daily by users. At that time, the NHS guidelines and criteria for obtaining a PRC test only included two classical symptoms such as fever and persistent cough. The COVID symptom app went viral in the United Kingdom and, within a few weeks, 4 millions users had downloaded it to report their potential COVID symptoms [13]. Every morning participants were asked to report if they felt well and, if they did not, they were asked to tick the appropriate symptoms on a list of 19 including skin symptoms. The users also had access to a PCR test if the algorithms on the app predicted that their symptoms were suspicious of a COVID infection. The skin symptoms were divided into erythemato-papular (bumpy, crusty, and itchy red rash) or urticarial (shorter lived itchy and red wheals) or COVID digits (red or purple lesions on fingers or toes) (Fig. 2). To analyze the skin data, a period of 2 months covering May and June 2020 was selected including over 30,000 individuals logging daily at that time [14]. Of those who had a confirmed COVID infection with a positive PCR (over 2000 users), 8% had a rash. In those who had a combination of symptoms suggestive of COVID with the algorithms but no PCR confirmation, a similar percentage (8%) had skin manifestations. Skin could also be predictive of infection before the onset of other symptoms: in 17% of those with a positive PCR and a rash, the rash preceded all other COVID symptoms (Figs. 3 and 4). Furthermore, in 21% of those with a rash and positive PCR, the rash ended up being the only presentation. COVID infection would have been missed if the rash had not occurred. By June 2020, skin rashes were more predictive than fever [14]. A more detailed survey was sent to the participants with a rash with a more detailed questionnaire. This allowed to look at the timing of the rash, the duration and the association with other classical symptoms, as well as possible past history of skin diseases. Users were also asked to provide a photo of the rash if they wished. Over 3000 pictures were received in a short period of time. These were assessed by three independent dermatologists in the summer of 2020 which led to the creation of a website funded by Zoe Global Limited and the British Association of Dermatologists (www.covidskinsigns.com). This allowed healthcare workers and the lay public to have access to a

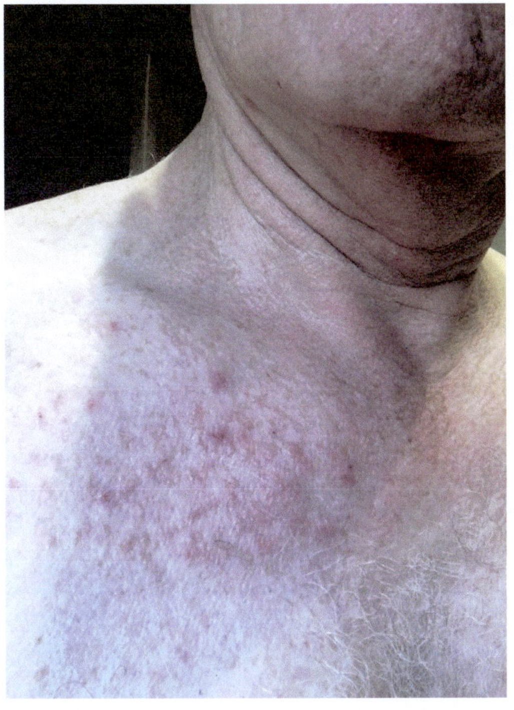

Fig. 3 Erythemato-papular eruption (lichenoid eruption) on the anterior chest. The most common COVID skin eruption

very informative gallery of pictures which helped to detect potential infection. The rashes were classified as below photographs of these types of rashes are to be found at www.covidskinsigns. com.

The most common rash reported on the COVID symptom app in the United Kingdom was an erythemato-papular rash (41% of all rashes) which was usually widespread often affecting wide areas of the torso and limbs and was very symptomatic with pruritus [14]. Patients often required potent topical steroids, as well as oral steroids in some cases as their quality of life was significantly affected. Less often, the rash was vesicular and could mimic chicken pox [15]. This was labelled as pseudo-chicken pox in early case reports. The papules could also be quite large and raised especially on the limbs. This type of rash occurred during but, more often, after the acute infection and the PCR by then was often negative. This confused a lot of dermatologists and patients about the potential link with COVID in early 2020. The mean duration was 14 days but could last for weeks. It could also

Fig. 4 Another example of an erythematous eruption but much more widespread

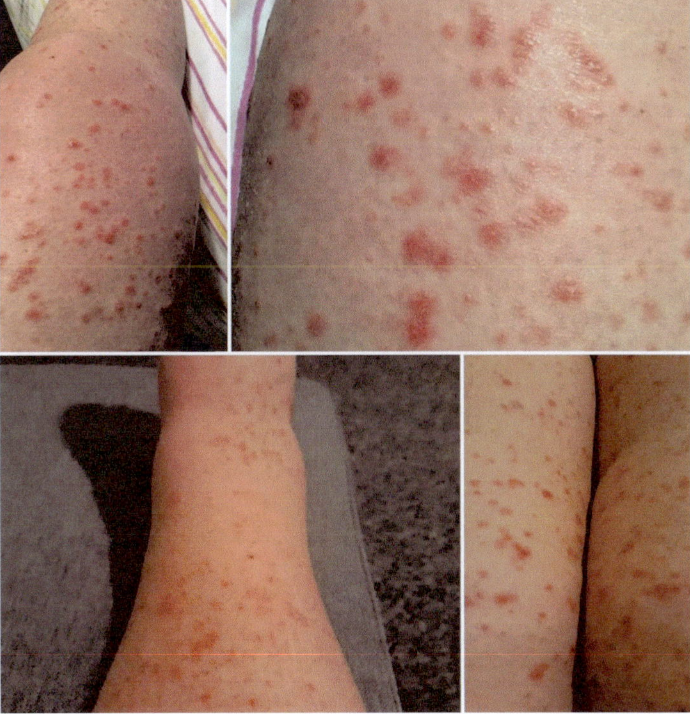

have a relapsing pattern with recurrent rashes at months interval which needed repeated courses of topical or oral corticosteroids. The affected areas could also leave some post-inflammatory pigmentation.

The second most common rash in the COVID symptom app was an urticarial rash (30% of the rashes) [14]. This again was usually more severe than previous cases of idiopathic urticaria and involved large body areas. The face could also be involved but cases of angioedema were not common. This rash could be seen before or during the acute phase of the infection so usually earlier than the erythemato-papular rash above. When occurring before other symptoms, it was helpful, as app users could be tested earlier and isolate to protect others. Urticaria also had a much shorter course than the erythemato-papular rash with a mean duration of 5 days. However, some cases had recurrent attacks over weeks. Patients were usually very symptomatic with severe pruritus and topical and/or oral steroids had to be used in many cases.

The third commonest rash was COVID digits which was described in the literature as pseudo-perniosis from mid-2020 [15]. This, as mentioned above, was really puzzling for dermatologists at the onset of the pandemic. 23% of the COVID suspected rashes on the COVID symptom app assessed with photos were COVID digits [14]. Patients presented with sore reddish and purplish papules or macules usually on the tips of the fingers/toes or on nail beds. These would heal with necrosis of the top layers of the epidermis over a few weeks and leave scaling at the site of the lesions. Lesions on the palms were less common and were more likely to be target lesions resembling erythema multiforme. The toes or fingers could be affected but toes were more commonly involved than fingers. This type of eruption could last for weeks and some patients did report relapse after re-infection, but in some cases, COVID digits recurred without any other symptoms many months after the acute infection. COVID digits were more common in children and young adults [16]. Research suggests that this is due to a better interferon and TNF response in younger individuals which led to a cytokine cascade targeting small blood vessels. Treatment was a bit empirical as the pandemic progressed. The weather was warm when the first lockdown occurred so warming the fingers or toes was not needed. Topical and oral steroids were used when the lesions were extensive and very symptomatic. Nifedipine and aspirin were also tried in some cases. However, most COVID digits occurred in individuals with a mild course and it is likely that many cases were underreported. The exact pathophysiology of COVID digits is still obscure but it appears that the virus damages small acral vessels with perivascular lymphocytic infiltrate and focal thrombosis, endothelial damage, and in many cases evidence of vasculitis [17]. Commercially available antibody to the viral spike protein of SARS-COV2 was detected in the cytoplasm of cutaneous dermal vessels [18]. Sars CoV-2 infects the host using the angiotensin converting enzyme 2 (ACE2) receptor, which is expressed in many tissues including endothelial cells.

Rashes of the head and neck were also seen in COVID positive patients. The rash often started around the eyes, anterior neck, and V of the neck (www.covidskinsigns.com). It was itchy and mimicked a photosensitive eruption. It could also last for weeks and need moderate to potent topical steroids. It was more common in women.

Regarding cutaneous vasculitis, this was quite a rare presentation, and as discussed above was more likely seen in hospitalized patients who had a lot of medication and organ failure which could also contribute to these presentations [6]. Cases of vasculitis in the community were rarer and were more likely to present on the lower legs at the sites of gravity. For patients in the community with mild COVID symptoms with vasculitic changes, investigations were recommended to rule out other causes [19].

Other skin presentations were observed over the last 2 years but were rarer. Pityriasis rosea was also seen more common and often coincided with a previous exposure to COVID (www.covidskinsigns.com). Reactivation of shingles was frequent and was also seen in children which was very unusual. Oral and genital involvement could be a very rare feature of COVID as stomatitis and vulvitis could present during or after COVID infection [20]. Some of the oral and genital presentations were thought to be herpetic but all investigations including viral swabs and serology were negative. The geographical tongue was described but this may not be specific to COVID itself and may be reported more often as individuals were more prone to report any changes. Exacerbation of previous dermatoses such as eczema and psoriasis were not uncommon as well as new cases of bullous pemphigoid. Rare cases of Stevens Johnson have also been linked to COVID infection.

Vaccination for COVID 19 started in Europe in January 2021 and skin reactions have also been reported after vaccines. A large study in Spain by Catala et al. looked at skin side effects of COVID vaccines with the use of eCRFs available to participating dermatology centres in Spain [21]. McMahon et al. in the United States also reported vaccination skin side effects via an international COVID registry (wwwaad.org/covidregistry) [22]. However, in this U.S. study, most cases received mRNA vaccine. The COVID Symptom Study app also collected side effects of COVID vaccines in over 170,000 subjects having had a first dose of the Pfizer vaccine and nearly 200,000, a first dose of the Astra Zeneca vaccine [23]. Skin reactions were reported in 1.1% of the mRNA vaccine and in 2.3% of the Astra Zeneca vaccine group. On the contrary, in the Spanish study, skin side effects were more common with the mRNA vaccines than the attenuated virus vaccines and were not that dissimilar to COVID infection apart from COVID digits which were much rarer. However, this could be explained by the very short follow-up of the Spanish study which could have missed COVID digits as these occur late even after vaccination. Urticarial reactions were slightly more common with vaccination than seen after infection where the erythemato-papular rash was the most common. Urticaria after vaccines was often affecting the neck and torso with a rapid onset usually after 24 h. 18% of the patients in the Spanish survey with urticaria had a past history of urticaria. COVID arm with swelling and redness at the site of vaccination was obviously specific to the vaccine and was common with the mRNA vaccines and often delayed to several days after the injection. It is important to note that this study will have picked up the most symptomatic cases who saw a dermatologist and many milder cases are likely to be under-reported. Cutaneous vasculitis after vaccination was rare but was still reported in 4% of the cases in the Spanish study. 11% of the cases with vaccination cutaneous side effects in the Spanish study had previous COVID infections but the authors did not report obvious differences in skin reactions in those who reported no previous COVID infection [21].

Long COVID and the skin is now becoming an important issue and dermatologists are aware that some individuals have recurrent skin eruptions which can last for months after an acute infection. These eruptions are more likely to be erythemato-papular followed by COVID digits and urticaria. Patients with pre-existing skin disease can also report that their condition is more difficult to control after COVID infection and these flares can last many months. Hair loss may also be a lasting complication of COVID and many women report phases of telogen effluvium which occur weeks after the acute infectious stage. Better data on the long-term impact of COVID on the skin will be available soon via databases such as the Zoe COVID symptom app (www.covid.joinzoe.com) and the American Association of Dermatology COVID registry (McMahon et al. 2021, www.aad.org/covidregistry), as well as the WHO [24].

References

1. Li Q, Guan X, Wu P, et al. Early transmission dynamics in Wuhan, China, of Novel coronavirus-infected pneumonia. N Engl J Med. 2020;382:1199–207. https://doi.org/10.1056/NEJMoa2001316.
2. Guan W, Hu Y, Liang WH, et al. Clinical characteristics of coronavirus disease 2019 in China. New Engl J Med. 2020 April 30;382(18):1708–20.
3. Recalcati S. Cutaneous manifestations in COVID-19: a first perspective. J Eur Acad Dermatol Venereol. 2020;34:e212. https://doi.org/10.1111/jdv.16387.
4. Duong TA, Velter C, Rybojad M, et al. Did Whatsapp® reveal a new cutaneous COVID-19 manifestation? J Eur Acad Dermatol Venereol. 2020;34 https://doi.org/10.1111/jdv.16534.

5. Marzano AV, Cassano N, Genivese G, et al. Cutaneous manifestations in patients with COVID-19: a preliminary review of an emerging issue. Br J Dermatol. 2020 Sep;183(3):431–42.

6. Casas C, Catala A, Carretero Hernandez G, et al. Classification of the cutaneous manifestations of COVID-19: a rapid prospective nationwide consensus study in Spain with 375 cases. Br J Dermatol. 2020;183:71. https://doi.org/10.1111/bjd.19163.

7. Fernandez-Nieto D, Ortega-Quijano D, Segurado-Miravalles G, et al. Comment on: cutaneous manifestations in COVID-19: a first perspective. Safety concerns of clinical images and skin biopsies. J Eur Acad Dermatol Venereol. 2020;34:e252. https://doi.org/10.1111/jdv.16470.

8. Freeman EE, McMahon DE, Lipoff JB, et al. The spectrum of COVID-19-associated dermatologic manifestations: an international registry of 716 patients from 31 countries. J Am Acad Dermatol. 2020;83:1118–29.

9. Fernandez-Nieto D, Jimenez-Cauhe J, Suarez-Valle A, et al. Characterization of acute acro-ischemic lesions in nonhospitalized patients: a case series of 132 patients during the COVID-19 outbreak. J Am Acad Dermatol. 2020;83(1):e61–3.

10. Landa N, Mendieta-Eckert M, Fonda-Pascual P, et al. Chilblain-like lesions on feet and hands during the COVID-19 pandemic. Int J Dermatol. 2020;59:739. https://doi.org/10.1111/ijd.14937.

11. Henry D, Ackerman M, Sancelme E, Finon A, Esteve E. Urticarial eruption in COVID-19 infection. J Eur Acad Dermatol Venereol. 2020:10.1111/jdv.16472. https://doi.org/10.1111/jdv.

12. Drew DA, Nguyen LH, Steves CJ, et al. Rapide implementation of mobile technology for real time epidemiology of COVID-19. Science. 2020, Jun 19;368(6497):1362–7.

13. Menni C, Valdes A, Freidin MB, et al. Real time tracking of self reported symptoms to predict COVID-19. Nat Med. 2020 Jul;26(7):1037–40.

14. Visconti A, Bataille V, Rossi N, Kluk J, Murphy R, et al. Diagnostic values of cutaneous manifestations of SARS-Cov-2 infection. Brit J Dermatol. 2021;184(5):880–7.

15. Marzano AV, Genovese G, Fabbrocini G, et al. Varicella-like exanthem as a specific COVID-19-associated skin manifestation: multicenter case series of 22 patients. J Am Acad Dermatol. 2020;83:280–5.

16. Freeman EE, McMahon DE, Lipoff JB, et al. Pernio-like skin lesions associated with COVID-19: a case series of 318 patients from 8 countries. J Am Acad Dermatol. 2020;83:486–92.

17. Colmenero I, Santonja C, Alonso-Riano M, et al. SARS-CoV-2 endothelial infection causes COVID-19 chilblains: histopathological, immunohistochemical and ultrastructural study of seven paediatric cases. Br J Dermatol. 2020;183:729–37.

18. Santoja C, Heras F, Nunez L, et al. Chilblain like lesion: Immunohistochemical demonstration of SARS-Cov2 spike proteinin blood vessel endothelium and sweat gland epithelium in a polymerase chain reactive-negative patient. Br J Dermatol. 2020 Oct;1834(4):778–80.

19. De Giorgi V, Recalcati S, Jia Z, et al. Cutaneous manifestations related to coronavirus disease 2019m (COVID-19): A retrospective study from China and Italy. J Am Acad Dermatol. 2020 Aug;83(2):674–5.

20. Martin Carreras-Presas C, Amaro Sanchez J, Francisco Lopez-Sanchez A, et al. Oral vesiculobullous lesions associated with SARS-Cov2 infection. Oral Dis. 2021 April;27(suppl):710–2.

21. Catala A, Munoz-Santos C, Casas G, et al. Cutaneous reactions after SARS-COV2 vaccination: a cross-sectional Spanish nationwide study of 405 cases. Br J Dermatol. 2022 Jan;186(1):142–52.

22. McMahon DE, Amerson E, Rosenbach M, et al. Cutaneous reactions reported after Moderna and Pfizer COVID-19 vaccination: a registry-based study of 414 cases. J Am Acad Dermatol. 2021;85:46–55.

23. Menni C, Klaser K, May A, et al. Vaccine side effects and SARS-Cov2 infection after vaccination in users of the COVID symptom study app in the UK: a prospective observational study. Lancet Infect Dis. 2021;21:939–49.

24. McMahon DE, Gallman AE, Hruza GJ, et al. Long COVID in the skin: a registry analysis of COVID-19 dermatological duration. Lancet Infect Dis. 2021;21:313–4.

Part III

Dermatoses Caused by Infection: Fungal Infections–Superficial Mycoses

Pityriasis Versicolor

Mariel Isa

Key Points

- Pityriasis versicolor is a superficial mycosis, worldwide distribution, caused by a yeast fungi of the genus *Malassezia* sp.
- Ultraviolet light Wood's Lamp is useful in many cases.
- Folliculitis considered a superficial inflammation of the hair follicle can be caused in some cases by fungi such as *Malassezia* sp..
- Treatment will depend directly on the affected area and the clinical variant. Topical or systemic treatment, alone or in combination, is used.

Introduction

Pityriasis versicolor is studied within the superficial mycoses, it has worldwide distribution and it is caused by yeast fungi of the genus *Malassezia* sp., dimorphic species, among which Malassezia furfur and *Malassezia globosa* stand out as the main isolated agents in humans. Many of these causative agents of P. versicolor have lipases and

M. Isa (✉)
Dermatology Professor at UASD, UNIBE and PUCMM, Dermatology Residency Co coordinator of the Instituto Dermatológico Dominicano y Cirugía de Piel Dr. Huberto Bogaert Díaz,
Santo Domingo, Dominican Republic

keratinases, enzymes that contribute to their virulence capacity [1–4].

It predominates in tropical areas, especially in the hottest and wettest months. It affects any age, with reports from a few days-old babies to elderly. It has no predominance of sex [1–4].

Synonymy

Tinea versicolor, Tinea flava, chromophytosis.

History

Pityriasis versicolor was considered a skin pathology since 1846 with E. Eichstedt who made the first reports of fungal origin, along with T. Sluyter called it as we know it today. By 1853, the parasite was named, considered a dermatophyte and was named *Microsporum furfur* by Charles-Phillipe Robin who then named the disease Tinea versicolor. By 1874, the levaduriform and non-dermatophytic nature was described by Louis Charles Malassez. In 1889, Henri Ernest Baillon created the genus *Malassezia* [2–4].

In 1904, the genre was changed and designated as *Pityrosporum* by R. Sabouraud. In later years, the names of *Pityrosporum ovale, Pityrosporum orbiculare* appeared. In the 1990s, it was possible to demonstrate similarity between *Malassezia*

W. Robles (ed.), *Skin Disease in Travelers*, Updates in Clinical Dermatology,
https://doi.org/10.1007/978-3-031-57836-6_8

Table 1 Morphologic characteristics of most common *Malassezia* species

Specie	Macroscopic morphology	Microscopic morphology	Associated pathologies
M. furfur	Convex opaque colonies, some rough or folded in appearance	Oval or spherical cells, elongated, with some filaments	Pityriasis versicolor, onychomycosis, folliculitis
M. globosa	Folded, slow growing, rough colonies	Spherical cells (3–8 μm in diameter). Short filaments can be observed	Pityriasis versicolor, folliculitis, seborrheic dermatitis, atopic dermatitis.
M. sympodialis	Bright colonies, flat or slightly convex, smooth	Globose small cells. With aspect of simpodial gemacion	Atopic dermatitis, seborrheic dermatitis, pityriasis versicolor
M. pachydermatis	Convex colonies, matt, smooth surface, cream or beige	Oval cells, small (2–4 μm in diameter), almost cylindrical, with broad-based in the formation of gems	Folliculitis, fungemia
M. restricta	Opaque and smooth colonies	Narrow base spherical cells	Seborrheic dermatitis, Pityriasis versicolor
M. slooffiae	Rough, folded colonies	Short, small, and cylindrical cells	Pityriasis versicolor, atopic dermatitis
M. obtusa	Flat colonies	Large, cylindrical levaduriform cells with filament formation capacity	Pityriasis versicolor

and *Pityrosporum*. In subsequent years, more species were identified, among which M. sympodialis in 1990, *M. globosa, M. restricta, M. obtusa,* and *M. slooffiae* in 1996 stand out [2, 3].

Today, more than 14 species of *Malassezia* are recognized. Table 1 [1–7].

Clinical Characteristics

Pityriasis versicolor lesions are characterized as presented as confluent macules or plaques, which can be hypo or hyperpigmented white, brown, or erythematous.

The lesions can be located in any part of the body but with preference for the trunk area in most cases, anterior and posterior thorax, neck, proximal areas of the upper extremities. In addition, cases are reported on the face, especially in children, infants, and athletes. There are few reports of other locations such as thighs and crotch, armpits, and genital areas [1, 4].

The hypopigmented cases are mainly caused by induced decrease in melanin due to the action of *Malassezia* on tyrosine by dicarboxylic acid and azelaic acid that has been proven to inhibit melanocyte dopa-tyrosinase. In addition, pitirial-

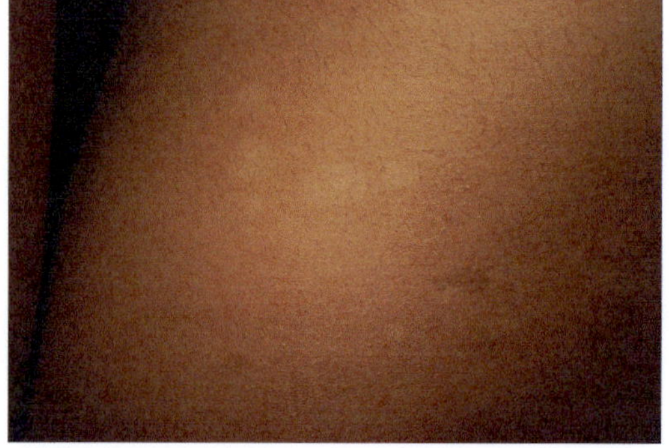

Fig. 1 Circumscribed, hypopigmented macules. Hypopigmented Pityriasis versicolor

actone and pitiriacitrin are mentioned as lipid metabolites that influence hypopigmentation. This variant is more characteristic of higher skin phototypes, mestizo, or brown skin and is probably the most common form of presentation in Latin America, places like Mexico, Brazil, Dominican Republic, and tropical countries report a large number of cases. The lesions usually present as multiple macules or hypopigmented plaques, alone or confluent as the cases progress, covered by an almost imperceptible furfury thin scale [2–5] (Figs. 1 and 2).

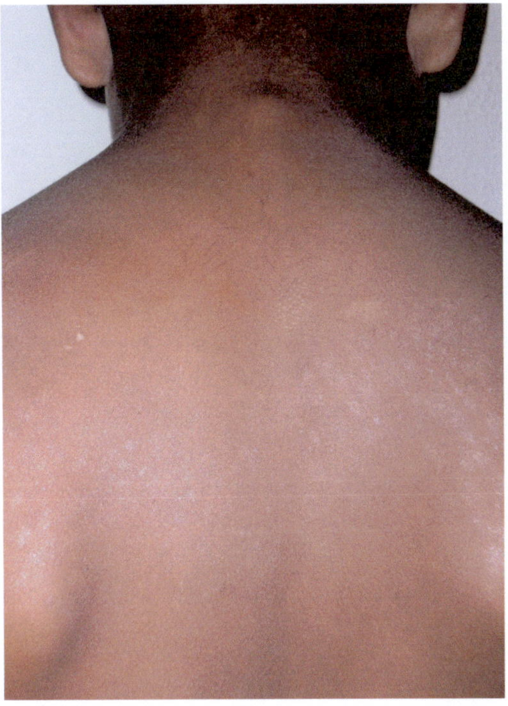

Fig. 2 Hypopigmented macules with pityriasiform desquamation

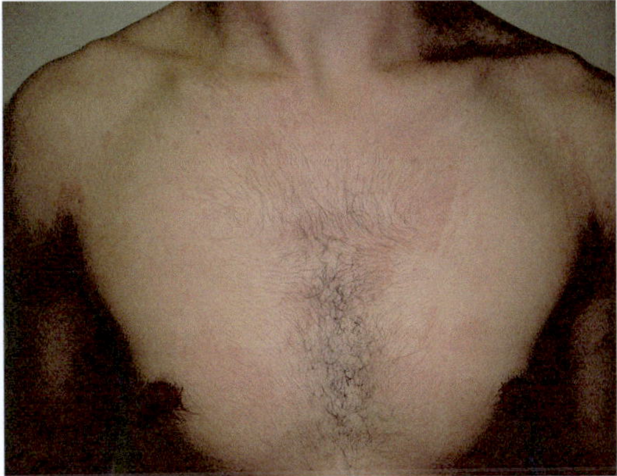

Fig. 3 Hyperpigmented (erythematous) plaques

In hyperpigmented cases, erythematous-squamous or brown-brown, gray-brown plaques can be observed with equal fine scaling on the surface. In general, these cases are attributed to an increase in the size of melanosomes due to multiple factors such as tryptophan and hyper-keratosis constituted by an increase in the corneal layer. This clinical form of presentation has been reported more in light skin, lower phototypes, however there are numerous reports in dark skin. [2, 3, 5, 8, 9] (Fig. 3).

Folliculitis considered a superficial inflammation of the hair follicle can be caused in some cases by fungi such as Malassezia, observed especially in young adults. The most frequent location is in the chest and entire back, although in some cases it spreads to the face, neck, and arms, being frequently confused with cases of acne where the presence of comedons and cases of bacterial folliculitis are always evident. It is characterized by presenting follicular-looking erythematous papules, small in size, with some pustules. Despite being observed in any type of patient, cases associated with immunosuppression have been reported, such as diabetic patients, HIV-AIDS, and in prolonged use of corticosteroids [1, 3, 10] (Figs. 4–6).

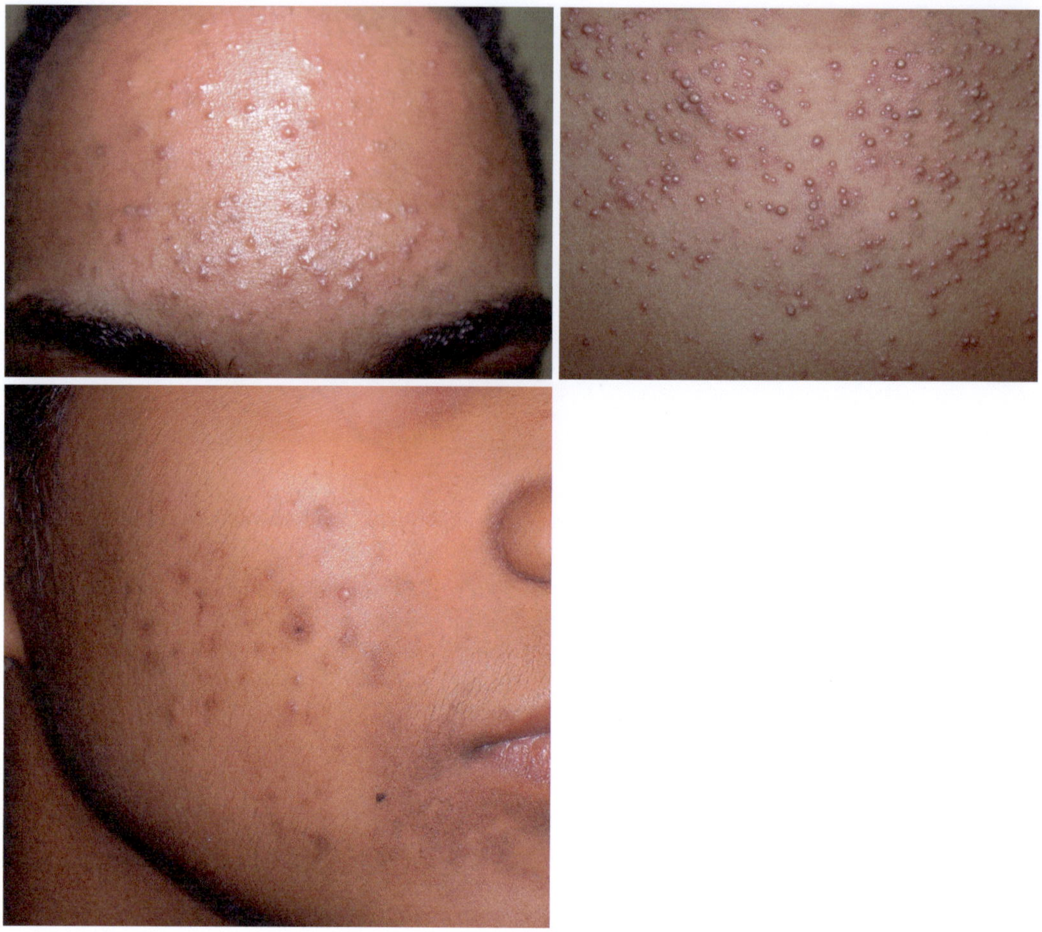

Fig. 4–6 Folliculitis form of Malassezia sp

Diagnosis

The diagnosis of Pityriasis versicolor is made based on the clinical findings of hypo or hyperpigmented macules in characteristic areas.

Ultraviolet light Wood's Lamp is useful in many cases a yellow-green fluorescence is observed in the lesions (Fig. 7).

Direct mycological examination is done by scraping the lesions, placing the sample on a slide and adding potassium hydroxide (KOH) in a concentration that varies from 10 to 40% or with adhesive tape applied in the lesions and in addition blue tint (Parker or Albert solution), typical thin filaments and spores with the appearance of "spaghettis with meatballs" can be observed (Fig. 8).

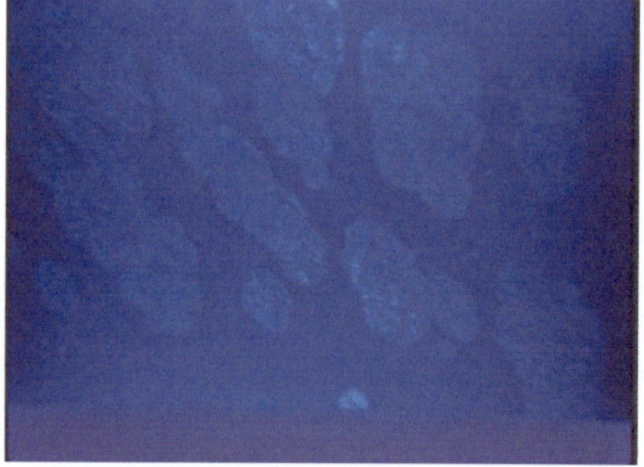

Fig. 7 *Malassezia* sp fluorescence seen with Wood lamp

The culture is carried out mainly in Sabouraud dextrose agar and Sabouraud plus antibiotics, adding long-chain fatty acids, oleic acid, glycerol

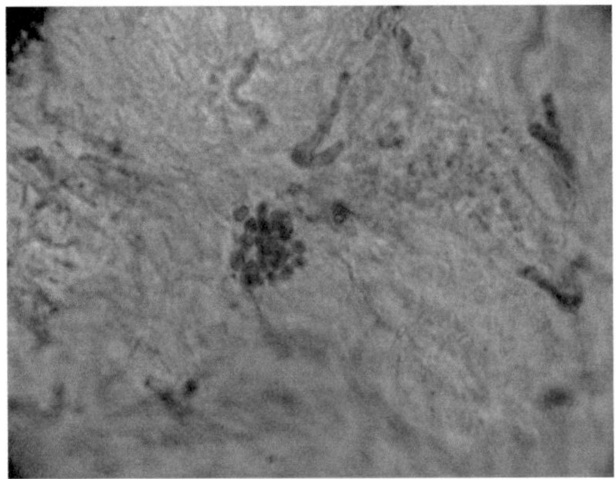

Fig. 8 Filaments and spores seen on direct mycological exam

monosterate, olive oil, since almost all the species are related to lipids. The optimal incubation is from 28 to 32. The colonies are fast growing that can be observed from 3 to 5 days [2, 3, 8].

M. furfur, which is the most frequently isolated agent, produces opaque, creamy-white, yellowish-white, mostly smooth, convex colonies and a cylindrical, elongated, spherical, or oval cell structure.

Differential Diagnosis

The differential diagnosis includes cases of hypopigmented mycosis fungoides that can be seen mostly in skin phototypes IV and V; with vitiligo that is easy to differentiate with ultraviolet light whose lesions look bright white. Pityriasis alba, Dotted leukoderma, and residual macules are also differential diagnosis. The hyperpigmented cases with Seborroeic dermatitis of the trunk; some cases of tinea corporis, Pityriasis rosea in the early stages or with a few lesions; most rarely with secondary syphilis, erythrasma, and undetermined leprosy [1–3, 7, 8, 11].

Treatment

Pityriasis versicolor is a non- or slightly pruritic process, can persist for a long time, and appear frequently towards the time of greatest heat and humidity.

Treatment will depend directly on the affected area and the clinical variant. Topical or systemic treatment, alone or in combination, is used.

20% sodium hyposulfite is one of the most commonly used topical treatment with excellent results, apply twice a day, salicylic acid-based solutions or soaps, 50% propylene glycol, sulfur preparations, cyclopyroxolamin, solutions based on 2% ketononazole, Whitfield ointment, sodium thiosulfite, tolnaftate, terbinafine cream or solution. For scalp, shampoos based on Zinc pyrithione 1%, ketonocazole 2%, among others. There are few reports of the use of calcineurin inhibitors such as tacrolimus and pimecrolimus alone or combined, especially in cases of facial disease or seborrheic dermatitis [1–4, 12].

Regarding systemic therapy, azole derivatives such as Itraconazole 100–200 mg/d can be used from 5 to 7 days, and treatment can be extended up to 14 days using 100 mg/d. Fluconazole from 150 to 300 mg weekly for up to 8 weeks. In folliculitis cases, azole derivatives can be used for a longer time and, depending on the therapeutic response, repeat schemes [1–7, 13].

Some recent reports mention the use of Narrow-band UVB phototherapy for its immunomodulatory effect, although studies with a larger number of patients are required [14].

References

1. Isa Isa R, Arenas R. Micosis superficiales, subcutáneas y pseudomicosis en República Dominicana. México: Graphimedic; 2009.
2. Arenas R. Micología Médica Ilustrada. 6th ed. Mexico: McGraw-Hill; 2019.
3. Bonifaz A. Micología Médica Básica. 4th ed. Mexico: McGraw-Hill; 2012.
4. Arenas R, Isa Isa R, Cruz AC. Pitiriasis versicolor en Santo Domingo, República Dominicana. Datos morfológicos de *Malassezia* spp. in vivo en 100 casos. Rev Iberoam Micol. 2001;18:29–32.
5. Giusiano G, Sosa M, Rojas F, Vanacore ST, Mangiaterra M. Prevalence of *Malassezia* species in pityriasis versicolor lesions in Northeast Argentina. Rev Iberoam Micol. 2010;27:71–4.
6. Isa Isa R, Cruz AC, Arenas R. Pitiriasis versicolor en lactantes. Estudio de 92 casos. Rev Iberoam Micol. 2001;18:109–12.
7. Ilahi A, et al. Real-time PCR identification of six *Malassezia* species. Curr Microbiol. 2017 Jun;74(6):671–7.

8. Isa Isa R, Cruz AC, Arenas R, et al. Pitiriasis versicolor en niños. Estudio epidemiológico y micológico de 797 casos estudiados en la República Dominicana. Med Cut Iber Lat Am. 2002;30(1):5–8.

9. Kallini JR, Riaz F, Khachemoune A. Tinea versicolor in dark-skinned individuals. Int J Dermatol. 2013;53(2):137–41.

10. Yi-Chiun T, Wang Jen-Yu W, Yu-Hung WY-J. Clinical differences in pediatric and adult *Malassezia* folicullitis: retrospective analysis of 321 cases over 9 years. Journ Am Acad Dermatol. 2019;81(1):278–80.

11. James AG, Abraham KH, Cox DS, Moore AE, Pople JE. Metabolic analysis of the cutaneous fungi *Malassezia globosa* and *M. restricta* for insights on scalp condition and dandruff. Int J Cosmet Sci. 2013;35:169–75.

12. Mussin J. Antifungal activity of silver nanoparticles in combination with ketoconazole against *Malassezia furfur*. AMB Express. 2019;9:13.

13. Pantazidou A, Tebruegge M. Recurrent tinea versicolor: treatment with itraconazole or fluconazole? Arch Dis Child. 2007;92(11):1040–2.

14. Balevi A, Üstüner P, Kalsi SA, Özdemir M. Narrowband UVB phototherapy: an effective and reliable treatment alternative for extensive and recurrent pityriasis versicolor. J Dermatolog Treat. 2018;29(3):252–5.

Dermatophyte Infections

Susan A. Howell and Alireza Abdolrasouli

Key Points

- Dermatophytes are a group of fungi special-ised to invade skin, hair and nail
- Species have evolved and become adapted to certain hosts, so infections can be anthropo-philic, zoophilic or geophilic in origin.

Introduction

Dermatophytes are a group of mould fungi that have the ability to invade keratinised tissue making them the primary cause of human superficial fungal skin, hair and nail infections worldwide. There are species that have evolved to live in specific ecological niches and are associated with human, animal or soil sources. Zoophilic and geophilic species can cause human infection, but anthropophilic species rarely infect animals. Human infections from anthropophilic species tend to be chronic with low levels of inflammation, whereas zoophilic or geophilic species tend to cause more aggressive and inflammatory infections. This might be explained in part by the difference in the human immune response to the fungus and any secreted metabolites between anthropophilic and zoophilic species and may reflect various levels of fungal adaptation to a host [1].

Dermatophyte infections occur worldwide, but there are differences in the geographic distri-bution of some species (Table 1). Infections tend to be more common in warm and humid environ-ments than in temperature climates and are also more prevalent in people with lower socio-economic conditions resulting in overcrowded housing with increased opportunity for transmis-sion. To develop a dermatophyte infection, there must be contact with a source (human, animal, soil, or environment) and an opportunity for inoc-ulation into the tissue (e.g. abrasion, contact with damaged tissue). Other risk factors include age, gender, general health, socioeconomic circum-stances and environment. Different risks may be associated with different clinical presentations, for example scalp infection is mostly associated with children and nail infection becomes more common with age [1, 2]. Therefore, the risks of travel could be related to exposure by travel to countries with a different environment, species and endemic infections or by migration bringing a different species to a non-endemic country.

S. A. Howell (✉)
Department of Mycology, St John's Institute of Dermatology, Viapath, St Thomas Hospital, London, UK
e-mail: sue.howell@viapath.co.uk

A. Abdolrasouli
Department of Medical Microbiology, Viapath, King's College Hospital, London, UK

Department of Infectious Diseases Epidemiology, Imperial College London, London, UK
e-mail: alireza.abdolrasouli@nhs.net

W. Robles (ed.), *Skin Disease in Travelers*, Updates in Clinical Dermatology, https://doi.org/10.1007/978-3-031-57836-6_9

Table 1. Dermatophyte species known to cause human infection

Genus and species	Previous name	Sites of infection	Source	Notes	Location
Trichophyton rubrum	–	All skin sites (rarely scalp), nails	Human	Common, ectothrix or endothrix hair invasion	Worldwide
Trichophyton interdigitale	–	Feet, nails, groin, body	Human	common	Worldwide
Epidermophyton floccosum	–	Feet, nails, groin, body	Human	common	worldwide
Trichophyton tonsurans	–	Scalp, body, occasionally nails	Human	Common, endothrix hair invasion	Worldwide
Trichophyton soudanense	–	Scalp	Human	Common, endothrix hair invasion	Africa, less common in Europe, USA, Australia, Brazil
Trichophyton violaceum	–	Scalp, body—exposed sites, occasionally nails	Human	Common, endothrix hair invasion	India, Pakistan, North Africa, Europe, Russia
Microsporum audouinii	–	Scalp, body	Human	Uncommon, ectothrix hair invasion—Wood's lamp positive	Europe, North America
Microsporum canis	–	Scalp, body	Cats, dogs	Common, ectothrix hair invasion—Wood's lamp positive	Worldwide
Trichophyton mentagrophytes	–	Scalp, face, body—exposed sites	Rodents, cats, dogs, sheep, horses, kangaroos	Common, ectothrix hair invasion	Worldwide
Trichophyton verrucosum	–	Scalp, face body—exposed sites	Cattle	Common, ectothrix hair invasion	Worldwide
Nannizzia gypsea	*Microsporum gypseum*	Scalp, face, body—exposed sites	Soil	Uncommon, ectothrix hair invasion	worldwide
Trichophyton concentricum	–	Body	Human	Rare	Pacific islands of Oceania, Central and South America, South East Asia
Trichophyton erinacei	–	Body—exposed sites, scalp, occasionally nails	Hedgehogs	Uncommon, ectothrix hair invasion	Europe, New Zealand
Trichophyton shoenleinii	–	Scalp	Human	Uncommon, favus, Wood's lamp positive	Eurasia and North Africa, Middle-East
Trichophyton quinkeanum	–	Scalp, body—exposed sites	Mice	Uncommon, ectothrix or endothrix hair invasion	Australia, possibly worldwide

(continued)

Table 1. (continued)

Genus and species	Previous name	Sites of infection	Source	Notes	Location
Microsporum ferrugineum	–	Scalp	Human	Common, ectothrix hair invasion—Wood's lamp positive	China, Japan, Asia, Russia, Eastern Europe, Africa
Nannizzia persicolor	*Microsporum persicolor*	Body—exposed sites	Voles, bats	Rare	Europe, Africa, Australia, North America
Nannizzia nana	*Microsporum nanum*	Body—exposed sites	Soil, pigs	Rare	Worldwide
Nannizzia fulva	*Microsporum fulvum*	Scalp, body—exposed sites	Soil	Uncommon to rare, ectothrix hair invasion	worldwide
Trichophyton terrestre	–	Generally considered a contaminant	Soil	Common	Worldwide
Trichophyton benhamiae	*Arthroderma benhamiae*	Scalp, body—exposed sites	Guinea pigs, rabbits, cats	Uncommon	Europe linked to pets in household
Lophophyton gallinae	*Microsporum gallinae*	Skin	Chickens, fowl	Rare, ectothrix hair invasion	Worldwide

Infections and Clinical Manifestations

Dermatophytes infect the non-living layers of the epidermis and rarely penetrate deeper into the tissue. The exception is Majocchi's granuloma and dermatophytic pseudomycetoma where the dermatophyte infects the hair follicle causing damage and leading to infection of the surrounding dermis. Deep dermatophytosis is a rare condition in which dermatophytes invade the deeper skin layers (dermis, subcutis) causing extensive lesions or even dissemination [3, 4]. Risk factors for invasive dermatophytosis include solid organ transplantation, HIV, CARD9 deficiency, and secondary immunodeficiencies such as immunosuppression and underlying disease [5, 6]. Superficial infections with dermatophytes are called tinea, and the common name is ringworm. There are many detailed descriptions of the clinical presentations at different body sites [7–11] so only a brief outline will be described here.

Skin in the skin, a typical presentation would be of an annular (ring-like) lesion with a slightly raised border and some signs of healing in the centre. The border would usually show evidence of scaling and some erythema (Fig 1). However,

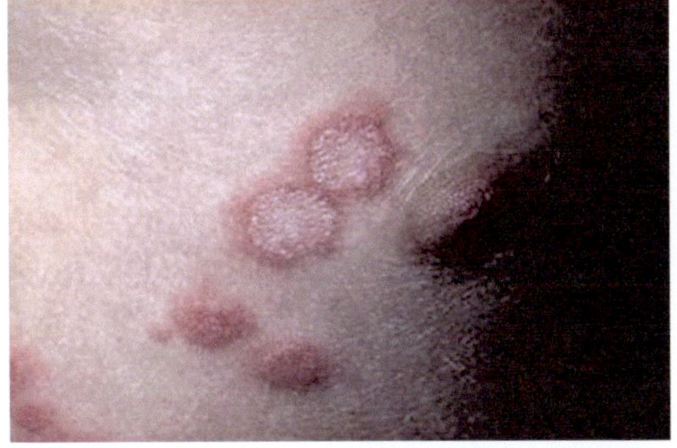

Fig. 1 Reprinted by permission from Springer Nature, Mycopathologia, Clinical forms of dermatophytosis, H. Degreef, © 2008 [12]. Tinea corporis caused by *Microsporum canis*

in skin folds (axillae, groin, web spaces) and hairy sites, this typical presentation may be lost and all that may be seen is a spreading area of scaling and erythema or discoloured skin.

Nail tinea unguium refers to infection caused by dermatophytes only, whereas onychomycosis is a generic term and includes all fungal causes of nail infection. The commonest nail presentation is distal/lateral where infection commences under the hyponychium and progresses towards the proximal nail fold. As the infection progresses, nail plate involvement occurs, and typical signs

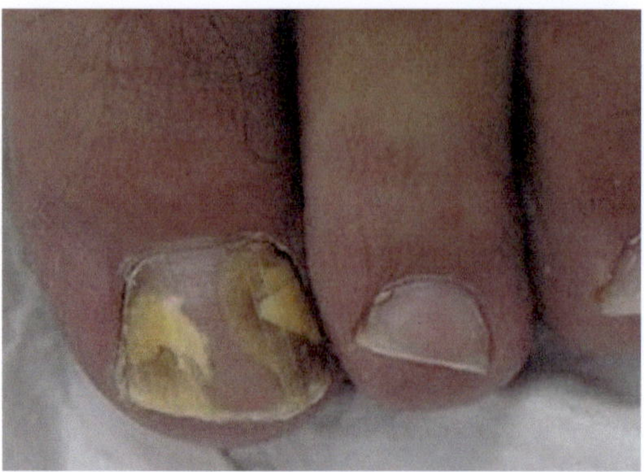

Fig. 2 Reprinted by permission from Springer Nature, Mycopathologia, Tinea ungium: diagnosis and treatment in practice, © 2017 [10]. Distal and lateral onychomycosis with dermatophytomas

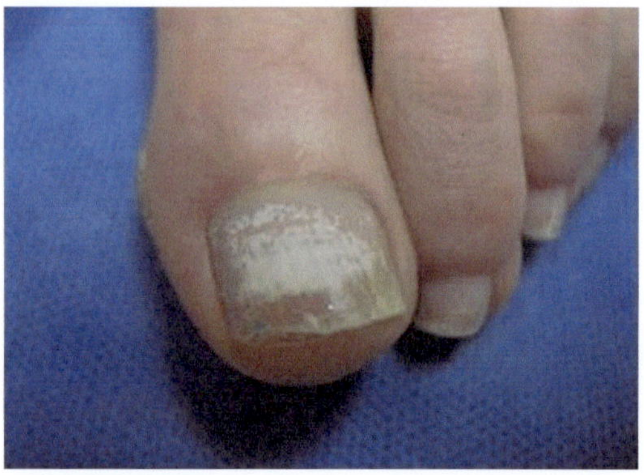

Fig. 3 Reprinted by permission from Springer Nature, Mycopathologia, Tinea ungium: diagnosis and treatment in practice, © 2017 [10]. Superficial white onychomycosis

are discolouration or streaking and hyperkeratosis (Fig 2). Other presentations include proximal and superficial white onychomycosis (Fig 3), the latter starts on the surface of the nail and progresses through the nail towards the nail bed.

Scalp tinea capitis initiates on the scalp skin and progresses to the hair follicle where the fungus penetrates the hair shaft. The infection of the hair may then progress to be either endothrix or ectothrix depending on the causative species. In endothrix infections, the fungus multiplies within the hair shaft making it very fragile and resulting in the hair breaking as it emerges from the scalp, leading to the black dot presentation. In ectothrix infections, the fungus forms a sheath around the hair shaft invading the outer cuticle layers only making it slightly less fragile, so hairs break slightly above the scalp surface. Both endothrix and ectothrix infections present with scaling and patches of hair loss, and there may be some erythema. In some patients, infection progresses to cause highly inflammatory lesions that are known as kerions. Favus infections are clinically distinct as they are associated with a scutula (cup shape) of infected skin debris around the base of the hair. The hairs are more likely to be longer as the fungus forms a weak endothrix infection that is characterised microscopically by the presence of air shafts where hyphae existed but are no longer visible.

Certain species of dermatophytes have a predilection to cause infections at certain body sites (Table 1). For example, *Trichophyton tonsurans*, *Trichophyton violaceum*, *Trichophyton soudanense*, *Microsporum audouinii* and *Microsporum canis* are mostly associated with scalp infections of children. Scalp infection of adults is much rarer due to the change in the composition and production of sebaceous lipids post puberty [7]. However, adults may develop skin lesions on areas in contact when cuddling an infected child.

Laboratory Diagnosis

Fungal infections of skin, hair and nail are traditionally diagnosed in the laboratory by microscopy and culture. Microscopic examination of tissue softened by treatment with potassium hydroxide solution is the gold standard, as visualisation of fungal structures in tissue confirms the presence of infection. The sensitivity of microscopy can be greatly enhanced by the use of a fluorescent microscope (Fig. 4a). Brightener

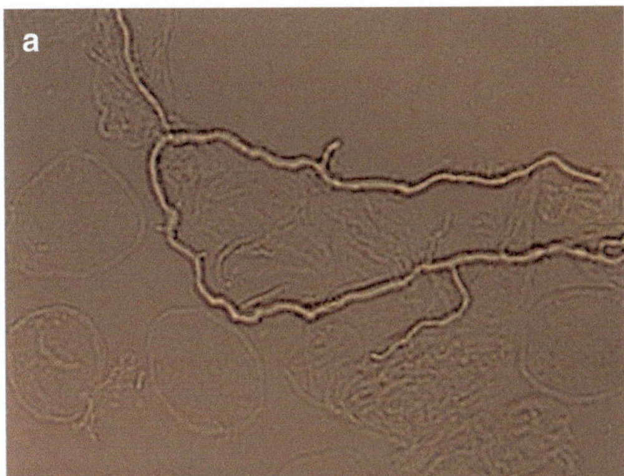

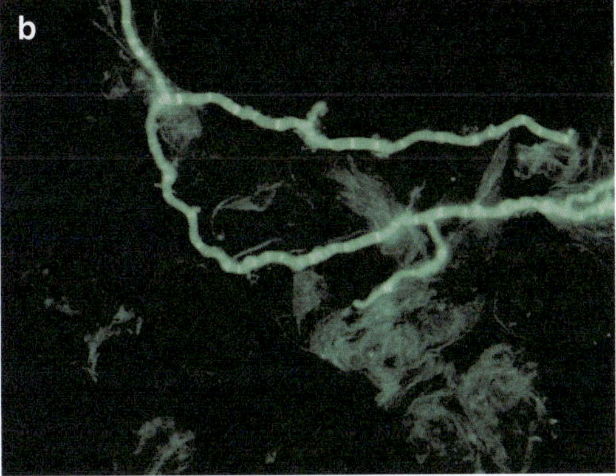

Fig. 4 (a, b) Fungal hyphae in a skin scraping seen by bright field microscopy (top) and the same field by fluorescence microscopy stained with Calcofluor white (bottom). Approximate magnification ×400

stains such as Blankophore or Calcofluor white added to the tissue suspension bind to chitin in the fungal cell wall and emit a greenish fluorescence under filtered UV light (Fig. 4b).

Culture of small pieces of skin, hair and nail on specific mycology media provides the causative organism(s) which can provide useful epidemiological information on the possible source, transmission and management for the patient. In routine diagnostic laboratories, fungi are identified using a combination of colony characteristics and microscopic features. Examples of four common species are shown in Fig. 5.

There are several commercially available molecular-based assays to directly detect a range of dermatophyte species in various clinical specimens. These methods have the advantage of faster turn-around-times, high-volume testing with some degree of automation and provide a species identification when fungal culture is negative. Culture failure is a known problem for nail samples where at least 30% of microscopy positive nails fail to grow a fungal pathogen in culture [13]. However, these molecular detection systems do not enable the detection of less common dermatophyte species or many of the non-dermatophyte causes of infection in skin, hair and nail samples.

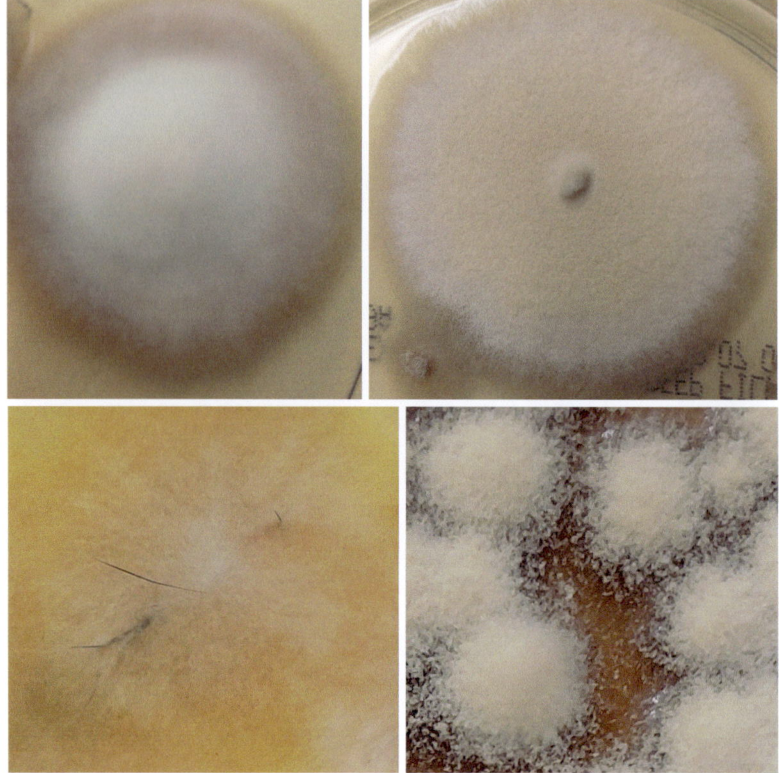

Fig. 5 Dermatophyte colonies on culture. Top row: *Trichophyton rubrum* (left), *T. interdigitale* (right). Bottom row: *Microscporum canis* (right), *T. tonsurans* (left)

Dermatophyte Taxonomy

Dermatophytes have been classically identified into three asexual genera *Trichophyton*, *Microsporum* and *Epidermophyton,* while species with sexual reproduction were placed in the genera *Arthroderma* and *Nannizzia*. While this morphological classification is useful in dermatology clinics and routine diagnostic mycology laboratories, it does not capture the true diversity of this group of fungi.

In 2013, a new nomenclature rule was introduced to fungal taxonomy, and under this system, one fungus has only one name [14]. As a result, the clinically important dermatophytes retained their familiar asexual names. However, molecular biology techniques applied to fungal taxonomy have provided a better understanding of the complex phylogenetic relationship of these fungi. A recent multilocus sequence analysis of type and reference strains of dermatophytes by de Hoog *et al.* [15] showed that *Trichophyton* is a polyphyletic genus and proposed a novel generic classification scheme containing seven genera: *Trichophyton*, *Epidermophyton*, *Nannizzia*, *Microsporum*, *Lophophyton*, *Paraphyton* and *Arthroderma*. Most of the anthropophilic and some zoophilic species remained in three older groups of *Trichophyton*, *Microsporum* and *Epidermophyton,* in contrast geophilic and some rare zoophilic dermatophytes are now classified in the remaining four genera (Table 1). Furthermore, under the new taxonomic scheme, novel geophilic species have been described such as *Arthroderma eboreum* and *Nannizzia aenygmaticum.*

Global Distribution of Commonest Dermatophyte Species

The frequency of disease and the causes of infection can vary considerably across the globe and even within continents [2, 9, 16–20]. Table 1 indicates the commonest dermatophyte species, their natural hosts, human body sites that are commonly infected, and the geographical locations where the species are commonly found. One species, *Trichophyton rubrum*, is widely recognised as the commonest cause of human dermatophytosis as it can infect almost all body sites (rarely the scalp) and has been isolated worldwide. This anthropophilic species is passed by contact with people with infection or from a contaminated environment where infected people have been, such as flooring, swimming pools and communal recreational facilities [9]. *Trichophyton interdigitale* is another common cause of foot, nail and groin infection, and there have been growing reports of it being linked to extensive tinea corporis originating from India [21]. The last anthropophilic species particularly linked to infections of feet, nails and groin is *Epidermophyton floccosum* but the incidence tends to be much lower that than of *T. rubrum* and *T. interdigitale* [19, 22].

T. tonsurans now predominates as the main cause of tinea capitis in urbanised areas in western Europe, the United States, South America and in parts of West Africa. This has been linked to the ease of anthropophilic transmission as this fungus can be isolated from fomites used by infected children, it may be passed around family members unless the whole family is screened and managed as a group, and there is an asymptomatic carrier state where there is a lack of clinical signs but the fungus is detected on culture [7, 23]. Other common causes are *T. soudanense*, *T. violaceum* and *M. audouinii* which have a higher incidence in the African and Indian subcontinents, but have been isolated from many other parts of the world [16]. *Trichophyton schoenleinii* is now rarely seen in Europe as the incidence of this infection has decreased over the last 50 years since the introduction of griseofulvin and improvements in living conditions. It is now only occasionally reported from Eastern Europe, Asia, Middle-East and Africa, and parts of China [24].

The commonest cause of zoophilic dermatophytosis is *M. canis* which has a worldwide distribution and is associated with contact with cats and dogs. Infection is usually of the scalp and exposed body skin sites, especially where these animals are kept as pet companions. A similar pattern of infection at the scalp and exposed body sites is seen with other zoophilic species (Table 1), and identification of the pathogen enables the animal source to be identified and treated to prevent recurrence. Some species of dermatophyte can be associated with rural occupations involving contact with animals or associated fomites [2] such as *Trichophyton verrucosum* infection of cattle farmers and *Nannizzia nana* amongst pig farmers. Although *Lophophyton gallinae* is a cause of a favus-like infection of chicken feathers and combs, it is not often transmitted to humans. *Trichophyton quinkeanum* infections have been reported from Australia and Hungary [2, 20] where there have been agricultural plagues of mice, which is the natural host for this species.

Trichophyton benhamiae is a cause of tinea capitis and tinea corporis linked to the ownership of pets (mostly rodents). The infection was first reported in Japan in 2002 and subsequently in Germany in 2011 [25] and has since then it has been reported in a number of countries in Europe. The link appears to be contact with infected pet guinea pigs with animals acquired from the pet trade [26].

Geophilic causes of infection tend to be due to *Nannizzia gypsea* and *Nannizzia fulva*, and these also are associated with infection of the scalp and exposed body sites. *Trichophyton terrestre* is generally viewed as a non-pathogenic dermatophyte.

Changes in Epidemiology due to Migration and Travel

As people travel, they carry with them any infections they have acquired. There has been a global change in the causes of tinea capitis that can be linked to population migration. *T. soudanense* and *T. violaceum* are endemic in parts of Africa and the Indian subcontinents, and these have been increasingly reported in Europe over the last couple of decades. More recently, there have been reports of cases being directly linked to migration [2, 27] and international adoption [28].

T. rubrum contains a variety of morphological variants and some have been associated with specific locations. *Trichophyton raubitschekii* has been reported from parts of Africa, Asia and the Mediterranean [29] but has been detected in Germany causing tinea corporis in patients that had travelled from Ghana and Cameroon [30].

Tinea imbricata, caused by *Trichophyton concentricum*, is generally only seen in people that live in the regions where this fungus is endemic (Table 1). It is believed that there may be a genetic predisposition amongst these populations [31], although infections have occasionally been reported from travellers to these regions too [32]. Tinea imbricata has a distinctive clinical presentation of concentric scaling rings which may affect the whole body surface, but rarely involving the palms, soles or nails. However, there have been case reports of *T. tonsurans* causing tinea corporis with a similar clinical presentation [33, 34], therefore travel to an endemic region should be considered when diagnosing tinea imbricata.

Dermatophyte Infections Transmitted by Sexual Contact

A newly recognised type of tinea infection, tinea genitalis, was suggested in 2015 [35] following a series of sexually transmitted dermatophyte infections of the genital region. The report from Switzerland included seven patients who had all travelled to South-East Asia and had sexual contact with other tourists or local sex workers. A common predisposing factor amongst six affected patients was shaving of the genital area. Clinical features included severe inflammation, scaly plaques and follicular pustules. The cause was identified as *T. interdigitale* and based on signature polymorphisms in the internal transcribed spacer (ITS) region of rDNA gene had a probable zoophilic origin despite lack of animal contact. A similar infection was reported in a patient in Australia who developed Majocchi's granuloma in the suprapubic region [36], and this infection was sexually transmitted to a partner in Australia.

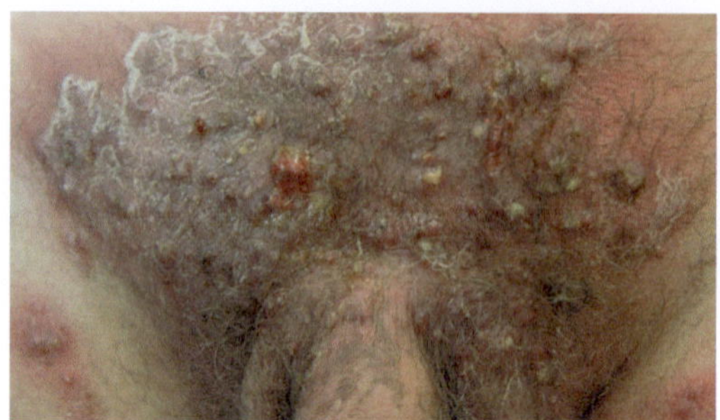

Fig. 6 Reprinted by permission from John Wiley & Sons, Journal der Deutschen Dermatologischen Gesellschaft, *Trichophyton mentagrophytes*—a new genotype of zoophilic dermatophyte causes sexually transmitted infections. C. Kupsch, Czaika V-A, C Deutsch, Y Graser, © 2019. [37]. A patient with an inflammatory infection caused by *Trichophyton mentagrophytes* type VII associated with sexual activity and intimate shaving, but no contact with animals

In Germany, 37 cases of sexually transmitted *Trichophyton mentagrophytes* infections were reported (Fig. 6), but in this report, most patients did not have a preceding history of travel [37].

Treatment and Prevention

Typical oral treatments for dermatophytosis use terbinafine, itraconazole, fluconazole or griseofulvin, and topical imidazoles and topical terbinafine are used for minor skin infections. The use of antifungal treatments has been thoroughly reviewed by Hay [38].

Oral treatment should be used for tinea capitis to ensure adequate penetration and persistence in the hair follicle, with topicals used as an adjunct. Griseofulvin is particularly useful against *Microsporum* scalp infections as treatment with terbinafine may require higher doses to be effective [7, 8]. Family members should be screened for infection to prevent recurrence and spread. Topical antifungal shampoos can be used as a precaution, but infection should always be treated orally if the patient's medical history permits.

Oral treatment is also recommended for tinea unguium as topical agents are usually most effective for very minor clinical signs of infection with no nail bed involvement or nail thickening.

For localized skin infections, topical treatment is usually effective, but if the infection is widespread or follicular, oral therapy should provide better outcomes. There are no agreed regimens to treat recalcitrant infections, but combinations of oral and topical agents using azoles and allylamines have been tried with variable outcomes.

Prevention of dermatophytosis relies on avoiding contact with a source of infection in the home or environment and receiving prompt diagnosis and treatment to prevent spread or recurrence. General actions that can be taken include wearing good fitting clothes and shoes to prevent skin and nail damage, wearing footwear and appropriate clothing when using communal and recreational facilities (e.g. swimming pools, showers, etc.), avoiding sharing clothes, towels, brushes and personal items with people with infection, regular washing of these items to reduce contamination of the environment, and monitoring pet health to prevent zoophilic infections.

Antifungal Resistance in Dermatophytes

Although dermatophytes can be tested for susceptibility to antifungal drugs using standard methods, in practice there remains technical difficulties with poorly sporing species and strains. Until recently, it was generally believed that resistance to antifungals was rarely encountered in dermatophytes, and treatment failures were linked to other complicating factors such as compliance or biofilm formation. Thus, antifungal susceptibility testing is not routinely performed and in clinical practice most cases are treated empirically.

Acquired resistance to commonly used antifungals is thought to arise as a result of selective pressure due to continuous exposure to antifungal agents, either through prolonged treatment in patients or the presence of antifungal agents in the environment [39]. The main mechanisms of drug resistance in pathogenic fungi include mutations in the genes encoding drug targets or their overexpression, overexpression of genes encoding multidrug transporter proteins, or a combination of these mechanisms.

Terbinafine resistance in *Trichophyton rubrum* and *Trichophyton interdigitale* has now been identified in clinical isolates in several countries in Europe, Asia, Middle East, and the United States. Resistance is usually associated with nonsynonymous point mutations (L393, F397, F415 and H440) in the gene encoding squalene epoxydase (SQLE) targeted by terbinafine. In a recent report from Switzerland, approximately 1% of *Trichophyton rubrum* isolates were found to be resistant to terbinafine [40].

A major concern is the recent emergence in India of a novel dermatophyte *Trichophyton indotiniae* (closely related *Trichophyton mentagrophytes* genotype VIII) [41] causing an epidemic of tinea cruris and tinea corporis with 30 to 70% of resistance amongst clinical isolates [21]. Several cases have been reported in Iran, and various European countries including Germany, Denmark, Poland, Belgium, Switzerland and France [42]. These cases are mainly amongst patients returning from the Indian subcontinent; thus, travel to or immigration from India is a risk factor. Direct human-to-human transmission is probable between family members [42], however, the possibility that the patients were infected from a common source cannot be excluded. Extensive lesions not responding to terbinafine therapy is a common clinical presentation, leading to persistent or recalcitrant infections that require other treatment strategies such as a switch to azole-based treatment. Terbinafine resistance in *Trichophyton indotiniae* is a result of point mutations in SQLE gene similar to those described previously, however, other amino acid substitutions (F397L, S395P, Q408L and S443P) have been detected amongst resistant strains [39]. There is currently no robust phenotypic test available to confidently differentiate this *Trichophyton indotiniae* from other members of the *Trichophyton mentagrophytes* complex in routine diagnostic laboratories, and sequence-based molecular approaches are needed for its accurate identification.

Itraconazole is widely used as the second-line treatment for many dermatophyte infections including those not responding to the first-line terbinafine therapy. The exact prevalence of itraconazole resistance amongst clinical isolates of *Trichophyton rubrum* or *Trichophyton interdigitale* causing onychomycosis and tinea pedis is largely unknown. Probably, overexpression of ATP-binding cassette (ABC) transporters, and major facilitator superfamily (MSF) transporters with up-regulation of multi-drug resistance genes (MDR1 and MDR2) lead to elevated minimum inhibitory concentration (MIC) of azole drugs in dermatophyte species [39].

Infections Resembling Dermatophytosis

Non-dermatophyte causes of nail infection can resemble tinea unguium as they may present with discolouration and hyperkeratosis. Many of these fungi (e.g. species of *Aspergillus*, *Fusarium*, *Scopulariopsis*) are found worldwide and are not travel associated. However, the prevalence of these infections does differ and factors such as climate and geography make mould and yeast infections more common in the Mediterranean and tropical countries [43] than in Western temperate countries.

Neoscytalidium species are naturally tree and plant pathogens found in tropical and subtropical countries in South America, West Indies and the Caribbean region, and also in the subcontinents of Africa, India and Asia [44]. Human infections in the United Kingdom and Europe have been linked to travel or migration [45–47].

Neoscytalidium species can cause onychomycosis and infections of the thicker skin of the feet and hands that resembles dermatophytosis, however, these infections do not generally spread to the thinner dorsal surfaces. In nail infections, paronychia or melanonychia may develop, something that is not usually seen with dermatophytes. Deeper infection is rare and mostly associated with immunocompromised patients. Treatment is difficult as these fungi are resistant in vitro to the commonly prescribed antifungals, although a combination of oral and topical nail lacquer for nail infection may give improvement [38, 44].

References

1. Gnat S, Nowakiewicz A, Lagowski D, Zieba P. Host- and pathogen-dependent susceptibility and predisposition to dermatophytosis. J Med Microbiol. 2019;68:823–36.
2. Segal E, Elad D. Human and zoonotic dermatophytoses: epidemiological aspects. Front Microbiol. 2021;12:713532.
3. Huang C, Peng Y, Zhang Y, Li R, Wan Z, Wang X. Deep dermatophytosis caused by *Trichophyton rubrum*. Lancet Infect Dis. 2019;19(12):1380.
4. Seçkin D, Arikan S, Haberal M. Deep dermatophytosis caused by *Trichophyton rubrum* with concomitant disseminated nocardiosis in a renal transplant recipient. J Am Acad Dermatol. 2004;51(5 Suppl):S173–6.
5. Lanternier F, Pathan S, Vincent QB, Liu L, Cypowyj S, Prando C, et al. Deep dermatophytosis and inherited CARD9 deficiency. N Engl J Med. 2013;369(18):1704–14.
6. Jachiet M, Lanternier F, Rybojad M, Bagot M, Ibrahim L, Casanova JL, Puel A, Bouaziz JD. Posaconazole treatment of extensive skin and nail dermatophytosis due to autosomal recessive deficiency of CARD9. JAMA Dermatol. 2015;151(2):192–4.
7. Hay RJ. Tinea capitis: current status. Mycopathologia. 2017;182:87–93.
8. Fuller LC, Barton RC, Mohd Mustapa MF, Proudfoot LE, Punjabi SP, Higgins EM. British Association of Dermatologists' guidelines for the management of tinea capitis 2014. Br J Dermatol. 2014;171:454–63.
9. Ilkit M, Durdu M. Tinea pedis: the etiology and global epidemiology of a common fungal infection. Crit Rev Microbiol. 2015;41(3):374–88.
10. Asz-Sigall D, Tosti A, Arenas R. Tinea unguium: diagnosis and treatment in practice. Mycopathologia. 2017;182:95–100.
11. Leung AKC, Lam JM, Leong KF, Hon KL. Tinea corporis: an updated review. Drugs in Context. 2020;9:2020-5-6.
12. Degreef H. Clinical forms of dermatophytosis (ringworm infections). Mycopathologia. 2008;166:257–65.
13. Onychomycosis HR. Literature review. Eur Acad Dermatol Venereol. 2005;19(1):1–7.
14. Hawksworth DL. A new dawn for the naming of fungi: impact of decisions made in Melbourne in July 2011 on the future publication and regulation of fungal names. IMA Fungus. 2011;2011(2):155–62.
15. de Hoog GS, Dukik K, Monod M, Pakeu A, Stubbe D, Hendrickx M, Kupsch C, Stielow JB, Freeke J, Göker M, Rezaei-Matehkolaei A, Mirhendi H, Gräser Y. Toward a novel multilocus phylogenetic taxonomy for the dermatophytes. Mycopathologia. 2017;182:5–31.
16. Rodriguez-Cerdeira C, Martinez-Herrera E, Szepietowski JC, et al. A systematic review of worldwide data on tinea capitis: analysis of the last 20 years. Eur Acad Dermatol Venereol. 2021;35:844–83.

17. Nweze EI, Eke IE. Dermatophytes and dermatophytosis in the eastern and southern parts of Africa. Med Mycol. 2018;56:13–28.
18. Seebacher C, Bouchara J-P, Mignon B. Updates on the epidemiology of dermatophyte infections. Mycopathologia. 2008;166:335–52.
19. Havlickova B, Czaika VA, Friedrich M. Epidemiological trends in skin mycoses worldwide. Mycoses. 2008;51(Suppl 4):2–15.
20. https://www.adelaide.edu.au/mycology/fungal-descriptions-and-antifungal-susceptibility/dermatophytes. Accessed 01 Jan 2022.
21. Nenoff P, Verma SB, Vasani R, Burmester A, Hipler UC, Wittig F, et al. The current Indian epidemic of superficial dermatophytosis due to *Trichophyton mentagrophytes*–a molecular study. Mycoses. 2019;62:336–56.
22. Borman AM, Campbell CK, Fraser M, Johnson EM. Analysis of the dermatophyte species isolated in the British Isles between 1980 and 2005 and review of worldwide dermatophyte trends over the last three decades. Med Mycol. 2007;45(2):131–41.
23. Ferguson L, Fuller C. Spectrum and burden of dermatophytes in children. J Infect. 2017;74:S54–60.
24. Gao Y, Zhan P, Hagen F, Menken SBJ, Sun J, Rezaei-Matehkolaei A, de Hoog S. Molecular epidemiology and in vitro antifungal susceptibility of *Trichophyton schoenleinii*, agent of tinea capitis favosa. Mycoses. 2019;62:466–74.
25. Nenoff P, Uhrlaß S, Krüger C, Erhard M, Hipler U-C, Seyfarth F, Herrmann J, Wetzig T, Schroedl W, Gräser Y. *Trichophyton* species of *Arthroderma benhamiae*–a new infectious agent in dermatology. J Dtsch Dermatol Ges. 2014;12(7):571–81.
26. Berlin M, Kupsch C, Stoelcker B, Heusinger A, Graser Y. German-wide analysis of the prevalence and the propagation factors of the zoonotic dermatophyte *Trichophyton benhamiae*. Journal of Fungi. 2020;6(3):161–72.
27. Ahmeen M. Epidemiology of superficial fungal infections. Clin Dermatol. 2010;28:197–201.
28. Markey RJ, Staat MA, Gerrety MJT, Lucky AW. Tinea capitis due to *Trichophyton soudanense* in Cincinnati, Ohio, in internationally adopted children from Liberia. Pediatr Dermatol. 2003;20(5):408–10.
29. Weitzman I, Summerbell RC. The dermatophytes. Clin Microbiol Rev. 1995;8(2):240–59.
30. Tietz H-J, Hopp M, Graser Y. First isolation of *Trichophyton raubitschekii* (syn. *T. Rubrum*) in Europe. Mycoses. 2002;45:10–4.
31. Pihet M, Bourgeois H, Mazière J-Y, Berlioz-Arthaudd A, Boucharaa J-P, Chabasse D. Isolation of *Trichophyton concentricum* from chronic cutaneous lesions in patients from the Solomon Islands. Trans R Soc Trop Med Hyg. 2008;102:389–93.
32. Veraldi S, Giorgi R, Pontini P, Tadini G, Nazzaro G. Tinea imbricata in an italian child and review of the literature. Mycopathologia. 2015;180:353–7.
33. Ouchi T, Nagao K, Hata Y, Otuka T, Inazumi T. *Trichophyton tonsurans* infection manifesting as multiple concentric annular erythemas. J Dermatol. 2005;32(7):565–8.
34. Hoque SR, Holden CA. *Trichophyton tonsurans infection* mimicking tinea imbricata. Clin Exp Dermatol. 2007;32:345–6.
35. Luchsinger I, Bosshard PP, Kasper RS, Reinhardt D, Lautenschlager S. Tinea genitalis: a new entity of sexually transmitted infection? Case series and review of the literature. Sexually Transmitted Infection. 2015;91:493–6.
36. Gallo JG, Woods M, Graham RM, Jennison AV. A severe transmissible Majocchi's granuloma in an immunocompetent returned traveller. Medical Mycology Case Reports. 2017;18:5–7.
37. Kupsch C, Czaika V-A, Deutsch C, Gräser Y. *Trichophyton mentagrophytes*–a new genotype of zoophilic dermatophyte causes sexually transmitted infections. J Dtsch Dermatol Ges. 2019;17(5):493–501.
38. Hay RJ. Therapy of skin, hair and nail fungal infections. J Fungi. 2018;4:99. https://doi.org/10.3390/jof4030099.
39. Monod M, Feuermann M, Yamada T. Terbinafine and itraconazole resistance in dermatophytes. In: Bouchara J-P, et al., editors. Dermatophytes and dermatophytoses. Springer Nature Switzerland; 2021. p. 414–32.
40. Yamada T, Maeda M, Alshahni MM, Tanaka R, Yaguuchi T, Bontems O, et al. Terbinafine resistance of *Trichophyton* clinical isolates caused by specific point mutations in the squalene epoxidase gene. Antimicrob Agents Chomether. 2017;61(7):e00115–7.
41. Tang C, Kong X, Ahmed SA, Thakur R, Chowdhary A, Nenoff P, et al. Taxonomy of the *Trichophyton mentagrophytes*/*T. Interdigitale* species complex harboring the highly virulent, multiresistant genotype *T. Indotineae*. Mycopathologia. 2021;186:315–26.
42. Dellière S, Joannard B, Benderdouche M, Mingui A, Gits-Muselli M, Hamane S, et al. Emergence of difficult-to-treat tinea corporis caused *by Trichophyton mentagrophytes* complex isolates, Paris, France. Emerg Infect Dis. 2022;28(1):224–8.
43. Iorizzo M, Piraccini B, Tosti A. New fungal nail infections. Curr Opin Infect Dis. 2007;20:142–5.
44. Machouart M, Menir P, Helenon R, Quist D, Desbois N. *Scytalidium* and scytalidiosis: What's new in 2012? Journal de Mycologie Medicale. 2013;23(1):40–6.
45. Hay RJ. *Scytalidium* infections. Curr Opin Infect Dis. 2002;15(2):99–100.
46. Arrese JE, Piérard-Franchimont C, Piérard GE. *Scytalidium dimidiatum* melanonychia and scaly plantar skin in four patients from the Maghreb: imported disease or outbreak in a Belgian mosque? Dermatology. 2001;202:183–5.
47. Miqueleiz-Zapatero A, Santa Olalla C, Buendía B, Barba J. Dermatomycosis due to *Neoscytalidium* spp. Scientific letter/Enferm Infec Microbiol Clin. 2017;35(2):127–36.

Tinea Nigra

Mariel Isa

Key Points

- *Hortaea werneckii* is a dematiaceous halophilic fungus with affinity to media with high salt concentration.
- The diagnosis is made based on the clinical and the mycological findings where septate pigmented hyphae are observed.
- Most patients tend to think it is a dirty looking residual stain.
- The most used treatment is topical antifungal or keratolytic therapies.

Introduction

Tinea nigra is a superficial mycosis contained within the group of superficial phaeohyphomycosis, caused by the fungus *Hortaea werneckii* (formerly *Exophiala werneckii* or *Phaeoannellomyces*) that affects the stratum corneum [1–3].

Hortaea werneckii is a dematiaceous fungus, halophilic, with affinity to media with high salt concentration. It is described in patients with hyperhidrosis processes. Traumatic inoculation is described as the probable mechanism of entry into the skin [2–4].

Synonymy

Keratomycosis nigricans, Epidermic cladosporiosis, pytiriasis nigra, black microsporiosis, superficial phaeohyphomycosis.

History

The first reports of the disease appear to be from Brazil in 1891 by Alejandro Cerqueira who describe it as keratomycosis nigricans palmaris. Multiple descriptions have occurred over time, as has the name of the microorganism (Table 1) [2, 3, 5].

Tinea nigra has a worldwide distribution, in tropical and subtropical regions, mainly in areas

Table 1 Historical background of Tinea nigra

1891—Alejandro Cerqueira	Keratomycosis nigricans
1898—Montoya, Flores	Carate negro
1921—Werneck Parreiras Horta	*Cladosporium werneckii*
1984—K Nishimura y Miyaji	*Hortaea*
1985—Michael MgGinnis y Shell	*Phaeoannellomyces*
1992—Zalar y de Hoog	Halophilic fungus

M. Isa (✉)
Dermatology at UASD, UNIBE and PUCMM,
Dermatology Residency Co-coordinator of the
Instituto Dermatológico Dominicano y Cirugía de
Piel Dr. Huberto Bogaert Díaz,
Santo Domingo, Dominican Republic

with high salt concentration. Their greatest incidence is reported in Central and South America, countries such as Brazil, Venezuela, Panama, report several cases. There are reports from Europe, Africa, Asia and the United States [1–4].

Clinical Characteristics

The clinical lesion is characterized by the presence of a brown hyperchromic macule or plaque with well-defined borders and sometimes with a fine scale on the surface, mostly localized on the palms, predominantly unilateral. Bilateral cases have been described. The lesions are chronic and asymptomatic, just few reports of mild pruritus and usually affects young people and sometimes they heal spontaneously [2–6] (Fig. 1 and 2).

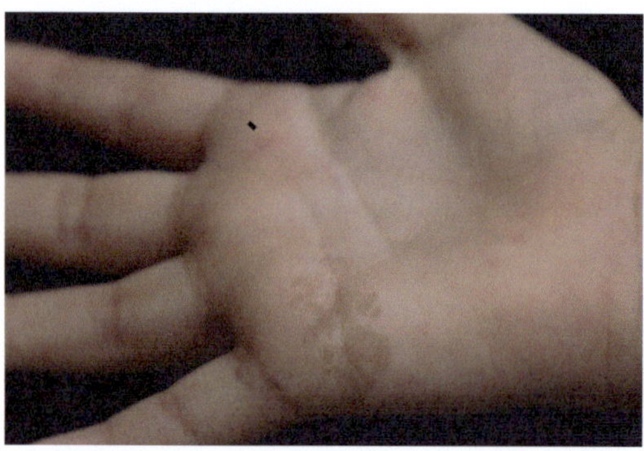

Fig. 1 Hyperpigmented brownish plaque on the right hand

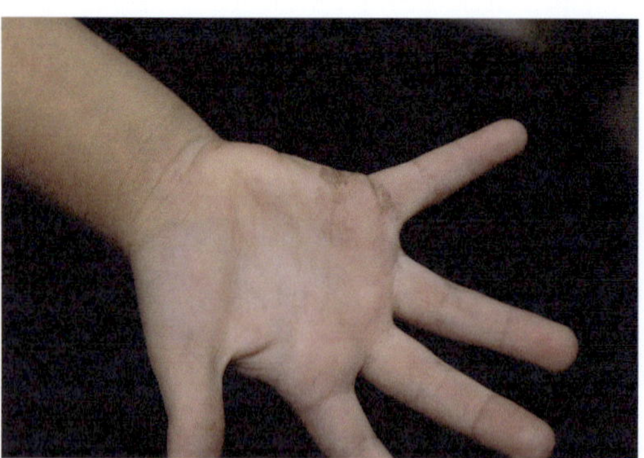

Fig. 2 Circumscribed, hyperpigmented plaque on the right hand

Diagnosis

The diagnosis is made through the mycological examination either by scraping the lesion with a direct examination with potassium hydroxide (KOH) of 10 to 20% or with the adhesive tape technique, where fungal elements (septate pigmented hyphae) are observed, light brown color, with hyaline ends and thick walls [1, 2, 4] (Fig. 3).

The culture is done in Saboreaud's dextrose agar alone or with antibiotics. The growth of the colonies varies from 2 to 4 weeks. Macroscopy shows creamy, yeast-like, shiny, blackish colonies Fig. 4.

The diagnosis is made based on the clinic and the mycological findings. Biopsy is not really necessary. Histopathological changes described mild hyperkeratosis and acanthosis at the epidermis and mild perivascular mononuclear infiltrate. In hematoxilin eoscin stain and periodic acid Schiff (PAS) stain, numerous pigmented hyphae can be seen at the level of the cornea layer [1, 2, 4, 5].

Dermoscopic patterns have been described for Tinea nigra, the presence of a blackish pigmentation, of irregular appearance, with spicules, without a pattern of networks or melanocytic ridges [2, 5].

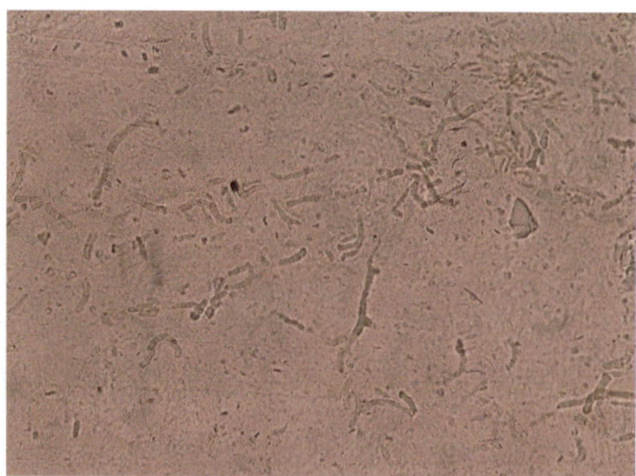

Fig. 3 Light brown color septate pigmented hyphae, with hyaline ends and thick walls

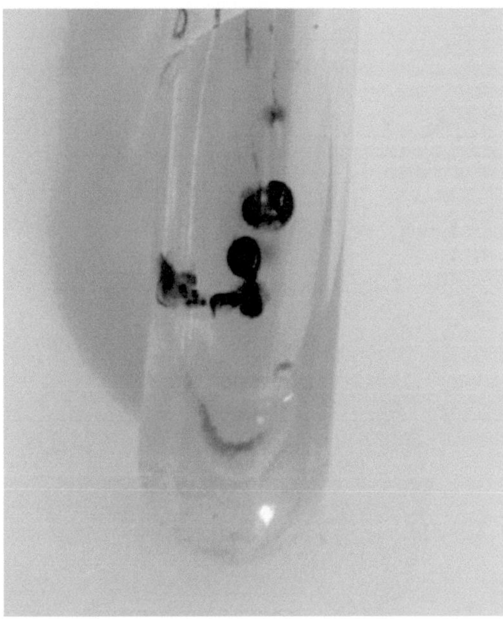

Fig. 4 Creamy, yeast-like, shiny, blackish colonies

Differential Diagnosis

Most patients tend to think it is a dirty looking residual stain. Nevi junction, malignant melanoma, contact dermatitis, dermatitis neglecta, drug reactions, among others, must be taken into consideration.

Treatment

The cases are mostly treated with topical antifungal or keratolytic therapies, due to the superficial nature of the condition. Withfield's ointment () is used twice a day for 7 to 15 days, retinoic acid, tincture of iodine 1%, solutions with salicylic acid 2–3%. Others like ketoconazole 2%, terbinafine 1%, cyclopyroxylamine 1%, bifonazole, butenafin 1%, clotrimazole, isoconazole, among others [1–3, 5, 6].

In case of requiring systemic treatment, the use of Itraconazole 100 mg daily for 15 days and terbinafine 250 mg is recommended [1, 2].

References

1. Arenas R. Micología Médica Ilustrada. 6th ed. Mexico: McGraw-Hill; 2019.
2. Bonifaz A. Micología Médica Básica. 4th ed. Mexico: McGraw-Hill; 2012.
3. Bonifaz A, et al. Tinea nigra by Hortaea werneckii, a report of 22 cases from Mexico. Stud Mycol. 2008;61:77–82.
4. Isa Isa R, Arenas R. Micosis superficiales, subcutáneas y pseudomicosis en República Dominicana. México: Graphimedic; 2009.
5. Rossetto A, Cruz R. Tinea nigra: successful treatment with topical butenafine. An Bras Dermatol. 2012 Nov-Dec;87(6):939–41.
6. Falcão E, Trope B, Martins N, Barreiros M, Ramos-e-Silva M. Bilateral tinea Nigra Plantaris with good response to Isoconazole cream: a case report. Case Rep Dermatol. 2015;7:306–10.

Part IV

Dermatoses Caused by Infection: Fungal Infections–Subcutaneous Mycoses

Mycetoma

Lucio Vera-Cabrera,
Jesus Alberto Cardenas-de la Garza (iD),
and Jorge Ocampo-Candiani

Abbreviations

TMP/SMX	Trimethoprim/sulfamethoxazole
AMPs	Antimicrobial peptides
HNPs	Human neutrophil peptides
hBD	Human beta-defensin

Key Points

- Mycetoma is an infection produced by soil inhabitants, either fungi or bacteria, and it is characterized by an increase of volume of the affected topographic site, generally the limbs, with production of subcutaneous channels which discharge a sero-purulent or sero-sanguinolent secretion containing the etiologic agents in form of microcolonies or grains.
- It is not transmissible from human to human and is mostly reported in tropical or subtropical regions of the world.
- Therapy consists of antimicrobials alone or in combination with surgical debridement of the lesions.
- The immune system is unable to eliminate the infection, and the disease may progress to produce extensive lesions or affect internal organs.
- Vaccines are in study, in order to help in those cases recalcitrant to the normal therapeutic schemes.

Introduction

Mycetoma is a chronic, granulomatous infection of the skin and subcutaneous tissue that may affect bone and underlying organs. It is caused by microorganisms living as saprophytes in the environment, including actinomycetals and fungi [1]. More than 56 different species of microorganisms associated with mycetoma have been reported. It is predominantly endemic in tropical and subtropical countries, including Mexico, Mali, Senegal, Sudan, Somalia, India, etc., although it has been reported worldwide [2–6]. Therapy of eumycetoma consists of the use of antifungals and surgery, while actinomycetoma cases are treated with antimicrobials given as combinations. The World Health Organization recognized mycetoma as a Neglected Tropical Disease in 2016. This has helped in obtaining disease recognition and access to research funding.

L. Vera-Cabrera (✉) · J. A. C.-d. la Garza ·
J. Ocampo-Candiani
Laboratorio Interdisciplinario de Investigación
Dermatológica, Servicio de Dermatología, Hospital
Universitario, U.A.N.L., Monterrey, Mexico
e-mail: lucio.veracb@edu.uanl.mx

W. Robles (ed.), *Skin Disease in Travelers*, Updates in Clinical Dermatology,
https://doi.org/10.1007/978-3-031-57836-6_11

History

Skeletons with lesions compatible to mycetoma infection have been identified from remains from the Byzantine empire (300–600 CE) in Asia and from the Tlatilco culture (1300–1100 BCE) in Mexico [7, 8]. The oldest written description of this infection dates back to the Atharva Veda, compiled around 1200–100 BCE, where it is described as "ant-hill foot" given the tortuous formation of subcutaneous sinus tracts [8, 9]. Gill reported in 1832 the first modern cases of the infection in field workers in Madurai in southeast India. Colebrook coined the term "Madura foot" in 1846. Later, Carter described its fungal etiology and renamed the entity as mycetoma. In 1913, Pinoy described the dual etiology of the disease separating it into actinomycetoma and eumycetoma [8].

Epidemiology

Mycetoma prevalence is higher, but not restricted to the "mycetoma belt" which comprises countries between the latitudes 15° south and 30° north. The countries with the highest incidence are Sudan, Mexico, Venezuela, and India. Overall, most cases are reported from Africa, Asia, and tropical and subtropical regions of America. Sporadic autochthonous cases from Australia, the United States, and Europe have been reported [10, 11]. The climate in endemic areas is primarily subtropical and tropical dry with an annual rainfall ranging from 50–1000 mm and low humidity. Actinomycetoma predominate in drier regions and are frequently seen in Mexico (*N. brasiliensis*), Argentina (*N. brasiliensis*), Senegal (*A. pelletieri*), and Niger (*S. somaliensis*). Eumycetoma cases predominate in India and Africa (Senegal, Sudan, Mali, and Somalia) where the dominant etiological agent is *M. mycetomatis* [1].

Pathogenesis

Fungi comprise more than 5 million species, they include species that kill plant tissue (necrotrophs) that derive nourishment from decaying organic matter (saprotrophs) or which live in mutual dependence with plants (mutualists), such as mycorrhizals. Pathogenic species are in the two first groups, without finding any plant mutualist described to date; it seems that the association with tissue destruction has selected species to become human pathogens [12].

Although traditionally it has been considered that mycetoma is produced by the pathogenic characteristics of the causative agents, it has recently been observed that genetic polymorphisms involved in neutrophil function are related to either the production of human mycetoma or its size, in the case of *M. mycetomatis* infection. IL-8 (CXCL8), its receptor CXCR2, thrombospondin-4, nitric oxide synthase, and complement receptor 1 have significant differences in mycetoma patients compared with geographically and ethnically matched controls. These findings open the possibility that certain individuals are predisposed to this infection [13].

The adaptive immune system is important for identifying invading exogenous antigens and to develop a response that can be triggered rapidly using memory cells to produce effector molecules. Patients with a weak adaptive immune system can present infections rarely seen in immunocompetent individuals, such as cutaneous cryptococcosis, pneumocystis pneumonia, candidiasis, etc. In subjects with an efficient immune system, infection by fungi will depend on the ability to grow at 37 °C, to penetrate the tissues, to be able to use tissue nutrients, and to overcome a hostile human immune system [12].

In mycetoma, the human host is not part of the ecological life cycle of the etiologic agents. Soil bacteria are predated by higher microorganisms, such as free-living amoebae; those able to survive phagocytosis by these microorganisms can prob-

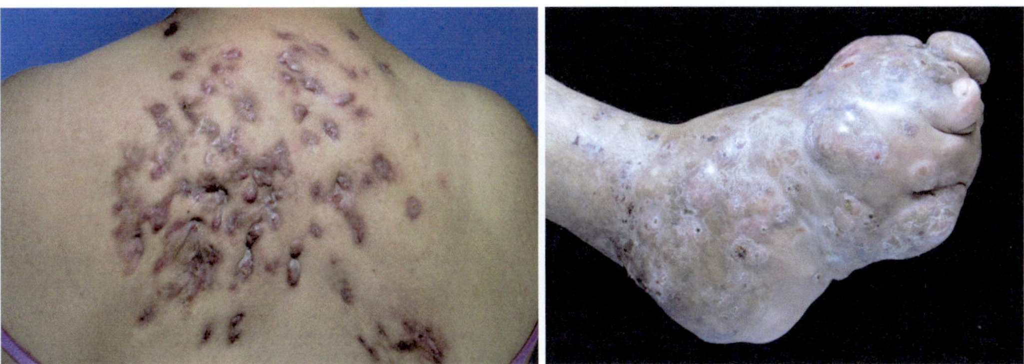

Fig. 1 Mycetoma of the back, (left) and on the foot, (right) caused by *Nocardia brasiliensis*. Notice the charcteristic triad of increase of volume, presence of fistulae, and granules of the etiologic agent

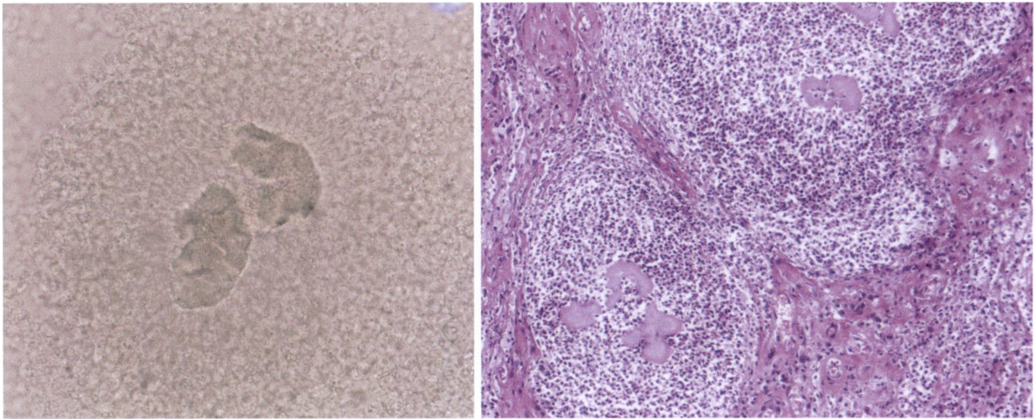

Fig. 2 Microscopic analysis of *N. brasiliensis* mycetoma. Left: Microscopic analysis of pus, showing the granules or microcolonies. Right: Histopathologic analysis show-ing the granules in the center of a Microabscessus with mixed inflammatory infiltrate (H&E)

ably survive the attack of professional human phagocytes such as macrophages and neutrophils once the infection is established in human tissue. Neutrophils are the first line of defense against skin infections. They destroy bacteria and other organisms by phagocytosis followed by intracellular digestion with lytic enzymes and antimicrobial peptides (AMPs). *N. brasiliensis* is the most frequently species of Nocardiae isolated from human mycetoma cases (Fig. 1). When evaluating the activity of human neutrophils AMPS, such as human alpha-defensins human neutrophil peptides (HNPs) 1–3, human beta-defensin (hBD)-3 and cathelicidin LL-37, *N. brasiliensis* is resistant to all of them, in contrast to species rarely isolated from mycetoma human cases, such as *N. farcinica*, *N. nova,* or *N. asteroides* [14]. Histopathological analysis of tissue from patients with *N. brasiliensis* mycetoma shows some characteristic features such as the presence of granules or microcolonies in the middle of micro-abscesses composed of a mixed inflammatory infiltrate, with abundant neutrophils surrounding the microcolonies. In contrast, in tissues of experimentally infected rats (*Rattus norvegicus*), that are resistant to the infection, or in BALB/c mice infected with attenuated strains of *N. brasiliensis*, granules in diverse stages of destruction are observed [15, 16]. It seems that some kind of activation or stimulation is needed to change the switch of inactive to active for neutrophils to destroy the *Nocardia* granules (Fig. 2).

An adaptive immune response is mounted after the establishment of mycetoma and a humoral antibody response is mounted against immunodominant antigens. In patients suffering from *M. mycetomatis* infection, low amounts of antibodies are formed, particularly against proteins of 45-, 60-, and 95-kDa [17]. However, only the latter seems to be specific of *M. mycetomatis*. In *N. brasiliensis*, three proteins of 24-, 26-, and 61-kDa have been described that react specifically against sera from infected patients. The 24–26-kDa complex has been used to develop an ELISA test that has been useful for diagnosis and prognosis of the infection. However, the presence of these antibodies does not correlate with a resistant status [18–20].

The immune response is divided into TH1 or cellular, TH2 or humoral, and TH17 or regulatory branches. The control of the immune response rests on the production of modulatory proteins denominated cytokines that produce the final outcome, either the elimination of the invading agent or the establishment of the infection. In patients infected with *M. mycetomatis*, higher levels of the Th-1 cytokines (IFN-γ, TNF-α, IL-1β, and IL-2) have been observed when patients are treated by surgical excision, compared to those patients subjected to antimicrobial therapy. In contrast, patients treated with surgical excision present lower quantities of Th-2 cytokines (IL-4, IL-5, IL-6, and IL-10) compared to those treated only with antimicrobials, suggesting that cell-mediated immunity may play a role in the pathogenesis of eumycetoma [21]. In *M. mycetomatis* infected patients, peripheral blood mononuclear cells (PBMC) stimulated with culture filtrate proteins of the same organisms produce normal levels of IFN gamma, TNF alfa and TGF beta [22]; however, high levels of IL-10, an interleukin associated to immunosuppression, were observed. By using a *N. brasiliensis* mycetoma model, it has been found that the establishment of a chronic infection, with no spontaneous cure, correlates with an increase of transforming growth factor β1 (TGF- β1) and interleukin-10 (IL- 10), which are cytokines known for their immunosuppressive effects. During early and chronic infections, these cytokines are elevated with increased TGF- β1 levels from days 3 to 30 and sustained IL-10 expression throughout infection compared to uninfected mice. In contrast, at 30 to 60 days post infection, IFN-γ production is decreased [23]. These experimental data confirm the importance of the cellular immune response and that a status of immunosuppression allows the installation and invasion of mycetoma etiologic agents.

Etiological Agents

More than 56 microorganisms have been reported to cause mycetoma [1]. Molecular sequencing techniques have improved precise etiological agent detection and recognition of new causative species, which was reported previously only as an unknown fungal isolate [24]. Around half of the cases worldwide correspond to eumycetomas and half to actinomycetomas. Distinction between fungal or bacterial etiology is of paramount importance to determine appropriate therapy.

M. mycetomatis is responsible for about 70% of all eumycetoma cases. Less prevalent fungal species include *Trematosphaeria* (*Madurella*) *grisea*, *Scedosporium boydii*, and *Falciformispora* (*Leptosphaeria*) *senegalensis*. Rarely, mycetoma cases produced by *Aspergillus*, *Acremonium*, *Curvularia*, *Cylindrocarpon*, *Fusarium*, *Phaeoacremonium*, and *Trichophyton* have been reported [1].

Regarding actinomycetomas, the most prevalent are *N. brasiliensis*, *A. madurae*, *A. pelletieri*, and *Streptomyces somaliensis*. *N. asteroides* was previously considered a somewhat common cause of actinomycetoma. Most of these isolates were likely misidentified and appear to belong to other *Nocardia* species including *N. otitidiscaviarum*, *N. harenae*, *N. wallacei*, and *N. takadensis* [1].

Clinical Manifestations

Mycetoma begins as painless nodule in an area of previous traumatism. It slowly progresses for months or years to form multiple nodules, fistulae, edema, and deformity. The nodules and fistulae drain a sero-purulent or sero-sanguinolent discharge containing the etiological agent grains. The classic mycetoma triad consists of painless subcutaneous mass, sinus formation, and discharge containing grains. The foot is the most common topography followed by the hands, arms, legs, and trunk. Men are three to four times more likely to get affected than women [2]. Agricultural workers and farmers are the most frequently affected. It may affect any age group but the most common decades are 20 to 40 years old. Bone involvement may lead to pathological fractures and pain. Infrequently, advanced infections may cause lung, central nervous system, gastrointestinal, or genitourinary affection. Clinically, eumycetoma and actinomycetoma are undistinguishable. Actinomycetoma tends to involve bone earlier, have more sinuses, and spread more rapidly than eumycetoma, perhaps due to the abundant number of proteases, peptidases, and caseinases encoded by its genome [25].

Diagnosis

The diagnostic approach in a patient with suspicion of mycetoma includes direct mycological examination of the grains, bacterial and fungal cultures, skin biopsy, and imaging methods (radiography, computed tomography, magnetic resonance imaging, and ultrasound). Direct mycological examination of the discharge with 10% potassium hydroxide may confirm the diagnosis by revealing grains. Color, morphology, and size of the grain suggest the etiological agent. Skin biopsies that include subcutaneous tissue for histopathology and cultures (bacterial, mycobacterial, and fungal cultures) should be obtained. Fine-needle aspiration cytology can also be employed. Histopathology reveals a granulomatous infiltrate surrounding the grains. PAS and Grocott's methenamine silver stain highlight the fungal hyphae. Gram, Kinyoun, and Ziehl-Neelsen stains may be used for actinomycete identification [1].

Discharge and biopsy specimens must be cultured in bacterial, mycobacterial, and fungal media. Samples must be preserved for at least 6–8 weeks as some agents grow slowly. Precise specie identification can be achieved with molecular techniques such as PCR analysis of tissue or culture. PCR has been demonstrated to be useful particularly when culture is negative, by isolating the grains, extracting the DNA, and identifying the etiologic agent by 16S RNA sequencing analysis. Another confirmatory analysis to identify fungal cultures consists of using ITS1-ITS4 primers [26–28]. In cases where RNA operon sequence analysis is not conclusive, multilocus sequencing is applied for a more precise identification or description of new etiologic agents. Sub-typing of isolates has been done with *M. mycetomatis* being able to identify 14 genotypes by variable number tandem repeat (VNTR analysis) [29]. This abundance of genotypes is expected, given that the source of the microorganisms is the soil where they have evolved freely and are not confined to a single host or environment as in human tuberculosis, leprosy or *H. pylori* where their evolution is slower (Table 1).

Table 1 Mycetoma: grain characteristics of main etiological agents

Etiological Agent	Grain characteristics
Actinomycetoma	
Nocardia brasiliensis	White-yellow, soft, oval, lobulated, or reniform small grains measuring 0.08–0.13 mm
Actinomadura madurae	White-yellow, soft, cartographic edges, large grains measuring 1–10 mm
Actinomadura pelletieri	Red-pink, hard, spherical, size 0.2–0.5 mm
Streptomyces somaliensis	White-yellow, hard, round-oval with smooth edges, size 0.5–2 mm
Eumycetoma	
Madurella mycetomatis	Black, hard, round, oval or lobulated, large grains measuring 0.5–5 mm
Trematosphaeria grisea	Black, variable consistency, round, oval or lobulated size 0.3–0.6 mm
Scedosporium boydii	White, soft, oval, reniform or multilobulated, size 1–2 mm

Table 2 Differential diagnosis of mycetoma

Botryomycosis	Chronic bacterial infection more common in immunocompromised hosts that present discharge with granules composed of bacterial clusters most commonly caused by *Staphylococcus aureus* and *Pseudomonas aeruginosa*
Actinomycosis	Subacute or chronic infection more commonly affecting the cervicofacial area that presents fistulae draining yellow "sulfur" granules. Caused by anaerobic filamentous bacteria usually of the *Actinomyces* genus
Tuberculosis	Cutaneous tuberculosis has a variable clinical picture and some cases of lupus vulgaris and tuberculosis verrucosa cutis may mimic mycetoma. Osteoarticular tuberculosis imaging is similar to mycetoma and present "rice bodies" that can be mistaken for mycetoma grains
Other mycoses	Chromoblastomycosis, sporotrichosis, blastomycosis, and cutaneous coccidioidomycosis
Tumors	Primary skin neoplasms including squamous cell carcinoma, basal cell carcinoma, Kaposi's sarcoma, and melanoma. Muscle and bone sarcomas. Metastases

Imaging methods are useful in the diagnosis and disease extent evaluation of mycetoma. In plain radiographs, periosteal reaction, erosions, and "punched out" lytic, lesions can be seen. Ultrasound detects hyperreflective echoes that correspond to the grains. The "dot-in-circle" sign can be appreciated and corresponds to a hyperechoic central area surrounded by hypoechoic tissue. Contrast-enhanced computed tomography is also useful to evaluate disease extent [30].

Contrast-enhanced magnetic resonance imaging is the most precise imaging method to evaluate bone, soft tissue, and internal organ involvement. The "dot-in-circle" sign is highly specific of mycetoma and consists of round, 2–5 mm hyperintense lesions surrounded by a low signal intensity surrounding border and a central focus of low intensity signal [31, 33].

Differential diagnosis of mycetoma varies depending on the geographic region, area affected, and disease evolution. Other infections such as botryomycosis, actinomycosis, osteomyelitis, cutaneous/osteoarticular tuberculosis, cocciodiodomycosis, phaeohyphomycosis, chromoblastomycosis, and sporotrichosis must be considered. Other differential diagnoses include primary skin cancer, soft tissue neoplasia, and metastasis (Table 2).

Treatment

The therapy of mycetoma depends on the fungal or bacterial etiology and disease severity. Eumycetoma therapy is based on antifungals and surgery. Actinomycetoma treatment consists of monotherapy or a combination of antibiotics. Overall, treatment response is better in actinomycetoma than in eumycetoma.

Eumycotic mycetoma therapy of choice is itraconazole 200–400 mg daily for 6 to 9 months followed by wide local excision [32]. Itraconazole should be continued after surgery until complete resolution. Eumycetoma cure rates are low (25–35%) and recurrence is common [33]. When possible, referral to a surgical center with experience in the treatment of mycetoma patients is recommended. Terbinafine 500–1000 mg daily as monotherapy or in combination with azoles has shown variable response. Posaconazole and voriconazole have shown efficacy in a few case reports and case series. Amphotericin B use is limited by its adverse effects. During antifungal therapy, liver function tests and drug interactions should be monitored periodically [32].

Actinomycetic mycetoma treatment evidence is limited and antibiotic regimens are based primarily on case series. Recommended therapy must be a combination of antimicrobials rather than relying on single drug to avoid resistance. Current mycetoma treatment consists of trimethoprim/sulfamethoxazole (TMP/SMX) in combination with amikacin administered in cycles. Each cycle consists of amikacin 15 mg/kg/day intramuscularly divided into two daily doses for 3 weeks, concomitant with TMP/SMX 8/40 mg/kg/day divided into two daily doses orally for 5 weeks. Audiometric and renal monitoring is necessary after each cycle. A total of 1 to 5 cycles can be administered depending on the clinical response. This scheme is particularly useful in extensive lesions, special topography like the head or neck, recalcitrant cases, or bone/internal organ involvement (). In localized cases secondary to *N. brasiliensis* involving the extremities without bone/internal organ involvement, TMP/SMX in combination with amoxicillin/clavulanic acid for 3–12 months is a useful alternative that does not require periodic laboratory monitoring. Impenem, meropenem, and linezolid represent second and third-line options in resistant cases. Other antibiotic combinations include dapsone, netilmicin, minocycline, rifampicin, and moxifloxacin [32]. Surgery is seldom required in actinomycetoma. A new antimicrobial of the oxazolidinone family, tedizolid (formerly DA-7218), has recently been accepted for clinical use. Linezolid, the first oxazolidinone on the market, has been observed to be active against *Nocardia*, however side effects such as myelosuppression, peripheral neuropathy, lactic acidosis, and serotonin syndrome have been observed [34]. Tedizolid is less toxic and highly active in vitro and in vivo. A few reports on patients have been published, observing excellent results [35, 36]. Its activity in mycetoma cases produced by *N. brasiliensis* or other actinomycetales is awaiting.

Few new antifungals have been described in recent years. Among them, 1,10-phenanthroline-5,6-dione based compounds which showed some in vitro action against *Phialophora verrucose* and fenarimol analogues which are active in vitro and in vivo against *M. mycetomatis* [37, 38]. The analysis of the in vivo antifungal effect is hindered by the lack of a subcutaneous model of infection resembling that of the human infection. Instead, an intra-peritoneal *M. mycetomatis* experimental infection in mice, and the use of *Galleria mellonella* larvae infections have been employed but the results are difficult to extrapolate to human infections [39, 40].

Vaccines

Given the low prevalence of mycetoma, a general use vaccine is not feasible. However, the use of whole cell vaccines or purified immunogenic antigens that could be used together with chemotherapy could be helpful in extensive, recalcitrant cases. Research has focused on the two main causative agents, *M. mycetomatis* and *N. brasiliensis*. A couple of immunogenic antigens from *M. mycetomatis*, a fructose-bisphosphate aldolase and a pyruvate kinase, have been reported [41]. By using the fructose-bisphosphate aldolase, three peptides that shown a potent binding affinity to B-cells and a very strong binding affinity to MHC II and MHC I alleles that have been designed using in silico systems [42]. However, they have not been tested in vivo.

In *N. brasiliensis*, an attenuated strain (NB-P200) has been obtained after 200 continuous subcultures [43]. Immunization with NB-P200 bacterial cells results in changes in the natural infection of experimental stablished *N. brasiliensis* mycetoma, inducing a decrease of lesions in experimental BALB/c infections [44].These results are promissory for future management of human mycetoma cases.

Conclusions

Mycetoma is a chronic, subcutaneous infection caused by aerobic actinomycetes or fungi. It predominantly affects countries between latitudes 15° south and 30° north including Mexico, Sudan, Venezuela, and India. Etiological agents vary widely between countries. Mycetoma usually affects the foot presenting slowly progressing firm edema, nodules, scars, and fistulae that drain serosanguinous or seropurulent material with the etiological agent grains. Diagnosis can be performed by direct mycological examination, cultures, biopsy, and imaging methods. Eumycetoma is treated with antifungals and surgery. Actinomycetoma therapy consists of antibiotic combinations usually consisting of TMP/SMX and amikacin.

References

1. Welsh O, Vera-Cabrera L, Salinas-Carmona MC. Cutaneous mycetoma. In: James WD, Elston D, editors. http://emedicine.medscape.com/article/1090932-overview#showall eMedicine Dermatology. St. Petersburg: eMedicine Corporation; 2018.

2. Lopez-Martinez R, Mendez-Tovar LJ, Bonifaz A, Arenas R, Mayorga J, Welsh O, et al. Update on the epidemiology of mycetoma in Mexico. A review of 3933 cases. Gac Med Mex. 2013;149(5):586–92.

3. Mahe A, Develoux M, Lienhardt C, Keita S, Bobin P. Mycetomas in Mali: causative agents and geographic distribution. Am J Trop Med Hyg. 1996 Jan;54(1):77–9.

4. Badiane AS, Ndiaye M, Diongue K, Diallo MA, Seck MC, Ndiaye D. Geographical distribution of mycetoma cases in Senegal over a period of 18 years. Mycoses. 2019 Nov 25;63:250. https://doi.org/10.1111/myc.13037.

5. Fahal A, Mahgoub el S, El Hassan AM, Abdel-Rahman ME. Mycetoma in The Sudan: an update from the Mycetoma research Centre, University of Khartoum, Sudan. PLoS Negl Trop Dis. 2015 Mar 27;9(3):e0003679. https://doi.org/10.1371/journal.pntd.0003679.

6. Dubey N, Capoor MR, Hasan AS, Gupta A, Ramesh V, Sharma S, et al. Epidemiological profile and spectrum of neglected tropical disease eumycetoma from Delhi. North India Epidemiol Infect. 2019;147:e294.

7. Mansilla-Lory J, Contreras-Lopez EA. Mycetoma in prehispanic Mexico. Review in the skeletical collection of Tlatilco culture. Rev Med Inst Mex Seguro Soc. 2009;47(3):237–42.

8. Venkatswami S, Sankarasubramanian A, Subramanyam S. The madura foot: looking deep. Int J Low Extrem Wounds. 2012;11(1):31–42.

9. Reis CMS, Reis-Filho EGM. Mycetomas: an epidemiological, etiological, clinical, laboratory and therapeutic review. An Bras Dermatol. 2018;93(1): 8–18.

10. Buonfrate D, Gobbi F, Angheben A, Marocco S, Farina C, Van Den Ende J, Bisoffi Z. Autochthonous cases of mycetoma in Europe: report of two cases and review of literature. PLoS One. 2014;9(6):e100590. https://doi.org/10.1371/journal.pone.0100590.

11. Lucas RE, Armstrong PK. Two cases of mycetoma due to *Nocardia brasiliensis* in Central Australia. Med J Aust. 2000 Feb 21;172(4):167–9.

12. Kohler JR, Hube B, Puccia R, Casadevall A, Perfect JR. Fungi that Infect Humans Microbiol Spectr. 2017;5:3. https://doi.org/10.1128/microbiolspec.FUNK-0014-2016.

13. van de Sande WW, Fahal A, Verbrugh H, van Belkum A. Polymorphisms in genes involved in innate immunity predispose toward mycetoma susceptibility. J Immunol. 2007 Sep 1;179(5):3065–74.

14. Rieg S, Meier B, Fahnrich E, Huth A, Wagner D, Kern WV, et al. Differential activity of innate defense antimicrobial peptides against Nocardia species. BMC Microbiol. 2010;10:61.

15. Vera-Cabrera L, Rodriguez-Quintanilla MA, Boiron P, Salinas-Carmona MC, Welsh O. Experimental mycetoma by Nocardia brasiliensis in rats. J Mycol Médicale. 1998;8:183–7.

16. Almaguer-Chavez JA, Welsh O, Lozano-Garza HG, Said-Fernandez S, Romero-Diaz VJ, Ocampo-Candiani J, et al. Decrease of virulence for BALB/c mice produced by continuous subculturing of Nocardia brasiliensis. BMC Infect Dis. 2011;11:290.

17. ELbadawi HS, Mahgoub E, Mahmoud N, Fahal AH. Use of immunoblotting in testing Madurella mycetomatis specific antigen. Trans R Soc Trop Med Hyg. 2016;110(5):312–6.

18. Salinas-Carmona MC, Vera L, Welsh O, Rodríguez M. Antibody response to Nocardia brasiliensis antigens in man. Zentralbl Bakteriol. 1992 Feb;276(3):390–7.

19. Vera-Cabrera L, Salinas-Carmona MC, Welsh O, Rodriguez MA. Isolation and purification of two immunodominant antigens from Nocardia brasiliensis. J Clin Microbiol. 1992;30(5):1183–8.

20. Salinas-Carmona MC, Welsh O, Casillas SM. Enzyme-linked immunosorbent assay for serological diagnosis of Nocardia brasiliensis and clinical correlation with mycetoma infections. J Clin Microbiol. 1993;31(11):2901–6.

21. Nasr A, Abushouk A, Hamza A, Siddig E, Fahal AH. Th-1, Th-2 cytokines profile among Madurella mycetomatis Eumycetoma patients. PLoS Negl Trop Dis. 2016;10(7):e0004862.

22. Elagab EA, Mukhtar MM, Fahal AH, van de Sande WW. Peripheral blood mononuclear cells of mycetoma patients react differently to Madurella mycetomatis antigens than healthy endemic controls. PLoS Negl Trop Dis. 2013;7(4):e2081. Published 2013 Apr 25. https://doi.org/10.1371/journal.pntd.0002081.

23. Rosas-Taraco AG, Perez-Linan AR, Bocanegra-Ibarias P, Perez-Rivera LI, Salinas-Carmona MC. Nocardia brasiliensis induces an immunosuppressive microenvironment that favors chronic infection in BALB/c mice. Infect Immun. 2012;80(7):2493–9.

24. Mhmoud NA, Santona A, Fiamma M, Siddig EE, Deligios M, Bakhiet SM, et al. Chaetomium atrobrunneum causing human eumycetoma: the first report. PLoS Negl Trop Dis. 2019;13(5):e0007276.

25. Vera-Cabrera L, Ortiz-Lopez R, Elizondo-Gonzalez R, Perez-Maya AA, Ocampo-Candiani J. Complete genome sequence of Nocardia brasiliensis HUJEG-1. J Bacteriol. 2012;194(10):2761–2. https://doi.org/10.1128/JB.00210-12.

26. Ahmed AA, van de Sande W, Fahal AH. Mycetoma laboratory diagnosis: review article. PLoS Negl Trop Dis. 2017;11(8):e0005638.

27. Arastehfar A, Lim W, Daneshnia F, van de Sande WWJ, Fahal AH, Desnos-Ollivier M, et al. Madurella real-time PCR, a novel approach for eumycetoma diagnosis. PLoS Negl Trop Dis. 2020;14(1):e0007845.

28. Mencarini J, Antonelli A, Scoccianti G, Bartolini L, Roselli G, Capanna R, et al. Madura foot in Europe: diagnosis of an autochthonous case by molecular approach and review of the literature. New Microbiol. 2016;39(2):156–9.

29. Lim W, Eadie K, Horst-Kreft D, Ahmed SA, Fahal AH, van de Sande WWJ. VNTR confirms the heterogeneity of Madurella mycetomatis and is a promising typing tool for this mycetoma causing agent. Med Mycol. 2019;57(4):434–40.

30. Guerra-Leal JD, Medrano-Danes LA, Montemayor-Martinez A, Perez-Rodriguez E, Luna-Gurrola CE, Arenas-Guzman R, et al. The importance of diagnostic imaging of mycetoma in the foot. Int J Dermatol. 2019;58(5):600–4.

31. van de Sande WW, Fahal AH, Goodfellow M, Mahgoub el S, Welsh O, Zijlstra EE. Merits and pitfalls of currently used diagnostic tools in mycetoma. PLoS Negl Trop Dis. 2014;8(7):e2918.

32. Welsh O, Salinas-Carmona MC, Cardenas-De la Garza JA, Rodriguez-Escamilla IM, Sanchez-Meza E. Current treatment of Mycetoma. Current treatment options. Infect Dis. 2018;10(3):389–96.

33. Welsh O, Vera-Cabrera L, Welsh E, Salinas MC. Actinomycetoma and advances in its treatment. Clin Dermatol. 2012;30(4):372–81.

34. Espinoza-González NA, Welsh O, de Torres NW, Cavazos-Rocha N, Ocampo-Candiani J, Said-Fernandez S, Lozano-Garza G, Choi SH, Vera-Cabrera L. Efficacy of DA-7218, a new oxazolidinone prodrug, in the treatment of experimental actinomycetoma produced by Nocardia brasiliensis. Molecules. 2008 Jan 11;13(1):31–40.

35. Matin A, Sharma S, Mathur P, Apewokin SK. Myelosuppression-sparing treatment of central nervous system nocardiosis in a multiple myeloma patient utilizing a tedizolid-based regimen: a case report. Int J Antimicrob Agents. 2017;49(4):488–92.

36. Giménez-Arufe V, Gutiérrez-Urbón J, Blanco-Aparicio M, Míguez-Rey E, Martín-Herranz MI. Nocardiosis pulmonar tratada con tedizolid. Farm Hosp. 2019;43(6):208–10.

37. Granato MQ, Goncalves DS, Seabra SH, McCann M, Devereux M, Dos Santos AL, et al. 1,10-Phenanthroline-5,6-Dione-based compounds are effective in disturbing crucial physiological events of Phialophora verrucosa. Front Microbiol. 2017;8:76.

38. Lim W, Melse Y, Konings M, Phat Duong H, Eadie K, Laleu B, et al. Addressing the most neglected diseases through an open research model: the discovery of fenarimols as novel drug candidates for eumycetoma. PLoS Negl Trop Dis. 2018;12(4):e0006437.

39. Ahmed AO, van Vianen W, ten Kate MT, van de Sande WW, van Belkum A, Fahal AH, et al. A murine model of Madurella mycetomatis eumycetoma. FEMS Immunol Med Microbiol. 2003;37(1):29–36.

40. Kloezen W, van Helvert-van PM, Fahal AH, van de Sande WW. A Madurella mycetomatis grain model in Galleria mellonella larvae. PLoS Negl Trop Dis. 2015;9(7):e0003926.

41. de Klerk N, de Vogel C, Fahal A, van Belkum A, van de Sande WW. Fructose-bisphosphate aldolase and pyruvate kinase, two novel immunogens in Madurella mycetomatis. Med Mycol. 2012;50(2):143–51.

42. Mohammed AA, ALnaby AM, Sabeel SM, AbdElmarouf FM, Dirar AI, Ali MM, Khandgawi MA, Yousif AM, Abdulgadir EM, Sabahalkhair MA, Abbas AE, Hassan MA. Epitope-based peptide vaccine against fructose-bisphosphate aldolase of Madurella mycetomatis using immunoinformatics approaches. Bioinform Biol Insights. 2018 Nov 12;12:1177932218809703.

43. Gonzalez-Carrillo C, Millan-Sauceda C, Lozano-Garza HG, Ortiz-Lopez R, Elizondo-Gonzalez R, Welsh O, et al. Genomic changes associated with the loss of Nocardia brasiliensis virulence in mice after 200 in vitro passages. Infect Immun. 2016;84(9):2595–606.

44. Garcia-Lozano JA, Garcia-Berlanga CC, Viveros-Rosado RT, Ocampo-Candiani J, Vargas-Villarreal J, Vera-Cabrera L. A novel experimental immunomodulatory therapy against Nocardia brasiliensis in a BALB/c murine model. Clin Exp Dermatol. 2019 Nov 14;45:544. https://doi.org/10.1111/ced.14139.

Chromoblastomycosis

Alexandro Bonifaz, Andrés Tirado-Sánchez, and Lorena Gordillo

Key Points

- Chromoblastomycosis is a chronic, orphan, neglected, occupational cutaneous and subcutaneous mycosis, caused by a group of dematiaceous fungi, and is characterized by verrucous nodules usually located in the lower limbs.
- It is the second most prevalent implantation mycosis in the world.
- The two most common etiological species are *Fonsecaea pedrosoi* and *Cladophialophora carrionii*.
- The disease is prevalent in tropical and subtropical climates; most reports come from Brazil; however, its frequency has increased due to returning travelers, aid workers, archaeologists, and immigrants.
- There are six clinical forms of chromoblastomycosis: nodular, tumoral, verrucous, cicatricial, plaque-type, and mixed form.
- The definite diagnosis is based on the demonstration of species of dematiaceous fungi on culture or histopathology.
- There are no clinical trials that determine the best option for treatment of chromoblastomycosis.
- The treatment includes physical therapies, systemic antifungals, and combined therapy.
- Early diagnosis of the disease is of paramount importance.

Chromoblastomycosis

Chromoblastomycosis (CBM), formerly known as chromomycosis, Fonseca disease, verrucous mycosis; is a chronic, orphan, neglected, occupational cutaneous, and subcutaneous mycosis caused by a group of melanized or dematiaceous (black) fungi. Verrucous nodules usually located in the lower limbs characterize CBM, resulting from traumatic implantation of fungi; it is the second most prevalent implantation mycosis globally [1–3].

Epidemiology

The disease is prevalent in tropical and subtropical climates. Most reports come from Brazil (mainly in the region of Amazonia); Madagascar, Costa Rica, and the Dominican Republic also report numerous cases [3]. In a smaller proportion, cases are reported from Cuba, Colombia, Guatemala, Honduras, Mexico (Oaxaca and Veracruz), Puerto Rico, and Venezuela. Some cases outside the Americas were reported in

A. Bonifaz (✉) · A. Tirado-Sánchez · L. Gordillo
Mycology Department, Dermatology Service,
Hospital General de México "Dr. Eduardo Liceaga",
Mexico City, Mexico

W. Robles (ed.), *Skin Disease in Travelers*, Updates in Clinical Dermatology,
https://doi.org/10.1007/978-3-031-57836-6_12

Australia, Congo, southern China, the Czech Republic, Romania, Eastern Germany, and Malaysia. The United States, France, Finland, Russia, and Japan have several reported cases outside the tropical zone [2, 4]. (Fig. 1).

Black fungi causing CBM have been isolated from soil, various plants, and wood pulp. Most strains, mainly *F. pedrosoi*, live in humid and warm climates with a temperature ranging between 25 and 30 °C, and an average rainfall of 800–1500 mm per year [3, 5]; in contrast, the cases produced by *C. carrionii* and *C. yegresii* correspond to semi-desert areas of cacti, reporting in the state of Falcón, Venezuela, and some areas of Madagascar and Australia [5, 6].

Infection usually occurs among immunocompetent adults between the ages of 20 and 40, and there are few reports among children, mainly in endemic regions [7]. Men are preferentially infected (ratio of 4:1), considered to be influenced by occupational issues and hormonal factors that may determine fungal adaptation. It is considered a common mycosis among rural workers (farmers and lumberjacks) [1, 3].

Ethio-Pathogenesis

The etiological agents of CBM are dimorphic, dematiaceous (pigmented) fungi, classified in the order *Chaetothyriales*, which are members of the *Herpotrichiellaceae* family (Table 1). The two most common etiological species are *Fonsecaea pedrosoi*, reported in warm and humid climates, and *Cladophialophora carrionii*, only reported in semi-desert climates [1, 8].

The disease is initiated by skin trauma (in only 33.8% of the cases in predisposed subjects, such as immunosuppression, diabetes mellitus), through which the conidia and hyphae penetrate, primarily through wood chips [9]; probable transmissions through cacti have also been reported. Its evolution is usually chronic, and the first clinical manifestation occurs at the inoculation site as a small nodule, which slowly grows to form extensive verrucous plaques [10].

Esterre et al. [11] consider that fibrosis produced in the dermis and subcutaneous cell tissue

is essential for developing CBM, probably because black fungi produce pyridinoline, a substance that induces cross-linking compounds of collagen fibers. It is essential to mention that most cases have significant fibrosis, causing low drug penetration. CBM is undoubtedly the most subcutaneous of the deep mycosis; only sporadic cases with bone involvement have been previously reported, as well as spreading to other organs, including CNS [1, 7, 12].

Specific histocompatibility antigens, including HLA-A29, may promote disease development. Among other virulence factors, fungal dimorphism, the capacity for morphological and biochemical changes, and melanin production are particularly important because pigmented fungi are difficult to phagocytize compared with non-melanized species [13–15]. The clinical types of CBM could be related to the cytokine profile, mainly tumor necrosis factor–α, interleukin 10 (IL10), as well as the inability of *Toll*-like receptors to recognize pathogens [16].

There is little information on the immune mechanisms involved in the development of CBM; various methods have detected specific antibodies against the two most common species. The most critical role of immunity is undoubtedly the tissue cell response, particularly the neuroprotective Th2 immune response (IL10) with ineffective humoral involvement and the polymorphonuclear, responsible for primary defense mechanisms; complement system activation (C5a) may influence neutrophil migration. It should be noted that the majority of patients with the disease are immunocompetent, and the infection is considered to be due to constant exposure to the etiological agent [17, 18].

Clinical Manifestations

CBM is a polymorphic condition; although there are many clinical classifications, we focus on the proposed by Queiroz-Telles et al. [12], which includes five clinical forms: nodular, tumor-like, verrucous, cicatricial, plaque-type; a mixed form is also described (Table 2). The most common location is on the limbs, more commonly the

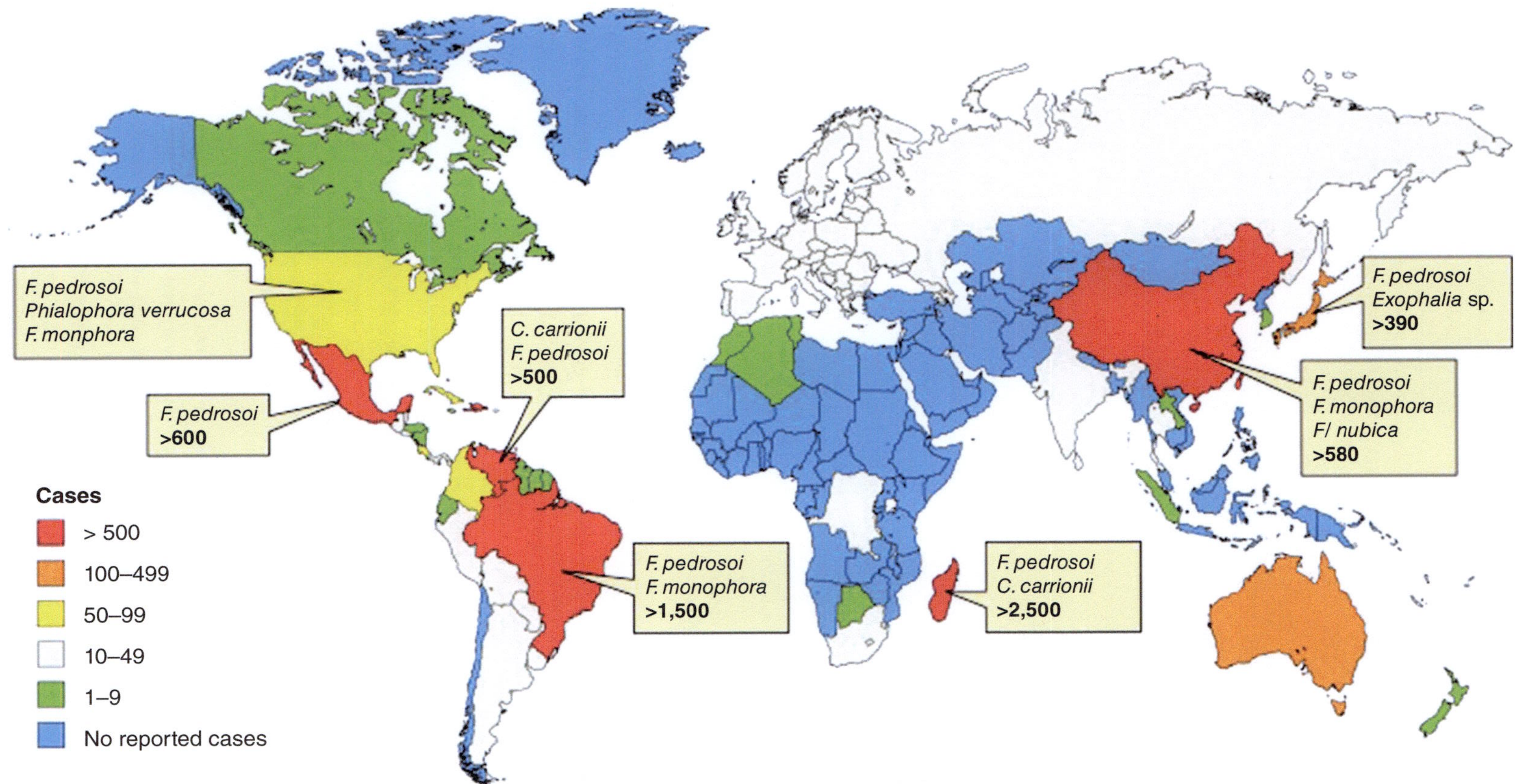

Fig. 1 Global distribution of chromoblastomycosis based on reported case series. Reproduced with permission: *Clin Microbiol Rev. 2017 Jan; 30* (1): *233–276. doi:* https://doi.org/10.1128/CMR.00032-16

Table 1 Main chromoblastomycosis etiologic agents

Agent
Fonsecaea pedrosoi[a]
Fonsecaea compacta
Fonsecaea monophora
Fonsecaea nubica
Phialophora verrucosa
Cladophialophora carrionii[a]
Cladophialophora yegresii
Rhinocladiella aquaspersa
Rhinocladiella similis
Exophiala jeanselmei
Exophiala dermatitidis
Exophiala spinifera

[a]Most common

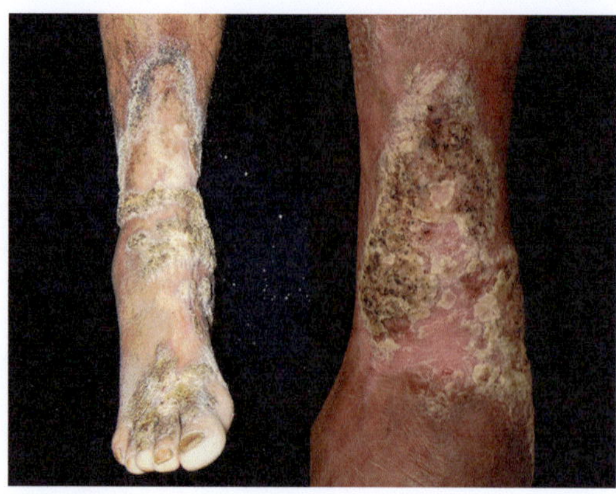

Fig. 2 Chromoblastomycosis in leg and forearm (black spots characteristic of the disease are observed)

Table 2 Clinical manifestations of chromoblastomycosis

Clinical type	Clinical description
Nodular	Moderately raised, soft, dull to pink violaceous growth. Surface smooth, verrucous, or scaly. It may gradually become tumoral
Tumoral	Tumor-like masses, prominent, papillomatous, sometimes lobulated; 'cauliflower like'. Surface partly or entirely covered with epidermal debris and crusts. More exuberant on lower extremities
Verrucous	Hyperkeratosis is an outstanding feature—Verrucous lesions. Frequently encountered along the border of the foot
Cicatricial	Non-elevated lesions enlarge by peripheral extension with atrophic scarring; healing usually occurs at the center. It may show an annular, arciform or serpiginous configuration. It tends to cover extensive areas of the body
Plaque	Slightly elevated, with variously sized and shaped areas of infiltration. Reddish to violaceous, presenting a scaly surface with marked lines of cleavage. Usually observed on the higher portions of the limbs

These types may be mixed in some patients

lower limbs (70–80%), predominating on the dorsal aspect of the feet; it also occurs on the trunk and exceptionally on the head (face and scalp) [1–4, 12, 19].

The most common clinical forms include nodular, tumor-like, and verrucous type; the first appears after one or several months of fungal implantation in the form of a slow-growing, small nodule that extends superficially, developing erythematous and scaly plaques with intense itching. Itchiness may lead to dissemination by autoinoculation and contiguous spread. Initial lesions slowly spread and present asymmetrical and unilateral, forming erythematous and scaly nodules; about a year later, it manifests as large verrucous or vegetative plaques, covered with large scale ulcers, crusts, and cellular debris (multiple black spots, representing transepidermal elimination of the fungus). The size of the lesions is variable; as the disease progresses, it leaves verrucous, exophytic, cauliflower-like areas (tumor-like lesions). Disease duration ranges from 20 days to 30 years. The symptoms may vary according to the severity; most patients complain of itchiness and local pain [1–4, 12]. The severity of the disease includes three stages: mild (solitary lesions <5 cm), moderate (several lesions <15 cm), and severe (extensive cutaneous regions affected, adjacent or non-adjacent) [12] (Fig. 2).

Less often, CBM occurs in a flattened and superficial form, similar to psoriasis or tinea corporis, occasionally with some satellite lesions. The cicatricial type is a chronic stage of CBM, usually seen in nodular or tumor-like forms; as the disease progresses, it leaves severe scarring. Lymphostasis is commonly seen, mainly due to disease spreading to the entire limb and developing *elephantiasis nostra*. Other complications

Table 3 Differential diagnosis of chromoblastomycosis

Group	Subgroup	Disease
Infectious diseases	Fungi	Paracoccidioidomycosis
		Blastomycosis
		Sporotrichosis (fixed)
		Coccidioidomycosis
		Phaeohyphomycosis
		Candidiasis (granulomatous type)
		Dermatophytosis (chronic tinea)
	Bacteria	Tuberculosis (verrucosa cutis and lupus vulgaris)
		Leprosy
		Syphilis (tertiary)
		Nocardiosis
		Ecthyma
		Atypical mycobacteriosis (*M.marinum, M.fortuitum*)
	Protozoa	Leishmaniasis
		Rhinosporidiosis
Non-infectious diseases	Inflammatory	Psoriasis
		Sarcoidosis
		Lupus erythematosus (tumidus)
		Lichen planus (hyperthropic)
		Lichen simplex
	Neoplastic	Lymphoma
		Sarcoma
		Squamous cell carcinoma
		Keratoacanthoma

include bacterial infections that cause ulcers, exudate, foul odor and pain, ankyloses, and malignant transformation (squamous cell carcinoma and melanoma) [1–4, 12].

Cases affecting periosteum and bone are rare, and hematogenous or lymphatic spread to the brain is observed in severely immunosuppressed patients [1–4, 12].

The main differential diagnosis includes tuberculosis verrucosa cutis and lupus vulgaris as well as verrucous conditions such as sporotrichosis, cutaneous leishmaniasis, non-tuberculous mycobacteriosis, hypertrophic lichen planus, and several neoplasms (squamous cell carcinoma, lymphoma, keratoacanthoma, and sarcomas).

Tinea corporis, psoriasis, Bowen's disease, sarcoidosis, chronic lupus erythematosus, mycetoma, leprosy, lobomycosis, protothecosis, rhinosporidiosis, botryomycosis, paracoccidioidomycosis, coccidioidomycosis, blastomycosis, ecthyma, halogenoderma, and tertiary syphilis are also differential diagnoses (Table 3) [19–22].

Diagnosis

A conclusive or definitive diagnosis is based on the demonstration of dematiaceous fungi on culture or histopathology [23–25]. Fresh or direct examinations are the most commonly used diagnostic methods; skin scraping with a scalpel for direct microscopy and culture is sensitive. The collected sample should be placed between slides with 20–40% KOH and observed under the microscope for keratin clearance after 10 to 20 min. The parasitic forms called muriform or fumagoid cells (also called Medlar sclerotes) are usually observed; these are cells of 4–10 μm, solitary or clustered, brown, thick walls, with double membranes divided by a central partition. Its reproductive form is through binary fission. Occasionally, it is also possible to observe thick, tabicated, dark filaments from clusters of muriform cells; this occurs in severe keratotic cases. It is important to note that all CBM-causing species form muriform cells which are different from

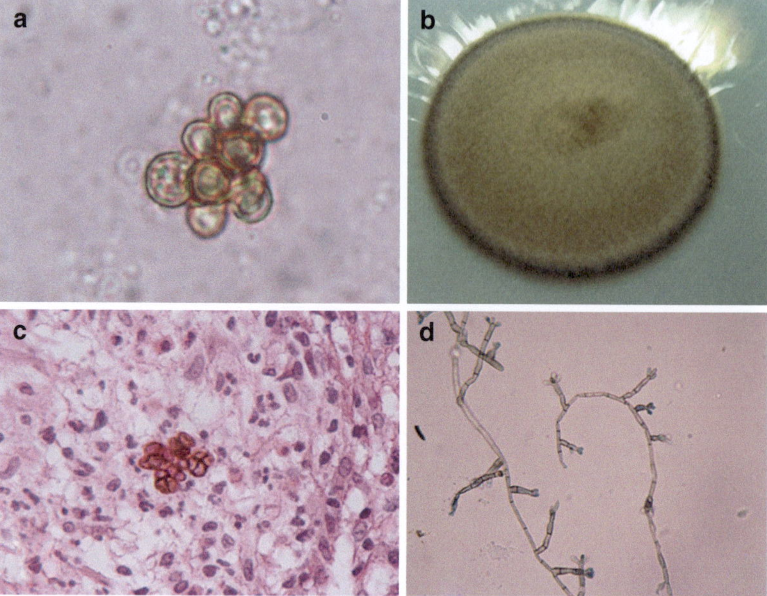

Fig. 3 Mycological aspects. (**a**) Muriform cells on direct examination (KOH, 60×). (**b**) Cultivation of *F. pedrosoi* (Sabouraud dextrose agar). (**c**) Muriform cells on biopsy (H&E, 40×). (**d**) Direct examination of *Fonsecaea pedrosoi* (Cotton blue, 40×)

cases of *phaeohyphomycosis* because the latter has dark filaments and blastoconidia [1, 4].

Culture in Sabouraud dextrose agar media with and without antibiotics is a specific diagnostic method. It is incubated at 25–28 °C. Most CBM-producing slow-growing species and colonies are macroscopically similar; colony growth manifests at 10 days, with peaks between 30 and 40 days [1, 4, 12]. The macro colonial and micromorphology of the colonies has already been described in the etiology section.

The two most common CBM-causing species include *Fonsecaea pedrosoi* (95%) in warm and humid climates and *Cladophialophora carrionii* in semi-arid climates. Another technique for diagnosis is the histopathology, which shows a suppurative, mixed granuloma. Hyperkeratosis with parakeratosis and irregular marked acanthosis at the epidermis level often develop pseudo-epitheliomatous hyperplasia (similar to other mycoses). In the superficial and middle dermis, a granulomatous reaction consisting of lymphocytes, epithelioid cells, Langhans-type giant cells, and foreign body cells are usually observed; muriform cells, also known as sclerotic, fumagoid, or Medlar bodies, are seen by the use of hematoxylin and eosin and with Ziehl-Neelsen and Wade-Fite stains, in small microabscesses or inside giant cells. No other stains are usually required because the fungus contains a dark brown pigment [23, 24]. (Fig. 3).

Histopathological examination is necessary to enhance positive culturing, thus reducing bacterial contamination and helping to evaluate criteria for interruption of the treatment [23].

Immunological tests, not necessarily required for CBM diagnosis, include serology, precipitins, and antibodies fixing the complement; however, it has been observed that the extracted antigens cross-react with pathogenic fungi like *S. schenckii* and other contaminant dematiaceous fungi, including *Cladosporium* and *Alternaria*, decreasing the importance of this test as a diagnostic tool in CBM. Delayed sensitivity determination is variable when an intradermal antigen is used and lacks diagnostic utility [26–28].

PCR amplification techniques of the rDNA internal transcriber spacer (ITS) region, with genetic sequences specific to each species, e.g., for the distinction between *Fonsecaea* and *Phialophora* species, translation elongation factor 1α or a partial β tubulin gene (βT2) may help in species identification from biological samples (infected tissue) and culture [29–31].

Table 4 Main therapeutic options for chromoblastomycosis

Physical methods	Chemotherapy	Combinations
Standard surgery	Calciferol (vitamin D3)	Itraconazole + cryosurgery[a]
Thermotherapy	5-fluorocytosine	Terbinafine + cryosurgery[a]
Cryosurgery[a]	5-fluorouracil	Itraconazole + terbinafine
Local heat (dry)	Thiabendazole	Itraconazole + terbinafine + dry heat
Mohs surgery	Amphotericin B	
CO$_2$ laser therapy	Ketoconazole	
	Fluconazole	
	Itraconazole[a]	
	Posaconazole	
	Terbinafine[a]	

[a]Most commonly used therapies

Treatment

There is no consensus guideline to determine the best option to treat CBM. Treatment selection and their effectiveness are highly variable, depending on several aspects (Table 4). Esterre and Queiroz-Telles [32] proposed three variables that determine the efficacy of CBM treatment: the etiological agent (*C. carrionii* and *P. verrucosa* are less sensitive to antifungal drugs than *F. pedrosoi*), the severity and the extent of the disease, and drug selection. Other variables include condition patient's comorbidities, the physician experience, and patient immunological status [1–3].

The clinical cure is a complete resolution of the disease, often leaving scars. Mycological cure involves the absence of the etiological agent on direct examination or culture [33, 34].

Physical Treatments

If the condition is mild and limited, or if systemic therapy has been used, traditional surgical removal and curettage with electrodessication are the most valuable options in well-circumscribed lesions. The best physical method is cryosurgery with liquid nitrogen, recommended especially in small, limited cases, not affecting joints, without lymphatic involvement, and usually in a single session, but can be performed by areas at different times; this method is recommended in association with systemic treatment (itraconazole and terbinafine), to prevent lymphatic spread. Local heat (45–50 °C) is effective for small and localized lesions, mainly associated with *F. pedrosoi*. Dry heat is preferred instead of wet heat (used in sporotrichosis), which may favor spreading of the lesion [35–37].

Mohs surgery and iontophoresis are no longer used. Photodynamic therapy is helpful when combined with systemic antifungal chemotherapy [38].

Systemic Treatment and Antifungal Chemotherapy

Calciferol (vitamin D3) and supersaturated potassium iodide (KI) had inconclusive results about their efficacy in CBM; the former should be used at doses of 600,000 IU per week evaluated every 2 months. The latter is used at 3–6 g/day, as in sporotrichosis [1, 4].

5-fluorocytosine (5FC) showed acceptable results in CBM, although the results may vary according to the consulted literature; it is prescribed at doses of 100–150 mg/kg; one of its drawbacks is that, like other drugs, severe cases do not entirely cure and small areas may remain active [4, 12].

Amphotericin B has been used intravenously, intra-arterial, and intra-lesion; the results are usually good; however, it may cause secondary side effects such as kidney disease and cardiotoxicity, arteritis, and necrosis, mainly related to long-term use. The disease often relapses after discontinuation of therapy [31, 36]. Other treatment options with inconsistent results include thiabendazole, ketoconazole, imiquimod, and carbon dioxide laser photocoagulation [37].

Itraconazole is a triazole derivative successfully employed with better results than previous therapies, recommended at high doses (continuous or pulsed) of 200–400 mg/day. Hepatic evaluation should be performed during treatment due to the toxic effect. This treatment may be used as monotherapy or associated with other therapies, particularly with cryosurgery. Sensitivity to itraconazole of agents related to CBM has been reported in several studies. No standard methods to test susceptibility are available for CBM-related melanized agents or do not predict clinical response [39–42].

Terbinafine is also one of the most used antifungals against CBM; it is used at doses between 250 and 500 mg/day. Some successful reports are at low doses (250 mg/day); however, the most appropriate dose is 500 mg/day. It is currently considered one of the most effective and best-tolerated therapies against CBM; this is probably because of its fungicide mechanism antifibrotic properties and does not involve cytochrome P-450 oxidase, resulting in the absence or minimal drug interactions [43, 44].

Other triazoles: Therapeutic successes with fluconazole have been reported at doses of 200–400 mg/day [44], and recently, some cases treated with posaconazole with acceptable results have been reported; however, there is no experience in large cohort of cases [45].

Combined Therapy: Several case reports of combined therapy, particularly cryosurgery with itraconazole or terbinafine are available in the literature. These combinations are useful in severe or recalcitrant cases. Other proposed combinations include itraconazole with 5FC. Treatment usually starts with itraconazole or terbinafine until the maximum reduction of the lesions, observed between 8 and 12 months, then cryosurgery or even surgery is used in one or more sessions. The results are variable and mainly depend on the disease extent.

Cure rates with antifungal drugs range from 15 to 80%. In most severe CBM, cure rates are considerably low, with high relapse rates [1–4, 12].

Control and Prevention

Because as rural workers, mostly farmers, are the most affected group with CBM, the most appropriate prophylactic measure is the use of closed footwear, which would prevent injuries that inoculates the fungus. If the condition has already developed, the early diagnosis of the disease is of paramount importance since the therapeutic options and the results are better than in advanced disease [4]. There are no available vaccines for implantation mycoses, including CBM.

References

1. Bonifaz A, Vázquez-González D, Perusquía-Ortiz AM. Subcutaneous mycoses: chromoblastomycosis, sporotrichosis and mycetoma. J Dtsch Dermatol Ges. 2010;8:619–27.
2. Queiróz AJR, Pereira Domingos F, Antônio JR. Chromoblastomycosis: clinical experience and review of literature. Int J Dermatol. 2018;57:1351–5.
3. Brito AC, Bittencourt MJS. Chromoblastomycosis: an etiological, epidemiological, clinical, diagnostic, and treatment update. An Bras Dermatol. 2018;93:495–506.
4. Burks JB, Wakabongo M, McGinnis MR. Chromoblastomycosis. A fungal infection primarily observed in the lower extremity. J Am Podiatr Med Assoc. 1995;85:260–4.
5. Queiroz-Telles F, de Hoog S, Santos DW, Salgado CG, Vicente VA, Bonifaz A, Roilides E, Xi L, Azevedo CM, da Silva MB, Pana ZD, Colombo AL, Walsh TJ. Chromoblastomycosis. Clin Microbiol Rev. 2017;30:233–76.
6. Bonifaz A, Carrasco E, Saúl A. Chromoblastomycosis: clinical and mycological experience of 51 cases. Mycoses. 2001;44:1–7.
7. Perez-Blanco M, Hernandez Valles R, Garcia-Humbria L, Yegres F. Chromoblastomycosis in children and adolescents in the endemic area of the falcon state, Venezuela. Med Mycol. 2006;44:467.
8. De Hoog GS, Queiroz-Telles F, Haase G, Fernandez-Zeppenfeldt G, Attili Angelis D, Gerrits Van Den Ende AH. Black fungi: clinical and pathogenic approaches. Med Mycol. 2000;38(Suppl 1):243–5.
9. Yang CS, Chen CB, Lee YY, Yang CH, Chang YC, Chung WH, Lee HE, Hui RC, Chuang YH, Hong HS, Sun PL. Chromoblastomycosis in Taiwan: a report of 30 cases and a review of the literature. Med Mycol. 2018;56:395–405.
10. Agarwal R, Singh G, Ghosh A, Verma KK, Pandey M, Xess I. Chromoblastomycosis in India: review of 169 cases. PLoS Negl Trop Dis. 2017;11:e0005534.
11. Esterre P, Inzan CK, Ramarcel ER, Andriantsimahavandy A, Ratsioharana M, Pecarrere JL, Roig P. Treatment of chromomycosis with terbinafine: preliminary results of an open pilot study. Br J Dermatol. 1996;134(Suppl 46):33–6.
12. Queiroz-Telles F, Esterre P, Perez-Blanco M, Vitale RG, Salgado CG, Bonifaz A. Chromoblastomycosis:

an overview of clinical manifestations, diagnosis, and treatment. Med Mycol. 2009;47:3–15.

13. Marques SG, Silva Cde M, Saldanha PC, Rezende MA, Vicente VA, Queiroz-Telles F, Costa JM. Isolation of *Fonsecaea pedrosoi* from the shell of the babassu coconut (Orbignya phalerata Martius) in the Amazon region of Maranhao Brazil. Nippon Ishinkin Gakkai Zasshi. 2006;47:305–11.

14. Tsuneto LT, Arce-Gomez B, Petzl-Erler ML, Queiroz-Telles F. HLA-A29 and genetic suceptibility to cromoblastomicosis. J Med Vet Mycol. 1989;27:181–5.

15. Gomez BL, Nosanchuk JD. Melanin and fungi. Curr Opin Infect Dis. 2003;16:91–6.

16. Leeyaphan C, Hau C, Takeoka S, Tada Y, Bunyaratavej S, Pattanaprichakul P, Sitthinamsuwan P, Chaiprasert A, Sasajima Y, Makimura K, Watanabe S. Immune response in human chromoblastomycosis and eumycetoma–focusing on human interleukin-17A, interferon-gamma, tumour necrosis factor-alpha, interleukin-1 beta and human beta-defensin-2. Mycoses. 2016;59:751–6.

17. Gimenes VM, Criado PR, Martins JE, Almeida SR. Cellular immune response of patients with chromoblastomycosis undergoing antifungal therapy. Mycopathologia. 2006;162:97–101.

18. Oberto-Perdigon L, Romero H, Perez-Blanco M, Apitz-Castro R. An ELISA test for the study of the therapeutic evolution of chromoblastomycosis by *Cladophialophora carrionii* in the endemic area of falcon state, Venezuela. Rev Iberoam Micol. 2005;22:39–4.

19. Tirado-Sánchez A, González GM, Bonifaz A. Endemic mycoses: epidemiology and diagnostic strategies. Expert Rev Anti-Infect Ther. 2020;18(11):1105–17.

20. Lupi O, Tyring SK, McGinnis MR. Tropical dermatology: fungal tropical diseases. J Am Acad Dermatol. 2005;53:931–51.

21. Bandyopadhyay A, Majumdar K, Gangopadhyay M, Banerjee S. Cutaneous Chromoblastomycosis mimicking tuberculosis Verrucosa Cutis: look for copper pennies! Turk Patoloji Derg. 2015;31:223–5.

22. Minotto R, Bernardi CD, Mallmann LF, Edelweiss MI, Scroferneker ML. Chromoblastomycosis: a review of 100 cases in the state of Rio Grande do Sul, Brazil. J Am Acad Dermatol. 2001;44:585–9.

23. Uribe JF. Histopathology of chromoblastomycosis. Mycophatologia. 1989;105:1–6.

24. Batres E, Wolf JE, Rudolph AH, Knox JM. Transepithelial elimination of cutaneous chromomycosis. Arch Dermatol. 1978;114:1231–2.

25. Yaguchi T, Tanaka R, Nishimura K, Udagawa S. Molecular phylogenetics of strains morphologically identified as *Fonsecaea pedrosoi* from clinical specimens. Mycoses. 2007;50:255–60.

26. Ventura-Flores R, Failoc-Rojas V, Silva-Díaz H. Chromoblastomycosis: clinical and microbiological characteristics of a neglected disease. Rev Chilena Infectol. 2017;34:404–7.

27. Iwatsu T, Miyaji M, Taguchi H, Okamoto S. Evaluation of skin test for chromoblastomycosis using anti-gens prepared from culture filtrates of Fonsecaea pedrosoi, Phialophora verrucosa, Wangiella dermatitidis and Exophiala jeanselmei. Mycopathologia. 1982;77:59–64.

28. Garcia Marques S, Silva PE, Cde M, Aparecida Resende M, Moura Silva AA, Mendes Caldas Ade J, Lopes Costa JM. Detection of delayed hypersensitivity to Fonsecaea pedrosoi metabolic antigen (chromomycin). Nippon Ishinkin Gakkai Zasshi. 2008;49:95–101.

29. de Andrade TS, Cury AE, de Castro LG, Hirata MH, Hirata RD. Rapid identification of Fonsecaea by duplex polymerase chain reaction in isolates from patients with chromoblastomycosis. Diagn Microbiol Infect Dis. 2007;57:267–72.

30. De Hoog GS, Attili-Angelis D, Vicente VA, Van Den Ende AH, Queiroz-Telles F. Molecular ecology and pathogenic potential of *Fonsecaea* species. Med Mycol. 2004;42:405–16.

31. De Hoog GS, Nishikaku AS, Fernandez-Zeppenfeldt GD, Padín-González C, Burger E, Badali H, et al. Molecular analysis and pathogenicity of the *Cladophialophora carrionii* complex, with the description of a novel species. Stud Mycol. 2007;58:219–34.

32. Esterre P, Queiroz-Telles F. Management of chromoblastomycosis: novel perspectives. Curr Opin Infect Dis. 2006;19:148–52.

33. Restrepo A. Treatment of tropical mycoses. J Am Acad Dermatol. 1994;31(3 Pt 2):S91–102.

34. Bonifaz A, Paredes-Solís V, Saúl A. Treating chromoblastomycosis with systemic antifungals. Expert Opin Pharmacother. 2004;5:247–54.

35. Hira K, Yamada H, Takahashi Y, Ogawa H. Successful treatment of chromomycosis using carbon dioxide laser associated with topical heat applications. J Eur Acad Dermatol Venereol. 2002;16:273–5.

36. Huang TH, Lan CE. Cutaneous chromoblastomycosis effectively treated with local heat monotherapy. Clin Exp Dermatol. 2019;44:461–2.

37. Bonifaz A, Martínez-Soto E, Carrasco-Gerard E, Peniche J. Treatment of chromoblastomycosis with itraconazole, cryosurgery and combination of both. Int J Dermatol. 1997;36:542–7.

38. Yang W, Zhang W, Luo J, Chen J, Tan Y, Lei X. 5-aminolevulinic acid-based photodynamic therapy associated with Itraconazole successfully treated a case of chromoblastomycosis. Photodiagn Photodyn Ther. 2019;101589:101589.

39. Restrepo A, González A, Gomez Y, Arango M, de Bedout C. Treatment of chromoblastomycosis with itraconazole. Ann N Y Acad Sci. 1988;544:504–16.

40. Kumarasinghe SP, Kumarasinghe MP. Itraconazole pulse therapy in chromoblastomycosis. Eur J Dermatol. 2000;10:220–2.

41. Gupta AK, Taborda PR, Sanzovo AD. Alternate week and combination itraconazole and terbinafine therapy for chromoblastomycosis caused by *Fonsecaea pedrosoi* in Brazil. Med Mycol. 2002;40:529–34.

42. Bonifaz A, Saul A, Paredes-Solis V, Araiza J, Fierro-Arias L. Treatment of chromoblastomycosis with terbinafine: experience with four cases. J Dermatolog Treat. 2005;16:47–51.
43. Xibao Z, Changxing L, Quan L, Yuqing H. Treatment of chromoblastomycosis with terbinafine: a report of four cases. J Dermatolog Treat. 2005;16:121–4.
44. Yu RY, Gao L. Chromoblastomycosis successfully treatment with fluconazole. Int J Dermatol. 1994;33:716–9.
45. Negroni R, Tobon A, Bustamante B, Shikanai-Yasuda MA, Patino H, Restrepo A. Posaconazole treatment of refractory eumycetoma and chromoblastomycosis. Rev Inst Med Trop Sao Paulo. 2005;47:339–46.

Sporotrichosis

Regina Casz Schechtman, Leonardo Lora Barraza,
Felipe da Costa, Miguel Ceccarelli Calle,
and Marcelo Zuniga

Key Points

- Sporotrichosis is a subacute or chronic infection caused by the fungal genus *Sporothrix*.
- This fungus is classified into two clades. Clade IIa includes isolates from the Americas. Clade IIb isolates are restricted to South America.
- Its distribution depends on exposure, regardless of race or gender.
- The zoonotic disease became a public health concern of international proportion.
- The thermo-dimorphic ability from *Sporothrix* spp. is perhaps its most important virulence factor.
- The clinical manifestations are divided into a cutaneous (localized and benign form) and extracutaneous disease (usually disseminated).
- The hypersensitivity immune response to the fungus occurs mainly in zoonotic sporothricosis.

- The diagnostic gold standard is the isolation of the fungus *Sporothrix* spp. in mycological culture.
- Drug treatment with itraconazol demonstrates good therapeutic effects.

Introduction

Sporotrichosis is a subacute or chronic infection caused by the fungal genus *Sporothrix* (Order Ophiostomatales), occurring preferably in tropical and subtropical regions, and is considered the most frequent subcutaneous mycosis in Latin America, where it is endemic.

The Sporothrix genus comprises a group of thermo-dimorphic pathogens that is normally associated with plant organic matter or decaying matter in hot and humid climate regions. Some of the agents that belong to the Sporothrix complex can cause disease in humans and other mammals.

Historically, the first recognized species was *S. schenckii*, however lately, recent changes in the nomenclature and taxonomy of *Sporothrix* were done, leading to a better understanding of the disease. New species were described based on the phenotypic and molecular characteristics of the *Sporothrix* complex: *S. globosa*, a globally distributed fungus, *S. brasiliensis*, the species related to the zoonotic epidemic in Brazil, *S.*

R. C. Schechtman (✉) · L. L. Barraza · F. da Costa · M. C. Calle · M. Zuniga
Instituto de Dermatologia Professor Rubem David Azulay, Santa Casa de Misericordia do Rio de Janeiro, Rio de Janeiro, Brazil

Pontifical Catholic University Rio de Janeiro, Rio de Janeiro, Brazil
e-mail: fdacosta@ug.uchile.cl

W. Robles (ed.), *Skin Disease in Travelers*, Updates in Clinical Dermatology,
https://doi.org/10.1007/978-3-031-57836-6_13

mexicana, initially limited to Mexico and *S. chilensis* among others.

Epidemiology

In 1898, Benjamin Schenck isolated this agent for the first time. However, Smith identified it as "Sporotricha" [1]. Finally, Howard confirmed the dimorphic nature of this fungus in 1961 [2]. *Sporothix schenckii* sensu lato strains heterogeneity was then described in 1979 by Kwon-Chung, who identified that isolated from fixed cutaneous and lymphocutaneous clinical forms differed in growth at 37 °C and virulence in animal models also [3]. This observation was later confirmed thanks to molecular tool essays as polymerase chain reaction (PCR) of DNA topoisomerase II gene and M13 PCR fingerprinting of S. schenckii isolates [4, 5].

Using phenotypic characteristics and sequence analysis of three protein-encoding loci, Marimon et al. described six species. Three of them were clinically common species under *S. schenckii* (*S. globose, S. brasiliensis,* and *S. luriei*), the rest were classified as environmental fungi (*S. albicans, S. Mexicana,* and *S. schenckii* sensu stricto [6, 7].

Currently, it is known that Sporothrix species differ in their geographical distribution. S. shenckii sensu stricto has been isolated from Europe (the United Kingdom, France), Africa (South Africa), and Asia (China, Japan), the Americas (Argentina, Brazil, Colombia, Mexico, Peru, the United States, etc.). Sporothrix schenckii sensu stricto is also classified into two clades, wherein clade IIa represents a homogenous clade that includes isolates from South America (Bolivia, Colombia, Peru) and North American isolates. Clade IIb isolates, on the other hand, are geographically restricted to South America, particularly Peru and Argentina [8]. *S. globosa* is distributed worldwide and has been described in the United States, Latin America (Guatemala, Colombia, Mexico), Europe (Italy, Spain, the United Kingdom), and Asia (China, India, Japan) [9].

Sporothrix luriei has been described from three human infections in Africa, Europ,e and Asia and a canine infection in Brazil [33, 38, 59]. Sporothrix mexicana has been recovered from the environment in Australia, Mexico, and Portugal, reported as an occasional cause of human infections [10, 63].

Although its prevalence is unknown since it' is not a reportable disease in most countries, it has been reported in the United States, Latin America (Brazil, Colombia, Guatemala, Mexico, Peru), Asia (China, India, Japan), and Australia [11]. Since it can affect anyone, its distribution depends on exposure, regardless of race or gender. For example, in some countries such as Uruguay, it has been more prevalent among males and armadillo hunters [8]; in Japan and India, it is more prevalent in female whose occupation is farming [12, 13].

Since 1950, sporotrichosis has been well-known subcutaneous mycosis in Brazil. By the 1960s, it was recognized as the second most prevalent cause of fungal infection in endemic areas such as Para state (Brazilian north region). In 1966, 56 cases were detected in a 5-years' retrospective study [14]. Almost 15 years later, another paper was published (1973–1978) with eight cases in the Amazon state (north region of Brazil), but Sporotrichosis was still considered to be the most prevalent subcutaneous mycosis [15].

In the following two decades around 1998, the number of felines infected by *Sporothrix* sp. has raised significantly, followed by a huge increase in human cases in the poorest areas of Rio de Janeiro state, Brazil. Both prevalence were incremented exponentially with time. By 2001, Sporotrichosis was considered to be an emergent zoonosis. Researchers from Fundação Oswaldo Cruz (FIOCRUZ) reported an epidemic behavior of the mycosis. Barros et al. compared the raising numbers of cases between the 1987 and 1998 decade (only 17 cases were notified) and compared with other 66 cases in a short period of 2 years. Most of these cases presented with the lymphocutaneous form (66.7%), followed by the fixed cutaneous form (24.2%) and some disseminated forms of the disease (6%) [16, 17].

In 2008, it was reported a case-series with 255 individuals, including 94 patients and 161 healthy household contacts in Rio de Janeiro state. It was demonstrated that zoonotic sporotrichosis presented with a more polymorphic spectrum of clinical presentations with 23.4% of disseminated cutaneous forms and a unique case of the palpebral lesion and conjunctival involvement [18].

Rio de Janeiro state has remained the major focus area in the last decade, since the first reports of zoonotic sporotrichosis cases in humans 20 years ago. In 2010, a 10-year review of 804 human cases of sporotrichosis (1998–2008) was published. Over 1500 felines were diagnosed with cutaneous sporotrichosis. Most of the human cases were women aged 40–49 years, engaged in domestic duties from deprived social strata. For this reason, zoonotic sporotrichosis could be considered a neglected infectious disease with atypical clinical presentation [19, 20].

Recently, an increment was reported in Recife (Brazilian northeastern region) on infected felines. 59 domestic cats have been confirmed to be infected, leading to an outbreak of human cases [21]. In 2015, at Sao Paulo state, Marques and cols performed a 10-years' cross-sectional retrospective study (from 2003 to 2013) on sporotrichosis and 25 cases were detected [22]. In 2018, at the Brazilian Dermatology Association Meeting, eight posters and two oral communications were presented on sporotrichosis, all of them connected to the zoonotic contact and presenting with atypical clinical features (hypersensitivity reactions, disseminated forms with high mortality), due to *Sporothrix brasiliensis*. It's important to stress out that the majority of the human cases reported were from different regions of the Brazilian territory (Southeast: Minas Gerais, Espírito Santo and São Paulo; South: Santa Catarina, Rio Grande do Sul; Central region: Brasilia, Northeast: Pernambuco). We then realize that there is an increase in human zoonotic sporotrichosis cases in Brazil [23].

Small sporotrichosis outbreaks have been reported worldwide [24]. In some latitudes due to occupational accidents or life style, for example, in South Africa it as reported more than 3000 gold mine workers contaminated by *S. schenckii* sensu lato, which probable origin were pit props used to maintain roofs of the mines [25]. This tendency has been pointed in other studies where male patients outnumber females at a rate of 3:1 for the same reasons [26]. In Latin American countries such as Guatemala, anglers got infected as a result of injuries involving contaminated fish [27], on the other hand, in Peru, it was observed that children have three times higher incidence compared with adults, due to activities such as playing in crop fields and dirty floors in house [28, 29]. In the United States, Florida reported nine cases among 65 employees of a garden center (incidence rate of 14%), acquired by traumatic contact with sphagnum moss for a period of 20 h/week [30]. In Wisconsin and other 14 states, an important number of forest workers involved in packaging pine seedlings in sphagnum moss were also infected in the same period, this data was tracked by two nurseries in Pennsylvania [31].

In Asia, China reported a unique outbreak in 15 infants, whose absence of traumatic or contact with any animal led to the hypothesis that contaminated cornstalks stacked by families for cooking and heating during winter season were the contamination source [32]. On the other hand, this mycosis is rare in Europe, after the First World War [33]. Sporadic cases have been observed in travelers, archaeologists, aid workers and immigrants [34]. Around Mediterranean region (particularly in southern Italy), sporothrix schenckii var. lurei and sensu lato had been reported last decades in humans and from commercial garden soils [35, 36]. A case of sporotrichosis of the feet due to *S. mexicana* was diagnosed in Portugal in 2009, presumably acquired while traveling abroad in Malaysia [37], and recently, the first autochthonous case from Portugal was reported, caused by *S. globosa* [38, 63].

Sporotrichosis is rarely seen on the British Isles and almost inexistent in the rest of European continent; few cases were recorded prior to 1911 and 16 cases from 1911 to 1968 [39, 63]. Before the Great War, France had a considerable number of cases, experimenting a declined tendency afterward [40]. Recently, an autochthonous case in a man was reported due to occupational contact with soil [41]. Finally, two cases of Mediterranean sporotrichosis have been reported in Cataluña province [42, 24].

Transmission

There are two ways to acquire the cutaneous disease, both by traumatic inoculation of the propagules through the skin. The classic clinical presentation known as "the Rose Gardener's disease" is transmitted by plant debris and the atypical "zoonotic disease" is caused by animal transmission. The zoonotic disease had acquired capital importance because of its treacherous outbreak, leading to a public health concern of international proportion. The small outbreaks from classic saprophytic route, in which the species *S. schenckii* and *S. globosa* prevail are under control. On the other hand, the number of outbreaks caused by horizontal-animal transmission (cat-cat and then, cat-human) is still increasing (Table 1).

Table 1 Difference between the classical and the zoonotic transmission of sporotrichosis

Sporotrichosis Different aspects	Classical "Rose Gardener Disease"	Atypical zoonotic disease
Sporothrix species	*S. schenkii, S. globosa*	*S. brasiliensis*
Vectors	Soil or organic matter	Cat-cat, cat-humans
Typical manifestation	Small ulcers in the extremities with lymphangitis	Not distinctive, more aggressive behavior, hypersensitivity phenomenon
Progression	Typical sporotrichoid	Nonspecific pattern
Systemic involvement	Rare	Not rare
Treatment	Itraconazole, Terbinafine, Amphotericine	Itraconazole, Terbinafine, Amphotericine (longer courses, higher dosage, multidrug therapy could be necessary)
Prognosis	Good	Variable according to host–parasite interactions

Physiopathology

The thermo-dimorphic ability from *Sporothrix* spp. is perhaps the most important virulence factor of the fungus. It presents a filamentous form at environmental temperature and develops a yeast-like form inside the mammal host or in vitro at 35–37 °C, which is remarkably very close to the physiologic temperature of the individuals. Thus, it may be an evolutionary adaptation of the fungus in order to survive.

The thermic conversion occurs efficiently among the species that cause the disease, particularly with *S. brasiliensis* and *S. globosa*. Otherwise, the environmental and saprophytic species (i.e., *S. inflata* and *S. mexicana*) demonstrate no ability of transformation from filamentous into yeast-like cells.

Another virulence factor is the presence of melanin. It could represent a protection mechanism from the host's natural defenses as well as inducing resistance to antifungal drugs such as amphotericin, itraconazole, and terbinafine.

Finally, the relationship between the pathogen properties and the host immune system is essential. It has been established that cell-mediated immune response is responsible for eliminating or controlling the infection. There is an antibody production against the Sporothrix's cell wall that is clinically evident in cellular immunosuppressed patients, like the HIV infected group. The immunosuppressed host presents with a disseminated and severe form of the disease.

Clinical Presentation

Classically, the clinical manifestations were divided into a cutaneous (localized and benign form) and extracutaneous disease (usually disseminated). More recently and considering the new pathogenic species, described in the last decade, and its clinical manifestations, Orofino-Costa et col. have proposed a new classification which also includes the hypersensitivity immune response to the fungus, more frequently seen when there is a zoonotic transmission of the disease, mainly erythema multiforme, erythema

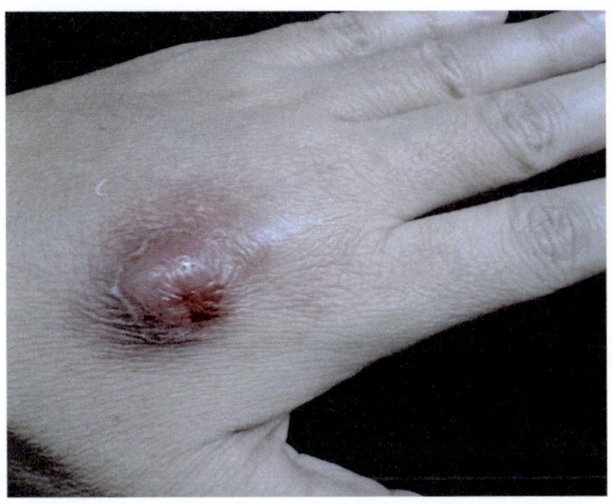

Fig. 1 Lymphocutaneous Form—Inoculation site: erythematous papule or nodule above the traumatic site of infection. It may ulcerate and drain a purulent discharge

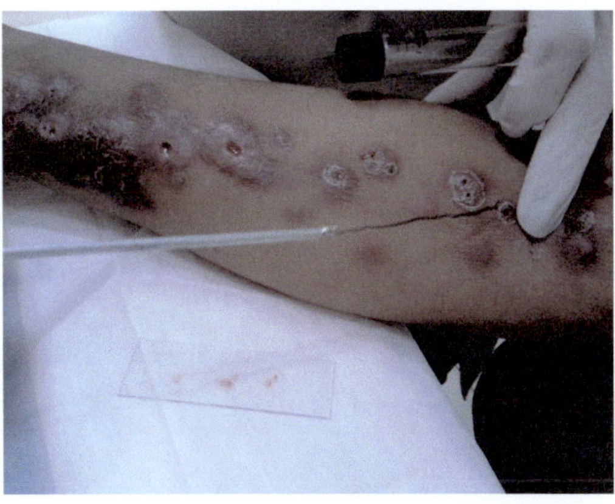

Fig. 2 The cutaneous-lymphatic presentation with "sporotrichoid pattern". Nodules present along the lymphatic flow. Those nodules may ulcerate and fistulize establishing a gumma

nodosum, and sweet syndrome [43, 44, 45] (Table 1).

The lymphocutaneous form is by far the most common presentation, described in 80% of patients. Initially, the lesion develops as an erythematous papule or nodule above the traumatic site of infection, the inoculation site. It may ulcerate and drain a purulent discharge (Fig. 1). By the next few weeks, the disease progresses and new nodules will develop along the lymphatic flow. Those nodules may ulcerate and fistulize establishing a *gumma*. The cutaneous-lymphatic presentation with "sporotrichoid pattern" is commonly associated with the infection caused by the *S. schenckii* and *S. globosa* species (Fig. 2).

In endemic areas, the sporotrichoid pattern can be misdiagnosed as leishmaniasis. In 1944, Azulay R and Cols. classified leishmaniasis and sporotrichosis, as "the large ulcer with little lymphangitis" and "the little ulcer with large lymphangitis," respectively [46]. Nowadays, this clinical presentation is no longer typical because of the diversity of new clinical presentations related to the emergent species of *Sporothrix* sp.

The second most common manifestation is the fixed cutaneous form. The individual develop an

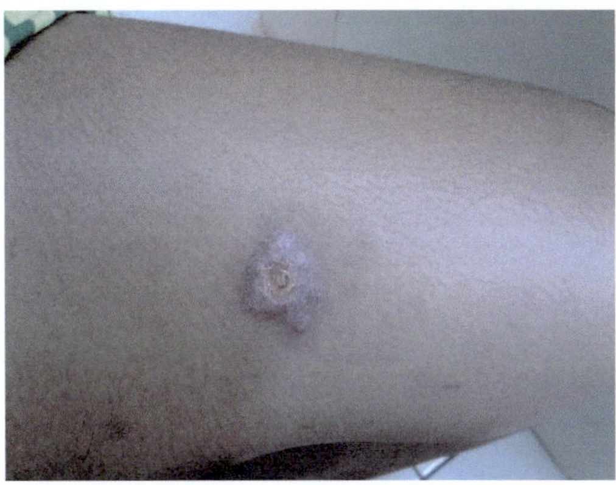

Fig. 3 Fixed cutaneous form. An isolated cutaneous lesion without lymphatic progression. It may present with ulceration, vegetation, or can acquire a verrucous or erythematous scaly surface

isolated cutaneous lesion without lymphatic progression. It may present with ulceration, vegetation, or can acquire a verrucous or erythematous scaly surface (Fig. 3). Multiple cutaneous lesions can occur without systemic involvement, and it is probably secondary to multiple inoculations sites.

The disease can also affect mucous membranes, especially the eyes, causing conjunctivi-

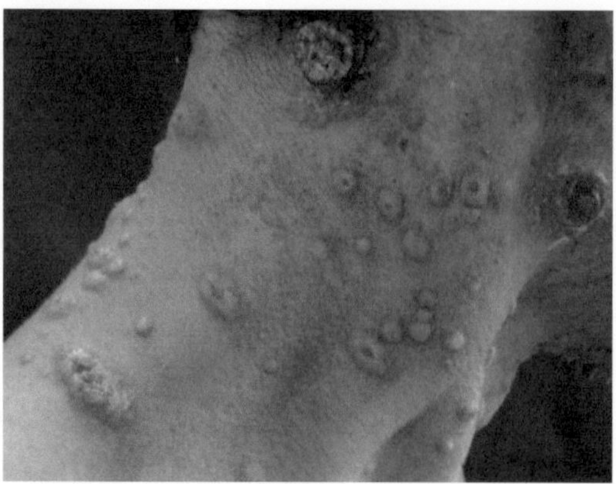

Fig. 4 Disseminated cutaneous sporothricosis (in an alcoholic and immunossupressed patient)

Systemic sporotrichosis is rare and affects mainly bones and joints. Mucous membrane compromise is possible, it is a serious infection, involves internal organs, and there may be fungemia. Extra cutaneous disseminated sporotrichosis affects a variety of organs, mainly lungs and central nervous system. Pulmonary involvement causes two types of presentations, a chronic and asymptomatic presentation similar to tuberculosis, and an acute presentation with massive adenopathy, abundant expectoration, dyspnea, and fatigue [62]. Central nervous system involvement can manifest as meningoencephalitis and hydrocephalus. Other affected organs include sinuses, liver, kidney, eyes, genitalia, and heart [50, 55].

tis, episcleritis, uveitis, choroiditis, and retrobulbar lesions, among others. Sporotrichosis is a frequent infectious cause of Parinaud syndrome. It is characterized by the concomitant compromise of the ocular mucosa and local lymphadenopathy.

Cutaneous disseminated sporotrichosis, also called hematogenous sporotrichosis [47], is uncommon and found in approximately 1–4% of cases. The disseminated cutaneous form is characterized by three or more lesions in at least two anatomical areas. After inoculation into the skin, hematogenous spread occurs. Typical disseminated disease (Fig. 4) occurs in immunocompromised patients, especially in HIV seropositive [48], as well as in other conditions, such as alcoholism [49], hepatitis C, haematological malignancies (leukemia and lymphomas), pregnancy, organ transplant, malnutrition, and corticosteroid treatment [50, 51]. In immunocompromised patients, the cutaneous disseminated form is usually associated with infections due to S. brasiliensis in Rio de Janeiro, Brazil [52, 53].

Differential diagnosis especially includes pyoderma gangrenosum [60], and other diseases such as Sweet's syndrome, mycobacteriosis, sarcoidosis [61], and cutaneous leishmaniasis [54].

Diagnosis

The diagnosis is based on clinical suspicion and confirmed by laboratory tests. The gold standard is the isolation of the fungus *Sporothrix* spp. in mycological culture from the infected tissue collected directly from the affected skin, deep biopsies, blood, sputum, or cerebrospinal fluid.

It is possible, but less frequent, to search for the presence of the fungus under KOH 10% preparation, directly from the patient's specimen. The classical aspect is a yeast-like structure, oval or elongated, known as "cigar-shaped bodies." On the other hand, in culture at 26° (the filamentous form), it presents a hyaline, delicate, and branched septate hyphae and conidiophores produced at the tip of the conidia, arranged as a daisy-flower or "flowery patterns." The histopathologic examination under Giemsa stain can also confirms the diagnosis.

Recently, there are promising new diagnostic techniques, such as PCR, that proved to be simple, high throughput, sensitive, and accurate for diagnosing sporotrichosis. ELISA test detecting characterized antigen's specific antibody has been efficient, such as *Sporothrix schenckii* Con

A-Binding Fraction (SsCBF), a cell wall antigen from *S. schenckii* yeast phase. Tests performed in serum samples from both human patients and felines with diverse clinical sporotrichosis forms. There is an effective clinical–serological correlation which allows therapeutic monitoring, helping to discern between therapy suspension or not [56].

Recently, an exoantigen isolated from *S. schenckii* filamentous form was used in the ELISA test, with sensitivity 97% and 89% specificity reported when evaluating different patient's serum samples. Another *Sporothrix spp* cell wall antigens have been studied as new biomarkers for diagnosis of infection, the 60 kDa and 70 kDa glycoproteins, identified as 3-carboxy-muconate cyclase of the *Sporothrix* proteome, as glycoforms and isoforms. Such glycoproteins seem to behave as a virulence factor expressed in the most virulent strains, contributing to fungus adherence and immunomodulation. mAb P6E7 produced antibodies against gp70 caused in vivo protection through passive immunization of mice infected with *S. schenckii*. Therefore, this component is considered to be a strong candidate for sporotrichosis therapeutic vaccine. Even though these tests are not commercially available, they can be found in certain research centers where sporotrichosis is endemic, such as Brazil [56].

Treatment

Endemic sporotrichosis has been a therapeutic challenge in Brazil. Drug treatments such as azoles, among this group Itraconazole, had shown good therapeutic effects and benefits such as its posology and less side effects than other options such as saturated potassium iodide solution or terbinafine [57, 58] (Ferreira, CP. et al. 2012; De Santis M, 2009).

Physiological characteristics, disadvantages, and other fits about these medications are displayed on Table 2.

Table 2 Pharmacological features and specific considerations about the main antifungal treatments for sporotrichosis treatment

Treatment	Posology	Management	Benefits	Disadvantages
Itraconazole	100 mg per day Or 200 mg per day for consensus	One pill after lunch or dinner. *If there's no improvement after 2 months: Two pills a day or consider changing medication	Fewer side effects. Posology	Pharmacological interactions (Statins) Financial cost
Terbinafine	250 mg per day	One pill per day *If there's no improvement after two months: Two pills a day or consider changing medication	Posology	Financial cost
Saturated potassium iodide solution 100 ml KI+ 70 ml H$_2$O	40 to 50 drops, three times a day. Or 20 to 25 drops twice a day	Starting with five drops per take, increasing one drop per day until reaching target dose	Financial cost	Gastrointestinal tract alteration, coryza, skin rash, metallic taste and thyroid dysfunction

References

1. Schenck BR. On refractory subcutaneous abscess caused by a fungus possibly related to the Sporotricha. Bull Johns Hopkins Hosp. 1898;9:286–90.
2. Howard DH. Dimorphism of Sporotrichum schenckii. J Bacteriol. 1961;81:464–9.
3. Kwon-Chung KJ. Comparison of isolates of Sporothrix schenckii obtained from fixed cutaneous lesions with isolates from other types of lesions. J Infect Dis. 1979;139:424–31.
4. Kanbe T, Natsume L, Goto I, et al. Rapid and specific identification of Sporothrix schenckii by PCR targeting the DNA topoisomerase II gene. J Dermatol Sci. 2005;38:99–106.
5. Galhardo MC, DeOliveira RM, Valle AC, et al. Molecular epidemiology and antifungal susceptibility patterns of Sporothrix schenckii isolates from a cat-transmitted epidemic of sporotrichosis in Rio de Janeiro, Brazil. MedMycol. 2008;46:141–51.
6. Marimon R, Gene J, Cano J, et al. Molecular phylogeny of Sporothrix schenckii. J Clin Microbiol. 2006;44:3251–6.
7. Marimon R, Gene J, Cano J, Guarro J. Sporothrix luriei: a rare fungus from clinical origin. Med Mycol. 2008;46:621–5.
8. Rodrigues AM, Bagagli E, de Camargo ZP, de Moraes Gimenes Bosco S. Sporothrix schenckii sensu stricto isolated from soil in an armadillo's burrow. Mycopathologia. 2014;177:199–206.
9. Yu X, Wan Z, Zhang Z, Li F, Li R, Liu X. Phenotypic and molecular identification of Sporothrix isolates of clinical origin in Northeast China. Mycopathologia. 2013;176:67–74.
10. Rodrigues AM, de Melo Teixeira M, de Hoog GS, et al. Phylogenetic analysis reveals a high prevalence of Sporothrix brasiliensis in feline sporotrichosis outbreaks. PLoS Negl Trop Dis. 2013;7: e2281.
11. Barros, MB. de Almeida Paes R, Schubach AO. Sporothrix schenckii and sporotrichosis. Clin Microbiol Rev 2011; 24: 633–654.
12. Fukushiro R. Epidemiology and ecology of sporotrichosis in Japan. Zentralbl Bakteriol Mikrobiol Hyg A. 1984;257:228–33.
13. Bhutia PY, Gurung S, Yegneswaran PP, et al. A case series and review of sporotrichosis in Sikkim. J Infect Dev Ctries. 2011;5:603–8.
14. Domingos-Silva, J. Casos de esporotricose no Para An Bras Dermatol, vol. 41, n 4. 1966.
15. Talhari S, Gadelha AR, Cunha MGS. Micoses profundas, Estudo dos casos diagnosticados em Manaus estado do Amazonas, de 1973-1978. An Bras Dermatol. 1980;55:3.
16. Lopes JO, Alves SH, Mari CR, et al. Epidemiology of sporotrichosis in the central region of Rio Grande do Sul. Rev Soc Bras Med Trop. 1999;32(5):541–5., set-out.
17. Freitas DF, Valle AC, Almeida-Paes R, Bastos F, Galhardo MC. Zoonotic Sporotrichosis in Rio de Janeiro, Brazil: A protracted epidemic yet to be curbed. Clin Infect Dis. 2010;50:452–3.
18. Barros MB, Pacheco-Schubach T, Gutierrez-Galhardo M, Oliveira-Schubach A, Fialho-Monteiro P, Santos-Reis R, Zancopé-Oliveira R, Santos-Lazéra M, Cuzzi-Maya T, Moita-Blanco T, Feldman-Marzochi K, Wanke B. Sporotrichosis: an emergent zoonosis in Rio de Janeiro. Mem Inst Oswaldo Cruz, Rio de Janeiro. 2001;96(6):777–9.
19. Barros MB, Schubach AO, Schubach TMP, Wanke B, Lambert-Passos SR. An epidemic of sporotrichosis in Rio de Janeiro, Brazil: epidemiological aspects of a series of cases. Epidemiol Infect. 2008;136:1192–6.
20. Schubach A, Schubach TM, Barros MB, Wanke B. Cat-transmitted sporotrichosis, Rio de Janeiro, Brazil. Emerging infectious diseases. 2005;11(12):1952–4. https://doi.org/10.3201/eid1112.040891.
21. Silva GM, Howes JC, Adria C. Surto de esporotricose felina na região metropolitana do Recife Pesq. Vet Bras. 2014;38(9):1767–71.
22. Marques GF, Martins AL, Sousa JM, Brandão LS, Wachholz PA, Masuda PY. Characterization of sporotrichosis cases treated in a dermatologic teaching unit in the State of São Paulo—Brazil, 2003–2013. An Bras Dermatol. 2015;90(2):273–5.
23. Brazilian Dermatology Society (SBD). Anais do 73° congresso Brasileiro de dermatologia. Listagem de trabalhos (e-pôster e Comunicações orais). 2018. Curitiba, PN.
24. Chakrabarti A, Bonifaz A, Gutierrez-Galhardo MC, Mochizuki T, Li S. Global epidemiology of sporotrichosis. Med Mycol. 2015 Jan;53(1):3–14.
25. Helm MAF, Berman C. The clinical, therapeutic and epidemiological features of the sporotrichosis infection on the mines. In: Sporotrichosis infection on mines of the Witwatersrand. Proceedings of the Transvaal Mine Medical Officers' Association, Dec 1944. Johannesburg, South Africa: The Transvaal Chamber of Mines; 1947. p. 59–67.
26. Vismer HF, Hull PR. Prevalence, epidemiology and geographical distribution of Sporothrix schenckii infections in Gauteng, South Africa. Mycopathologia. 1997;137:137–43.
27. Mayorga R, Caceres A, Toriello C et al. An endemic area of sporotrichosis in Guatemala. Sabouraudia 1978; 16: 185–198 [in Spanish].
28. Neyra E, Fonteyne PA, Swinne D, et al. Epidemiology of human sporotrichosis investigated by amplified fragment length polymorphism. J Clin Microbiol. 2005;43:1348–52.
29. Lyon GM, Zurita S, Casquero J, et al. Population-based surveillance and a case-control study of risk

factors for endemic lymphocutaneous sporotrichosis in Peru. Clin Infect Dis. 2003;36:34–9.

30. Hajjeh R, McDonnell S, Reef S, et al. Outbreak of sporotrichosis among tree nursery workers. J Infect Dis. 1997;176:499–504.

31. Grotte M, Younger B. Sporotrichosis associated with sphagnum moss exposure. Arch Pathol Lab Med. 1981;105:50–1.

32. Song Y, Yao L, Zhong SX, et al. Infant sporotrichosis in Northeast China: a report of 15 cases. Int J Dermatol. 2011;50:522–9.

33. Alberici F, Paties CT, Lombardi G, et al. Sporothrix schenckii var luriei as the cause of sporotrichosis in Italy. Eur J Epidemiol. 1989;5:173–7.

34. Bonifaz A, Vázquez-González D. Sporotrichosis: an update. G Ital Dermatol Venereol. 2010 Oct;145(5):659–73.

35. Cafarchia C, Sasanelli M, Lia RP, et al. Lymphocutaneous and nasal sporotrichosis in a dog from southern Italy: case report. Mycopathologia. 2007;163(75–79):119.

36. Criseo G, Romeo O. Ribosomal DNA sequencing and phylogenetic analysis of environmental Sporothrix schenckii strains: comparison with clinical isolates. Mycopathologia. 2010;169:351–8.

37. Dias NM, Oliveira MM, Santos C, Zancope-Oliveira RM, Lima N. Sporotrichosis caused by Sporothrix mexicana. Portugal Emerg Infect Dis. 2011;17:1975–6.

38. Oliveira DC, Lopes PG, Spader TB, et al. Antifungal susceptibilities of Sporothrix albicans, S. brasiliensis, and S. luriei of the S. schenckii complex identified in Brazil. J Clin Microbiol. 2011;49: 3047–9.

39. Symmers WS. Sporotrichosis in Ireland. Ulster Med J. 1968;37:85–101.

40. Mariat F. Ecology of Sporothrix schenckii and of Ceratocystis stenoceras in Corsica and Alsace. French provinces free of sporotrichosis Sabouraudia. 1975;13:217–25. [in French]

41. Magand F, Perrot JL, Cambazard F, Raberin MH, Labeille B. Autochthonous cutaneous sporotrichosis in France. Ann Dermatol Venereol. 2009;136:273–5. [in French]

42. Ventin M, Ramirez C, Ribera M, et al. A significant geographical area for the study of the epidemiological and ecological aspect of Mediterranean sporothricosis. Mycopathologia. 1987;99:41–3.

43. Gutierrez-Galhardo MC, Barros MBL, Schubach A, Cuzzi T, Schubach TMP, Lazéra MS, Francesconi-Do-Valle ACF. Erythema multiforme associated with sporotrichosis. J eur acad dermatol venereolol. 2005;19:507–9.

44. Gutierrez-Galhardo MC, De Oliveira Schubach A, De Lima Barros M, Blanco TC, Cuzzi-Maya T, Schubach TM, Dos Santos Lazéra M, Francesconi do Valle AC. Erythema nodosum associated with sporotrichosis. Int J Dermatol. 2002;41:114–6.

45. Freitas DF, Valle AC, Cuzzi T, Brandão LG, Zancopé-Oliveira RM, Galhardo MC. Sweet syndrome associated with sporotrichosis. Br J Dermatol. 2012;166(1):212–3.

46. Azulay RD, Azulay DR, Azulay-Abulafia, L. Dermatologia. 6th ed. Chapter 45. P. 512. Guanabara-Koogan Ed. Rio de Janeiro. 2015.

47. Mahajan VK. Sporotrichosis: an overview and therapeutic options. Dermatol Res Pract. 2014;2014:272376. https://doi.org/10.1155/2014/272376.

48. Moreira JAS, Freitas DFS, Lamas. The impact of sporotrichosis in HIV-infected patients: a systematic review. Infection. 2015;43:267.

49. Benvegnú AM, Stramari J, Dallazem LND, Chemello RML, Beber AAC. Disseminated cutaneous sporotrichosis in patient with alcoholism. Rev Soc Bras Med Trop. 017;50(6):871–873. https://doi.org/10.1590/0037-8682-0281-2017

50. Espinoza-Hernández CJ, Jesús-Silva A, Toussaint-Caire S, Arenas R. Disseminated sporotrichosis with cutaneous and testicular involvement. Actas Dermosifiliogr. 2014;105(2):204–6.

51. Bonifaz A, Tirado-Sánchez A. Cutaneous disseminated and extracutaneous sporotrichosis: current status of a complex disease. J Fungi (Basel). 2017;3(1):6. https://doi.org/10.3390/jof3010006.

52. Almeida-Paes R, de Oliveira MM, Freitas DF, do Valle AC, Zancopé-Oliveira RM, Gutierrez-Galhardo MC. Sporotrichosis in Rio de Janeiro, Brazil: Sporothrix brasiliensis is associated with atypical clinical presentations. PLoS Negl Trop Dis. 2014;8(9):e3094. Published 2014 Sep 18. https://doi.org/10.1371/journal.pntd.0003094

53. Gutierrez-Galhardo MC, Do Valle AC, Fraga BL, Schubach AO, De Siqueira Hoagland BR, Monteiro PC, De Lima Barros MB. Disseminated sporotrichosis as a manifestation of immune reconstitution inflammatory syndrome. Mycoses. 2010;53:78–80.

54. Saeed L, Weber RJ, Puryear SB, et al. Disseminated cutaneous and osteoarticular sporotrichosis mimicking pyoderma gangrenosum. Open Forum Infect Dis. 2019;6(10):ofz395. Published 2019 Sep 9. https://doi.org/10.1093/ofid/ofz395

55. Bonifaz A, Tirado-Sanchez A, Paredes-Solis V, et al. Cutaneous disseminated sporotrichosis: clinical experience of 24 cases. J Eur Acad Dermatol Venereol. 2018;32:e77–9.

56. Orofino-Costa R, de Macedo PM, Rodrigues AM, Bernardes-Engemann AR. Sporotrichosis: an update on epidemiology, etiopathogenesis, laboratory and clinical therapeutics. An Bras Dermatol. 2017;92(5):606–20.

57. De Santis M, Di Gianantonio E, Cesari E, Ambrosini G, Straface G, Clementi M. First trimester itraconazole exposure and pregnancy outcome: a prospective cohort study of women contacting teratology information services in Italy. Drug Saf. 2009;32(3):239–44.

58. Ferreira CP, do Valle ACF, Freitas DFS, Reis R, Galhardo MCG. Pregnancy during a sporotrichosis epidemic in Rio de Janeiro, Brazil. Int J Gynecol Obstet. 2012;117(3):294–5.

59. Ajello L, Kaplan W. A new variant of Sporothrix schenckii. Mykosen. 1969;12:633–44.
60. Byrd DR, El-Azhary RA, Gibson LE, Roberts GD. Sporotrichosis masquerading as pyoderma gangrenosum: case report and review of 19 cases of sporotrichosis. J Eur Acad Dermatol Venereol. 2001;15:581–4.
61. Yang DJ, Krishnan RS, Guillen DR, Schmiege LM, Leis PF, Hsu S. Disseminated sporotrichosis mimicking sarcoidosis. Int J Dermatol. 2006;45:450–3.
62. Padhye AA, Kaufman L, Durry E, et al. Fatal pulmonary sporotrichosis caused by Sporothrix schenckii var. luriei in India. J Clin Microbiol. 1992;30:2492–4.
63. De Oliveira MM, Verissimo C, Sabino R, et al. First autochthone case of sporotrichosis by Sporothrix globosa in Portugal. Diagn Microbiol Infect Dis. 2014;78:388–90.

Part V

Dermatoses Caused by Infection: Fungal Infections–Deep Mycoses

Blastomycosis

Mahreen Ameen

Key Points

- Blastomycosis is a chronic suppurative granulomatous fungal infection.
- It is an endemic mycosis that is most prevalent in the North American continent.
- It is acquired by inhalation leading to asymptomatic or respiratory infection.
- Extrapulmonary infection is more likely in the immunocompromised and most commonly affects the skin but can also affected the central nervous system (CNS).
- Itraconazole is the drug of choice for the treatment of non-CNS infection that is not life-threatening and 6–12 months of treatment is normally required.

Blastomycosis is a rare endemic mycosis that can lead to a systemic, granulomatous fungal infection. The aetiolgical agents are *Blastomyces dermatitidis* and *Blastomyces gilchristii*, which belong to a group of dimorphic fungi that can affect both immunocompetent, as well as immunocompromised individuals. Blastomycosis is primarily a pulmonary infection, and the skin is the most common extra-pulmonary organ involved.

M. Ameen (✉)
Royal Free Hospital NHS Foundation Trust, London, UK

Mycology

Blastomyces spp. are thermally dimorphic fungi that undergo a reversible morphological change between hyphae at 22—25 °C and yeast at 37 °C. Therefore, they grow as a filamentous mold in the environment and as a yeast in human tissues. At 25 °C, the mycelial form grows as a fluffy white mold while at 37 °C it grows as a brown folded yeast. In the environment, it reproduces asexually with small conidia that are 2–10 μm in diameter. In infected cells, Blastomycosis dermatitidis is seen as budding yeast cells that are relatively large at 8–10 μm in diameter.

The yeast have a unique form amongst the dimorphic fungi and are characterized by a broad-based bud and doubly refractile cell walls. The mycelial form is characterized by septate hyphae that produce asexual spores. The morphology of the mycelial form is not distinct from other fungi and therefore requires transition to the yeast or molecular confirmation for identification [1–3].

Epidemiology and Pathogenesis

This is an endemic mycosis that is most prevalent in the North American continent, particularly in the states that border Mississippi and

Ohio rivers, near the Great Lakes region and southeastern parts of the United States. It is also endemic in four Canadian provinces from Quebec to Saskatchewan [4–6]. In endemic regions, blastomycosis is not uniformly distributed. *Blastomyces* generally reside in forested areas with decaying vegetation and rotting wood located near water sources. *Blastomyces* can also grow in bird guano. Epidemics within endemic regions have been reported relating to occupational or recreational activities in wooded areas along waterways that disrupt soil. Rarely autochthonous cases of culture-proven blastomycosis have been reported outside of North America in Africa and India and hence the term 'North American blastomycosis' is now obsolete [7]. The incidence of blastomycosis is probably higher than the number of reported cases as those infected can be asymptomatic or have subclinical infection.

Blastomycoisis affects all ages and ethnicities. However, it is more common in males probably because of occupational and recreational exposures. It also has a higher incidence in certain ethnic groups such as the Hmong populations in Wisconsin [8].

Knowledge of the geographic distribution and epidemiological risks is important for including blastomycosis in the differential diagnosis in patients with pulmonary infections.

When human activity disrupts soil, *Blastomyces* conidia become aerosolized. They can then be inhaled by human hosts and pass into the lower respiratory tract. The conidia may be phagocytized and killed by alveolar macrophages and neutrophils resulting in asymptomatic infection. However, conidia may also evade host immune responses surviving phagocytosis and germinate to yeast [9]. *Blastomyces* yeast have thick walls which make them more resistant to host defences and pathogenic to lung tissue resulting in symptomatic pulmonary disease. After infection has resolved, human hosts develop cell-mediated immunity, which can last for 2 years or longer [10].

Clinical Manifestations

Blastomycosis is associated with a spectrum of disease ranging from asymptomatic infection to an acute or chronic pneumonia. Onset of symptoms can occur from 3 weeks to 3 months after inhalation of mycelial fragments or spores.

Asymptomatic infection is believed to occur in 50% of infected individuals. If symptomatic, initial symptoms of blastomycosis in immunocompetent individuals are flu-like and usually resolve within a few days. Often symptoms may be so mild that infection can go undiagnosed. Pneumonia can be acute or chronic. Acute pulmonary blastomycosis may be mild and can be mistaken for other lower respiratory tract infections including bacterial acquired pneumonia. Undiagnosed or untreated acute pulmonary blastomycosis can progress to chronic pneumonia and symptoms may include fever, night sweats, chronic cough, hemoptysis, malaise, and weight loss. Because of the non-specific clinical features of chronic blastomycosis, delayed diagnosis is common unless blastomycosis is considered in the differential diagnosis when patients present with skin lesions as well or fail to respond to antibacterial therapy [3, 11].

Some patients may develop rapidly progressive infection presenting with acute respiratory distress syndrome (ARDS). This is associated with a high mortality, sometimes greater than 50%, which usually occurs when the diagnosis of blastomycosis-induced ARDS is delayed. ARDS occurs more commonly in immunocompromised individuals or the elderly [12–14].

Extrapulmonary disease can occur in 25–40% of patients after hematogenous dissemination from the lungs. *Blastomyces* can disseminate to any organ of the body. The skin is the most common site of extrapulmonary disease. Primary cutaneous blastomycosis is rare. It can occur due to direct inoculation after trauma to the skin [15]. Cutaneous lesions begin as papulopustular lesions, which then evolve into vegetative and verrucous plaques. This can progress with central clearing or ulceration and result in scarring. Violaceous nodules and plaques have also been described. Cutaneous lesions may be associated with local lymphangitis or lymphadenopathy. Cutaneous blastomycosis can rarely present with draining sinus tracts or ulcers from underlying osteomyelitis. Skin lesions can occur on any body site but are more commonly located on exposed body areas such as the head and limbs. Erythema nodosum, although associated with other endemic mycoses, is uncommon in association with *Blastomyces* infection [3, 16–18].

After skin, dissemination to the bone occurs in 25% of extrapulmonary cases. Bony lesions usually affect the lower spine and pelvis and are typically lytic. Bony lesions can be painful and can be associated with cutaneous ulcers, abscesses, or draining sinus tracts. Contiguous extension can result in septic arthritis. Bony lesions can mimic malignancy, and progressive bony destruction can result in pathologic fractures [3, 19].

The central nervous systemic (CNS) is affected in 5–10% of immunocompetent infected individuals, and infection can result in intracranial or epidural abscess or meningitis. Extrapulmonary infection can also affect the genitourinary system resulting in orchitis, epididymitis, and prostatitis [20, 21].

Disseminated infection occurs more commonly in the immunocompromised such as organ transplant recipients, those with HIV infection, malignancy and those receiving treatment with tumor necrosis factor-alpha inhibitors. The immunocompromised are at high risk of CNS involvement and severe pulmonary disease such as ARDS [22–27].

Unlike other opportunistic infections, such as cryptococcosis and histoplasmosis, blastomycosis is an uncommon opportunistic infection with HIV immunosuppression. It usually occurs with CD4+ T-lymphocyte counts <200 cells/mm^3. CNS involvement occurs in 40% of HIV co-infected cases. Reactivation of latent blastomycosis infection is common in HIV infected individuals. Mortality is high with advanced HIV immunosuppression [28].

Investigations

Investigations usually include chest radiography although there are no radiographic features that are specific and diagnostic for blastomycosis. Radiographic features may include nodules, masses, interstitial disease, consolidation, and cavitation and may mimic bacterial pneumonia, tuberculosis, or malignancy. If CNS involvement is suspected, lumbar puncture and cerebrospinal analysis is performed. Definitive diagnosis is established by direct visualization of the characteristic thick-walled, broad-based budding yeasts by direct examination of tissue, or the isolation of *Blastomyces* in culture. Specimens for direct microscopy in 10% KOH can be skin scrapings, pus from skin lesions, sputum, bronchoalveolar lavage, gastric washings, or biopsy tissue from any lesion. Gomori methenamine silver (GMS) or periodic acid-Schiff (PAS) stains can help visualize characteristic *Blastomyces* yeast. In contrast, they are not well visualized with either Gram stain or haematoxylin and eosin stain [29]. Organisms can be difficult to identify in skin biopsies as they are often within histiocytes. Histopathology of infected tissues reveals a pyogranulomatous response without caseation and pseudoepitheliomatous hyperplasia. The most sensitive method for diagnosing blastomycosis is culture, which typically takes 5–10 days but can take up to 30 days depending on the density of organisms in the specimen. Bony involvement can be assessed by radionuclide bone scans, computed tomography scans, or magnetic resonance imaging. Serology to exclude HIV co-infection is recommended [30, 31].

Treatment

Although acute blastomycosis in the immunocompetent host may be mild and self-limiting, all diagnosed cases are treated in order to prevent extrapulmonary dissemination and the risk of any future reactivation. The choice of treatment is generally guided by the extent of infection, CNS involvement, the host immune status, and pregnancy.

Itraconazole is the drug of choice for mild to moderate pulmonary or non-CNS disseminated infection that is not life threatening. The recommended dose is an initial loading dose of 200 mg three times a day for 3 days followed by 200 mg once or twice daily for 6–12 months. It is recommended that serum itraconazole levels is measured 2 weeks after commencement of treatment in order to ensure adequate drug exposure. Ketoconazole (400–800 mg daily) and fluconazole (400–800 mg daily) are second-line agents as they have lower efficacy against *Blastomyces*. Furthermore, long-term treatment with ketoconazole may be associated with adverse effects. The new generation of azoles, voriconazole, posaconazole, and isavuconazole have demonstrated activity against *B. dermatitidis* [30, 32, 33].

Voriconazole has been successfully used in the treatment of CNS blastomycosis as high voriconazole concentrations can be achieved in the CSF and brain tissue. Voriconazole has also been used as salvage therapy in patients who were intolerant to other drugs [32].

Amphotericin B has been the treatment of choice for those who have failed on treatment with azoles, for those with severe pulmonary or disseminated infection, in the immunocompromised and in pregnancy. Either the lipid formulation (3–5 mg/kg/day) or amphotericin deoxycholate (0.7–1 mg/kg/ day) is given for 1–2 weeks or until there is clinical improvement. After an initial response to amphotericin B, step-down therapy to an azole is recommended. This is usually itraconazole at a loading dose and then 200 mg twice daily for 6–12 months. In the immunocompromised, itraconazole is given for 12 months or until immunosuppression is reversed [30].

Liposomal amphotericin B is recommended for CNS infection as it achieves CNS penetration and is better tolerated with prolonged therapy. For CNS infection, it is usually given at a dose of 5 mg/kg/day for 4–6 weeks. This is followed by an oral azole, which is given for at least 12 months or until there is resolution of CNS abnormalities. Either fluconazole 800 mg daily, itraconazole 200 mg two to three times daily or voriconazole 200–400 mg twice daily can be given [30].

Blastomycosis can be a diagnostic challenge. Delayed diagnosis is not uncommon even in endemic areas if patients present with non-specific clinical features. However, blastomycosis should be considered when there is simultaneous pulmonary and cutaneous infection. It should also alert suspicion in any illness following risk of exposure to *Blastomyces,* in cases of pneumonia that fail to resolve, and ARDS. The treatment of blastomycosis can be problematic when long courses of drug therapy are required, which can be associated with adverse effects.

References

1. Lopez-Martinez R, Méndéz-Tovar LJ. Blastomycosis. Clin Dermatol. 2012;30(6):565–72.
2. Castillo CG, Kauffman CA. ∙ Miceli MH ∙. Blastomycosis. Infect Dis Clin North Am 2016;30(1):247–264.
3. McBride JA, Gauthier GM, Klein BS. Clinical manifestations and treatment of blastomycosis. Clin Chest Med. 2017;38(3):435–49.
4. Chapman SW, Lin AC, Hendricks KA, Nolan RL, Currier MM, Morris KR, Turner HR. Endemic blastomycosis in Mississippi: epidemiologic and clinical studies. Semin Respir Infect. 1997;12(3):219–28.
5. Klein BS, Vergeront JM, Weeks RJ, Kumar UN, Mathai G, Varkey B, Kaufman L, Bradsher RW, Stoebig JF, Davis JP. Isolation of *Blastomyces dermatitidis* in soil associated with a large outbreak of blastomycosis in Wisconsin. N Engl J Med. 1986;314(9):529–34.
6. Morris S, Brophy J, Richardson SE, Summerbell R, Parkin PC, Jamieson F, Limerick B, Wiebe L, Ford-Jones EL. Blastomycosis in Ontario, 1994–2003. Emerg Infect Dis. 2006;12:274–9.
7. Baily GG, Robertson VJ, Neill P, Garrido P, Levy LF. Blastomycosis in Africa: clinical features, diagnosis, and treatment. Rev. Infect Dis. 1991;13(5):1005–8.
8. Roy M, Benedict K, Deak E, Kirby M, et al. A large community outbreak of blastomycosis in Wisconsin with geographic and ethnic clustering. Clin Infect Dis. 2013;57(5):655–62.
9. Sterkel AK, Mettelman R, Wüthrich M, Klein BS. The unappreciated intracellular lifestyle of *Blastomyces dermatitidis*. J Immunol. 2015;194(4):1796–805.
10. Klein BS, Bradsher RW, Vergeront JM, Davis JP. Development of long-term specific cellular immunity after acute *Blastomyces dermatitidis* infection: assessments following a large point source outbreak in Wisconsin. J Infect Dis. 1990;151(1):97–101.
11. Seitz AE, Younes N, Steiner CA, Prevots DR. Incidence and trends of blastomycosis-associated

hospitalizations in the United States. PLoS One. 2014;9(8):e105466.

12. Lemos LB, Baliga M, Guo M. Acute respiratory distress syndrome and blastomycosis: presentation of nine cases and review of the literature. Ann Diagn Pathol. 2001;5(1):1–9.

13. Meyer KC, McManus EJ, Maki DG. Overwhelming pulmonary blastomycosis associated with the adult respiratory distress syndrome. N Engl J Med. 1993;329(17):1231–6.

14. Schwartz IS, Embil JM, Sharma A, Goulet S, Light RB. Management and outcome of acute respiratory distress syndrome caused by blastomyosis: a retrospective case series. Medicine. 2016;95(18):e3538.

15. Larson DM, Eckman MR, Alber RL, Goldschmidt VG. Primary cutaneous (inoculation) blastomycosis: an occupational hazard to pathologist. Am J Clin Pathol. 1983;79(2):253–5.

16. Smith JA, Riddell J IV, Kauffman CA. Cutaneous manifestations of endemic mycoses. Curr Infect Dis Rep. 2013;15(5):440–9.

17. Brick KE, Drolet BA, Lyon VB, Galbraith SS. Cutaneous and disseminated blastomycosis: a pediatric case series. Pediatr Dermatol. 2013;30(1):23–8.

18. Mason AR, Cortes GY, Cook J, Maize JC, Thiers BH. Cutaneous blastomycosis: a diagnostic challenge. Int J Dermatol. 2008;47(8):824–30.

19. Saccente M, Abernathy RS, Pappas PG, Shah HR, Bradsher RW. Vertebral blastomycosis with paravertebral abscess: report of eight cases and review of the literature. Clinc Infect Dis. 1998;26(2):413–8.

20. Bariola JR, Perry P, Pappas PG, et al. Blastomycosis of the central nervous system: a multicenter review of diagnosis and treatment in the modern era. Clin Infect Dis. 2010;50(6):797–804.

21. Seo R, Oyasu R, Schaeffer A. Blastomycosis of the epididymis and prostate. Urology. 1997;50(6):980–2.

22. Gauthier GM, Safdar N, Klein BS, Dr A. Blastomycosis in solid organ transplant recipients. Transpl Infect Dis. 2007;9(4):310–7.

23. Grim SA, Proria L, Miller R, et al. A multicenter study of histoplasmosis and blastomycosis after solid organ transplantation. Transpl Infect Dis. 2012;14(1):17–23.

24. Barocas JA, Gauthier GM. Peritonitis caused by *Blastomyces dermatitidis* in a kidney transplant recipient: case report and literature review. Transpl Infect Dis. 2014;16(4):634–41.

25. Smith JA, Kauffman CA. Endemic fungal infections in patients receiving tumour necrosis factor-alpha inhibitor therapy. Drugs. 2009;69(11):1403–15.

26. Pappas PG. Blastomycosis in the immunocompromised patient. Semin Respir Infect. 1997;12(3):243–51.

27. Smith RJ, Boos MD, Burnham JM, McKay EM, Kim J, et al. Atypical cutaneous blastomycosis in a child with juvenile idiopathic arthritis on infliximab. Pediatrics. 2015;136(5):e1386–9.

28. Pappas PG, Pottage JC, Powderly WG, et al. Blastomycosis in patients with the acquired immunodeficiency syndrome. Ann Intern Med. 1992;116(10):847–53.

29. Saccente M, Woods GL. Clinical and laboratory update on blastomycosis. Clin Microbiol Rev. 2010;23(2):367–81.

30. Chapman SW, Dismukes WI, Proia LA, et al. Infectious Diseases Society of America Clinical practice guidelines for the management of blastomycosis: 2008 updated by the Infectious Disease Society of America. Clin Infect Dis. 2008;46(12):1801–11.

31. Fang W, Washington L, Kumar N. Imaging manifestations of blastomycosis: a pulmonary infection with potentialdissemination. Radiographics. 2007;27(3):641–55.

32. Ta M, Flowers SA, Rogers PD. The role of voriconazole in the treatment of central nervous system blastomycosis. Ann Pharmacother. 2009;43(10):1696–700.

33. Proia LA, Harnisch DO. Successful use of posaconazole for treatment of blastomycosis. Antimicrob Agents Chemother. 2012;56(7):4029.

Coccidioidomycosis

Yul W. Yang and David J. DiCaudo

Key Points

- Travelers to areas of Arizona, California, and other arid regions of North, Central, and South America are at risk of acquiring coccidioidomycosis through airborne inhalation of spores from the soil.
- Coccidioidomycosis primarily affects the lungs and produces respiratory disease mimicking bacterial pneumonia, but severity of disease varies widely from asymptomatic infection to fulminant disease and death.
- Cutaneous manifestations are very common in coccidioidomycosis and are often florid.
- Most cutaneous manifestations are immunologically mediated reactions, including an acute exanthem, Sweet syndrome, interstitial granulomatous dermatitis, and erythema nodosum. Dissemination of organisms to the skin occurs in less than 1% of infected patients and is the most severe cutaneous manifestation.
- Diagnosis of coccidioidomycosis is established by serology, histology, or culture, in the appropriate clinical context.
- Treatment depends upon the severity of infection. An infectious disease specialist is recommended for patients requiring systemic treatment.

Introduction

Coccidioidomycosis, also known as "Valley Fever," is a fungal infection endemic to arid regions of western Canada through Central and South America, and is especially prevalent in the desert areas of the southwestern United States [1] (Fig. 1). Coccidioidomycosis has been reportable in the United States since 1995, with an estimated 150,000 cases annually [2]. Arizona and California have the highest known incidence rates in the world, and Arizona has more reported cases than all other states combined [3]. The exact endemic prevalence in other countries is less elucidated due to lack of public health reporting, recognition, and available laboratory diagnosis [4]. The highly endemic areas in the southwestern United States are popular tourist destinations for visitors from around the globe, with an estimated 5.89 million international visitors to Arizona alone in 2018 (https://tourism.az.gov/international-research/). Coccidioidomycosis has been reported in travelers originating from distant continents [5, 6]. Infections have been reported even after very brief visits, with symptoms occurring weeks after exposure.

Coccidioidomycosis is primarily an infection of the lungs; however, there are a variety of distinctive and often florid cutaneous manifestations, which are important clues to the diagnosis. In non-endemic areas, knowledge of coccidioido-

Y. W. Yang · D. J. DiCaudo (✉)
Mayo Clinic, Scottsdale, AZ, USA
e-mail: yang.yul@mayo.edu; dicaudo.david@mayo.edu

W. Robles (ed.), *Skin Disease in Travelers*, Updates in Clinical Dermatology,
https://doi.org/10.1007/978-3-031-57836-6_15

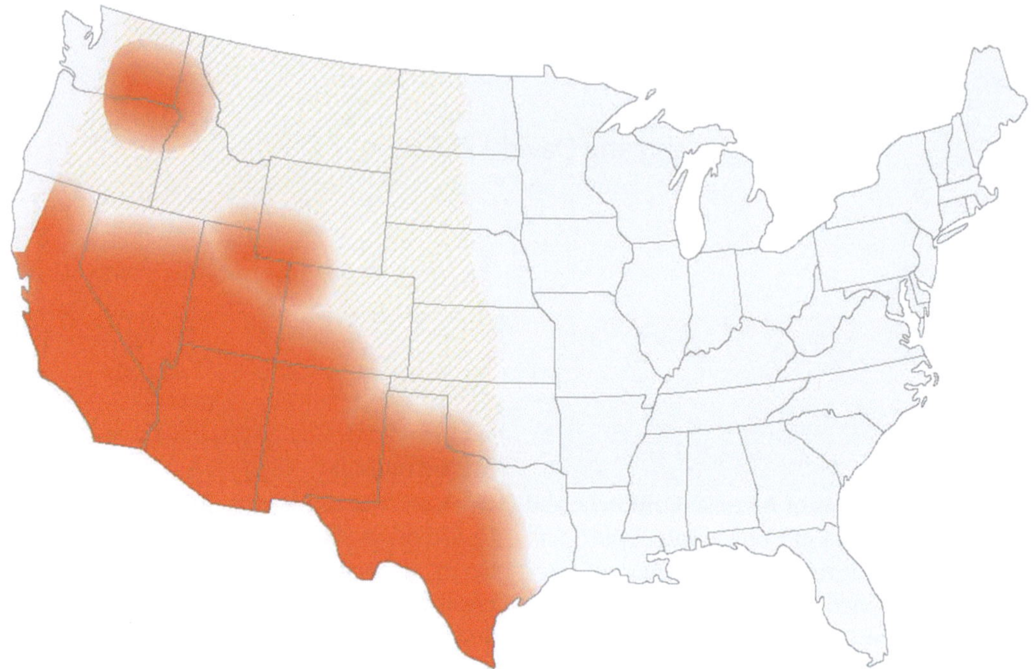

Fig. 1 Estimated endemic areas with coccidioidomycosis in the United States. This map shows CDC's current estimate of where the fungi that cause coccidioidomycosis (Valley Fever) live in the environment in the United States. Darker shading shows areas where *Coccidioides* is more likely to live. Diagonal shading shows the potential range of *Coccidioides*. The disease is also common in northern Mexico, including areas along the U.S. border, as well as parts of Central and South America. (Source: CDC, accessed online February 10, 2020, in the public domain, available on the agency website for no charge. The use of this material does not imply endorsement by CDC, ATSDR, HHS or the United States Government of the information in this article.) https://www.cdc.gov/fungal/diseases/coccidioidomycosis/maps.html

mycosis is important for rapid recognition and appropriate treatment of returning travelers.

Pathogenesis

The causative organisms are *Coccidioides* species, *C. immitis and C. posadasii,* which have different geographic distributions, but produce essentially identical diseases. *Coccidioides* sp. are dimorphic fungi, existing in a mycelial (hyphal) form in the soil and in a spherule form in living tissues. Nearly all infections originate in the lungs and are acquired directly from the environment through the inhalation of airborne arthroconidia. The infection occurs widely in humans, horses, dogs, cats, rodents, other mammals, and reptiles in endemic areas [7].

Direct person-to-person transmission or animal-to-person transmission rarely, if ever, occurs.

The soil-dwelling organism releases arthroconidia that are carried by the wind and suspended in the air, especially during natural events or human activities that disrupt the soil. Clusters of new infections have been reported after earthquakes, dust storms, archaeological excavations, military drills, construction, and recreational activities [8]. However, most infected persons have no recollection of a specific exposure to excessive airborne dust. The organism remains airborne for prolonged periods and may infect individuals whenever the arthroconidia are inhaled. In highly endemic areas, coccidioidomycosis may comprise 24% of newly diagnosed community acquired pneumonias [9, 10].

Clinical Features

With rare exceptions, coccidioidomycosis originates in the lungs. Remarkably, most patients are asymptomatic or develop only a mild, self-limited upper respiratory infection, which may be undiagnosed and unrecognized. However, many patients develop symptoms of pneumonia, ranging from mild to extremely severe and potentially fatal. After an incubation period of 1–4 weeks, patients may develop fever, cough, night sweats, fatigue, and arthralgia. The symptoms mimic a bacterial pneumonia or influenza and are frequently misdiagnosed [2].

Host factors have an extremely important effect on the clinical course of coccidioidomycosis. While most patients are asymptomatic or develop mild illness, other patients may progress to severe pulmonary disease, dissemination, and even death. Multiple risk factors have been identified, including immunosuppression (such as from HIV, cancer, organ transplantation, chemotherapy), pregnancy, and ethnicity [11].

Cutaneous Manifestations

Coccidioidomycosis produces a variety of striking cutaneous manifestations, which may be broadly grouped into two categories: reactive and organism-specific [12–14]. Reactive cutaneous eruptions are very common and are produced by the immune response to the pulmonary infection. These include acute exanthem, Sweet syndrome, interstitial granulomatous dermatitis, and erythema nodosum. Patients may develop one or multiple reactive cutaneous manifestations or may have none. In organism-specific manifestations, the fungal spherules are directly identifiable in the skin. This latter category is almost always due to blood borne dissemination of the organisms from the lungs to the skin. Primary cutaneous infection, due to direct traumatic inoculation into the skin, is extremely rare.

Acute Exanthem

The exanthem of coccidioidomycosis is an unusually florid generalized eruption, which develops suddenly during the first week of the illness (Fig. 2) [15]. The eruption may sometimes develop even before systemic symptoms and may be the patient's chief complaint. Patients present with widespread, broad, symmetrical, pink or red patches, often with sharply demarcated borders on the trunk and extremities. As they can appear annular and targetoid, the exanthem is frequently misdiagnosed clinically as erythema multiforme. Involvement of the palms and soles is common. Pruritus is variably present and may be severe. Early reports in the literature of erythema multiforme associated with coccidioidomycosis likely represented cases of acute exanthem. In contrast to erythema multiforme, the histopathology of the acute exanthem is nonspecific, showing mild spongiosis or minimal interface changes, without the numerous necrotic keratinocytes of erythema multiforme [15].

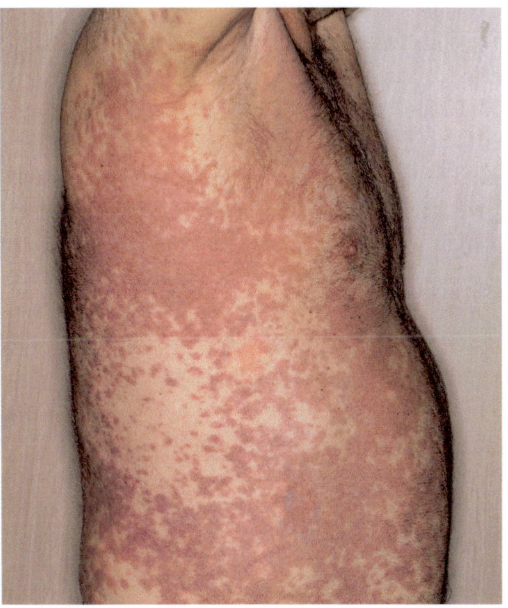

Fig. 2 Acute exanthem of coccidioidomycosis. Widespread, confluent dusky red macules and patches

The exanthem of coccidioidomycosis is frequently misdiagnosed clinically. Because coccidioidomycosis mimics bacterial pneumonia, patients often receive antibiotic therapy, and the exanthem may be mistaken for an allergic drug reaction. The exanthem of coccidioidomycosis may also mimic a viral exanthem, allergic contact dermatitis, or erythema multiforme, as described above.

Sweet Syndrome

Sweet syndrome is a distinctive neutrophilic cutaneous eruption, which may occur as a reactive sign of underlying systemic diseases, especially due to respiratory infection, autoimmune conditions, or malignancy [16]. Viral pneumonia and myeloid malignancies are especially well recognized causes. In endemic areas, pulmonary coccidioidomycosis is a common cause of Sweet syndrome and often occurs early in the course of the illness (Fig. 3). The first reported case was described in a French tourist who had visited northern Mexico [17]. Subsequent reports from endemic areas have confirmed the association with coccidioidomycosis [18].

Patients present with pink or red, tender papules and plaques, often with pustular features. Fever, arthralgia, and peripheral blood neutrophilia are typically associated. Sweet syndrome may be particularly severe in patients with coccidioidomycosis and may present with widespread annular, pustular plaques with bullous features. Typical skin biopsy findings of Sweet syndrome include a diffuse, band-like neutrophilic dermal infiltrate with leukocytoclastic debris and marked subepidermal edema [18].

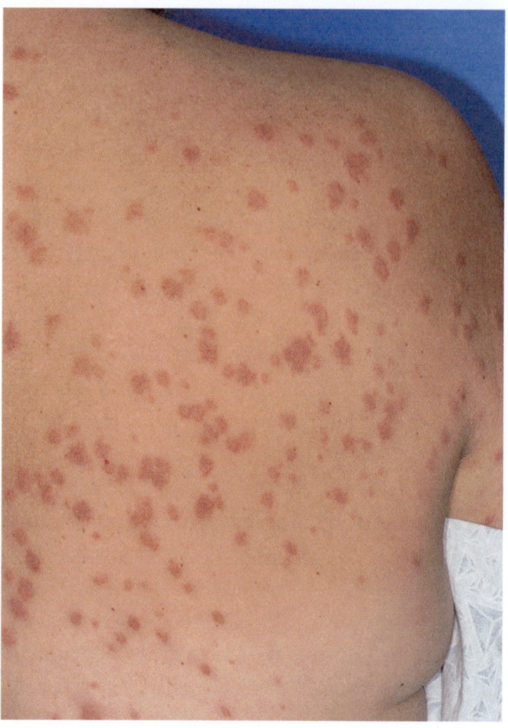

Fig. 3 Sweet syndrome associated with coccidioidomycosis. Edematous pink papules and plaques. Skin biopsy confirmed neutrophilic dermal inflammation without microorganisms

one report [21]. Patients present with pink papules and plaques, which range from few to numerous. Pruritus is variable. The plaques may be strikingly annular and may resemble granuloma annulare both clinically and histopathologically. Interstitial histiocytes form palisading infiltrates in the dermis and are sometimes associated with multinucleate giant cells or neutrophils. As with other reactive cutaneous manifestations, no organisms are present in the skin.

Interstitial Granulomatous Dermatitis

Interstitial granulomatous dermatitis similarly occurs as a reactive manifestation in a broad range of systemic diseases, especially autoimmune diseases [19]. Pulmonary coccidioidomycosis is a common cause in endemic areas [20], which has been reported to last up to 9 years in

Erythema Nodosum

Erythema nodosum is a panniculitis which is commonly induced by a variety of causes including infections (streptococcus, Yersinia, tuberculosis), sarcoidosis, medications, and inflammatory bowel disease [22]. In endemic areas, erythema nodosum has been recognized as a sign of coccidioidomycosis for many decades. The first reports of "Valley Fever" from the San Joaquin Valley of California were patients with coccidioidomycosis, presenting with the classic triad of fever, cough, and erythema nodosum [23]. Erythema nodosum differs from other reactive cutaneous manifestations, in that it tends to erupt later in the clinical course, typically several weeks after the onset of systemic symptoms. Erythema nodosum is considered to be a good prognostic sign in patients with coccidioidomycosis, because it implies a strong, cell-mediated immune response to the organisms in the lungs. The favorable prognostic significance has been specifically demonstrated in pregnant patients with coccidioidomycosis [24].

Erythema nodosum typically presents with tender deep nodules on the anterior shins and ankles and may be associated with arthralgia. The appearance is often sufficiently distinctive to diagnose clinically without biopsy confirmation. Skin biopsy typically demonstrates granulomatous septal panniculitis with widened fibrotic septa and prominent multinucleate giant cells. No fungal organisms are seen.

Disseminated Coccidioidomycosis

Extrapulmonary dissemination of coccidioidomycosis occurs in less than 1% of patients. Nearly any organ may be affected, and the skin, bones, and meninges are the most common sites [2]. Even when widespread, disseminated coccidioidomycosis may result in a range of outcomes, from lack of symptoms to fulminant and potentially fatal illness. The organisms may persist as a nidus of infection in the skin after the lung infection appears to have cleared, and in some instances, there may be no clinical or radiographic evidence of a preceding lung infection. Disseminated skin lesions may be detected in asymptomatic patients during skin cancer screening and has reported as an incidental finding in a patient who had previously traveled to an endemic area [25].

On exam, disseminated cutaneous coccidioidomycosis has been described as papules, macules, pustules, vesicles, nodules, ulcers, verrucous growths, or cysts. The majority of affected patients present with more than one lesion [26]. Given the wide breadth of reported clinical presentations, biopsies are crucial in diagnosing disseminated cutaneous coccidioidomycosis. Microscopic examination reveals distinctive fungal spherules associated with granulomatous inflammation. The organisms are visible on routine hematoxylin eosin-stained sections and are accentuated with fungal stains.

Primary Cutaneous Coccidioidomycosis

Primary cutaneous coccidioidomycosis is extremely rare. Even isolated single nodules of coccidioidomycosis in the skin are more likely to have originated from dissemination. Nevertheless, well-documented cases of primary cutaneous infection have been reported [27]. The infection occurs from direct traumatic inoculation of organisms into the skin, especially in agricultural workers. Laboratory technicians have been reported to develop cutaneous infections from accidental exposure [28–30].

The most common findings have been verrucous plaques or granulomatous nodules [27]. The localized infection may give rise to sporotrichoid pattern of spread along lymphatic pathways, and regional lymphadenopathy may occur.

Diagnosis

Diagnosis of coccidioidomycosis should be strongly considered in patients with recent travel to endemic areas, presenting with pulmonary symptoms and cutaneous manifestations as described above. Coccidioidomycosis may be confirmed by multiple diagnostic methods including serology, microscopic identification, and culture.

Serologic testing is routinely performed in patients with suspected coccidioidomycosis. Currently, the commonly used serologic tests only detect the antibody-based immune response to coccidioidomycosis and do not detect the actual organism itself. For this reason, early infection may yield negative serologic results for weeks, while awaiting antibody generation. When the diagnosis of coccidioidomycosis is considered, repetition of serologic testing in several weeks may be beneficial, if initial results are negative. In addition, it should be recognized that immunocompromised hosts are less likely to show serologic positivity, while remaining at higher risk for dissemination [31].

Enzyme immunoassay (EIA) is useful for serologic testing of coccidioidomycosis, but lacks optimal sensitivity and specificity. Recent studies of commercial EIA against a composite clinical standard found a 53.1–69.4% sensitivity and a 95.4–96.7% specificity for IgG, and a 34.7–57.1% sensitivity and a 70.4–85.5% specificity for IgM [32]. There have been further variations reported between laboratories, based on the type of enzyme immunoassay [33].

As a result of these limitations in EIA testing, coccidioidomycosis frequently has serologic patterns that differ from the classic concept of IgM and IgG responses. For example, patients with acute coccidioidomycosis may sometimes develop detectable IgG antibodies without ever having had detectable IgM. This pattern may still support the diagnosis of acute infection in the appropriate clinical setting and should not be dismissed merely as evidence of remote exposure. It is important to note that resolution of active coccidioidomycosis typically results in negative serologies after a period of months to years [2]. Thus, an isolated positive IgG titer may likely represent an acute or recent infection. In addition, the relatively poor specificity of IgM indicates that an isolated positive IgM is of questionable significance in the absence of other confirmatory serologic tests.

In addition to enzyme immunoassays, complement fixation and immunodiffusion are other serologic antibody-based tests, which may be more specific. These methods are frequently used in addition to EIA for confirmation of the diagnosis. High quantitative complement fixation titers, especially if >1:32, are concerning for complicated infection such as dissemination [34].

Repeated testing of the antibody titer may be helpful in assessing the resolution of infection, while also monitoring the clinical symptoms and physical exam findings.

In some cases, *Coccidioides* sp. may be identified in histologic sections or may be cultured from sputum or tissue [2]. Histologic identification or positive culture offers a definitive diagnosis. From a dermatologic perspective, however, the common reactive cutaneous manifestations (acute exanthem, Sweet syndrome, interstitial granulomatous dermatitis, and erythema nodosum) are purely immunologically mediated, and biopsies of these eruptions do not reveal any organisms. In contrast, *Coccidioides* sp. may be definitively identified by microscopy or culture in skin specimens from disseminated or primary cutaneous infections. In histologic specimens from the skin or other organs, the organisms appear as thick-walled fungal spherules, which are distinguished from other fungi by their large size (10–80 microns). Mature spherules occasionally show formation of characteristic endospores (Fig. 4). Of note, *Coccidioides* sp. in fungal culture are highly infectious and may result in more significant organism exposure than found in nature. For this reason, mold cultures concerning for *Coccidioides sp* should be opened only in appropriate biological safety cabinets. Further recommendations after laboratory exposure have been published [35].

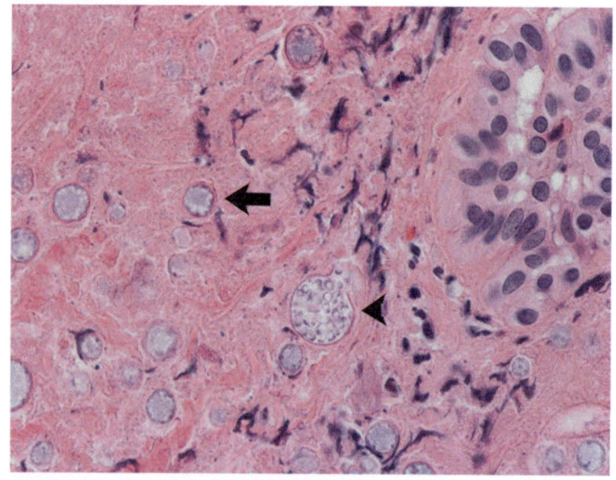

Fig. 4 Disseminated coccidioidomycosis involving the dermis (hematoxylin-eosin, 600×). Thick-walled fungal spherules (arrow). Large spherule containing endospores (arrowhead)

A delayed-type hypersensitivity skin test has also been recently approved in the United States [36], with sensitivity and specificity reportedly >98%. The test is performed by intradermal administration and is read 48 hours after placement. Actual clinical experiences have shown lower levels of sensitivity and specificity [37]. In contrast to serology, the delayed hypersensitivity test remains positive after initial infection, and thus is less useful than serology in distinguishing an acute infection from remote exposure.

Due to the pulmonary symptoms, many patients with coccidioidomycosis undergo various imaging studies during evaluation. Chest X-rays most commonly show consolidation. Other frequent radiologic findings include pulmonary nodules, central adenopathy, and pleural effusions. When clinically necessary, high resolution CT scans may be used to find more subtle abnormalities [38]. Although non-specific, the radiologic findings are a useful adjunct combined with additional testing.

The field of coccidioidomycosis testing is always changing and improving. Given the difficulty of diagnosis, we highly recommend collaboration with infectious disease specialists for all travelers who may have coccidioidomycosis. Consultations with infectious disease specialists from endemic areas may be helpful as well.

Treatment

Treatment of coccidioidomycosis in travelers may be initiated under the guidance of infectious disease specialists. Per 2016 Infectious Diseases Society of America Guidelines [2], uncomplicated coccidioidal pneumonia may or may not require systemic treatment in many individuals. However, some patients may warrant antifungal medications, such as those with disseminated disease, debilitating illness, extensive pulmonary involvement, or comorbidities/patient characteristics (age, African/Filipino ancestry, diabetes, immunosuppression, etc.)

The treatment of reactive cutaneous eruptions (acute exanthem, Sweet syndrome, interstitial granulomatous dermatitis, erythema nodosum) is directed toward relief of symptoms. As noted above, reactive cutaneous eruptions are immune mediated, and fungal organisms are not seen in the skin. If asymptomatic, dermatologic treatment is not required, as the rashes should improve as the coccidioidomycosis resolves. If symptomatic, we typically prescribe mid-potency topical corticosteroids (triamcinolone). We do not routinely prescribe systemic glucocorticoids, due to theoretical concern of inhibiting the immune response against the organism [11]. However, a brief course of systemic glucocorticoids may be considered on a case-by-case basis, with the advice of an infectious disease specialist.

Conclusion

Coccidioidomycosis is a pulmonary fungal infection that is very common in popular tourist destinations of the desert southwest. Through airborne exposure from the environment, travelers are at risk of infection during their visit, and the onset of symptoms may occur after returning home. Cutaneous manifestations of coccidioidomycosis are seen very commonly and are often florid. In combination with the travel history, these striking cutaneous findings may be helpful clues to the diagnosis.

References

1. Brown J, Benedict K, Park BJ, Thompson GR 3rd. Coccidioidomycosis: epidemiology. Clin Epidemiol. 2013;5:185–97.
2. Galgiani JN, Ampel NM, Blair JE, Catanzaro A, Geertsma F, Hoover SE, et al. 2016 Infectious Diseases Society of America (IDSA) clinical practice guideline for the treatment of coccidioidomycosis. Clin Infect Dis. 2016;63(6):e112–46.
3. McCotter OZ, Benedict K, Engelthaler DM, Komatsu K, Lucas KD, Mohle-Boetani JC, et al. Update on the epidemiology of coccidioidomycosis in the United States. Med Mycol. 2019;57(Suppl_1):S30–40.
4. Laniado-Laborin R, Arathoon EG, Canteros C, Muniz-Salazar R, Rendon A. Coccidioidomycosis in Latin America. Med Mycol. 2019;57(Suppl_1):S46–55.
5. Subedi S, Broom J, Caffery M, Bint M, Sowden D. Coccidioidomycosis in returned Australian travellers. Intern Med J. 2012;42(8):940–3.

6. Diaz JH. Travel-related risk factors for coccidioidomycosis. J Travel Med. 2018;25(1)

7. Johnson L, Gaab EM, Sanchez J, Bui PQ, Nobile CJ, Hoyer KK, et al. Valley fever: danger lurking in a dust cloud. Microbes Infect. 2014;16(8):591–600.

8. Freedman M, Jackson BR, McCotter O, Benedict K. Coccidioidomycosis outbreaks, United States and worldwide, 1940-2015. Emerg Infect Dis. 2018;24(3):417–23.

9. Valdivia L, Nix D, Wright M, Lindberg E, Fagan T, Lieberman D, et al. Coccidioidomycosis as a common cause of community-acquired pneumonia. Emerg Infect Dis. 2006;12(6):958–62.

10. Kim MM, Blair JE, Carey EJ, Wu Q, Smilack JD. Coccidioidal pneumonia, Phoenix, Arizona, USA, 2000-2004. Emerg Infect Dis. 2009;15(3):397–401.

11. Odio CD, Marciano BE, Galgiani JN, Holland SM. Risk factors for disseminated coccidioidomycosis, United States. Emerg Infect Dis. 2017;23(2)

12. DiCaudo DJ. Coccidioidomycosis: a review and update. J Am Acad Dermatol. 2006;55(6):929–42. quiz 43-5

13. DiCaudo DJ. Coccidioidomycosis. Semin Cutan Med Surg. 2014;33(3):140–5.

14. Garcia Garcia SC, Salas Alanis JC, Flores MG, Gonzalez Gonzalez SE, Vera Cabrera L, Ocampo CJ. Coccidioidomycosis and the skin: a comprehensive review. An Bras Dermatol. 2015;90(5):610–9.

15. DiCaudo DJ, Yiannias JA, Laman SD, Warschaw KE. The exanthem of acute pulmonary coccidioidomycosis: clinical and histopathologic features of 3 cases and review of the literature. Arch Dermatol. 2006;142(6):744–6.

16. Nelson CA, Noe MH, McMahon CM, Gowda A, Wu B, Ashchyan HJ, et al. Sweet syndrome in patients with and without malignancy: a retrospective analysis of 83 patients from a tertiary academic referral center. J Am Acad Dermatol. 2018;78(2):303–9 e4.

17. Holemans X, Levecque P, Despontin K, Maton JP. First report of coccidioidomycosis associated with sweet syndrome. Presse Med. 2000;29(23):1282–4.

18. DiCaudo DJ, Ortiz KJ, Mengden SJ, Lim KK. Sweet syndrome (acute febrile neutrophilic dermatosis) associated with pulmonary coccidioidomycosis. Arch Dermatol. 2005;141(7):881–4.

19. Peroni A, Colato C, Schena D, Gisondi P, Girolomoni G. Interstitial granulomatous dermatitis: a distinct entity with characteristic histological and clinical pattern. Br J Dermatol. 2012;166(4):775–83.

20. DiCaudo DJ, Connolly SM. Interstitial granulomatous dermatitis associated with pulmonary coccidioidomycosis. J Am Acad Dermatol. 2001;45(6):840–5.

21. Mangold AR, DiCaudo DJ, Blair JE, Sekulic A. Chronic interstitial granulomatous dermatitis in coccidioidomycosis. Br J Dermatol. 2016;174(4):881–4.

22. Blake T, Manahan M, Rodins K. Erythema nodosum - a review of an uncommon panniculitis. Dermatol Online J. 2014;20(4):22376.

23. Hirschmann JV. The early history of coccidioidomycosis: 1892-1945. Clin Infect Dis. 2007;44(9):1202–7.

24. Arsura EL, Kilgore WB, Ratnayake SN. Erythema nodosum in pregnant patients with coccidioidomycosis. Clin Infect Dis. 1998;27(5):1201–3.

25. Rance BR, Elston DM. Disseminated coccidioidomycosis discovered during routine skin cancer screening. Cutis. 2002;70(1):70–2.

26. Carpenter JB, Feldman JS, Leyva WH, DiCaudo DJ. Clinical and pathologic characteristics of disseminated cutaneous coccidioidomycosis. J Am Acad Dermatol. 2010;62(5):831–7.

27. Tortorano AM, Carminati G, Tosoni A, Tintelnot K. Primary cutaneous coccidioidomycosis in an Italian Nun Working in South America and review of published literature. Mycopathologia. 2015;180(3–4):229–35.

28. Doucette J, Trimble JR. Primary cutaneous coccidioidomycosis; report of a case of a laboratory infection. AMA Arch Derm. 1956;74(4):405–10.

29. Carroll GF, Haley LD, Brown JM. Primary cutaneous coccidioidomycosis: a review of the literature and a report of a new case. Arch Dermatol. 1977;113(7):933–6.

30. Sorensen RH, Cheu SH. Accidental cutaneous Coccidioidal infection in an immune person. A case of an exogenous reinfection. Calif Med. 1964;100:44–7.

31. Blair JE, Coakley B, Santelli AC, Hentz JG, Wengenack NL. Serologic testing for symptomatic coccidioidomycosis in immunocompetent and immunosuppressed hosts. Mycopathologia. 2006;162(5):317–24.

32. Grys TE, Brighton A, Chang YH, Liesman R, Bolster LaSalle C, Blair JE. Comparison of two FDA-cleared EIA assays for the detection of Coccidioides antibodies against a composite clinical standard. Med Mycol. 2018;57:595.

33. Khan S, Saubolle MA, Oubsuntia T, Heidari A, Barbian K, Goodin K, et al. Interlaboratory agreement of coccidioidomycosis enzyme immunoassay from two different manufacturers. Med Mycol. 2019;57(4):441–6.

34. McHardy IH, Dinh BN, Waldman S, Stewart E, Bays D, Pappagianis D, et al. Coccidioidomycosis complement fixation titer trends in the age of antifungals. J Clin Microbiol. 2018;56(12)

35. Stevens DA, Clemons KV, Levine HB, Pappagianis D, Baron EJ, Hamilton JR, et al. Expert opinion: what to do when there is Coccidioides exposure in a laboratory. Clin Infect Dis. 2009;49(6):919–23.

36. Wack EE, Ampel NM, Sunenshine RH, Galgiani JN. The return of delayed-type hypersensitivity skin testing for coccidioidomycosis. Clin Infect Dis. 2015;61(5):787–91.

37. Mafi N, Murphy CB, Girardo ME, Blair JE. Coccidioides (spherulin) skin testing in patients with pulmonary coccidioidomycosis in an endemic regiondagger. Med Mycol. 2019;58:626.

38. Jude CM, Nayak NB, Patel MK, Deshmukh M, Batra P. Pulmonary coccidioidomycosis: pictorial review of chest radiographic and CT findings. Radiographics. 2014;34(4):912–25.

Histoplasmosis

Ricardo Negroni and Fernando Antonio Messina

Key Points

- Classical histoplasmosis is a systemic mycosis endemic in the American continent, its etiologic agent is the dimorphic fungus *Histoplasma capsulatum* var. *capsulatum.*
- The source of infection is the soil with acid pH, rich in organic materials, with bat or bird droppings, in temperate and humid zones. Microconidiae are the infective elements.
- Lungs are the portal of entry and the majority of the infections is asymptomatic or presents a mild respiratory disease.
- More severe cases are observed in persons who inhaled a great amount of spores and clinically are like pneumonia or acute respiratory distress.
- Travelers from non-endemic areas are at risk to get an acute respiratory histoplasmosis when they are in endemic zones and enter in a bat cave or participate in outdoor activities with ground removing or get in contact with bat or avian guano, these infections frequently appear as outbreaks.

- Progressive disseminated histoplasmosis is observed in patients with some deficit of cell mediated immunity, like HIV infection, lymphomas, auto immune disorder treated with corticosteroids or in transplant recipients.
- Immigrants from endemic areas, who suffered some of these predisposing factors, may present a disseminated histoplasmosis when they are living in a non-endemic zone. Fever, anemia, loss of weight, hepatosplenomegaly, and skin or mucous membrane lesions are most common clinical manifestations.
- Histoplasmosis diagnosis is based on the fungus finding in histopathology, its isolation in cultures, positive serologic tests searching for specific antibodies, or by the detection of *Histoplasma* antigens in urine.
- Amphotericin B and itraconazole are most frequently antifungal drugs used in this systemic mycosis.

Introduction

Classical histoplasmosis is a systemic mycosis due to the dimorphic fungus *Histoplasma capsulatum* var.*capsulatum.* It lives in the soil as mold and grows as budding yeast in human and animal tissues [1–3].

Histoplasmosis has been registered in 60 countries, but it is more prevalent in the middle-

R. Negroni (✉)
Buenos Aires University School of Medicine,
Mycology Unit of the Francisco J. Muñiz Infectious
Diseases Hospital, Buenos Aires, Argentina

F. A. Messina
Mycology Unit of the Francisco J. Muñiz Infectious
Diseases Hospital, Buenos Aires, Argentina

W. Robles (ed.), *Skin Disease in Travelers*, Updates in Clinical Dermatology,
https://doi.org/10.1007/978-3-031-57836-6_16

east section of U.S.A and in Latin America [4, 5]. The infection is produced by the inhalation of microconidiae of the mycelial form of the fungus and the lung is the portal of entry. Most of the infections in immunocompetent hosts are asymptomatic or course as mild and self-limited respiratory diseases [4, 6, 7]. The severity of the clinical manifestations of these infections is related to the amount of microconidiae inhaled [5–8].

Chronic progressive pulmonary histoplasmosis is observed in men above 50 years of age with chronic obstructive pulmonary disease [5, 9, 10].

Disseminated progressive histoplasmosis occurs in patients with cell-mediated immunity failures. The course of the infections is related to the severity of the immunity alterations [10–13]. Acute or subacute forms are often detected in HIV-positive patients with low TCD_{4+} cells counts as well as in those suffering lymphomas or other malignant diseases. Less frequently, disseminated histoplasmosis is observed in children under 1 year of age [10–12, 16]. The chronic disseminated histoplasmosis is more frequent in men above 53 years of age and the most important predisposing factors are: a mild deficit of cell-mediated immunity observed in patients with type II diabetes, the use of low doses of corticosteroids or non-steroids anti-inflammatory agents, alcoholism, and chronic smoking [4, 6, 10–12].

Histoplasmosis is more prevalent in the American Continent from Canada to Argentina. Most of the endemic areas are located along the great river valleys with temperate and humid climate. In these zones 20–80% of adults react to histoplasmin skin test as a consequence of asymptomatic or mild and self-limited respiratory infections. Autochthonous cases have also been registered in Africa, Australia, India, China, and the Far East [13–15].

Histoplasma capsulatum has been isolated from the ground in the endemic regions, especially from rich soil with high nitrogen concentration, acid pH, and bat or bird excreta. Some "epidemic spots" have been recorded inside and outside the endemic zones. These are character-ized by heavy soil contamination with *Histoplasma capsulatum* and may produce small outbreaks of respiratory infections. These outbreaks appear after cleaning pigeons or hen houses or entering caves or mines where bats have nested or after any action which leads to disturbance of the soil where black birds or pigeons have roosted. *H. capsulatum* may infect bats, which are able to spread the fungus to new places inside or outside the endemic regions [16, 17].

Natural infections with *H. capsulatum* have been detected in several animal species, especially in rodents and dogs [4, 6, 8].

Histoplasmosis is not usually transmitted from man to man or from animal to man, but a few cases of this mycosis has been recorded in liver transplant recipients who received the liver from an infected person [4, 6, 10, 15].

Histoplasma capsulatum mycelial form, also called saprophytic form, grows at 28 °C in several culture media as Sabouraud dextrose-agar and dextrose-potatoes-agar. After 15 days of incubation it presents cottony aerial mycelia, white to tan in color. Microscopically vegetative mycelium consists in hyaline, septate, branched hyphae. Two types of conidiae are observed: Macroconidiae are spherical or pear shape, 10–25 μm in diameter, with a thick cell wall covered by digit form tubercles and microconidiae which are spherical or pyriform, with smooth thin walls, 2 or 5 μm in diameter, sessile or borne on short sporophores [1, 4, 6, 8].

H. capsulatum yeast form develops in rich culture media as brain heart infusion-agar with 5% rabbit blood at 37 °C. After 4–5 days incubation colonies are visible as whitish, wrinkled, 2–3 mm in diameter, moist, glossy and creamy consistency growth. Microscopically, small single budding yeasts, 3–5 μm in diameter, are observed. The yeast form is also found in animal tissues as small yeast-like spherical or oval elements, with a thin cell wall which does not take aniline stains which was mistaken for a capsule. The majority of these yeasts are inside the macrophages or giant cells in the granulomas. In the smears stained with Giemsa or Wright techniques the cell wall does not take up the stain and appears as a clear halo. The cytoplasm has a single distinct mass, half-moon shaped, darker than the rest of the cytoplasm and placed at the opposite side of the bud. In the histopathological preparations these yeast-like elements stain red with periodic acid Schiff (PAS) and dark brown or black with Grocott methenamine-silver technique [2, 4, 6, 8, 18].

H. capsulatum sexual reproduction follows the heterothallic conjunction of compatible mating types (+) and (−). They are paired in poor culture media, such as yeast extract-agar or soil extract-agar at 28 °C for several weeks. The young cleistothecia are globose, 100–150 μm in diameter; they become irregularly stellate with age because of the radiated, spinal peridial hyphae. Asci are club to pear shape, 3–5 × 10–15 μm in diameter and contain 8 oval ascospores. This sexual (teleomorphic) form is called *Ajellomyces capsulatus* [2, 6, 8].

There are three varieties of *Histoplasma capsulatum: H. capsulatum var. capsulatum, H. capsulatum var. duboisii,* the etiological agent of African histoplasmosis and *H. capsulatum* var. *farcinimosum,* which produces epizootic lymphangitis in horses and mules in southern and central Europe, North of Africa, the Middle East, and Southern Asia [1, 6, 8].

Molecular biology techniques have allowed the identification of seven phylogenetic species of *H. capsulatum* var. *capsulatum* [4, 19].

The infection is produced by the inhalation of *H. capsulatum* microconidiae which penetrate in the airway until the pulmonary alveoli where they are phagocytized but not lysed by the alveolar macrophages. Inside the alveolar macrophages microconidiae transform into yeast like budding elements. In this phase of the infection, the yeast-like elements are able to survive and grow inside the phagolysosomes of macrophages [2, 4, 6, 10].

The initial stage of the inflammatory response involves polymorphonuclear neutrophils, which are able to decrease the growth of *H. capsulatum* by a mechanism not related to nitric oxide, but these cells did not reach the infection control. In the early part of the infection, macrophages per-mit the rapid reproduction of *H. capsulatum* yeasts, when they are numerous they are liberated and captured by other macrophages and by dendritic cells. Dendritic cells are in charge of *H. capsulatum* antigens presentation to the CD_{4+} lymphocytes giving way to the acquired specific cell-mediated immunity. In immunocompetent hosts, the activation of cell-mediated immunity produces Th_1 cytokines that effectively dominate the progress of the infection. In this stage of the infection, the macrophages become activated by the action of INF-γ, IL_2, $IL_{12,}$ and TNF-α and they are able to kill yeasts by nitric oxide activity. Other cytokines such as IL_1 and CSF-GM also aid to contain the infection. Maturation of cell-mediated immunity turns evident 2 or 3 weeks after the infective contact by the production of compact epithelioid cell granulomas in the affected tissues. The histoplasmin skin test turns positive and the blastogenic response of lymphocytes to the specific antigens becomes evident [4, 6, 10, 15].

The important role of TCD_4+ cells in the defensive mechanisms against histoplasmosis is clearly seen in AIDS-patients. Other cells are also important in infection control: NK lymphocytes are able to kill extracellular yeast cells, but the mechanism is not completely clear; TCD_{17} lymphocytes produce $IL_{17,}$ which has an important role in polymorphonuclear neutrophils chemotaxis during the initial phase of the infection [10, 12].

The primary pulmonary infection progresses initially by contiguity through the lung, then it moves to the mediastinal lymph nodes and finally to the blood stream. This hematogenous dissemination is asymptomatic in the majority of the cases and *H. capsulatum* yeast cells colonize the reticuloendothelial system. In immunocompetent hosts, the infection progresses to a latent stage which probably persists for lifetime. This latent stage is characterized by the presence of compact epithelioid cell granulomas with caseous center containing live yeasts inside. They can be detected in lungs, lymph nodes, liver, and spleen. Over time, these granulomas are surrounded by a collagen fibrosis, which later gets calcified [3, 5, 6, 9].

Traveler's Histoplasmosis

Travelers usually present the symptomatic primary respiratory histoplasmosis. The majority of them lives in non-endemic regions and acquires the infection in the endemic zones. These patients present a febrile respiratory self-limited syndrome. Most cases occur in clusters of individuals who acquire the infection in a common source heavily contaminated with bat or bird excreta. There is often a group history of participation in activities that expose them to the infection, especially spelunkers or volunteers involved in cleaning tasks or old buildings rehabilitation. An increasing number of clustered cases in travelers have been reported in the literature, largely due to a rise in international travels and to greater rates of ecotourism [20, 21]. Histoplasmosis is responsible for 70% of mycoses in travelers, followed by coccidioidomicosis [20].

Another possibility is observed this mycosis in immigrants who come from endemic areas to live in a non-endemic zone and present a reactivation of a latent *Histoplasma* infection due to different causes of immunodeficiency, especially AIDS, auto-immunological disorders, organs transplantation, etc. These patients usually suffer a subacute disseminated histoplasmosis with several organs involved and a severe outcome [22].

The diagnosis of histoplasmosis in non-endemic areas is a serious challenge for clinicians.

In this chapter, we present the clinical manifestations and treatment of primary infection and subacute disseminated histoplasmosis.

Primary Respiratory Histoplasmosis

More than 95% of the infections are asymptomatic or present mild self-limited flu-like respiratory symptoms. The course of the primary infection depends upon the number of inhaled microconidiae as well as on previous clinical and immune state of the host. The incubation period varies between 3 days and 3 weeks and after 1 month patients improve. Primary infection is retrospectively recognized by finding calcified nodules in lung, lymph nodes and spleen, and the positive histoplasmin skin test. These calcifications appear in a quarter of those infected 1 or 2 years after the infection [4–6, 16].

The clinical manifestations of the severe cases are similar to those produced by acquired community pneumonia. The symptoms observed are fever, asthenia, myalgia, headache, night sweat, weight loss, dry cough, dyspnea, chest pain, and hepatomegaly. Chest radiographs frequently show bilateral diffuse pulmonary infiltrates and hiliar and mediastinal adenomegalies [4–6, 8].

Computer Tomography (CT) scan exams often show micronodular diffuse bilateral intersticiopathy with reticulonodular patterns and hiliar or mediastinal adenopathies (Fig. 1). Some patients develop an adult acute respiratory distress, but fatal outcome is rare [4, 6, 15]. This syndrome is usually observed in the histoplasmosis outbreak.

Approximately 6% of these acute infections present clinical manifestations related to hypersensitivity such as erythema nodosum or multiphorm, polyarthritis, pleural, or pericardial effusion [1–3, 10].

Independently of the severity of these diseases they tend to remit spontaneously after 4–6 weeks. Sequelae of the primary infection are bilateral interstitial pulmonary fibrosis and nodules which calcify overtime. In severe cases, calcifications are also seen in hiliar and mediastinal lymph nodes, liver, and spleen [6, 8, 10, 13].

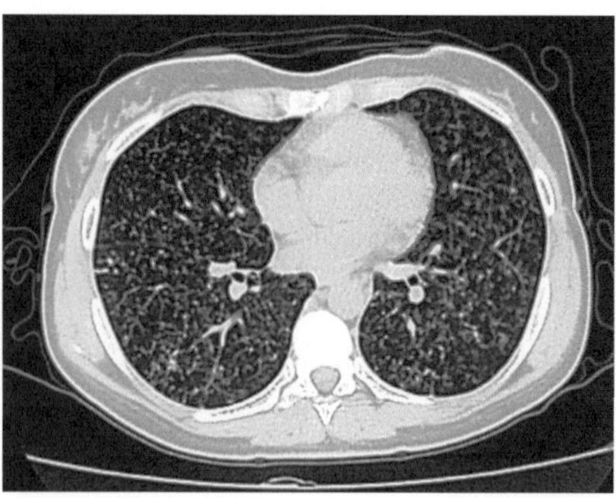

Fig. 1 Chest CT scan of a patient with a severe subacute primary infection of histoplasmosis which presents reticulonodular interstitial lesions of the lungs

Three or four weeks after infection serological tests searching for antibodies against *H. capsulatum* antigens become positive. The specific antibodies can be demonstrated by immunodiffusion reactions (ID), counterimmunolectrophoresis (CIE), complement fixation test (CFT), and ELISA for IgM, but only the first three are sufficiently specific. These serological tests become positive only in moderate or severe infections. Antibody titers are proportional to fungal burden and tend to diminish after primary infection remission [3, 4, 8, 9].

Skin test with histoplasmin becomes positive 3 weeks after the first infective contact and vanishes 2 or 3 years later if a new infection does not occur [4, 10, 14].

Histoplasma capsulatum is rarely isolated from bronchoalveolar lavage, blood cultures, or urine samples in the most severe cases during the first 2 weeks of evolution.

In high endemic areas, some cases of acute pulmonary re-infections have been registered, but it is very rare in travelers [5, 6, 15].

Subacute Disseminated Form

AIDS constitutes the most important risk factor for this clinical form. In South America, more than 90% of the cases are HIV-positive patients with CD_{4+} cell counts below 150/µl [12, 13, 15, 23].

Histoplasmosis is associated with an estimated tenfold increase in frequency when HIV-positive patients of endemic zones and those of non-endemic zones are compared [12, 23]. After HAART introduction, the incidence of histoplasmosis in these patients decreased from 5% of cases requiring hospitalization to 2.5% [24]. In other endemic areas a higher proportion of AIDS related histoplasmosis is observed, in Indianapolis (U.S.A), 27% of the HIV-positive patients requiring hospitalization suffer this mycosis, this disease is also a very common in Guyana and Guatemala [25–27].

Clinical manifestations are those of other severe infectious processes: prolonged fever, weight loss, asthenia, anorexia, diarrhea, vomit-

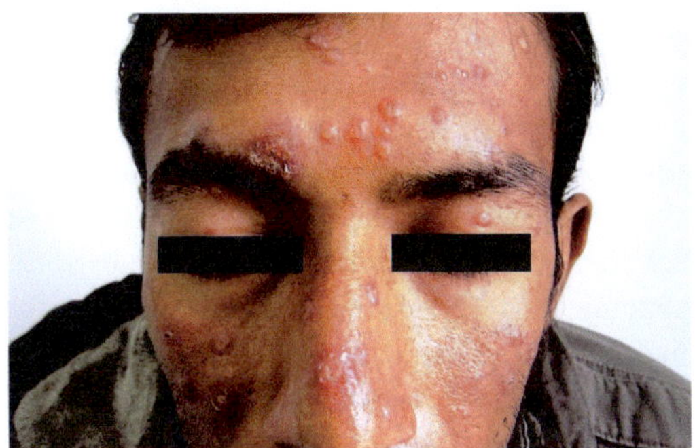

Fig. 2 Moluscoid papules and ulcerated skin lesions in a patients suffering subacute disseminated histoplasmosis related to AIDS

ing, hepatosplenomegaly, multiple adenomegalies, pancytopenia, cough with mucopurulent or bloody expectoration, dyspnea, skin and mucous membrane lesions. In Latin America, skin and mucous membrane lesions appear in 80% of these patients. On the other hand, they are less frequently observed in U.S.A, only in 6% of the cases [10, 12, 15, 23, 24].

Skin lesions are usually multiple and exhibit a wide spectrum of clinical aspects. More frequently they manifest as small papules, 3–4 mm in diameter, with an ulcer at the vertex, covered with scabs, and located on various parts of the body (Fig. 2). Other skin lesions are large ulcers with a granulomatous base and sharp edges; vegetated ulcers, nodules, diffuse hypodermitis, moluscoid papules, or lupoid lesions are less frequently seen [12, 24, 25].

Mucosal alterations are located on the oropharynx, on the larynx, and on the penis. They appear like ulcers, with a red fundus, covered by yellowish-white secretions. They are less common than the cutaneous lesions [12].

Chest X-ray and CT scan studies show disseminated micronodular intersticiopathy on both lungs as well as bilateral diffuse shadows. Pleural attack is very rare [10, 12, 15, 23].

Few patients with subacute disseminated histoplasmosis present central nervous system compromise. It manifests as a meningoencephalitis with focal sings due to basal nuclei of the brain compromised [10, 11, 23]. Encephalic magnetic resonance shows focal lesions on the basal nuclei of the brain. Cerebrospinal fluid presents increased proteins level and discrete lymphocytic pleocitosis (50–100 cells/µl) [10, 12, 25]. *H. capsulatum* is rarely isolated from CSF cultures.

Gastrointestinal attack is observed. The most common clinical manifestations are diarrhea, abdominal pain and stomachaches, hematemesis, melena, digestive ulcers, and intestinal perforation with very serious peritonitis. Ulcers of the stomach and the gut are often detected by endoscopic studies [12, 15, 24, 25].

Bone lesions are rarely detected. They are more often located in the long bones and can be seen in radiology examinations as osteolytic images [10].

Abdominal ultrasonography and CT scan frequently show heterogeneous hepatomegaly, homogeneous splenomegaly, and abdominal and retroperitoneal adenopathies [23].

Complementary laboratory studies reveal acceleration of the erythrocyte sedimentation rate, thrombocytopenia, anemia, and elevation of hepatic enzymes levels (especially alkaline phosphatase).

Due to the low counts of CD_4 + cells these patients often present other associated diseases especially tuberculosis and *Candida* esophagitis [10, 12, 23].

Disseminated histoplasmosis is detected in less than 1% of solid organs transplant recipients. Previous CMV infection is an important risk factor for mycoses [28]. These patients present clinical signs and symptoms similar to those exhibited by cases with AIDS-related histoplasmosis. Skin nodules, gummas, and diffuse hypodermitis are often detected [29–31]. These lesions frequently evolve to big ulcers [10, 12].

Histoplasmosis is a late complication of solid organs transplantations and a decrease in its incidence has been detected, probably due to the less aggressive immunosuppression therapy [15, 25].

Subacute histoplasmosis is also observed in patients under treatment with blockers of TNF-α and inhibitor of calcineurin. These drugs are used in chronic intestinal inflammatory disease, rheumatoid arthritis, and dermatomyositis. The clinical manifestations observed in these patients are less severe than those present in AIDS related histoplasmosis. Nodular necrotizing hypodermitis is often detected [32–35].

In patients with skin or mucous membranes lesions, Tzanck's cytodiagnosis test is a very useful diagnostic method. In Argentina, approximately 80% of disseminated histoplasmosis in HIV-positive cases cytodiagnosis test is the first diagnostic evidence for histoplasmosis (Fig. 3). The clinical sample is obtained by scraping the base of the ulcers and preparing smears on slides which are stained by Giemsa technique. Biopsies from different tissues such as skin, mucous membrane, lymph nodes, and bone marrow are also very useful [36]. Blood cultures by lysis-centrifugation technique have shown to be very effective in AIDS patients. *H. capsulatum* was isolated in 75% of the cases and in 20% of them it was the first diagnostic element [37]. The

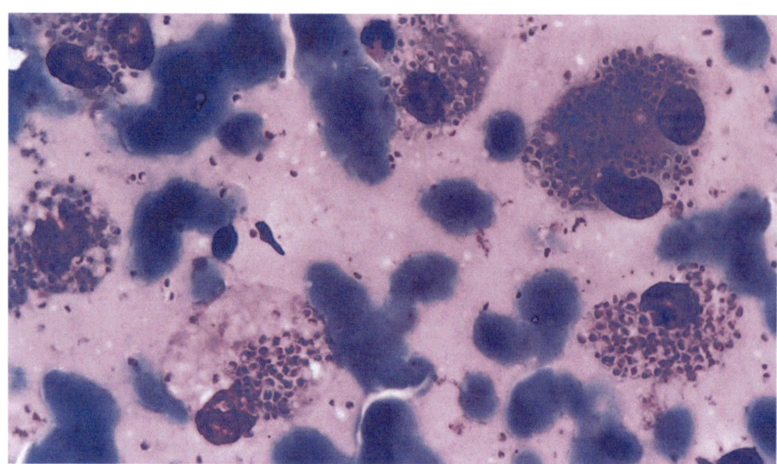

Fig. 3 Tzanck's cytodiagnosis showing yeast-like elements of *Histoplasma capsulatum* inside macrophages, clinical samples obtained from skin papule of an HIV-positive patient with disseminated histoplasmosis, ×1000 Giemsa stain

microscopic examination of the leukocyte layer of the hematocrit (buffy coat) and the bronchoalveolar lavage culture are useful diagnostic tools [23, 25].

Serological studies searching for antibodies yield frequent false-negative results in AIDS patients, ID, CIE, and CFT are positive in only 30% of these cases. ELISA technique increases the positive results to 75%, but cross reactions with other fungal antigens have frequently been observed with this method [10, 12, 15, 23].

Histoplasma antigenemia and antigenuria have been detected in patients with subacute disseminated forms by radioimmunoassay and ELISA techniques. An ELISA test, searching for *H. capsulatum* galactomannan in urine has recently been validated as a very useful diagnostic procedure [38–41]. Molecular biology methods are also used in the diagnosis of subacute disseminated histoplasmosis, nested PCR and real time PCR are often employed for *H. capsulatum* detection in blood or biopsies, but commercial kits are not available in most of the endemic areas [42].

Histoplasmin skin test is usually negative in these patients [12].

Treatment

Azolic compounds such as itraconazole, ketoconazole, fluconazole, voriconazole, posaconazole, and isavuconazole as well as the polyenic antibiotics amphotericin B are active in vitro and in vivo against *H. capsulatum* [1, 2, 4, 6, 15].

Symptomatic primary infections do not usually require antifungal treatment excepting those cases that do not present spontaneous remission within 4–6 weeks after the infection or in immunocompromised patients. These cases are usually treated with itraconazole by oral route at a daily dose 200 mg during 3 months. Severe acute pneumonitis with marked respiratory insufficiency requires mechanical respiratory assistance as well as corticosteroids in doses equivalent to 60 or 80 mg/day of prednisone. During steroids treatment, patients should receive intravenous amphotericin B and after

patients recovery the schedule treatment is changed to oral itraconazole at daily doses of 200 or 400 mg [10, 14, 15].

Hypersensitivity reactions such as erythema nodosum, arthritis, pericarditis, and pleurisy are treated with non-steroid anti-inflammatory drugs and, in serious cases, with corticosteroids. Antifungal protection is mandatory in these patients [6, 13].

Itraconazole is the treatment of choice in mediastinal granulomas and it should be administered in a daily dose of 400 mg during 18 months. There is not any effective treatment for mediastinal fibrosis [6, 13, 15].

In patients with subacute disseminated histoplasmosis deoxychollate amphotericin B in dose of 0.7 mg/Kg/day or liposomal amphotericin B in dose of 3 mg/Kg/day are the treatments of choice, especially for the patients presenting diarrhea and emesis, for persons receiving drugs which interact with itraconazole and for those suffering serious clinical manifestations. Itraconazole is indicated in less severe cases [10, 12, 23, 43, 44]. During the first 3 or 4 days of treatment with itraconazole doses of 600 mg/day are required to achieve rapidly effective tissue concentration. After these days 400 mg/day is usually administered. In AIDS patients, a secondary prophylaxis is indicated after the initial part of the treatment, for prophylaxis itraconazole at a daily dose of 200 mg is the treatment of choice and it is maintained until the patient presents two CD_{4+} cell counts with >150 cells/µl [45]. Posaconazole has been successfully used in few patients with disseminated histoplasmosis who did not response or did not tolerate itraconazole and amphotericin B [46].

Histoplasma meningitis is difficult to treat. Liposomal amphotericin B in a daily dose of 5 mg/Kg during 6 weeks is the treatment of choice, followed by oral itraconazole in a dose of 400 mg/day during 12 months in order to avoid relapses [47, 48]. Fluconazole does not seem to be more effective than itraconazole in this *Histoplasma* meningitis [15]. Due to the risk of hydrocephalus, ventricular-atrial or peritoneal shunts are frequently required. Intratecal administration of amphotericin B is not used due to its severe side effects.

Summaries of Five Studies as Examples of Histoplasmosis in Travelers and Immigrants

We are presenting herewith the summaries of five studies as examples of histoplasmosis in travelers and immigrants.

In May 2001, there was a histoplasmosis outbreak in 15 people resident in 4 states of U.S.A who had participated in a geo-biology community college class trip to Nicaragua. The participants' median age range was 38 years (18–61); 57% were women. During their trip they visited a biological research station and 14 of them entered a small cave which had been used as silver mine. They stayed there for 10 min and saw flying bats and bat guano on the ground. All of them acquired histoplasmosis infection. 86% of them suffered symptomatic infections and the diagnosis was made based on serological tests searching for antibodies and antigenuria. The clinical samples were obtained 2–3 weeks after the exposure. Five patients presented a febrile respiratory illness which required hospital assistance. All the infections were self-limited and the patients did not receive antifungal treatment [21].

Between 2000 and 2011, 23 cases of imported histoplasmosis in travelers were identified in Israel. Their median age was 31 years (19–66) and 74% were males. All but one had acquired the infection in Central or South America and only one had been infected during his trip to Ohio River in Illinois, U.S.A. Nine cases had visited a cave with bats in Guatemala and all of them presented symptomatic infections. Other 13 cases had visited different bat caves in Central America and 1 patient had probably acquired the infection in the hollow of a tree trunk in the Bolivian Amazon jungle. All the cases were immunocompetent persons. These patients were divided into two groups: 14 were symptomatic cases, 13 presented fever, and 10 also complained of respiratory manifestations, cough, dyspnea, and chest pain. Lungs X-ray and CT scan studies showed nodular lesions without calcification or diffuse infiltrative shadows. Hiliar adenomegalies were seen in few cases. The diagnosis of histoplasmosis was based on specific serological reactions searching for antibodies, positive ID tests for M and H bands, and CFT with titers >1:32 and the detection of *H. capsulatum* galactomannan in urine in one case. The second group was nine asymptomatic persons who were diagnosed during the evaluation of incidental radiological findings or because of travel patterns, as they had suffered a previous histoplasmosis. Most of them presented multiple calcified nodules in the lungs without hiliar adenopathies or lymph node calcifications. Serological tests were positive in only two cases [49].

In March 2001, the Pennsylvania Department of Health was notified of a cluster of acute febrile respiratory illness among student-travelers who had been to Acapulco, Mexico. Within 2 weeks, 21 students were examined in various health care centers. They presented an acute illness characterized by fever, chills, dry cough, chest pain, and headache. Two of them were hospitalized. Chest radiographs showed diffuse infiltrates in both lungs and hiliar lymphadenopathy suggestive of acute histoplasmosis. A transbronchial lung biopsy specimen from a student hospitalized in Missouri was obtained and the histopathology study showed intracellular yeasts compatible with *H. capsulatum.*

CDC carried out a telephone survey among people who had been to Acapulco between March and May 2001. The case definition was based on the signs and symptoms mentioned above. The laboratory-confirmed case was defined by the presence of some of the following findings: H or M bands on ID or a titer 1:32 on CFT on either acute or convalescent serum specimens or a four-fold increase in titers between acute and convalescent-phase sera in American travelers.

A total of 262 travelers met the case definition, of whom 245 were student travelers from various states of U.S.A. 191 individuals completed the questionnaire. 122 of them presented a febrile respiratory illness compatible with the case definition. The median age was 21 and 112 provided serum specimens for serological tests. 75 cases met the laboratory confirmed case definition. All of them had stayed at the same hotel in Acapulco during the outbreak.

The hotel environmental study led to the conclusion that a possible source of infection was the organic material which was found in the utility shaft in the central stairwell. The maintenance work in this place of the building, which had been done after a fire in January 2001, permitted the aerosolization of dust contaminated with *H. capsulatum* spores. Another possibly infected place was a planter containing large pot plants, located on the eighth floor. It was broken and soil from the broken planters, which had come from a local chicken farm, was dispersed [50].

This was the most important acute histoplasmosis outbreak suffered by travelers.

A meta-analysis that studied 71 publications, including 814 cases with possible, probable, or proven histoplasmosis infection acquired during travels, has recently been published. The majority of patients were European young adult males who had been to Central or South America for tourism or professional activities and had visited caves with bat droppings or participated in outdoor activities (Fig. 3). Most of them belonged to 47 clusters of travelers. They presented fever, chills, sweat, headache, body pain, dry cough, dyspnea, anorexia, asthenia, and weight loss. Digestive symptoms were frequent, especially diarrhea and vomiting. Rheumatic syndrome was detected in 11% of the cases. The main clinical manifestation was migrating arthritis. A few cases with neurological signs or symptoms were seen, headache and alterations of mental status being the most common manifestations. Only one case of disseminated progressive histoplasmosis with multiorganic involvement and fatal evolution was observed.

Chest X-ray and CT scan studies often showed bilateral disseminated nodular infiltrates or reticulonodular intersticiopathy as well as mediastinal adenopathies.

According to the evidences of active histoplasmosis, patients were divided into three groups: Proven cases, when the patient presented compatible signs and symptoms of acute histoplasmosis together with epidemiological data, and *H. capsulatum* was seen in cytological or histopathological studies of bronchoalveolar lavage or in biopsies or the fungus was isolated in cultures of these specimens. Probable cases with compatible clinical and epidemiological data, which also presented positive serological tests with histoplasmin as well as positive skin tests with this antigen, but *H. capsulatum* could not be seen or isolated from clinical samples (in some of these cases the diagnosis was made by positive antigenuria, using a specific test searching for *H. capsulatum* galactomannan) and finally, possible cases that were those that only presented clinically and epidemiologically compatible findings. Two thirds of the studied cases belonged to the proven and probable groups.

Sixty-seven percent of these persons received antifungal treatment. Most of them were treated with oral itraconazole in doses between 200 mg to 400 mg/day for 3–6 months. Other cases were initially treated with intravenous amphotericin B and, after 7–10 days, this treatment was changed to itraconazole. More than 95% of the cases presented a good clinical response to these treatments and were cured without important sequelae [20].

Histoplasmosis incidence in Spain has increased in recent years, mainly due to the presence of immigrants from Latin America and a high frequency of travels to this continent for tourism and cooperation. Four cases suffering subacute disseminated histoplasmosis were studied at a medical center in Pamplona, Navarra, Spain. All of them were immigrants from South America, of whom three were males and one female. Three of them were HIV positive and one suffered dermatomyositis under immunosuppressive treatment. The laboratory diagnosis of histoplasmosis was made by histological and microbiological studies, by cultures and PCR directly on the clinical samples obtained from the patients' lesions. They did not have skin lesions, but they presented fever, weight loss, anemia, hepatosplenomegaly, and adenomegalies in different parts of the body. All of them were treated with intravenous liposomal amphotericin B. Three had a good clinical response to the treatment and one died due to the rapid outcome of the mycosis [22].

References

1. Arenas R. Histoplasmosis. En: Arenas R. Micología Médica Ilustrada. 4° Edición. México: McGraw-Hill Interamericana; 2011. p. 192–202.
2. Bonifaz A. Histoplasmosis. En: Bonifaz A. Micología Médica Básica. 4° Edición. México: McGraw-Hill Interamericana; 2012. p. 279–96.
3. George RB, Penn RL. Histoplasmosis. In: Sarosi GA, Davies SF, editors. Fungal diseases of the lung. 2nd ed. New York: Raven Press Ldt; 1993. p. 39–50.
4. Deepe GE. Histoplasma capsulatum. In: Mandell GL, Bennett JE, Dolin R, editors. Mandell, Douglas, Bennett. Enfermedades Infecciosas. Principios y práctica. Séptima Edición. Barcelona: Elsevier España; 2012. p. 3299–313.
5. Goodwin JE, Lloyd R, Des PR. Histoplasmosis in normal host. Medicine. 1980;60:231–66.
6. Kauffman CA. Histoplasmosis. In: Kauffman CA, Pappas PG, Sobel JD, Dismukes WE, editors. Essential in clinical mycology. New York: Springer; 2011. p. 321–36.
7. Alsip S, Dismukes W. Approach to the patients with suspected histoplasmosis. In: Remington JS, Swartz MN, editors. Current topics in infectious diseases. New York: McGraw-Hill; 1986. p. 254–96.
8. Kwon-Chung KJ, Bennett JE. Histoplasmosis. In: Kwon- Chung KJ, Bennett JE, editors. Medical mycology. Philadelphia: Lea & Febiger; 1992. p. 464–513.
9. Negroni R. Histoplasmosis. In: Hay RJ. Tropical fungal infections. Bailliere's Clin Trop Med Commun Dis. 1989;4:169–83.
10. Negroni R. Clinical spectrum and treatment of classic histoplasmosis. Rev Iberoamer Micol. 2000;17:159–67.
11. Goodwin JE, Shapiro JL, Thurman GH, Thurman SS, Des PR. Disseminated histoplasmosis. Clinical and pathologic correlations Medicine. 1980;59:1–33.
12. Negroni R, Arechavala AI, Maiolo EI. Histoplasmosis clásica en pacientes inmunocomprometidos. Medina Cutánea Ibero- Latino- Amicana. 2010;38:59–69.
13. Wheat LJ, Kauffman CA. Histoplasmosis. In: Walsh T, Rex J (Editors). Fungal infections. Part II. Recent advances in diagnosis, treatment and prevention of endemic and cutaneous mycoses. Infect Dis Clin N Am. 2003;16:17:1–9.
14. Kauffman CA. Histoplasmosis. Clin Chest Med. 2009;30:17–225.
15. Wheat LJ, Azar MM, Bahr NC, Sec A. Histoplasmosis. Infect Dis N Am. 2016;30:207–27.
16. Negroni R, Dure R, Ortiz-Naredo A, Maiolo EI, Arechavala A, Santiso G, Iovannitti C, Ibarra-Camou B, Canteros CE. Brote de histoplasmosis en la Escuela de Cadetes de la Base Aérea de Morón, Provincia de Buenos Aires. República Argentina Rev Argent Microbiol. 2010;42:254–26.
17. Sanchez Alemán MA. Histoplasmosis, la micosis del viajero. Enf Inf Microbiol. 2009;29:111–6.
18. Salfelder K, de Liscano TR, Sauerteig E. Histoplasmosis capsulati. In: Atlas of fungal pathology, current histopathology series, 17. Kluwer Academic Publisher: Dordrecht; 1990. p. 73–97
19. Muñiz MM, Pizzini CV, Peralta JM, Reiss E, Zancopé-Oliveira RM. Genetic diversity of *Histoplasma capsulatum* strains isolated from soil, animals and clinical specimens in Rio de Janeiro state, Brazil, by a PCR-based random amplified polymorphic DNA assay. J Clin Microbiol. 2001;39:4487–94.
20. Staffolani S, Buonfrate D, Angheben A, Gobbi F, et al. Acute histoplasmosis in immunocompetent travelers a systemic review of literature. BMC Infect Dis. 2018;18:673–86.
21. Weinberg M, Weeks J, Lance-Parker S, Taeger M, et al. Severe histoplasmosis in travelers to Nicaragua. Emerg Infect Dis. 2003;9:1322–5.
22. Navascués A, Rodríguez I, Reparaz J, Salvo S, Gil-Setas A, Martínez Peñuela JM. Detección de cuarto casos de histoplasmosis en Navarra. Rev Iberoamer Micol. 2011;28:194–7.
23. Negroni R, Micosis asociadas al sida. En: Benetucci J. SIDA y enfermedades asociadas. 3rd ed. Buenos Aires: FUNDAI; 2008. p. 325–51.
24. Corti M, Negroni R, Esquivel P, Villafañe MF. Histoplasmosis diseminada en pacientes con sida: Análisis epidemiológico, clínico, microbiológico e inmunológico de 26 pacientes. Enfermedades Emergentes. 2004;6:8–15.
25. Kauffman CA. Diagnosis of histoplasmosis in immunosuppressed patients. Curr Opin Infect Dis. 2008;2008(21):421–5.
26. Huber F, Nacher M, Aznar C, Pierre-Demar M, El Guedi M, Vaz T, et al. AIDS-related *Histoplasma capsulatum var capsulatum* infection: 26 years' experience of French Guiana. AIDS. 2008;22:1047–53.
27. Samayoa B, Roy M, Ahlquist Cleveland A, Medina, Dalia N, et al. High mortality and coinfection in a prospective cohort of human immunodeficiency virus/ acquired immune deficiency syndrome patients with Histoplasmosis in Guatemala. Am J Trop Med Hyg. 2017;97(1):42–8.
28. La Rocco MT, Burgert M. Fungal infections in the transplant recipient and laboratory methods for diagnosis. Rev Iberoamer Micol. 1997;14:143–6.
29. Peddi VR, Hariharan S, First MR. Disseminated histoplasmosis in renal allograft recipients. Clin Transpl. 1996;10:160–5.
30. Marques SA, Hozumi S, Camargo RMP, Carvalho MFC, Marques ME. Histoplasmosis presenting as cellulitis 18 years after renal transplantation. Med Mycol. 2008;46:725–8.

31. Silveira FP, Husain S. Fungal infections in solid organ transplantation. Med Mycol. 2007;46:725–8.
32. Gundacker ND, Baddley JW. Fungal infections in the era of biologic therapy. Curr Clin Micro Rpt. 2015;2:76–83.
33. Luckett K, Dummer JS, Miller G, Hester S, Thomas L. Histoplasmosis in patients with cell-mediated immunodeficiency: human immunodeficiency virus, organ transplantation and tumoral necrosis- α inhibitor. Open Forum of Infectious Diseases. Oxford University Press; 2014. p. 116. https://doi.org/10.1093/ofid7OFU.
34. Olson T, Bongarzt T, Cowson C, Roberts GD, Orenstein R, Matterson EC. Histoplasmosis infection in patients with rheumatoid arthritis, 1998-2009. BCM Infect Dis. 2011;11:145–53.
35. Vergidis R, Avery RK, Wheat LJ, Dotson JL, Assi MA, et al. Histoplasmosis complicating tumoral necrosis factor-α therapy: a retrospective analysis of 98 cases. Clin Infect Dis. 2015;61:409–17.
36. Arechavala A, Robles AM, Negroni R, Bianchi TA. Valor de los métodos directos e indirectos de diagnóstico en las micosis sistémicas asociadas al sida. Rev Med Trop Sao Paulo. 1993;35:163–9.
37. Bianchi MH, Robles AM, Vitale R, Helou S, Arechavala A, Negroni R. Usefulness of blood culture in the diagnosing HIV-related systemic mycoses: evaluation of a manual lysis-centrifugation method. Med Mycol. 2000;32:77–80.
38. Gomez BL, Figueroa JL, Hamilton AJ, Diez S, Rojas M, Tobon AM, et al. Detection of the 70-kilodalton *Histoplasma capsulatum* antigen in serum of histoplasmosis patients: correlation between antigenemia and therapy during follow-up. J Clin Microbiol. 1999;37:675–80.
39. Lindsley MD, Holland HL, Bragg SL, Hurst SF, Wannemuchler KA, Morison CJ. Production and evaluation of reagents for detection of *Histoplasma capsulatum* antigenuria by enzyme immunoassay. Clin Vaccine Immunol. 2007;14
40. Arechavala AI, Bianchi MH, Messina FA, Romero M, Negroni R, Santiso G. Usefulness of an ELISA kit for the detection of *Histoplasma capsulatum* in patients with AIDS. Rev Pat Trop. 2017;46:135–45.
41. Caceres DH, Samayoa BF, Medina NG, Tobon AM, Guzman BJ et al. Multicenter validation of commercial antigenuria reagents to diagnose progressive disseminated histoplasmosis in people living with HIV/AIDS in Two Latin American Countries. J Clin Microbiol. 2018;56: e1950–17. https://doi.org/10.1128/JCM.01950-17
42. Bracca A, Tosello ME, Girardini JE, Amigot SL, Gomez C, Serra E. Molecular detection of *Histoplasma capsulatum var capsulatum* in human clinical samples. J Clin Microbiol. 2003;41:1753–5.
43. Negroni R, Robles AM, Arechavala AI, Taborda A. Itraconazole in human histoplasmosis. Mycoses. 1989;23:123–30.
44. Negroni R, Taborda A, Robles AM, Arechavala AI. Itraconazole in the treatment of histoplasmosis associated with AIDS. Mycoses. 1992;35:281–7.
45. Negroni R, Messina FA, Arechavala AI, Santiso GM, Bianchi MH. Eficacia del tratamiento y de la profilaxis secundaria en la histoplasmosis asociada al sida. Experiencia del Hospital de Infecciosas Francisco J, Muñiz de la ciudad de Buenos Aires Rev, Iberoamer Micol. 2017;34:94–8.
46. Restrepo A, Tobón A, Clark B, Graham DR, et al. Salvage treatment of histoplasmosis with posaconazole. J Infect. 2007;54:319–27.
47. Esteban I, Minces P, De Cristofano A, Negroni R. Histoplasmosis del sistema nervioso central en una paciente pediátrica inmunocompetente. Arch Argent Pediatr. 2016;114:e 171- e 174.
48. Negroni R, Robles AM, Arechavala A, Iovannitti C, Helou S, Kaufman L. Chronic meningoencephalitis due to *Histoplasma capsulatum*. Usefulness of serodiagnostic procedures in diagnosis. Serodiagnosis & Immunotherapy. 1995;7:84–8.
49. Segel M, Rozenman J, Lindsley MD, Tamar L, et al. Histoplasmosis in Israeli travelers. Am J Trop Med Hyg. 2015;92:1168–72.
50. Morgan J, Cano MV, Flikin DR, Phelan M, et al. A large outbreak of histoplasmosis among American travelers associated with a hotel in Acapulco, Mexico. Am J Trop Med Hyg. 2003;69:663–9.

Talaromycosis Caused by *Talaromyces marneffei*

Updated Epidemiology, Clinical Manifestations, Diagnosis and Therapeutics Strategies

Cunwei Cao, Liyan Xi, and Yuping Ran

Key Points

- Talaromycosis caused by thermally dimorphic fungus *Talaromycosis marneffei* is endemic in tropical countries and regions of Asia, particularly in Southeast Asia. It has been increasingly diagnosed well beyond its original endemic areas recently.
- The infection is significant to individuals with advanced HIV disease who have a CD4 count <100 cells/mm^3 and individuals with congenital or other acquired immunodeficiency.
- Talaromycosis usually has atypical presentations, skin lesions can be a single or first-episode symptom of *T. marneffei* infection and have a strong suggestive role in the diagnosis of this disease.

- Diagnosis the infection mainly bases on traditional microscopy with staining methods and mycological culture, as well as antigen or antibody detection, molecular detection, and dermoscopic examination.
- Amphotericin B is the first-line to initial antifungal treatment, other antifungal drugs such as voriconazole and itraconazole showed good anti-talaromycosis activity.

The latest updates on talaromycosis should shed light on how to control this fatal endemic mycosis.

Brief Introduction

Talaromyces marneffei, formerly known as *Penicillium marneffei*, is an important pathogenic thermally dimorphic fungus, which is endemic across a narrow band of tropical countries of South and Southeast Asia [1–6]. The fungus was first isolated in 1956 from the hepatic lesions of a bamboo rat (*Rhizomys sinensis*) in South Vietnam [7]. In 1959, Researcher G. Segretain formally described the mycology characteristic of the fungus and named it as *Penicillium marneffei* in honor of Hubert Marneffe, director of Pasteur Institute in Indochina [8]. Taxonomically, it was originally classified into the Deuteromycotina, *Hyphomycetes, Penicillium* Subgenus

C. Cao
Department of Dermatology and Venereology,
The First Affiliated Hospital of Guangxi Medical
University, Nanning, Guangxi, China

L. Xi
Department of Dermatology, Sun Yat-sen Memorial
Hospital, Sun Yat-sen University, Southern Medical
University, Guangzhou First People's Hospital, South
China University of Technology,
Guangzhou, Guangdong, China
e-mail: xiliyan@mail.sysu.edu.cn

Y. Ran (✉)
Department of Dermatovenereology, West China
Hospital of Sichuan University,
Chengdu, Sichuan, China

W. Robles (ed.), *Skin Disease in Travelers*, Updates in Clinical Dermatology,
https://doi.org/10.1007/978-3-031-57836-6_17

Biverticillium according to its morphology characteristic [8]. Based on phylogenetic and phenotypic analyses, *T. marneffei* was re-classified in 2011 as a member of the family *Trichocomaceae*, order *Eurotiales*, class *Eurotiomycetes*, division *Ascomycota* [9]. This microorganism is the only thermally dimorphic pathogen in more than 200 species of *Talaromyces* and can cause systemic mycosis. Sixty years after the discovery of the pathogen, talaromycosis due to *T. marneffei* was eventually recognized as a significant infectious complication in HIV/AIDS patients and subjects with other immune defects, which was reported not only among patients residing in endemic areas but also in individuals who had traveled to these endemic areas [2].

Epidemiology and Ecology of *T. marneffei* Infection

Endemic Regions

T. marneffei is an AIDS-defining illness in South and Southeast Asia, ranking just after tuberculosis and cryptococcosis [2, 10]. The endemic regions of the fungal disease include Northern Thailand, Vietnam, Northern India, Cambodia, Malaysia, Indonesia, Myanmar, Bangladesh, Laos, Southern China, Hong Kong, and Taiwan areas [4–6, 11–16] (Fig. 1). Travel-related talaromycosis is being increasingly recognized in non-endemic areas such as Australia, Belgium, France, Germany, Japan, the Netherlands, Oman, Ouagadougou, Sweden, Switzerland, Togo, the United Kingdom and the USA [17–25]. In China, the highest incidence areas of *T. marneffei* are Guangxi, Yunnan, Guangdong [4, 26]. As the floating population number increases year by year, the disease has traveled far beyond the original epidemic area, and the other 21 provinces and cities have reported cases successively in China [27–29]. Thus, the current evidence strongly indicates an expansion of the known endemic regions. Lasker and Ran analyzed polymorphic microsatellite markers (PMM) for typing the isolates from China and Thailand, identified distinct allele combinations, suggesting the potential geographic

isolation of populations. Due to the high discriminatory power, reproducibility, and potential for high throughput, PMM analysis may provide a suitable typing method for epidemiologic and surveillance investigations of *T. marneffei* [30].

Ecology and Transmission

Subsequent studies showed that four species of bamboo rats (*Rhizomys sinensis*, *R. pruinosus*, *R. sumatrensis*, and *Cannomys badius*) were important enzootic reservoirs of *T. marneffei* [31–36]. All of them are common in hilly and mountainous areas in Southeast Asia and inhabit underground [37, 38]. Researches have revealed that infection in *R. pruinosus* has a high prevalence in Guangdong and Guangxi Province, of China [37, 39], while infection in *R. sumatrensis* and *C. badius* showed higher prevalence in northern Thailand [36] and India [40]. The distribution of bamboo rats species is generally in accordance with the distribution of *T. marneffei* [2, 35, 41], and multi-locus genotypes show that *T. marneffei* isolates from humans are similar or identical to those infecting bamboo rats [39]. A study shows that among the internal organs of the infected rats, the lungs had the highest positivity, next in decreased order of frequency was the liver. Nevertheless, none of the cultures from the intestine, lymph node, and embryo or amniotic fluid yielded the fungus [35, 37]. An investigation found that approximately 13% of nasal swabs from outdoor dogs in Chiang Mai, Thailand were positive when tested by PCR, but culture results were negative [42]. Besides, *T. marneffei* has been positively detected in soil samples in Thailand, including an elephant camps, a bat cave, and temple grounds [43]. However, having a pig, poultry, or cattle farms and owning pets also were not risk factors for infection [38], and there is no evidence of direct animal-to-human transmission. Although *T. marneffei* has been isolated from bamboo rat feces and soil samples within or surrounding wild bamboo rat's burrow, there is no detection in the artificial farm of bamboo rats. Interestingly, a study demonstrated that *T. marneffei* can survive in sterile soil for

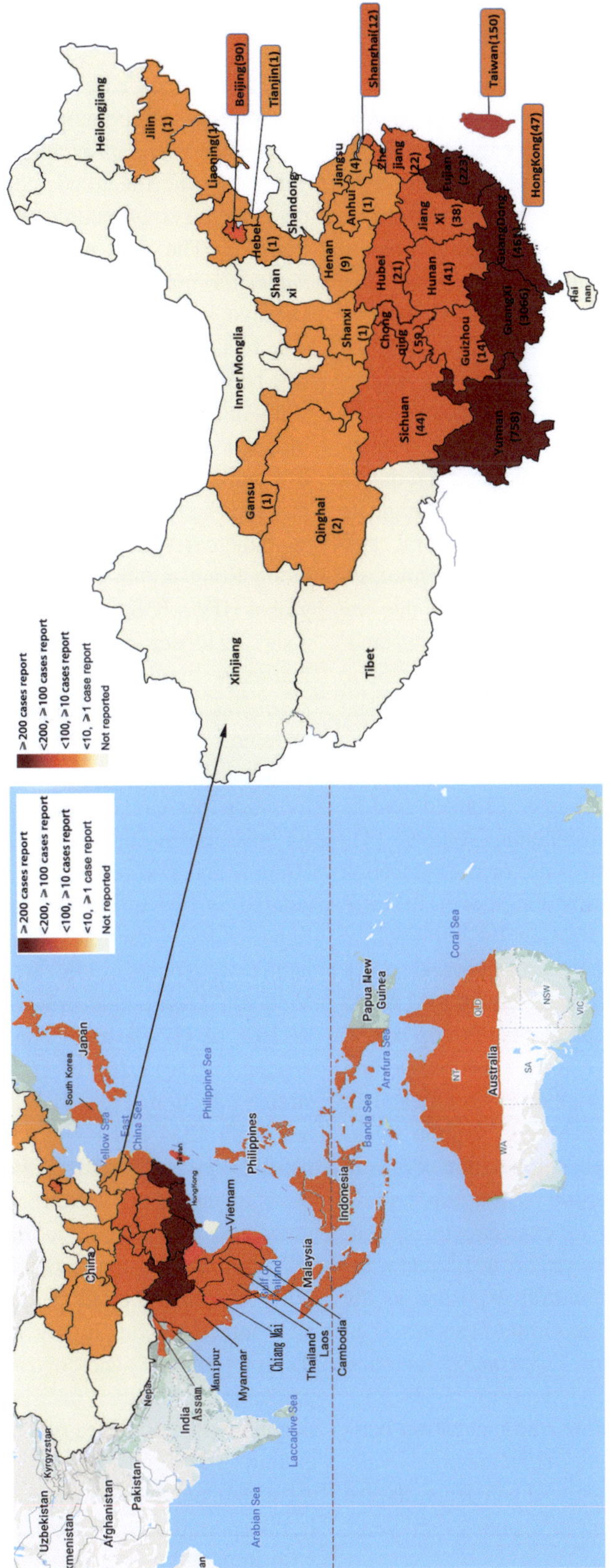

Fig. 1 Geographical distribution of *Talaromyces marneffei* infection in Southeast Asia

several weeks, but can survive for only a few days in nonsterile soil [44], and a research performed by Elizabeth et al. suggesting that survivability in the soil was limited when faced with natural fungal competitors may explain it [43]. In addition, previous studies found that *T. marneffei* was present in occasional bamboo rat burrows and only the samples collected from burrows of *R. sumatrensis* and *R. pruinosus* showed positive for *T. marneffei* [33, 36, 37]. As data showed by Huang, He et al., *T. marneffei* can be isolated from the soil and the bamboo root nearby the burrow, but was not recovered in the bamboo petiole, the leaves and the debris of food from the surrounding areas [37]. So, more research is required to ascertain the specific conditions that regulate the growth of *T. marneffei* in soils in natural environments [43]. Collectively, these epidemiological data suggest humans and bamboo rats are exposed to an as-yet-undiscovered common environment reservoir of infection, in which bamboo rats may be exploited by *T. marneffei* to expand its biomass and biogeography [37, 39].

A laboratory study supports that bamboo rats become infected by inhaling aerosolized conidia originating from environmental sources [41] rather than by fecal-oral route or transplacental crossing and an experimental model in mice reproduced systemic infection by intratracheal instillation of the organism that confirmed it [45]. Studies in Thailand [38] and Vietnam [46] found that more *T. marneffei* infections develop during a rainy season. However, there is no compelling evidence indicating that other environmental or climatological factors including bamboo thickets, forests, precipitation, temperature, or wind are associated with infection by *T. marneffei* [38, 46]. Therefore, history of exposure to or consumption of bamboo rats was not a risk factor for infection; instead, agricultural exposure to the soil during the rainy season [38, 47] serves as an important risk factor for *T. marneffei* infection and can be predicted by humidity levels [46]. According to the literature, the incubation periods of infection with *T. marneffei* are highly variable, which could be 1–3 weeks in acute disease or reactivation of a latent infection several years after exposure [20, 46].

Epidemiology in Subpopulations

The first human case of *T. marneffei* infection occurred as a laboratory-acquired infection in 1959 when Segretain accidentally pricked his finger with a needle filled with *T. marneffei* and developed a small nodule at the site of inoculation [8]. The first natural human case of *T. marneffei* infection was reported in 1973 by DiSalvo and collaborators, the patient was an American minister with Hodgkin's disease who had been living in Southeast Asia [31]. Twelve years later, indigenous cases of *T. marneffei* infection were reported from the Guangxi region in southern China in 1985, these cases were observed between 1964 and 1983 [32]. Additional sporadic cases were reported from Thailand and Hong Kong within the 1980s [7, 9]. When the global HIV-AIDS pandemic arrived in southeast Asia, incidence rate of *T. marneffei* infection markedly increased. From 1988, cases of *T. marneffei* infection started being observed in patients with advanced HIV infection. Over three decades, talaromycosis changed from a rare infection to a leading HIV-associated opportunistic infection in Southeast Asia. In Thailand and Hong Kong, *T. marneffei* infection has been considered as one of the top three AIDS-defining opportunistic infections, alongside tuberculosis and cryptococcosis. In Southern China and Vietnam, *T. marneffei* infection accounts for up to 16% of HIV-hospital admissions and is the second leading cause of HIV-associated bloodstream infections [12–14]. HIV infected individuals with CD4 cell count <100 cells/µL are at particular risk and make up the majority of infections in regions of endemicity [15]. It is also associated with a higher mortality rate than most HIV-associated complications in Southern China [16]. In recent decades, improved treatment of HIV infection with highly active antiretroviral therapy (HAART) and control of the HIV/AIDS epidemic with other measures have led to a decline in the incidence of *T. marneffei* infection among HIV-infected patients. However, an increasing number of *T. marneffei* infections have been reported among non-HIV-infected patients with impaired cell-mediated immunity [17, 18].

Anti-interferon-gamma autoantibody-associated immunodeficiency is associated with severe or persistent infections caused by *T. marneffei* in adult non-HIV-infected patients [18, 19]. The affected patients have high-titer serum neutralizing anti-IFN-γ autoantibodies that inhibit STAT1 phosphorylation and IL-12 production, leading to a severely compromised Th1 response [48]. Talaromycosis caused by *T. marneffei* was also reported in other secondary immunodeficiency conditions, such as autoimmune diseases requiring corticosteroids and/or other immunosuppressive therapy, solid or haematological malignancies, solid organ or haematopoietic stem cell transplantation, and use of novel target therapy such as monoclonal antibodies against CD20 and kinase inhibitors [4, 32, 49–57].

In literature, the proportion of *T. marneffei* infection in children is about 6–7.5%, age ranged from 3 months to 16 years [27, 58]. Unlike the previous reports with most HIV-infected pediatric cases, recent studies showed most pediatric patients were HIV-negative [59]. *T. marneffei* infection in these HIV-negative children were usually associated with various forms of immune-related underlying diseases and primary immunodeficiency (PIDs), such as idiopathic CD4 lymphopenia, leukemia, hyper-IgM syndrome, hyper-IgE syndrome, mutations in CYBB, CD40L, or gain-of-function mutation in STAT1/STAT3 pathway, resulting in a functional defect of the IFN-γ and IL-17 immune response [58, 60–63].

Thus, the epidemiology in subpopulations of *T. marneffei* infection has changed during the past three decades. *T. marneffei* infection is nowadays not solely limited to HIV-infected patients. This suggests that disseminated talaromycosis should be an indicator to look for underlying primary immunodeficiency after excluding secondary causes.

Clinical Manifestations

Talaromycosis would present various degrees of severity depending on the underlying immunocompromising condition and the timing of diagnosis. In early stage, *T. marneffei* infection could only involve single organ, such as cornea or lungs, presented focal symptoms without systemic involvement [21, 64]. Disseminated infections were usually associated with HIV/AIDS patients or immunosuppressed HIV-negative patients with the pathogen isolated from more than one body site (noncontiguous) or from blood or bone marrow. The symptoms and signs of disseminated *T. marneffei* infection are non-specific and develop over weeks to months, including fevers, cough, weight loss, fatigue, abdominal distension, diarrhea, hepatosplenomegaly, and lymphadenopathy, which often misdiagnose as tuberculosis, or other invasive mycoses, makes differential diagnosis problematic. Central nervous system involvement is an emerging syndrome in *T. marneffei* infected HIV-positive patients, presented with an acute onset of altered mental status with confusion, agitation, or depressed consciousness, and the case-fatality rate in these kind of patients was about 80% [65, 66].

Cutaneous manifestation is an important aspect of any disease for the clinicians to get a correct diagnosis. Accounting for 65–85% *T. marneffei* infected patients occurred skin lesions. It often becomes the first sign to attract attention in disseminated cases and has a strong suggestive role in the diagnosis of this disease [4, 67]. Characteristic lesions are papules with central necrosis, predominantly located on the face, mouth, and upper trunk (Fig. 2) [4, 67, 68].

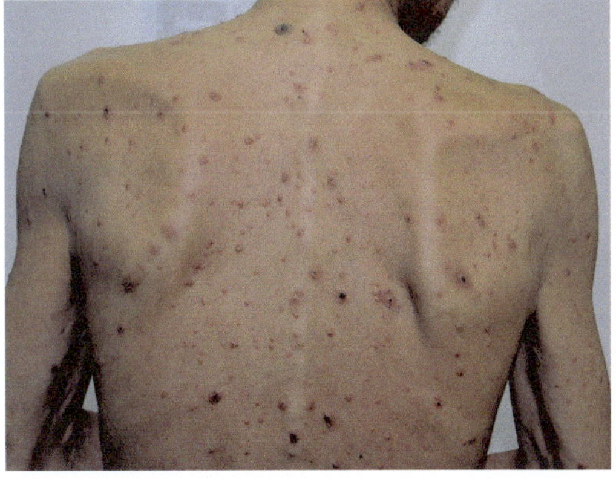

Fig. 2 A typical disseminated *Talaromyces marneffei* infection in AIDS patient presented with extensive characteristic cutaneous papules with central necrosis, nodules, ulcers, and crusts, predominantly located on face, mouth, and upper trunk

Also, papules, pustules, nodules, subcutaneous abscesses, cysts, or ulcers can also occur. All of these eruptions were caused by *T. marneffei* direct through blood circulation disseminated infection. However, reactive rashes were recently recognized association with *T. marneffei* infection, such as Sweet's syndrome, erythema nodosum, exanthematous pustulosis, as well as pustular psoriasis, which can occur in non-HIV patients who suffered from adult-onset immunodeficiency syndrome due to anti-IFN-γ autoantibodies. Whereas, erythematous nodules, verrucous lesions, or erythematous plaques have been reported as unmasking IRIS in *T. marneffei*-associated immune reconstitution inflammatory syndrome (IRIS) in patients starting HAART [68, 69].

According to the literature, when compared to HIV-infected patients, *T. marneffei* infected in HIV-negative patients usually have a longer diagnostic interval, a higher percentage of dyspnea, are significantly older, less likely to have fever, splenomegaly, and umbilicated skin lesions, and more likely to have Sweet's syndrome and osteoarticular lesions. The non-HIV-infected patients also had higher leukocyte, CD4 lymphocyte, and platelet counts, lower alanine transaminase level and blood culture-positive rate [29, 49].

Diagnosis

Susceptibility Risk Factors of *T. marneffei* Infection

A patient with the following susceptibility risk factors should be suspected of talaromycosis: (1). The individuals with fever, weight loss, fatigue, hepatosplenomegaly, lymphadenopathy, respiratory abnormalities and don't respond to antibiotic treatment; (2). The individuals with advanced HIV disease who have a CD4 count <100 cells/mm^3; or with a primary immunocompromised condition, such as anti-IFN-γ autoantibodies associated adult-onset immunodeficiency syndrome, mutations in CYBB, CD40L, or gain-of-function mutation in the STAT1/STAT3 pathways associated pediatric talaromycosis; or with secondary immunodeficiency conditions other than HIV (e.g., autoimmune diseases requiring corticosteroids and/or other immunosuppressive therapy, solid or hematological malignancies, solid organ or hematopoietic stem cell transplantation, and novel target therapies such as monoclonal antibodies against CD20 and kinase inhibitors); (3). Individual resident in endemic areas or with history of travel to the endemic regions.

Diagnosis by Staining Methods and Cultures

Direct microscopic examination, mycological culture, and histopathology are traditional gold standard diagnostic methods which could identify *T. marneffei* from clinical specimens. Microscopic examination of a direct smear of bone marrow aspirates, touch smear of skin biopsy, lymph node aspirate, or broncho alveolar lavage fluid (BALF) can lead to rapid presumptive diagnosis [2, 10, 70]. In patients with heavy fungemia, the organisms may be seen on the peripheral blood smear [71]. In the histopathological examination of tissue sections, *T. marneffei* presents as yeast-like cells distributed within and outside macrophages and histiocytes, 2–6 µm in diameter with oval, round, elongated, sausage-like shapes, divide by fission [10]. Transmission electron microscopic observation of the infected tissue showed oval yeast cells were phagocytosed within distended histocytes, and some had a typical septum [72] (Fig. 3). The cross-wall formation can differentiate yeast cells of *T. marneffei* from those of *Histoplasma capsulatum*, which also appear as intracellular yeasts. The histopathological characteristic of *T. marneffei* infected tissues manifested as granulomatous, suppurative reaction and non-reactive necrosis. Staining methods Giemsa, Wright, GMS, periodic acid-Schiff stains, as well as optical brighteners (calcofluor white) could be used for staining the direct smears microscopic examination (Fig. 4). Whereas, Grocott methenamine silver or PAS stain would be preferable for histopathological examination.

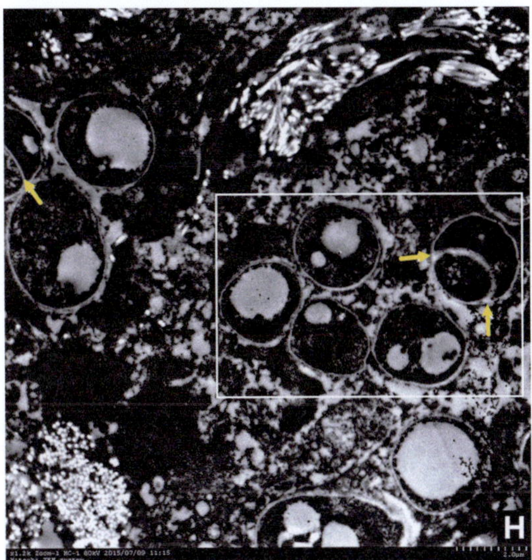

Fig. 3 Transmission electron microscopic observation of the oval yeast cells were phagocytosed within distended histocytes. Note the transverse septum shown by the arrows. This is the characteristic ultrastructure of *Talaromyces marneffei* yeast cells inside histocytes

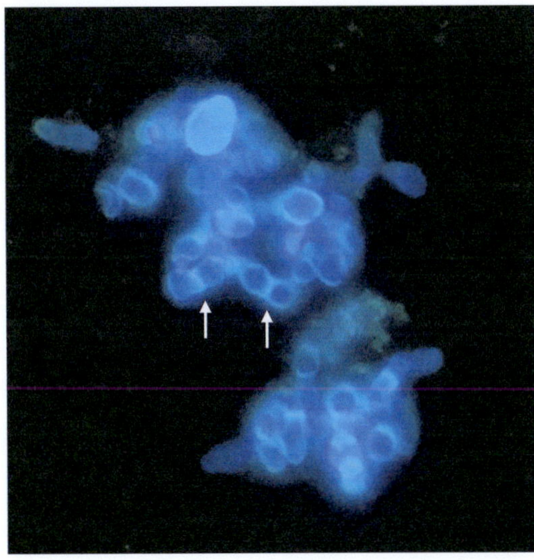

Fig. 4 Calcofluor white staining the direct smears microscopic examination of broncho alveolar lavage fluid (BALF), the arrowheads highlight the midline septum in a dividing yeast cell characteristic of *Talaromyces marneffei* (×1000)

Mycological culture to isolate *T. marneffei* from all tissues or body fluids could provide a definitive diagnosis of talaromycosis. The high sensitivity samples are bone marrow (100%), skin biopsy (90%), and blood (76%), respectively [73]. Identification of *T. marneffei* is based upon the morphology of the colony, the organism microscopic morphology, and its mold-to-yeast conversion when transferred from 25 °C to 37 °C [74]. When cultured *T. marneffei* on Sabouraud dextrose agar medium at 37 °C, yeast-like colonies developed. Under microscopy, septated sausage-like yeast cells could be seen; when cultured on Sabouraud dextrose agar medium at 25 °C, the *T. marneffei* colony is velvety pink-white or yellow-green and producing diffusible red pigment in the culture medium (Fig. 5). However, there are other *Talaromyces* or related *Penicillium* species may produce similar pigments and exhibit similar morphological and colonial appearances at 25 °C [75–77]. Morphology observation using optical microscopy and scanning electron microscopy showed septate hyphae with branched or unbranched conidiophores with secondary branches. Phialides grouped in brush-like clusters (penicilli) at the end of conidiophores are arranged in whorls; flask-shaped phialides bearing unbranched chains of smooth or rough, and round to ovoid conidia (2–3 μm diameter) are also seen. When cultured at 37 °C on brain-heart infusion or blood agar or upon entering the human body, conidia convert to the pathogenic yeast phase divide by fission [78]. Cultures would take 3–14 days to grow and to demonstrate temperature-regulated dimorphism, resulting in diagnostic delay and raised mortality, particularly in patients without skin lesions [79]. A comparative analysis of gene expression in mycelial- and yeast-phase *T. marneffei* cells using high-throughput DNA microarrays. A total of 1884 differentially expressed genes with annotations in the gene ontology (GO) database were identified between *T. marneffei* mycelial and yeast cells. These differentially expressed genes mainly belong to 18 categories in the organism's ontology, including reproduction, immunity, metabolism, signaling, etc. Bioinformatics suggests that these differentially expressed genes may help explain the resistance to adverse environments and the virulence of *T. marneffei* [80].

Fig. 5 When cultured *T. marneffei* on Sabouraud dextrose agar (SDA) at 37 °C, yeast-like colonies developed (**a**). Under microscopy, the arrowheads indicate the transverse septum of the sausage-like yeast cells (**c**, ×400); at 25 °C, the colony is velvety pink-white or yellow-green and producing diffusible red pigment into the medium (**b**). Under microscopy, septate hyphae with branched or unbranched conidiophores with secondary branches. Phialides grouped in brush-like clusters (penicilli) at the end of conidiophores are arranged in whorls (in cycle) (**d**, ×400)

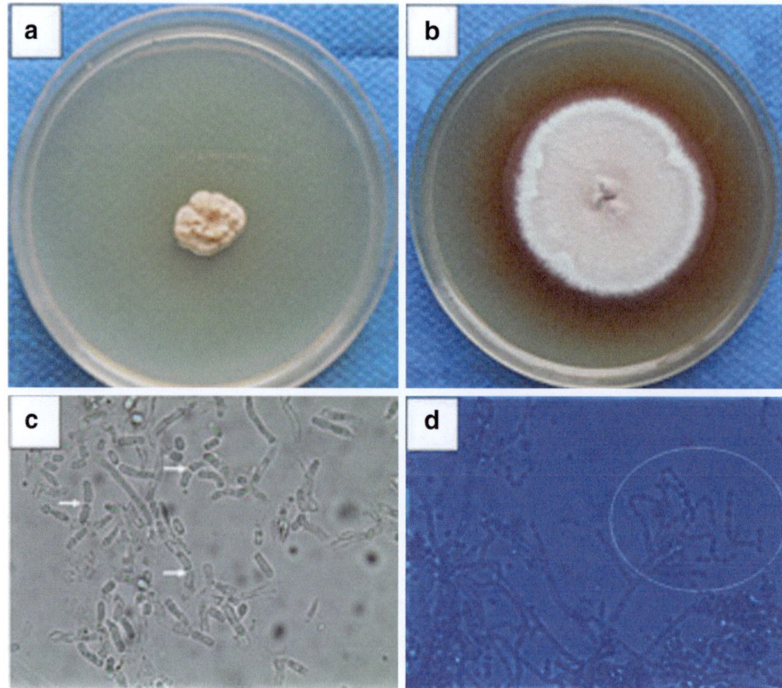

Non-culture-Based Diagnostic Methods

The methods for detecting certain special components of *T. marneffei*, such as an antigen, antibody, DNA fragment or protein have been developed to diagnose talaromycosis rapidly.

Antigen or Antibody Detection

Mp1p is a special secreted cell wall mannoprotein which was found to be useful for the serological diagnosis of *T. marneffei* infection. The monoclonal-antibody-based Mp1p antigen detection ELISA was developed. Evaluation of the test revealed high specificity (100%) and did not cross-react with other fungi [67]. It could detect *T. marneffei* from many kinds of clinical samples, such as sera, plasma, and urine. A prospective study was performed on 521 symptomatic hospitalized AIDS patients followed over 6 months in Vietnam, the assay detected infection up to 16 weeks before cultures turning positive, was superior to cultures when from the same patients with a combined sensitivity of 98% (compared to cultures of 84% in 80 talaromycosis patients),

and had a specificity of 96%. Urine samples yielded the highest sensitivity and specificity, followed by plasma and serum samples [81]. The other retrospective study in southern China showed that the same assay could detect *T. marneffei* Mp1p antigen in 9.4% of 8131 banked serum samples from HIV patients in outpatient clinics [48]. These data demonstrate that the Mp1p ELISA is highly accurate as a rapid diagnostic tool and has the potential as a screening tool to identify sub-clinical infections for early treatment to prevent talaromycosis. A commercial Mp1p ELISA (by Wantai Beijing) was approved in 2018 in China for clinical use. Meanwhile, the anti-Mp1p antibody was also used in an ELISA-based method for the detection of the mannoprotein Mp1p in the serum of patients [82], which has variable sensitivities, ranging from 30% to 80%, in HIV patients with talaromycosis. The combined antibody and antigen tests for the diagnosis of *T. marneffei* infection had a sensitivity of 88% (23 of 26), with a positive predictive value of 100% and a negative predictive value of 96% [26, 53]. However, the sensitivity of both methods used in no-HIV is limited.

Several additional serologic methods have been developed as a screening tool for diagnosis *T. marneffei* infection. The commercial Platelia *Aspergillus* galactomannan assay cross-reacts with *T. marneffei* and has a sensitivity ranging from 73% to 81% in patients with or without HIV, especially in patients with fungemia (95%), at a cut-off index of 0.5 [49, 83]. A commercial β-d-glucan antigen detection test that can also be useful as a screening tool and adjunct to diagnosis *T. marneffei* infection [84, 85].

Molecular Detection

Several PCR-based assays (e.g., nested-PCR, TaqMan real time PCR, multiplex ligation-dependent probe amplification, loop-mediated isothermal amplification), targeting the ribosomal DNA (ITS1-5.8S-ITS2, 18S), or the MP1 gene have been developed to detect *T. marneffei* in clinical samples including whole blood, plasma or paraffin-embedded tissue [73, 86–90]. Evaluation of the tests revealed a high diagnostic specificity of the assay (100%), while diagnostic sensitivity ranged from 67 to 86%, respectively. These assays provide useful tools for the rapid diagnosis of *T. marneffei* infection [49, 54, 55]. However, they have been tested in small sample sizes, and none has been prospectively validated or commercially developed for clinical use.

All these methods require the physician to suspect the pathogen before examination, which might limit the application clinically. Next-generation sequencing based on metagenomics (mNGS) has been successfully applied in the diagnosis of disseminated *T. marneffei* infection, which does not depend upon prior assumptions from the physicians and provides a new technique for rapid etiological diagnosis [90]. mNGS availability is limited especially in the resource-limited settings. Overall, it might be prudent to use a combination of several methods to achieve the highest diagnostic yield [91].

Matrix-Assisted Laser Desorption/ Ionization-Time Of Flight (MALDI-TOF) Method

The MALDI-TOF is a rapid and reliable approach for the identification of a variety of pathogenic fungi and has recently been used for accurate discrimination *T. marneffei* isolates from morphologically similar, nonpathogenic relatives. The cultured specimens could be identified by MALDI-TOF based on either an in-house database generated from institution's *T. marneffei* clinical strain collection [29, 56] or the comprehensive NIH MDL Mold Library [57]. The MALDI-TOF represents a rapid and reliable tool for downstream fungal identification, eliminating the need to demonstrate thermal dimorphism and can be performed by relatively inexperienced operators; however, the current cost of the MALDI-TOF machine is likely to be prohibitive in resource-limited settings.

Dermoscopic Examination

On polarized dermoscopic examination, four types of skin lesion could be observed in *T. marneffei* infection patients: molluscum-like, folliculitis-like or acne-like, xanthoma-like rashes and ulcers that were pervaded by hemispherical papules, nodules, and ulcers. One significant characteristic feature on dermoscopic examination was central necrosis, known as a "Jade Pendant" sign. Papules or nodules with an umbilicated notch centrally were analogous to molluscum contagiosum; papules or nodules with scabs in the middle and hairs grown in or around were similar to folliculitis or acne; yellowish papules or nodules without any scabs, umbilicated notch with hairs had a smooth surface resembling xanthoma. Additionally, different vessels buried inside or around the lesion was another characteristic feature. Punctiform, tufted, lumbricoid, and hairpin vessels appeared irregularly in almost every lesion and were considered to be caused by capillary hyperplasia and telangiectasia. Evenly distributed hemispherical papules or nodules with visible central necrosis and irregular vessels are typical lesions of this disease [68]. The dermoscopic appearance which may aid in early diagnosis *T. marneffei* infection and help in distinguishing it from similar appearing entities such as cutaneous histoplasmosis, blastomycosis, and leishmaniasis. Under dermoscopy, histoplasmosis has arborizing telangiectasias on the periphery of the lesion and superficial scaling. Blastomycosis shows overlapping pink-colored papillomatous structures and irregular vessels whereas leishmaniasis is characterized by burst star-whitish appearance and hairpin vessels. Clinically, if a patient exhibits central necrotic papules or nodules with irregular vessels, along with biopsy revealing dermal capillaries infiltrated by yeast cells, should be suspected for disseminated *T. marneffei* infection.

Imaging Examinations

Chest CT scan or X-ray findings are broad and include infiltrates or nodules, focal lung consolidation, ground-glass shadows diffuse miliary lesions, nodular bump. Some cases combined with enlarged hilar or mediastinum lymph nodes, pleural effusion, and cavity lesion. Rare case involving the main trachea, causing subsequent structural damage to the tracheal cartilage, severe tracheostenosis, and tracheal absence. Osteolytic lesions mainly occur in non-HIV patients, involving bones have moth-eaten pattern destruction, periosteal proliferation, fracture, and surrounding soft-tissue swelling [92, 93]. Abdominal ultrasounds frequently show markedly enlarged liver and spleen and intraabdominal lymph node enlargement.

In Vitro Drug Susceptibility, Therapeutics Strategies, and Prevention

In Vitro Drug Susceptibility

At present, no guideline is available for *in vitro* antifungal susceptibility testing of *T. marneffei*. The common antifungal susceptibility testing methods for *T. marneffei* include broth microdilution method (The Clinical and Laboratory Standards Institute microdilution method (CLSI M27-A3)) or E-test. Studies using different methods showed that most of azole antifungal agents had high activity against *T. marneffei*, low MICs for itraconazole ($\leq$0.008 µg/ml), voriconazole (<0.063 µg/ml) and posaconazole (<0.002 µg/ml), while MIC intermediate to high for fluconazole (0.3–7.9 µg/ml). Amphotericin B showed

intermediate antifungal activity (0.25–1.0 µg/ml); whereas the MICs of anidulafungin and caspofungin were 2–8 µg/ml, micafungin was >8 µg/ml, indicated [94–97], suggesting that echinocandins may be less effective against *T. marneffei* [59, 60]. These MICs generally correlate with good anti-talaromycosis activity observed for itraconazole and amphotericin B and correlate with poor clinical efficacy for fluconazole in clinical practice [45].

Additionally, traditional herbs, like berberine, were found to have *in vitro* antifungal activity against *T. marneffei*, especially in combination with antifungal agents [98].

Therapeutic Strategies in Talaromycosis with or Without HIV-Infected

Amphotericin B deoxycholate (D-AmB) is the first-line initial antifungal treatment for severe *T. marneffei* infection. International guidelines recommend for talaromycosis in HIV-infected patients is: D-AmB; 0.6–1.0 mg/kg per day for 2 weeks, followed by itraconazole 400 mg per day for 10 weeks, then with itraconazole 200 mg per day as secondary prophylaxis until CD4 counts are >100 cells per µL for at least 6 months [99, 100]. Liposomal amphotericin B (L-AmB) at 3–5 mg/kg per day is effective and better tolerated than D-AmB. However, the drug is not available in a resource-limited situation [101]. Voriconazole is an effective therapeutic option for disseminated talaromycosis, given 6 mg/kg BID for 1 day, 4 mg/kg BID for 10–14 days, followed by oral voriconazole 200 mg BID for 12 weeks in HIV patients. It has been reported that voriconazole is effective in the treatment of patients who did not respond to an initial amphotericin B therapy [102, 103]. Considering it can be administered by the oral route or by using intravenous-to-oral step-down therapy, voriconazole has the potential to be more convenient than the currently recommended treatment regimen. In a multicenter open-label, non-inferiority trial comparing itraconazole (600 mg per day for 3 days, followed by 400 mg per day, for 11 days) with standard D-AmB initial therapy in HIV-infected talaromycosis patients reported mortality after 2 weeks is 7.4% and 6.5%, and after 6 months is 21.0% and 11.3%, respectively. The study indicated D-AmB was superior to itraconazole as initial treatment for talaromycosis [104].

For prevention, HIV-infected people living or traveling in endemic areas, primary prophylactic treatment with itraconazole is recommended when the CD4 cell count is less than 100/mm^3. Itraconazole can be taken orally for 200 mg once a day until CD4 cell count >100/ mm^3 and more than 6 months [98].

At present, the standard recommendation regarding the appropriate duration of treatment and prophylaxis of *T. marneffei* among HIV-uninfected patients is unavailable. In literature, the duration of treatment was significantly longer in HIV-uninfected patients compared to HIV-infected patients, and some cases may require lifelong treatment.

Special Population: Treatment of Non-HIV *T. marneffei* Infection in Children

Clinical experience with the treatment of non-HIV *T. marneffei* pediatric patients is limited. Studies showed when treated with voriconazole 7 mg/kg twice per day, for at least 12 days, followed by oral for at least 13 weeks, 70–80% children had a complete response to therapy at primary and long-term follow-up assessment [92, 102]. No adverse events were recorded during and after the treatment. D-AmB 1 mg/kg/d has been used for *T. marneffei* infected children, but the nephrotoxic side effects are significant. Regarding the dose-dependent nephrotoxicity and electrolyte imbalance related to D-AmB treatment, pharmacokinetics and pharmacodynamics study has been used to evaluate the association between D-AmB exposure and response in the treatment of taralomycosis [105].

Despite antifungal therapy, case fatality rates among adult patients with or without HIV-infected are 20%, 29.4%, respectively. Whereas, mortality in the pediatric patients with talaromycosis could be up to 55% [56], higher than the adult patients, due to underlying immunodeficiency and delated treatment.

Summary and Conclusions

In the last decades, great progress has been made on investigation and understanding the epidemiology, susceptible population, pathogenesis, clinical characteristics, diagnosis, and treatment of talaromycosis. Talaromycosis remains a significant infectious complication for patients with HIV/AIDS and other immunodeficiencies. The disease is increasingly diagnosed well beyond its original endemic areas. There is an urgent need for the development of rapid and affordable point-of-care diagnostic tests. More clinical studies are also needed to define the best therapeutic options for the management of talaromycosis patients.

References

1. Cao C, Xi L, Chaturvedi V. Talaromycosis (Penicilliosis) due to T*alaromyces (Penicillium) marneffei:* insights into the clinical trends of a major fungal disease 60 years after the discovery of the pathogen. Mycopathologia. 2019;184(6):709–20.
2. Vanittanakom N, Cooper CR Jr, Fisher MC, Sirisanthana T. *Penicillium marneffei* infection and recent advances in the epidemiology and molecular biology aspects. Clin Microbiol Rev. 2006;19(1):95–110.
3. Ustianowski AP, Sieu TP, Day JN. *Penicillium marneffei* infection in HIV. Curr Opin Infect Dis. 2008;21(1):31–6.
4. Hu Y, Zhang J, Li X, Yang Y, Zhang Y, Ma J, Xi L. *Penicillium marneffei* infection: an emerging disease in mainland China. Mycopathologia. 2013;175(1–2):57–67.
5. Imwidthaya P. Update of *Penicillosis marneffei* in Thailand. Mycopathologia. 1994;127(3):135–7.
6. Tsang CC, Lau SKP, Woo PCY. Sixty years from Segretain's description: what have we learned and should learn about the basic mycology of *Talaromyces marneffei*? Mycopathologia. 2019;184(6):721–9.
7. Capponi M, Segretain G, Sureau P. Penicillosis from Rhizomys sinensis. Bull Soc Pathol Exot Filiales. 1956;49(3):418–21.
8. Segretain G. *Penicillium marneffei n.sp.*, agent of a mycosis of the reticuloendothelial system. Mycopathol Mycol Appl. 1959;11:327–53.

9. Samson RA, Yilmaz N, Houbraken J, Spierenburg H, Seifert KA, Peterson SW, Varga J, Frisvad JC. Phylogeny and nomenclature of the genus *Talaromyces* and taxa accommodated in *Penicillium subgenus* Biverticillium. Stud Mycol. 2011;70(1):159–83.

10. Liyan X, Changming L, Xianyi Z, Luxia W, Suisheng X. Fifteen cases of penicilliosis in Guangdong, China. Mycopathologia. 2004;158(2):151–5.

11. Yuen KY, Wong SS, Tsang DN, Chau PY. Serodiagnosis of *Penicillium marneffei* infection. Lancet. 1994;344(8920):444–5.

12. Jayanetra P, Nitiyanant P, Ajello L, Padhye AA, Lolekha S, Atichartakarn V, Vathesatogit P, Sathaphatayavongs B, Prajaktam R. *Penicilliosis marneffei* in Thailand: report of five human cases. Am J Trop Med Hyg. 1984;33(4):637–44.

13. Deng ZL, Connor DH. Progressive disseminated penicilliosis caused by *Penicillium marneffei*. Report of eight cases and differentiation of the causative organism from Histoplasma capsulatum. Am J Clin Pathol. 1985;84(3):323–7.

14. Cao C, Bulmer G, Li J, Liang L, Lin Y, Xu Y, Luo Q. Indigenous case of disseminated histoplasmosis from the *Penicillium marneffei* endemic area of China. Mycopathologia. 2010;170(1):47–50.

15. Ranjana KH, Priyokumar K, Singh TJ, Gupta CC, Sharmila L, Singh PN, Chakrabarti A. Disseminated *Penicillium marneffei* infection among HIV-infected patients in Manipur state, India. J Infect. 2002;45(4):268–71.

16. Tsui WM, Ma KF, Tsang DN. Disseminated *Penicillium marneffei* infection in HIV-infected subject. Histopathology. 1992;20(4):287–93.

17. Liu MT, Wong CK, Fung CP. Disseminated *Penicillium marneffei* infection with cutaneous lesions in an HIV-positive patient. Br J Dermatol. 1994;131(2):280–3.

18. Antinori S, Gianelli E, Bonaccorso C, Ridolfo AL, Croce F, Sollima S, Parravicini C. Disseminated *Penicillium marneffei* infection in an HIV-positive Italian patient and a review of cases reported outside endemic regions. J Travel Med. 2006;13(3):181–8.

19. Castro-Lainez MT, Sierra-Hoffman M, Adams R, Howell A, Hoffman-Roberts H, Fader R, Arroliga AC, Jinadatha C. *Talaromyces marneffei* infection in a non-HIV non-endemic population. IDCases. 2018;12:21–4.

20. Julander I, Petrini B. *Penicillium marneffei* infection in a Swedish HIV-infected immunodeficient narcotic addict. Scand J Infect Dis. 1997;29(3):320–2.

21. De Monte A, Risso K, Normand AC, Boyer G, L'Ollivier C, Marty P, Gari-Toussaint M. Chronic pulmonary penicilliosis due to *Penicillium marneffei*: late presentation in a french traveler. J Travel Med. 2014;21(4):292–4.

22. Patassi AA, Saka B, Landoh DE, Kotosso A, Mawu K, Halatoko WA, Wateba MI, Adjoh K, Tidjani O, Salmon D, et al. First observation in a non-endemic country (Togo) of *Penicillium marneffei* infection in a human immunodeficiency virus-infected patient: a case report. BMC Res Notes. 2013;6:506.

23. Pautler KB, Padhye AA, Ajello L. Imported *penicilliosis marneffei* in the United States: report of a second human infection. Sabouraudia. 1984;22(5):433–8.

24. Surja SS, Adawiyah R, Houbraken J, Rozaliyani A, Sjam R, Yunihastuti E, Wahyuningsih R. *Talaromyces atroroseus* in HIV and non-HIV patient: a first report from Indonesia. Med Mycol. 2019. myz090. Online ahead of print;58:560.

25. Guiguemde KT, Sawadogo PM, Zida A, Cisse M, Sangare I, Bamba S. First case report of *Talaromyces marneffei* infection in HIV-infected patient in the city of Ouagadougou (Burkina Faso). Med Mycol Case Rep. 2019;26:10–2.

26. Jiang J, Meng S, Huang S, et al. Effects of Talaromyces marneffei infection on mortality of HIV/AIDS patients in southern China: a retrospective cohort study. Clin Microbiol Infect. 2019;25(2):233–41.

27. Guo J, Li BK, Li TM, Wei FL, Fu YJ, Zheng YQ, Pan KS, Huang CY, Cao CW. Characteristics and prognosis of *Talaromyces marneffei* infection in non-HIV-infected children in southern China. Mycopathologia. 2019;184(6):735–45.

28. Zheng J, Gui X, Cao Q, Yang R, Yan Y, Deng L, Lio J. A clinical study of acquired immunodeficiency syndrome associated *Penicillium marneffei* infection from a non-endemic area in China. PLoS One. 2015;10(6):e0130376.

29. Li HR, Cai SX, Chen YS, Yu ME, Xu NL, Xie BS, Lin M, Hu XL. Comparison of *Talaromyces marneffei* infection in human immunodeficiency virus-positive and human immunodeficiency virus-negative patients from Fujian, China. Chin Med J (Engl). 2016;129(9):1059–65.

30. Lasker BA, Ran Y. Analysis of polymorphic microsatellite markers for typing *Penicillium marneffei* isolates. J Clin Microbiol. 2004;42(4):1483–90.

31. Segretain G. Description d'une nouvelle espece de *Penicillium*: *Penicillium marneffei n.sp*. Bull Soc Mycol Fr. 1959;75:412–6.

32. DiSalvo AF, Fickling AM, Ajello L. Infection caused by *Penicillium marneffei*: description of first natural infection in man. Am J Clin Pathol. 1973;60(2):259–63.

33. Deng ZL, Yun M, Ajello L. Human *penicilliosis marneffei* and its relation to the bamboo rat (*Rhizomys pruinosus*). J Med Vet Mycol. 1986;24(5):383–9.

34. Gugnani H, Fisher MC, Paliwal-Johsi A, Vanittanakom N, Singh I, Yadav PS. Role of *Cannomys badius* as a natural animal host of *Penicillium marneffei* in India. J Clin Microbiol. 2004;42(11):5070–5.

35. Ajello L, Padhye AA, Sukroongreung S, Nilakul CH, Tantimavanic S. Occurrence of *Penicillium marneffei* infections among wild bamboo rats in Thailand. Mycopathologia. 1995;131(1):1–8.

36. Chariyalertsak S, Vanittanakom P, Nelson KE, Sirisanthana T, Vanittanakom N. *Rhizomys suma-*

trensis and *Cannomys badius*, new natural animal hosts of *Penicillium marneffei*. J Med Vet Mycol. 1996;34(2):105–10.

37. Huang X, He G, Lu S, Liang Y, Xi L. Role of *Rhizomys pruinosus* as a natural animal host of *Penicillium marneffei* in Guangdong, China. Microb Biotechnol. 2015;8(4):659–64.

38. Chariyalertsak S, Sirisanthana T, Supparatpinyo K, Praparattanapan J, Nelson KE. Case-control study of risk factors for *Penicillium marneffei* infection in human immunodeficiency virus-infected patients in northern Thailand. Clin Infect Dis. 1997;24(6):1080–6.

39. Cao C, Liang L, Wang W, Luo H, Huang S, Liu D, Xu J, Henk DA, Fisher MC. Common reservoirs for *Penicillium marneffei* infection in humans and rodents, China. Emerg Infect Dis. 2011;17(2):209–14.

40. Gugnani HC, Paliwal-Joshi A, Rahman H, Padhye AA, Singh TS, Das TK, Khanal B, Bajaj R, Rao S, Chukhani R. Occurrence of pathogenic fungi in soil of burrows of rats and of other sites in bamboo plantations in India and Nepal. Mycoses. 2007;50(6):507–11.

41. Imwidthaya P, Thipsuvan K, Chaiprasert A, Danchaivijitra S, Sutthent R, Jearanaisilavong J. *Penicillium marneffei*: types and drug susceptibility. Mycopathologia. 2001;149(3):109–15.

42. Chaiwun B, Vanittanakom N, Jiviriyawat Y, Rojanasthien S, Thorner P. Investigation of dogs as a reservoir of *Penicillium marneffei* in northern Thailand. Int J Infect Dis. 2011;15(4):e236–9.

43. Pryce-Miller E, Aanensen D, Vanittanakom N, Fisher MC. Environmental detection of *Penicillium marneffei* and growth in soil microcosms in competition with T*alaromyces stipitatus*. Fungal Ecol. 2008;1(1):49–56.

44. Joshi A, Gugnani H, Vijayan V. Survival of *Penicillium marneffei* in sterile and unsterile soil. J Med Mycol. 2003;13:211–2.

45. Kudeken N, Kawakami K, Kusano N, Saito A. Cell-mediated immunity in host resistance against infection caused by *Penicillium marneffei*. J Med Vet Mycol. 1996;34(6):371–8.

46. Bulterys PL, Le T, Quang VM, Nelson KE, Lloyd-Smith JO. Environmental predictors and incubation period of AIDS-associated *Penicillium marneffei* infection in Ho Chi Minh City, Vietnam. Clin Infect Dis. 2013;56(9):1273–9.

47. Chariyalertsak S, Sirisanthana T, Supparatpinyo K, Nelson KE. Seasonal variation of disseminated *Penicillium marneffei* infections in northern Thailand: a clue to the reservoir? J Infect Dis. 1996;173(6):1490–3.

48. Browne SK, Burbelo PD, Chetchotisakd P, Suputtamongkol Y, Kiertiburanakul S, Shaw PA, Kirk JL, Jutivorakool K, Zaman R, Ding L, et al. Adult-onset immunodeficiency in Thailand and Taiwan. N Engl J Med. 2012;367(8):725–34.

49. Kawila R, Chaiwarith R, Supparatpinyo K. Clinical and laboratory characteristics of *penicilliosis marneffei* among patients with and without HIV infection in northern Thailand: a retrospective study. BMC Infect Dis. 2013;13:464.

50. Lam KY, Cheung F, Yam LY, Lee CH, Fung KH. Atypical manifestations in a patient with systemic lupus erythematosus. J Clin Pathol. 1997;50(2):174–6.

51. Zhou F, Bi X, Zou X, Xu Z, Zhang T. Retrospective analysis of 15 cases of *Penicilliosis marneffei* in a southern China hospital. Mycopathologia. 2014;177(5–6):271–9.

52. Hart J, Dyer JR, Clark BM, McLellan DG, Perera S, Ferrari P. Travel-related disseminated *Penicillium marneffei* infection in a renal transplant patient. Transpl Infect Dis. 2012;14(4):434–9.

53. Woo PC, Lau SK, Lau CC, Chong KT, Hui WT, Wong SS, Yuen KY. *Penicillium marneffei* fungaemia in an allogeneic bone marrow transplant recipient. Bone Marrow Transplant. 2005;35(8):831–3.

54. Stathakis A, Lim KP, Boan P, Lavender M, Wrobel J, Musk M, Heath CH. *Penicillium marneffei* infection in a lung transplant recipient. Transpl Infect Dis. 2015;17(3):429–34.

55. Seo JY, Ma YE, Lee JH, Lee ST, Ki CS, Lee NY. A case of disseminated *Penicillium marneffei* infection in a liver transplant recipient. Korean J Lab Med. 2010;30(4):400–5.

56. Chan JF, Chan TS, Gill H, Lam FY, Trendell-Smith NJ, Sridhar S, Tse H, Lau SK, Hung IF, Yuen KY, et al. Disseminated infections with *Talaromyces marneffei* in non-AIDS patients given monoclonal antibodies against CD20 and kinase inhibitors. Emerg Infect Dis. 2015;21(7):1101–6.

57. Ramirez I, Hidron A, Cardona R. Successful treatment of pulmonary invasive fungal infection by *Penicillium non-marneffei* in lymphoblastic lymphoma: case report and literature review. Clin Case Rep. 2018;6(6):1153–7.

58. Lee PP, Chan KW, Lee TL, Ho MH, Chen XY, Li CH, Chu KM, Zeng HS, Lau YL. Penicilliosis in children without HIV infection-are they immunodeficient? Clin Infect Dis. 2012;54(2):e8–e19.

59. Sirisanthana V, Sirisanthana T. Disseminated *Penicillium marneffei* infection in human immunodeficiency virus-infected children. Pediatr Infect Dis J. 1995;14(11):935–40.

60. Han XJ, Su DH, Yi JY, Zou YW, Shi YL. A literature review of blood-disseminated *P. marneffei* infection and a case study of this infection in an HIV-negative child with comorbid eosinophilia. Mycopathologia. 2019;184(1):129–39.

61. Lin WC, Dai YS, Tsai MJ, Huang LM, Chiang BL. Systemic *Penicillium marneffei* infection in a child with common variable immunodeficiency. J Formos Med Assoc. 1998;97(11):780–3.

62. Fan H, Huang L, Yang D, Lin Y, Lu G, Xie Y, Yu J, Zhang D. Pediatric hyperimmunoglobulin E syn-

drome: a case series of 4 children in China. Medicine (Baltimore). 2018;97(14):e0215.

63. Lee PP, Mao H, Yang W, Chan KW, Ho MH, Lee TL, Chan JF, Woo PC, Tu W, Lau YL. *Penicillium marneffei* infection and impaired IFN-gamma immunity in humans with autosomal-dominant gain-of-phosphorylation STAT1 mutations. J Allergy Clin Immunol. 2014;133(3):894–896 e895.

64. Anutarapongpan O, Thanathanee O, Suwan-Apichon O. *Penicillium* keratitis in a HIV-infected patient. BMJ Case Rep. 2016:bcr2016216139.

65. Le T, Huu Chi N, Kim Cuc NT, Manh Sieu TP, Shikuma CM, Farrar J, Day JN. AIDS-associated *Penicillium marneffei* infection of the central nervous system. Clin Infect Dis. 2010;51(12):1458–62.

66. Noritomi DT, Bub GL, Beer I, da Silva AS, de Cleva R, Gama-Rodrigues JJ. Multiple brain abscesses due to *Penicillium spp* infection. Rev Inst Med Trop Sao Paulo. 2005;47(3):167–70.

67. Chan JF, Lau SK, Yuen KY, Woo PC. *Talaromyces (Penicillium) marneffei* infection in non-HIV-infected patients. Emerg Microbes Infect. 2016;5:e19.

68. Xu X, Ran X, Pradhan S, Lei S, Ran Y. Dermoscopic manifestations of *Talaromyces (Penicillium) marneffei* infection in an AIDS patient. Indian J Dermatol Venereol Leprol. 2019;85(3):348–50.

69. Sudjaritruk T, Sirisanthana T, Sirisanthana V. Immune reconstitution inflammatory syndrome from *Penicillium marneffei* in an HIV-infected child: a case report and review of literature. BMC Infect Dis. 2012;12:28.

70. Chaiwun B, Khunamornpong S, Sirivanichai C, Rangdaeng S, Supparatpinyo K, Settakorn J, Ya-in C, Thorner P. Lymphadenopathy due to *Penicillium marneffei* infection: diagnosis by fine needle aspiration cytology. Mod Pathol. 2002;15(9):939–43.

71. Othman J, Brown CM. *Talaromyces marneffei* and dysplastic neutrophils on blood smear in newly diagnosed HIV. Blood. 2018;131(2):269.

72. Hua X, Zhang R, Yang H, Lei S, Zhang Y, Ran Y. Primary oral *Penicillium marneffei* infection diagnosed by PCR-based molecular identification and transmission electron microscopic observation from formalin-fixed paraffin-embedded tissues. Med Mycol Case Rep. 2012;2:15–8.

73. Supparatpinyo K, Khamwan C, Baosoung V, Nelson KE, Sirisanthana T. Disseminated *Penicillium marneffei* infection in Southeast Asia. Lancet. 1994;344(8915):110–3.

74. Cao C, Li R, Wan Z, Liu W, Wang X, Qiao J, Wang D, Bulmer G, Calderone R. The effects of temperature, pH, and salinity on the growth and dimorphism of *Penicillium marneffei*. Med Mycol. 2007;45(5):401–7.

75. Hoog S, Guarro J, Gené J, Ahmed S, Al-Hatmi A, Figueras M, Vitale R. Atlas of clinical fungi, vol. 1; 2019.

76. Frisvad JC, Yilmaz N, Thrane U, Rasmussen KB, Houbraken J, Samson RA. *Talaromyces atroroseus*, a new species efficiently producing industrially relevant red pigments. PLoS One. 2013;8(12):e84102.

77. Yilmaz N, Houbraken J, Hoekstra ES, Frisvad JC, Visagie CM, Samson RA. Delimitation and characterisation of *Talaromyces purpurogenus* and related species. Persoonia. 2012;29:39–54.

78. Liao X, Ran Y, Chen H, Meng W, Xiang B, Kang M, Xiong Z, Zhuang J, Peng X, Deng C, et al. Disseminated *Penicillium marneffei* infection associated with AIDS, report of a case. Zhonghua Yi Xue Za Zhi. 2002;82(5):325–9. (in Chinese)

79. Le T, Wolbers M, Chi NH, Quang VM, Chinh NT, Lan NP, Lam PS, Kozal MJ, Shikuma CM, Day JN, et al. Epidemiology, seasonality, and predictors of outcome of AIDS-associated *Penicillium marneffei* infection in Ho Chi Minh City, Vietnam. Clin Infect Dis. 2011;52(7):945–52.

80. Lin X, Ran Y, Gou L, He F, Zhang R, Wang P, Dai Y. Comprehensive transcription analysis of human pathogenic fungus *Penicillium marneffei* in mycelial and yeast cells. Med Mycol. 2012;50(8):835–42.

81. Shi N, Kong J, Wang K, Cao C. Coinfection with *Talaromyces marneffei* and other pathogens associated with acquired immunodeficiency. JAMA Dermatol. 2019.1532 Online ahead of print.

82. Wang YF, Cai JP, Wang YD, Dong H, Hao W, Jiang LX, Long J, Chan C, Woo PC, Lau SK, et al. Immunoassays based on *Penicillium marneffei* Mp1p derived from Pichia pastoris expression system for diagnosis of penicilliosis. PLoS One. 2011;6(12):e28796.

83. Li H, Sang J, Li R, Liu Y, Zhang J. Disseminated *Penicillium marneffei* infection with verrucoid lesions in an AIDS patient in Beijing, a non-endemic region. Eur J Dermatol. 2010;20(3):378–80.

84. Yoshimura Y, Sakamoto Y, Lee K, Amano Y, Tachikawa N. *Penicillium marneffei* infection with beta-D-glucan elevation: a case report and literature review. Intern Med. 2016;55(17):2503–6.

85. Huang YT, Hung CC, Liao CH, Sun HY, Chang SC, Chen YC. Detection of circulating galactomannan in serum samples for diagnosis of *Penicillium marneffei* infection and cryptococcosis among patients infected with human immunodeficiency virus. J Clin Microbiol. 2007;45(9):2858–62.

86. Hien HTA, Thanh TT, Thu NTM, Nguyen A, Thanh NT, Lan NPH, Simmons C, Shikuma C, Chau NVV, Thwaites G, et al. Development and evaluation of a real-time polymerase chain reaction assay for the rapid detection of *Talaromyces marneffei* MP1 gene in human plasma. Mycoses. 2016;59(12):773–80.

87. Lu S, Li X, Calderone R, Zhang J, Ma J, Cai W, Xi L. Whole blood nested PCR and real-time PCR amplification of *Talaromyces marneffei* specific DNA for diagnosis. Med Mycol. 2016;54(2):162–8.

88. Zeng H, Li X, Chen X, Zhang J, Sun J, Xie Z, Xi L. Identification of *Penicillium marneffei* in paraffin-embedded tissue using nested PCR. Mycopathologia. 2009;168(1):31–5.

89. Zhang JM, Sun JF, Feng PY, Li XQ, Lu CM, Lu S, Cai WY, Xi LY, de Hoog GS. Rapid identification and characterization of *Penicillium marneffei* using multiplex ligation-dependent probe amplification (MLPA) in paraffin-embedded tissue samples. J Microbiol Methods. 2011;85(1):33–9.

90. Li X, Zheng Y, Wu F, Mo D, Liang G, Yan R, Khader JA, Wu N, Cao C. Evaluation of quantitative real-time PCR and platelia galactomannan assays for the diagnosis of disseminated *Talaromyces marneffei* infection. Med Mycol. 2020;58(2):181–6.

91. Zhu YM, Ai JW, Xu B, Cui P, Cheng Q, Wu H, Qian YY, Zhang HC, Zhou X, Xing L, et al. Rapid and precise diagnosis of disseminated *T. marneffei* infection assisted by high-throughput sequencing of multifarious specimens in a HIV-negative patient: a case report. BMC Infect Dis. 2018;18(1):379.

92. Zeng W, Qiu Y, Lu D, Zhang J, Zhong X, Liu G. A retrospective analysis of 7 human immunodeficiency virus-negative infants infected by *Penicillium marneffei*. Medicine (Baltimore). 2015;94(34):e1439.

93. Qiu Y, Zhang J, Liu G, Zhong X, Deng J, He Z, Jing B. A case of *Penicillium marneffei* infection involving the main tracheal structure. BMC Infect Dis. 2014;14:242.

94. Lei HL, Li LH, Chen WS, Song WN, He Y, Hu FY, Chen XJ, Cai WP, Tang XP. Susceptibility profile of echinocandins, azoles and amphotericin B against yeast phase of *Talaromyces marneffei* isolated from HIV-infected patients in Guangdong, China. Eur J Clin Microbiol Infect Dis. 2018;37(6):1099–102.

95. Lau SK, Lo GC, Lam CS, Chow WN, Ngan AH, Wu AK, Tsang DN, Tse CW, Que TL, Tang BS, Woo PC. *In vitro* activity of posaconazole against *Talaromyces marneffei* by broth microdilution and Etest methods and comparison to itraconazole, voriconazole, and anidulafungin. Antimicrob Agents Chemother. 2017;61(3):e01480–16.

96. Liu D, Liang L, Chen J. *In vitro* antifungal drug susceptibilities of *Penicillium marneffei* from China. J Infect Chemother. 2013;19(4):776–8.

97. Sekhon AS, Garg AK, Padhye AA, Hamir Z. *In vitro* susceptibility of mycelial and yeast forms of *Penicillium marneffei* to amphotericin B, fluconazole, 5-fluorocytosine and itraconazole. Eur J Epidemiol. 1993;9(5):553–8.

98. Luo H, Pan KS, Luo XL, Zheng DY, Andrianopoulos A, Wen LM, Zheng YQ, Guo J, Huang CY, Li XY, et al. *In vitro* susceptibility of berberine combined with antifungal agents against the yeast form of *Talaromyces marneffei*. Mycopathologia. 2019;184(2):295–301.

99. Kaplan JE, Benson C, Holmes KK, Brooks JT, Pau A, Masur H, Centers for Disease C, Prevention, National Institutes of H, America HIVMAotIDSo: Guidelines for prevention and treatment of opportunistic infections in HIV-infected adults and adolescents: recommendations from CDC, the National Institutes of Health, and the HIV Medicine Association of the Infectious Diseases Society of America. MMWR Recomm Rep 2009, 58(RR-4):1–207; quiz CE201–204.

100. Supparatpinyo K, Perriens J, Nelson KE, Sirisanthana T. A controlled trial of itraconazole to prevent relapse of *Penicillium marneffei* infection in patients infected with the human immunodeficiency virus. N Engl J Med. 1998;339(24):1739–43.

101. Iribarren JA, Rubio R, Aguirrebengoa K, Arribas JR, Baraia-Etxaburu J, Gutierrez F, Lopez Bernaldo de Quiros JC, Losa JE, Miro JM, Moreno S et al. Prevention and treatment of opportunistic infections and other coinfections in HIV-infected patients: May 2015. Enferm Infecc Microbiol Clin. 2016;34(8):516 e511–18.

102. Ouyang Y, Cai S, Liang H, Cao C. Administration of voriconazole in disseminated *Talaromyces (Penicillium) marneffei* infection: a retrospective study. Mycopathologia. 2017;182(5–6):569–75.

103. Supparatpinyo K, Schlamm HT. Voriconazole as therapy for systemic *Penicillium marneffei* infections in AIDS patients. Am J Trop Med Hyg. 2007;77(2):350–3.

104. Le T, Kinh NV, Cuc NTK, Tung NLN, Lam NT, Thuy PTT, Cuong DD, Phuc PTH, Vinh VH, Hanh DTH, et al. A trial of itraconazole or amphotericin B for HIV-associated Talaromycosis. N Engl J Med. 2017;376(24):2329–40.

105. Le T, Ly VT, Thu NTM, Nguyen A, Thanh NT, Chau NVV, Thwaites G, Perfect J, Kolamunnage-Dona R, Hope W. Population pharmacodynamics of amphotericin B deoxycholate for disseminated infection caused by *Talaromyces marneffei*. Antimicrob Agents Chemother. 2019;63(2):pii: e01739-18.

Part VI

Dermatoses Caused by Bites or Stings

Insect Bites

Elizabeth Salazar-Rojas

Key Points
- Insect bite reactions depend on the type of insect but mainly on the patient's response.
- Secondary infection (impetigo or cellulitis), severe allergic reactions and vector-borne diseases are well known complications of insect bites and clinicians should be aware, recognise and treat them.
- Treatment may include oral antihistamines, topical steroids and oral or topical antibiotics.

Introduction

Insect bites and infestation are common reasons for consultation to dermatologists and general practitioners. Among them, fleas and bed bugs bites are more common in children, whilst mosquito bites are more common in young people and are prevalent in tropical or subtropical territories.

Incidence

The incidence is unknown because the vast majority do not produce severe clinical manifestations and therefore they are not reported. Summer is the time of the year with the highest incidence with more people affected. Physicians must exclude severe manifestations by considering vector-borne diseases, anaphylaxis and secondary infections (such as impetigo, cellulitis or lymphangitis) [1].

The transmission of vector-borne diseases is very important in developing countries or tropical/subtropical areas. However due to globalisation, these diseases have been introduced in Europe; it is to be considered that the host, the vector and the pathogen must adapt or switch to suitable conditions to cause infection [2].

The bites of insects such as mosquitoes, bedbugs and fleas are generally not painful because the bite is done with a piercing mouthpart that

E. Salazar-Rojas (✉)
Hospital Angeles del Pedregal, Mexico City, Mexico

W. Robles (ed.), *Skin Disease in Travelers*, Updates in Clinical Dermatology,
https://doi.org/10.1007/978-3-031-57836-6_18

penetrates the skin with slight trauma [3]. Human sweat contains organic compounds with a specific odour produced by microflora which causes specific attraction to mosquitoes. Mosquito bites may have a higher incidence in certain conditions, populations and age: pregnancy, alcohol ingestion, large body size, male gender and increasing age in children [4].

Horseflies, blackflies and midges create a hole in the skin and lick the blood from the wound producing pain, local reaction and other general symptoms such as edema and dizziness. If the individual has never been bitten, the saliva proteins will start an immune reaction that will make the individual sensitive to further bites; other contents of the saliva include anticoagulants, vasodilators and digestive enzymes. A regular exposure to insect bites may lead to desensitisation [1].

Tick bites are in general not painful so the individual may not even be aware of the bite but the tick may still be attached to the skin.

Diagnosis requires:

1. Clinical features (detailed history and presentation).
2. Outdoor activities, travels or animal contact.
3. Affection of related individuals.

Clinical Findings

In general, the bites appear as multiple or single papules surrounded by small or big areas of swelling or erythema may present depending on the host

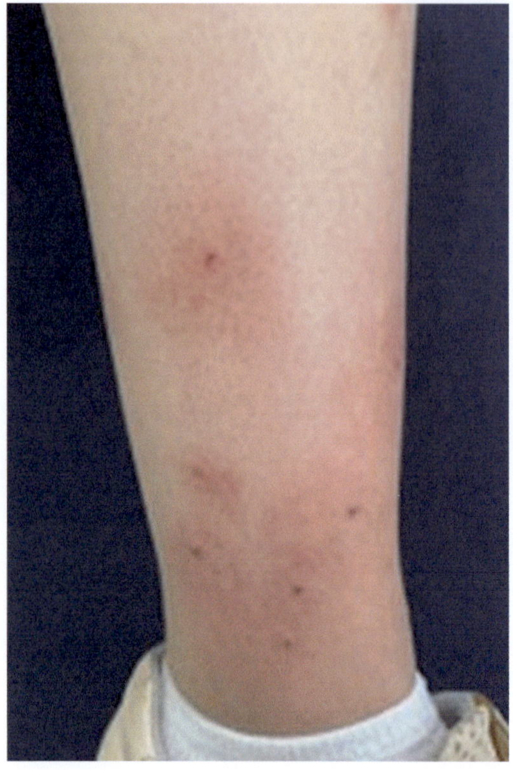

Fig. 1 Patient with multiple excoriated papules with surrounding erythema secondary to an exposition to grass fleas in legs (uncovered skin)

immune response. They may cause pruritus, pain or be completely asymptomatic. Other inflammatory changes like urticaria, bruising or blisters may emerge. The lesions can last for a few hours or days, but the most exasperating and most common cause of consultation is pruritus, therefore, the surrounding skin may have scratch marks as well (Fig. 1).

Table 1 List of insect and vector-borne diseases [12]

Vector	Disease
Mosquitoes – *Aedes aegypti* – *Aedes albopictus* – *Culex quinquefasciatus* – *Anopheles* – *Haemagogus*	Dengue, chikungunya, Yellow fever, Zika virus Chikungunya, dengue, West Nile virus Lymphatic filariasis Malaria, lymphatic filariasis Yellow fever
Blackflies	Onchoceriasis
Fleas	Plague, Murine thypus, tungiasis, tularemia, cat scratch disease
Sandflies	Leishmaniasis
Lice	Thypus, Louse-borne relapsing fever
Ticks	Crimean-Congo haemorrhagic fever, tick-borne encephalitis, thypus, Lyme
Triatomine bugs	Chagas
Tsetse flies	Sleeping sickness
Mites	Rickettsial pox, scrub typhus

Tick Bites

A typical clinical finding of tick bites is erythema migrans. This is an expanding rash very commonly seen in the early stages of Lyme disease (caused by Borrelia burgdorferi). It may appear as an erythematous papule with an annular surrounding halo known as "bull's eye", which can start between 3 and 30 days (usually 7 days) after the tick bite. Other vector-borne diseases are listed on Table 1.

Mosquito Bites

A severe reaction to mosquito bites may cause Skeeter syndrome, defined as local inflammatory reaction with fever starting within hours after the bite, this syndrome can be misdiagnosed as bacterial infection or cellulitis [5].

Horsefly Bites

Cause by *Tabanus bovinus*, the skin lesions appear as multiple, erythematous, roundish, flattened, large painful plaques with a central point surrounded by satellite lesions. Of interest is a crossed allergenicity between wasp venom, mosquito and horsefly extracts causing a wasp-horsefly syndrome [6].

Midge Bites

Phlebotominae (sand fly) and *Simuliidae* (black fly) are important vectors for Leishmaniasis and Onchocerciasis, respectively [7]. Black flies are known as buffalo gnats or turkey gnats, their bites cause papules, erythematous wheals, induration and severe swelling of the affected area with adenopathy called "stiff neck" [8].

Bedbug Bites

There are two species of these blood parasites: *Cimex lecturarius* and *Cimex hemipterus*. They are flat insects (5–7 mm) that hide under mattresses as reddish stains or behind headboards, they can live for as long as 1 year with no food, they produce an specific sweet smell. The warmth and carbon dioxide of the human body attract these insects, their saliva contains anaesthetic, vasodilatory, anticoagulant and proteolytic compounds that allow them to feed for 5–10 min undetected. The common clinical findings are small erythematous papules or wheals in unclothed areas like the face, neck or extremities in a row or cluster [9].

Mite Bites

Mites are very small (0.5–2 mm) eight-legged arthropods, they cause itchy small spot bites on the skin near constrictive clothing like belts or sock lines. The larval form is called chigger, the skin lesions are caused by an allergic reaction to the chiggers saliva [10].

Flea Bites

Fleas are flightless jumping insects that survive as external parasites, humans are occasional hosts because they prefer dogs or cats. The typical lesions are small pruritic papules located in the ankles [10].

Spider Bites

There are two medically important spiders: the black widow (*Latrodectus mactans*) and the brown recluse (*Loxosceles reclusa*), specific treatment is require for these bites. The first one can be found worldwide, they live outdoors, the female is black with a classic red hourglass mark on the ventral abdomen. The bite is like a very strong pinprick, then the venom spreads containing α-*latrotoxin* producing a massive release of acetylcholine causing muscles spasms that may resolve in 48–72 h. Treatment includes benzodiazepines, strong pain killers and antivenom.

The Brown recluse spider or fiddleback is found in south-central United States and South America. They live indoors, have an inverted violin-shaped in their thorax and instead of having four pairs of eyes they have three pairs. The bite can be minimally painful with an erythematous halo and central necrosis, the venom has sphingomyelinase D which causes neutrophil activation. Treatment with dapsone and antihistamines may help, debridement is not recommended [10].

Ant Stings and Bites

There are more than 12,000 species of ants. Most ants are not aggressive. Red ants cannot sting but spray a venom with formic acid which cause burns. The most aggressive are fire ants of the genus *Solenopsis*, Chinese needle ants and samsum ants. Their venom contains piperidine alkaloids which causes painful, itchy papules and sterile pustules [11].

Ladybird Bites

The harlequin ladybird is the most aggressive, it is red or orange with multiple spots and a white typical spot on its head. The bite can be painful but harmless.

Flower Bug Bites

They are tiny, with an oval body. The bites can be painful and itchy, usually slow to heal.

Differential Diagnosis

Bee, fire ants, hornet or wasp stings, vegetation contact (poison ivy or giant hogweed), caterpillar reaction, erythema migrans. Other pathologies with similar manifestation are chicken pox, impetigo, shingles or bullous pemphigoid and pyoderma gangrenosum.

Treatment

The vast majority will develop minor symptoms or none, therefore they will require no treatment at all. Removing a visible sting or tick would be the first advice, then wash profusely with water and mild soap, patients must avoid scratching.

Over the counter drugs like antihistamines and mild pain killers may be used, as well as cool compresses or topical corticosteroids such as hydrocortisone 1% cream. Non-sedating antihistamines like cetirizine and loratadine are the most common drugs to treat pruritus. Topical or systemic antibiotics to treat *Staphylococcus aureus* may be needed for severe manifestations of secondary infection such as cellulitis or impetigo, cephalosporins or amoxicillin are frequently used.

Calamine is an anti-itch compound containing zinc and ferric oxide used to treat sting and bites because it gives a cooling sensation as it evaporates but has not proven to be better than corticosteroid creams.

Auto injections of epinephrine are available for patients with a history of severe allergic reaction to insect bites.

Outcome

Scars or post-inflammatory hyperpigmented spots may appear as seen in Fig. 2.

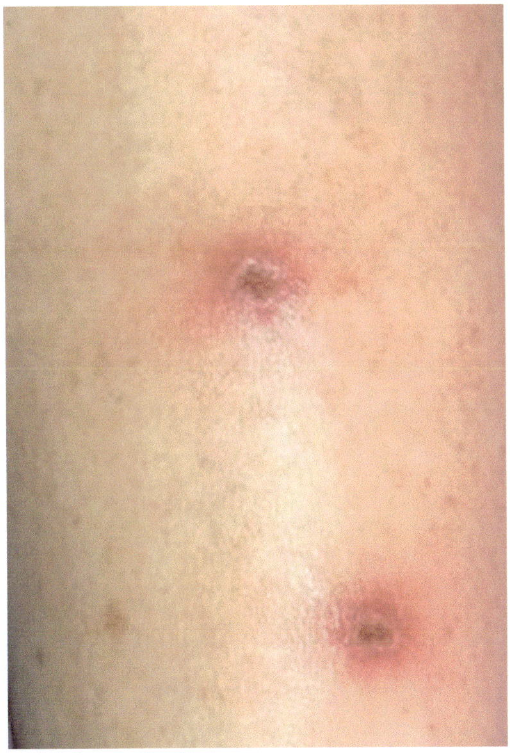

Fig. 2 Patient with atopic dermatitis presented with excoriated papules and surrounding erythema in her legs persisting 3 weeks after mosquito bites

Prevention

Knowing the local epidemiology of the disease and the special behaviour for the vector species like habitats, feeding preferences and seasons. For instance, to prevent yellow fever infection travellers to tropical or subtropical areas of Africa and South America must use insect repellent, wear long-sleeved shirts and long pants, avoid going outdoors after dusk, but mainly, get vaccinated [12].

One of the most efficient and cost-effective method to prevent mosquito, sandflies bites and triatomine bugs are insecticide-treated bed nets [12].

Housing modification using window screens/nets or fans/air conditioning keeps away mosquitoes effectively.

Insect repellents such as DDT (dichlorodiphenyltrichloroethane) which has the longest efficacy is used in agriculture and lasts from 6 to 12 months but its use is restricted. DEET (N,N-diethyltoluamide) 10–35% or picaridin 20% are very effective and last for almost 12 h, they can be used in pregnant (after first trimester) or breastfeeding women and in children over 2 months-old if an adult supervises application (no lips or hands). Lemon eucalyptus oil contains p-menthane-3,8-diol as an active ingredient, is less effective than DEET or picaridin but is the best of the natural repellents. [10] Citronella is less effective than DEET products, but adding vanillin to citronella oil could prolong the protection time [13].

Reducing vector-borne disease may be possible by suppressing mosquito populations with novel methods like a sterile insect technique (SIT) with both irradiated or chemically treated males, an incompatible insect technique (IIT) using a bacteria named *Wolbachia* or various genetic modification strategies carrying a transgene that causes larvae death before reaching the pupal stage are promising strategies [14].

References

1. Wilcock, J., Etherington, C., Hawthorne, K., & Brown, G. Insect bites. BMJ. 2020;m2856.
2. Semenza JC, Suk JE. Vector-borne diseases and climate change: a European perspective. FEMS Microbiol Lett. 2018;365(2).

3. Management of insect bites. Where's the evidence. Drug Ther Bull. 2012;50(4):45–8.

4. Singh S, Mann BK. Insect bite reactions. Indian J Dermatol Venereol Leprol. 2013;79(2):151–64.

5. Simons FE, Peng Z. Skeeter syndrome. J Allergy Clin Immunol. 1999;104(3 Pt 1):705–7.

6. Veraldi S, Esposito L. Skin lesions caused by Tabanus bovinus bites. J Travel Med. 2017;24(5):10.

7. Maroli M, Khoury C. Prevenzione e controllo dei vettori di leishmaniosi: attuali metodologie [Prevention and control of leishmaniasis vectors: current approaches]. Parassitologia. 2004;46(1–2):211–5.

8. Goddard J, Stewart P, Deerman H, Nations TM, Varnado WC. Development and resolution of cutaneous lesions caused by black Fly bites (Diptera: Simuliidae). Am J Med. 2018;131(10):e415–6.

9. Studdiford JS, Conniff KM, Trayes KP, Tully AS. Bedbug infestation. Am Fam Physician. 2012;86(7):653–8.

10. Juckett G. Arthropod bites. Am Fam Physician. 2013;88(12):841–7.

11. Hoffman DR. Ant venoms. Curr Opin Allergy Clin Immunol. 2010;10(4):342–6.

12. World Health Organization. A global brief on vector-borne diseases. World Health Organization; 2014. https://apps.who.int/iris/handle/10665/111008. Accessed Sept 11, 2020.

13. Kongkaew C, Sakunrag I, Chaiyakunapruk N, Tawatsin A. Effectiveness of citronella preparations in preventing mosquito bites: systematic review of controlled laboratory experimental studies. Trop Med Int Health. 2011;16(7):802–10.

14. Flores HA, O'Neill SL. Controlling vector-borne diseases by releasing modified mosquitoes. Nat Rev Microbiol. 2018;16(8):508–18.

Tick-Borne Infections

Dirk M. Elston

Key Points

- Ticks carry a variety of diseases including rickettsial fevers, monocytic ehrlichiosis, anaplasmosis, babesiosis, tularemia, borrelioses, tick-borne encephalitides, and tick typhus.
- Ticks may transmit more than one pathogen at a time.
- Most bacterial tick-borne illnesses respond to doxycycline.

Introduction

Both hard and soft ticks are important disease vectors. The family Ixodidae contains the hard ticks, identified by their hard dorsal scutum, which covers the entire body of the male but only a small portion of the female to allow engorgement (Figs. 1 and 2). This family contains ticks of the genera *Dermacentor, Ixodes, Amblyomma, Haemaphysalis, Hyalomma, Rhipicephalus*. The family Argasidae, the soft ticks, have a soft cuticle and retroverted mouthparts. They include *Ornithodoros, Argas,* and *Otobius* ticks. Both hard and soft ticks have the developmental stages of egg, larva, nymph, and adults. Larvae have 6 legs, nymphs have 8 legs like the adults but are smaller and sexually immature. Argasid ticks live in close association with their hosts and take multiple blood meals from the same host. In contrast, ixodid ticks are questing ticks that attach to a different host during each stage of the life cycle.

D. M. Elston (✉)
Department of Dermatology, Dermatologic Surgery
Medical University of SC, Charleston, SC, USA
e-mail: elstond@musc.edu

W. Robles (ed.), *Skin Disease in Travelers*, Updates in Clinical Dermatology,
https://doi.org/10.1007/978-3-031-57836-6_19

Fig. 1 Female *Ixodes scapularis* tick. Note that the inornate scutum is small to allow for engorgement. Ixodes ticks are characterized by an anterior anal groove

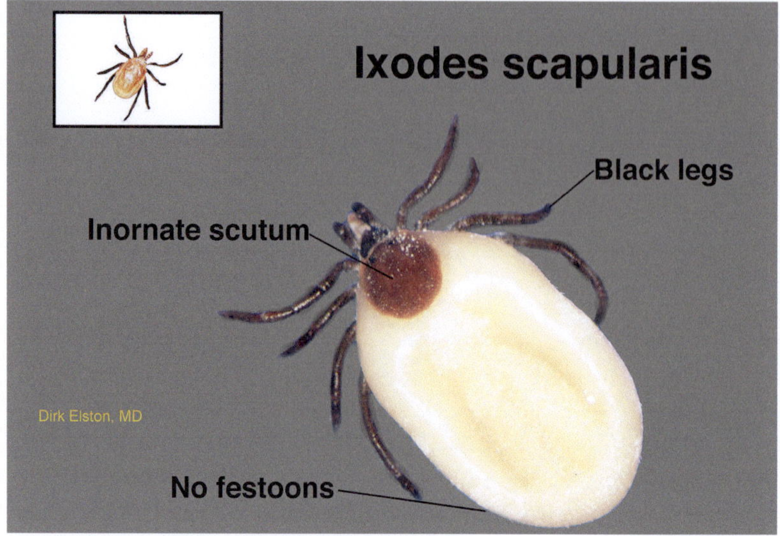

Fig. 2 Male *Dermacentor variabilis* tick. Dermacentor ticks have a highly ornate scutum, prominent eyes, and festoons

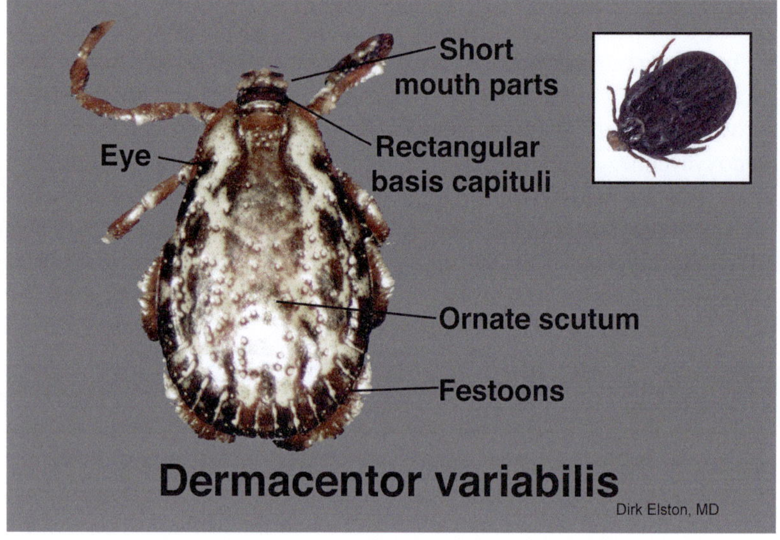

Tick Bite Reactions and Infestation

Dermacentor ticks tend to attach to the upper body and are an important cause of tick paralysis. Removal of the tick generally results in prompt recovery, but as they are often hidden by hair and not identified. Tick paralysis carries a 10% mortality rate with death from respiratory paralysis, and the tick identified post-mortem. *Ixodes* ticks tend to attach on the trunk, and *Amblyomma* ticks prefer the lower legs and genitals, often attaching by the hundreds. Infestations may be prevented by application of permethrin to clothing and tick repellents such as N,N-diethyl-m-toluamide (DEET). Tick inspections with prompt removal of the tick can prevent disease transmission as it takes 24–72 h of feeding before transmission occurs.

Histologically, tick bites are characterized by wedge-shaped necrosis with thrombosis of vessels and a polymorphous infiltrate with many eosinophils in older bites. The reaction tends to be extremely pruritic and persistent and often responds best to intralesional injections of triamcinolone. Secondary infection with *Staphylococcus aureus* and group A *Streptococcus* is common.

A-Galactoside Syndrome

The α-Gal syndrome presents with anaphylaxis to red meat (beef, lamb, and pork) or biologic agents that cross react with the saliva of *Amblyomma* ticks. It is characterized by an IgE antibody against the carbohydrate Galα1-3Galβ1-4GlcNAc-R (α-Gal) present in tick saliva. *Amblyomma* ticks often attach by the hundreds, and recurrent tick bites induce high levels of anti-α-Gal IgE antibodies that mediate hypersensitivity to red meat. The tick-borne pathogen *Anaplasma phagocytophilum* increases the level of tick α-Gal, which may increase the risk of developing the syndrome [1].

Tick-Borne Diseases

Tick-borne diseases are increasing in incidence and new pathogens are being recognized and ticks may transmit multiple pathogens simultaneously [1–5]. Table 1 summarized major tick-borne illnesses, presenting manifestations, vectors, and treatment. Individual diseases are discussed in more detail below.

Table 1 Tick-borne diseases

Disease	Tick vector	Organism	Diagnostic features	Treatment (Adults)	Alternative treatment (Adults)	Treatment (Children)	Alternative treatment (Children)
African tick bite fever	*Amblyomma hebraeum, Amblyomma variegatum, Amblyomma lepidum*	*Rickettsia africae*	Fever, often multiple eschars, maculopapular rash (may be vesicular), aphthous stomatitis	Doxycycline 100 mg PO or IV every 12 h until 3 days after apyrexia			
Anaplasmosis	*Ixodes scapularis, Ixodes pacificus, Ixodes ricinus, Ixodes persulcatus*	*Anaplasma phagocytophilum*	Morbilliform rash	Doxycycline 100 mg PO or IV every 12 h × 5–14 days	Tetraycycline 500 mg PO every 6 h × 5–14 days or Rifampin 300 mg PO every 12 h × 7–10 days	Doxycycline 2.2 mg/kg PO every 12 h × 5–14 days	Tetraycycline 25–50 mg/kg/day PO in 4 divided doses × 5–14 days or Rifampin 10 mg/kg PO every 12 h × 7–10 days
Astrakhan spotted fever	*Rhipicephalus sanguineus, Rhipicephalus pumilio*	*Rickettsia conorii caspia*	Fever, eschar, maculopapular rash, conjunctivitis	Doxycycline 100 mg PO or IV every 12 h until 3 days after apyrexia			
Australian spotted fever	*Haemaphysalis novaeguineae*	*Rickettsia marmionii*	Fever, eschar, morbilliform rash	Doxycycline 100 mg PO or IV every 12 h until 3 days after apyrexia			
Babesiosis	*Ixodes scapularis*	*Babesia microti*	Fever, petechiae, ecchymosis, jaundice	Atovaquone 750 mg PO every 12 h × 7–10 days and Azithromycin 500–1000 mg PO on day 1 then 250–1000 mg on subsequent 6–9 days +/− Exchange transfusion	Clindamycin 600 mg PO every 8 h (300–600 mg IV every 6 h) and quinine 650 mg PO every 6–8 h × 7–10 days +/− Exchange transfusion	Atovaquone 20 mg/kg (maximum 750 mg/dose) PO every 12 h × 7–10 days and Azithromycin 10 mg/kg (maximum 500 mg/dose) PO on day 1 then 5 mg/kg on subsequent 6–9 days +/− Exchange transfusion	Clindamycin 7–10 mg/kg (maximum 600 mg/ dose) PO or IV every 8 h and Quinine 8 mg/kg (maximum 650 mg/dose) PO every 8 h × 7–10 days +/− exchange transfusion

Crimean-Congo hemorrhagic fever	*Hyalomma* spp.	*Crimean-Congo Hemorrhagic Fever virus*	Hemorrhagic fever	Supportive Treatment, Ribavirin 30 mg/kg PO initial loading dose, then 15 mg/kg every 6 h × 4 days, and then 7.5 mg/kg every 8 h × 6 days			
Far eastern spotted fever	*Dermacentor silvarum*	*Rickettsia heilongjianji*	Eschar, morbilliform rash, lymphadenopathy	Doxycycline 100 mg PO or IV every 12 h until 3 days after apyrexia			
Flinders Island spotted fever	*Aponomma hydrosauri, Ixodes granulatus, Amblyomma cajennense*	*Rickettsia honei*	Fever, eschar, morbilliform rash (may be purpuric), lyphadenopathy	Doxycycline 100 mg PO or IV every 12 h until 3 days after apyrexia			
Human monocytic ehrlichiosis	*Amblyomma americanum, Dermacentor variabilis, Rhipicephalus*	*Ehrlichia chaffeensis*	Morbilliform rash	Doxycycline 100 mg PO or IV every 12 h × 5–14 days	Tetraycycline 500 mg PO every 6 h × 5–14 days or rifampin 300 mg PO every 12 h × 7–10 days	Doxycycline 2.2 mg/kg PO every 12 h × 5–14 days	Tetraycycline 25–50 mg/kg/day PO in 4 divided doses × 5–14 days or rifampin 10 mg/kg PO every 12 h × 7–10 days
Indian tick typhus	*Rhipicephalus sanguineus, Boophilus microplus, Haemaphysalis leachii*	*Rickettsia conorii indica*	Fever, eschar, morbilliform rash (may be purpuric)	Doxycycline 100 mg PO or IV every 12 h until 3 days after apyrexia			
Israeli spotted fever	*Rhipicephalus sanguineus*	*Rickettsia conorii israelensis*	Fever, eschar, morbilliform rash	Doxycycline 100 mg PO or IV every 12 h until 3 days after apyrexia			

(continued)

Table 1 (continued)

Disease	Tick vector	Organism	Diagnostic features	Treatment (Adults)	Alternative treatment (Adults)	Treatment (Children)	Alternative treatment (Children)
Japanese (oriental) spotted fever	*Ixodes ovatus, Dermacentor taiwanensis, Haemaphysalis longicornis, Haemaphysalis flava*	*Rickettsia japonica*	Fever, eschar, morbilliform rash	Doxycycline 100 mg PO or IV every 12 h until 3 days after apyrexia			
Lymphangitis-associated ricketsiosis	*Hyalomma asiaticum, Hyalomma truncatum**	*Rickettsia sibirica subspecies mongolitimonae*	Fever, multiple eschars, maculopapular rash, lymphangitis	Doxycycline 100 mg PO or IV every 12 h until 3 days after apyrexia			
Mediterranean spotted fever	*Rhipicephalus sanguineus, Rhipicephalus simus, Haemaphysalis leachii, Haemaphysalis punctaleachii*	*Rickettsia conorii*	Fever, single eschar, morbilliform rash	Doxycycline 200 mg PO every 12 h × 1 day (or 100 mg PO every 12 h until 1 day after apyrexia)	Tetracycline 500 mg PO every 6 h × 10 days or ciprofloxacin 750 mg PO every 12 h × 8 days (or until 1 day after apyrexia)	Doxycycline 4.4 mg/kg PO every 12 h × 1 day (or 2.2 mg/kg PO every 12 h until 1 day after apyrexia)	Clarithromycin 7.5 mg/kg/day PO in 2 divided doses x 7 days or Azithromycin 10 mg/kg PO daily × 3 days or chloramphenicol 50 mg/kg/day divided in four doses × 7 days (or until 1 day after apyrexia)
North Asian (Siberian) tick typhus	*Dermacentor nuttalli, Dermacentor marginatus, Haemaphysalis concinna, Dermacentor sinicus*	*Rickettsia sibirica*	Fever, eschar, rash (may be purpuric), lymphadenopathy	Doxycycline 100 mg PO or IV every 12 h until 3 days after apyrexia			
Powassan encephalitis	*Ixodes cookei, Dermacentor andersoni*	*Powassan encephalitis virus*	Encephalitis	Supportive treatment			

Q fever	*Dermacentor occidentalis, Amblyomma americanum, Haemaphysalis leporis-palustris, Ixodes dentatus, Otobius magnini, Rhipicephalus sanguineus, Haemaphysalis humerosa, Amblyomma triguttatum, others*	*Coxiella burnetti*	Fever, macules, petechiae, and purpura	Doxycycline 100 mg PO every 12 h × 15–21 days			
Queensland tick typhus	*Ixodes holocyclus, Ixodes tasmani*	*Rickettsia australis*	Fever, eschar, vesicular rash	Doxycycline 100 mg PO or IV every 12 h until 3 days after apyrexia			
Rocky Mountain spotted fever	*Dermacentor andersoni, Dermacentor variabilis, Rhipicephalus sanguineus, Amblyomma cajennense, Amblyomma aureolatum*	*Rickettsia rickettsii*	Fever, eschar rare, morbilliform rash (may be purpuric)	Doxycycline 100 mg PO or IV every 12 h until 3 days after apyrexia	Tetraycycline 500 mg PO (or 250 mg IV) four times daily (maximum dose 2 g/day) or chloramphenicol 50–75 mg/kg PO or IV four times daily (maximum dose 4 g/day) until 3 days after apyrexia	Doxycycline 2.2 mg/kg PO or IV every 12 h (if less than 45 kg) until 3 days after apyrexia	Chloramphenicol 12.5–25 mg/kg PO or IV every 6 h × 5–10 days until 3 days after apyrexia

(continued)

Table 1 (continued)

Disease	Tick vector	Organism	Diagnostic features	Treatment (Adults)	Alternative treatment (Adults)	Treatment (Children)	Alternative treatment (Children)
STARI	*Amblyomma americanum*	*Borrelia lonestari*	Erythema migrans-like (Lyme-like) erythematous annular rash	Doxycycline 100 mg PO every 12 h × 14–21 days	Amoxicillin 1000 mg PO every 8 h × 14–21 days or Azithromycin 500 mg PO every 12 h × 1 day then 500 mg PO daily × 4–9 days or Cefuroxime 500 mg PO every 12 h × 14–21 days	Amoxicillin 50 mg/kg PO every 8 h × 14–21 days	Azithromycin 20 mg/kg PO every 12 h × 1 day then 10 mg/kg PO daily × 4–9 days or Cefuroxime 30–40 mg/kg PO every 12 h × 14–21 days
Tick-borne encephalitis	*Ixodes ricinus, Ixodes persulcatus, Haemaphysalis concinna*	*Tick-borne Encephalitis virus subtype Western (European), Siberian, and Far-Eastern (Russian Spring-Summer Encephalitis)*	Encephalitis	Supportive treatment			
Tick-borne lymphadenopathy (TIBOLA), Dermacentor-borne necrosis and lymphadenopathy (DEBONEL)	*Dermacentor marginatus, Dermacentor reticulatus*	*Rickettsia slovaca*	Fever and rash rare, eschar, cervical lymphadenopathy	Doxycycline 100 mg PO or IV every 12 h until 3 days after apyrexia			

Tick-borne relapsing fever	*Orinithodoros parkeri*	*Borrelia parkeri*	Episodic fever, macular rash, eschar	Doxycycline 100 mg PO or IV every 12 h × 7 days	Tetraycycline 500 mg PO (or 250 mg IV) every 6 h × 7 days or Erythromycin 500 mg PO or IV every 6 h × 7 days or Chloramphenicol 500 mg PO or IV every 6 h × 7 days or Penicillin G 600,000 IU IV or IM daily × 7 days	Penicillin V 25–50 mg/kg/day (maximum 500 mg/dose) PO divided in four doses × 7 days or Penicillin G 25,000–50,000 IU/kg/day IM divided in 1 to 2 doses × 7 days or or Penicillin G 25,000–50,000 IU/kg/day IV divided into four doses × 7 days	Erythromycin 30–50 mg/kg/day (max 2 g/day) PO divided in 2–4 doses × 7 days
Tularemia	*Amblyomma americanum, Dermacentor andersoni, Dermacentor variabilis, Rhipicephalus sanguineus, Dermacentor reticulatus, Ixodes ricinus*	*Franciscella tularensis*	Fever, ulcerative papule, lymphadenopathy, eschar	Streptomycin 1 g IM every 12 h × 10 days or Gentimicin 5 mg/kg IM or IV once daily × 10 days	Doxycycline 100 mg IV every 12 h × 14–21 days or chloramphenicol 15 mg/kg IV every 6 h × 12–21 days or ciprofloxacin 400 mg IV every 12 h × 10 days	Streptomycin 15 mg/kg IM every 12 h (maximum 2 g/day) × 10 days or Gentimicin 2.5 mg/kg IM or IV every 8 h × 10 days	Doxycycline 2.2 mg/kg IV every 12 h (if weight < 45 kg) × 14–21 days or chloramphenicol 15 mg/kg IV every 6 h × 14–21 days or ciprofloxacin 15 mg/kg IV every 12 h × 10 days

Anaplasmosis and Human Monocytic Ehrlichiosis

Ehrlichia and *Anaplasma* are small intracellular Gram-negative organisms closely related to *Rickettsia*. Both produce febrile illness, especially in the spring and summer months into early fall. *Ehrlichia chaffeensis* is associated with monocytic ehrlichiosis (ME) and transmitted by a variety of ticks, most commonly *Amblyomma americanum, Dermacentor,* and *Rhipicephalus* ticks. *Ixodes scapularis* is the major vector for anaplasmosis (formerly human granulocytic ehrlichiosis). ME most commonly occurs in the south central and southeastern United States, in areas with large populations of white-tailed deer *(Odocoileus virginianus)*. The disease resembles a milder form of Rocky Mountain spotted fever (RMSF) and responds to tetracyclines. Following tick exposure, individuals develop an abrupt headache with fever, headache, and sometimes a rash which may be petechial, macular, or morbilliform and typically manifests 5 days after tick bite. Unlike RMSF, it is less likely to involve acral surfaces, but appears on the face, trunk, and extremities. Pancytopenia is common with thrombocytopenia (70–90%) and leukopenia (60–70%) occurring early in the course of illness. Elevated liver enzymes are common, but with appropriate treatment, most patients recover. The death rate is approximately 3%.

The diagnosis should be suspected in endemic areas when patients present with fever and a headache and all such patients should receive early treatment with a tetracycline. Treatment should not be delayed for definitive diagnosis which may require serological studies or Wright Giemsa staining of peripheral blood smears. Direct fluorescent antibody and polymerase chain reaction (PCR) tests can also be employed.

Anaplasmosis occurs in North America, Europe, and Asia. The ticks that transmit HGA are *Ixodes scapularis* in the eastern United States, *Ixodes pacificus* in the western United States, *Ixodes ricinus* in Europe, and *Ixodes persulcatus* in Asia. In the United States, the majority of cases occur in the upper Midwest states and New England where the vector is prevalent. The presentation is similar to ME with fever and severe headache. Lack of history of a tick bite should not prevent early treatment with doxycycline. Other symptoms include myalgia, malaise, nausea, cough, arthralgia, and anorexia. Co-infection with Lyme disease occurs as both diseases are transmitted by the same vector. Microscopic examination of peripheral blood may demonstrate the organisms in more than half of patients with Ehrlichiosis. Direct fluorescent antibody and PCR testing have also been employed.

Rocky Mountain Spotted Fever

RMSF is most common in the mid-Atlantic states and carries a significant death rate. The major determinant of outcome is time to initiation of tetracycline therapy and doxycycline should be prescribed for anyone in an endemic area who presents with fever and a headache regardless of the history of a tick bite. *Rickettsiae* are obligate intracellular coccobacilli that invade endothelial cells. In the western United States, *Rickettsia ricketsii* is transmitted by *Dermacentor andersoni*, whereas in the eastern United States, when most cases occur, the disease is transmitted by *Dermacentor variabilis*. *Rhicephalus* and *Amblyomma* ticks are also vectors of RMSF and the disease extends into Central and South America. *Rickettsia ricketssii* may be transmitted to humans as soon as 6–8 h after tick attachment, although 24 h is typically required for transmission. Five days following the tick exposure, most patients develop a petechial or morbilliform eruption that may begin on the palms and soles. Other symptoms include myalgia, nausea, and vomiting. Upward of 25% of infected individuals die without appropriate treatment. Direct fluorescent antibody and PCR testing are commonly employed. As titers may be delayed, treatment should never wait for definitive diagnosis. Doxycycline is the preferred treatment in both adults and children. *Rickettsiae* are susceptible to chloramphenicol and some fluoroquinolones but outcomes are worse than with tetracycline therapy. They are resistant to penicillins, cephalosporins, aminoglycosides, trimethoprim-sulfamethoxazole, and erythromycin.

American Tick Bite Fever

Rickettsia parkeri is carried by *Amblyomma* ticks and the illness is characterized by fever, headache, diffuse myalgias, and arthralgias. A characteristic eschar may be present as in other Rickettsial fevers. A petechial or morbilliform rash may appear on the trunk and extremities, including the palms and soles. As with other rickettsial diseases, doxycycline is the treatment of choice.

Mediterranean Fever (Boutonneuse Fever)

Mediterranean Fever is caused by *Rickettsia conorii* transmitted by dog ticks *Rhipicephalus sanguineus*. Although the disease is endemic to the Mediterranean, cases have occurred in Europe, Africa, and Asia. Closely related diseases include *Rickettsia conorii indica* (Indian Tick Typhus), *Rickettsia conorii israelensis* (Israeli Spotted Fever) and *Rickettsia conorii caspia rickettsia* (Astrakhan Fever). Cases occur mainly between July and September. In Africa, the ticks *Haemaphysalis leachi* and *Haemaphysalis punctaleachi* transmit *Rickettsia conorii*.

After an incubation period of 6 days (range 1–16 days), there is sudden onset of fever, headaches, chills, arthralgias, and myalgias, as in other rickettsial diseases. A generalized morbilliform eruption with an eschar at the site of the tick bite is characteristic. Gastrointestinal symptoms occur in approximately one third of patients. The diagnosis may be confirmed by direct fluorescent antibody, serology, or PCR assay.

African Tick Bite Fever

Rickettsia africae causes African Tick Bite Fever in both Africa and the Caribbean where ticks were transported on slave ships. The disease is transmitted by *Amblyomma* ticks that feed on cattle and wild game. After 6–7 days, individuals develop headache, myalgia, and rash, typically with a prominent eschar. Doxycyline therapy is preferred.

Other Spotted Fevers

Rickettsia japonica causes Japanese Spotted Fever, especially along the southwestern and central coast of Japan. The clinical presentation resembles other spotted fevers, with an eschar, fever, rash, and headache. *Rickettsia honei*, the causative agent of Flinders Island Spotted Fever, has been isolated in the Flinders Island, the Island of Tasmania, Thailand, and more recently in Texas. The vector is thought to be *Aponomma hydrosauri*, which feeds on reptiles. Typically, human infection occurs in the spring and summer, with sudden onset of fever, headache, arthralgias, myalgias, joint swelling, and cough followed by the development of a purpuric or morbilliform eruption. Flinders Island spotted fever is treated with oral doxycycline 200 mg daily for 7–10 days. *Rickettsia australis* causes Queensland Tick Typhus associated with *Ixodes holocyclus* and *Ixodes tasmani*. The majority of patients recall a tick bite and more than half develop an eschar. This spotted fever is treated similarly to other spotted fevers. Doxycycline (200 mg daily) is the preferred treatment, although quinolone antibiotics have been suggested as an alternative. The agent of Siberian Tick Typhus, *Rickettsia sibirica subspecies sibirica* has been isolated from *Dermacentor nuttalli*, *Dermacentor marginatus*, *Dermacentor silvarum*, and *Haemaphysalis concinna*. In China, infection with *Rickettsia sibirica subspecies sibirica* is referred to as North Asian tick typhus.

Tick-Borne Lymphadenopathy/ Dermacentor-Borne Necrosis Erythema Lymphadenopathy

Tick-borne lymphadenopathy is associated with eschar at the tick bite site and painful lymphadenopathy, caused by *Rickettsia slovaca* and transmitted by *Dermacentor marginatus*. *Rickettsia raoultii*, identified in *Ixodes* and *Dermacentor* ticks, may also be a cause. Dermacentor borne necrosis erythema lymphadenopathy syndrome is by *Dermacentor marginatus* and caused by *Rickettsia slovaca*. These diseases are seen most often in the pediatric population, often in southern or eastern Europe. Symptoms include headache, fever myalgia, confusion, and irritability. As with other rickettsial diseases, doxycycline is the preferred treatment, especially when symptoms are severe.

Lymphangitis-Associated Rickettsiosis

Lymphangitis-associated Rickettsiosis is caused by *Rickettsia sibirica mongolitimonae*, which is considered a subspecies of *Rickettsia sibirica*. It is transmitted by *Hyalomma* ticks in Africa, Asia, and Europe.

Q Fever

Coxiella burnetii causes Q fever and is transmitted by inhalation of contaminated aerosols, parenteral administration of infected blood transfusions, ingestion of contaminated milk, transplacentally, and by arthropod vectors. Q fever is typically acquired from occupational exposure to infected domestic animals such as sheep, cattle, and goats. Although *Coxiella burnetti* has been isolated from more than 40 species of tick, vector-borne transmission to humans is uncommon. Ticks in the United States include *Dermacentor andersoni, Dermacentor occidentalis, Amblyomma americanum, Haemaphysalis leporis-palustris, Ixodes dentatus*, and *Otobius magnini*. In addition to fever, headache, and myalgias, patients may experience hepatitis, myocarditis, pericarditis, or pneumonia. In the treatment of endocariditis associated with Q fever, doxycycline is not effective as a monotherapy and an infectious disease specialist should be consulted. Patients have been treated with combinations of a tetracycline with hydroxychloroquine or a fluoroquinolone.

Babesiosis

Babesia is an arthropod-borne parasite that infects erythrocytes with manifestations similar to malaria [6]. *Ixodes scapularis* is the primary vector for *Babesia microti* in the Northeastern

and midwestern United States. In one study, almost half of the affected patients did not recall a tick bite and diagnosis was often delayed due to the nonspecific nature of symptoms. Sixty-eight percent of the patients required hospitalization, with 21% requiring intensive care unit admission. Coinfection with Lyme, anaplasma, or both was noted in almost a third of the patients [7].

Patients may present with hepatomegaly and splenomegaly and signs of hemolytic anemia such as jaundice. Giemsa-stained peripheral blood smears may demonstrate intraerythroctyic parasites and PCR is available [8]. Clindamycin (600 mg four times per day) and quinine (650 mg three to four times per day) for 7–10 days is the standard treatment. Azithromycin and atovaquone may be as effective with a lower incidence of side effects. Atovaquone-proguanil has been effective in refractory cases in immunocompromised patients and ivermectin therapy is promising [9].

Tularemia

Francisella tularensis is a small, pleomorphic, aerobic, Gram-negative coccobacillus with a wide distribution. Almost half of all reported cases of tularemia were reported from Arkansas, Missouri, South Dakota, and Oklahoma. An arthropod-borne disease, Tularemia may be transmitted by ticks, deerfly, mites, and biting flies. The primary tick vectors *Amblyomma americanum, Dermacentor andersoni*, and *Dermacentor variabilis*. Tularemia may cause ulceroglandular, oculoglandular, oropharyngeal, typhoidal, and pneumonic syndromes. Serologic diagnosis is commonly employed and treatment is typically with streptomycin or other aminoglycosides, although chloramphenicol has also been used for neurologic disease and fluoroquinolones may have some efficacy.

Borrelioses

Tick-Borne Relapsing Fever is caused by *Borrelia hermsii, Borrelia turicatae,* and *Borrelia parker*. Tick-borne relapsing fever caused by Borrelia is transmitted by soft ticks of the genus *Ornithodorous*. Tick-borne relapsing fever presents with fever, headache, myalgia, arthralgia, nausea, and vomiting approximately 1 week after tick bite. An eschar may be present. As the fever defervesces, a morbilliform eruption may occur. Thrombocytopenia develops in more than one third of infected individuals and may be severe. Tetracyclines are considered the treatment of choice [10].

Lyme Disease and STARI

Borreliosis is present in much of the world, and both the spirochete and the vector influence disease manifestations. Acrodermatitis chronica atrophicans is more prevalent in central Europe. Lyme arthritis is most prominent in New England and the mid-Atlantic states and transmitted by *Ixodes* ticks. Southern Tick–Associated Rash Illness (STARI) presents similarly to Lyme disease as an expanding erythematous annular rash referred to a erythema migrans. This disease is caused by *Borrelia lonestari* and is transmitted by *Amblyomma americanum* in the southern and south central United States. STARI has been identified in Alabama, Missouri, Georgia, South Carolina, North Carolina, and Maryland. Lyme disease is more likely to progress to arthritic, cardiac, or neurological disease. Treatment guidelines for STARI are recommended as would be used in the treatment of Lyme disease: 10–30 days of oral doxycycline at 3 mg/kg in divided doses, amoxilcillin 500 mg three times daily, or cefuroxime 500 mg orally twice daily. A longer treatment duration is suggested if fever, a flu like illness, severe headache, or lymphadenopathy occur. Babesiosis, primarily a zoonotic disease, is transmitted to humans through the bite of Ixodes scapularis ticks or by blood transfusion. Co-infection with borrelioses has been reported [11].

Tick Borne Viruses

Ticks are responsible for transmitting a number of different viral diseases including Colorado Tick Fever, Tick Borne Encephalitis, Crimean-Congo Hemorrhagic Fever, Alkhurma Hemorrhagic Fever, Omsk Hemorrhagic Fever, and Powassan Encephalitis. Arboviruses may cause primarily encephalitis, hemorrhagic fever, or systemic febrile illness.

Colorado Tick Fever

Colorado tick fever (CTF) is endemic to the western United States and Canada where it is carried by rodents and other small mammals and transmitted by *Dermacentor andersoni*. It is caused by a coltivirus of the Reoviridae family. A variety of other ticks have also been implicated and CTF virus can be transmitted by exposure to infected animals and blood. Following an incubation period of 1–14 days, patients develop fever, headache, myalgia, chills, conjunctival injection, retroorbital pain, photophobia, and abdominal symptoms. Fever commonly relapses over the course of the disease. Central hepatitis, nervous system disease and disseminated intravascular coagulopathy may occur but most patients recover without sequelae. The accompanying rash may be morbilliform or petechial. Both serological testing and PCR are available.

Crimean-Congo Hemorrhagic Fever

Crimean-Congo hemorrhagic fever (CCHF) virus is a Nairovirus of the family Bunyaviridae. *Hyalomma* ticks are the principal vectors. Natural hosts of *Hyalomma* ticks include large herbivores, including camels, ostriches, hornbills, starlings, guinea fowl, and small mammals. CCHF occurs primarily in Africa, central and southwestern Asia, and to a lesser extent in Europe. As with tularemia, the disease may be spread by tick bite or contact with blood or meat from infected animals. After a 2–7 day incubation period fever, headache, chills, myalgia, arthralgia, photophobia, retro-orbital pain, and abdominal symptoms predominate. The hemorrhagic eruption may involve intertriginous sites and gut. Hepatitis may manifest with jaundice, hepatomegaly, and elevated liver enzymes. Thrombocytopenia and leukopenia may be noted. Case fatality ranges up to 60% and therapy is largely supportive. Ribavirin has also been used.

Eyach Virus

Eyach Virus transmitted by *Ixodes ricinus* causes encephalitis and polyradiduloneuritis in eastern and central Europe. Rabbits are the animal reservoir and treatment is largely supportive.

Tick-Borne Encephalitis

Tick-borne Encephalitis (TBE) virus is a flavivirus transmitted by *Ixodes* and *Haemaphysalis* ticks in Europe and Asia. After a 1–2 week incubation, patients present with fever, headache, myalgia, neurological, and abdominal symptoms. Thrombocytopenia and leukopenia may occur. Depending on the severity of the central nervous system manifestations, fatality may occur in up to 35% of patients. Clinical manifestations are thought to result from the host immune response to infection. Cytokines and chemokines associated with innate and Th1 adaptive immune responses are elevated in cerebrospinal fluid and are positively associated with disease severity [12].

Related diseases include the Louping virus in Britain and Langat virus in southeast Asia. In North America, the Powassan virus carried by *Ixodes cookie* and *Dermacentor* ticks causes a similar syndrome.

Severe Fever with Thrombocytopenia Syndrome

Severe fever with thrombocytopenia syndrome is an important emerging tick-borne infectious disease caused by a Phlebovirus and transmitted by *Haemaphysalis longicornis* [13]. The disease started in Asia but has spread to North America and the vector has spread. The most common presenting symptoms include severe fever, myalgia, and diarrhea [14].

Prevention of Tick-Borne Disease

Some vaccines are available, but tick repellents and acaricides are the mainstay of efforts at prevention. N,N-diethyl-3-methylbenzamide (DEET) is effec-tive against a broad range of arthropods, including ticks and picaridin have some efficacy as well, but both should be used in conjunction with permethrin-treated fabrics in areas where *Hyalomma* ticks are not endemic [15]. Permethrin mimics *Hyalomma* sexual pheromone and paradoxically attracts *Hyalomma* ticks that carry Congo-Crimean hemorrhagic fever, therefore the agent should be avoided in areas where these ticks are prevalent. Newer textile technology incorporates N-N-diethyl-m-toluamide, permethrin, cypermethrin, pyrethrum, picaridin, bioallethrin, citriodiol, and essential oils as well as some commonly used antimicrobial agents such as chitosan, zwitterionic compounds, silver and silver-based compounds, titanium dioxide nanoparticles, imidazolium salts, triclosan, and quaternary ammonium salts [16]. They may be useful for outdoor clothing, bed nets, tents, camping gear, and military uniforms and most survive multiple wash cycles. They offer protection against tick bites and arthropod-borne disease with less environmental impact.

DEET is the gold standard for insect repellents, with tremendous versatility and substantivity [17]. Other agents have been studied, IR3535, and botanicals [18]. It is generally safe, but toxicity has occurred with inhalation and misuse [19]. There have been very few lethal cases of DEET poisoning, usually due to deliberate overdoses. Studies in pregnant women found no effect on the developing fetus from proper use and its continued use as a repellent is endorsed by both the Centers for Disease Control and Prevention and the Environmental Protection Agency [20].

Removal of leaf litter and controlled burns can reduce the tick population and reduce the risk of tick-borne disease transmission [21, 22]. Bait stations can be used to treat deer and other host populations to control tick populations with less environmental impact than spraying insecticides.

References

1. Cabezas-Cruz A, Hodžić A, Román-Carrasco P, Mateos-Hernández L, Duscher GG, Sinha DK, Hemmer W, Swoboda I, Estrada-Peña A, de la Fuente J. Environmental and molecular drivers of the α-gal syndrome. Front Immunol. 2019;10:1210.

2. Stamm LV. Tick-borne diseases on the rise: an ounce of prevention is worth a pound of cure. Future Microbiol. 2019;14:833. https://doi.org/10.2217/fmb-2019-0148.

3. Bouchard C, Dibernardo A, Koffi J, Wood H, Leighton PA, Lindsay LR. N increased risk of tick-borne diseases with climate and environmental changes. Can Commun Dis Rep. 2019;45(4):83–9.

4. Rochlin I, Ninivaggi DV, Benach JL. Malaria and Lyme disease - the largest vector-borne US epidemics in the last 100 years: success and failure of public health. BMC Public Health. 2019;19(1):804.

5. Binder AM, Armstrong PA. Increase in reports of tick-borne Rickettsial diseases in the United States. Am J Nurs. 2019;119(7):20–1.

6. Rodriguez-Morales AJ, Bonilla-Aldana DK, Escalera-Antezana JP, Alvarado-Arnez LE. Research on Babesia: a bibliometric assessment of a neglected tick-borne parasite. F1000Res. 2018;7:1987.

7. Fida M, Challener D, Hamdi A, O'horo J, Abu Saleh O. Babesiosis: a retrospective review of 38 cases in the Upper Midwest. Open Forum Infect Dis. 2019;6(7)

8. Rucksaken R, Maneeruttanarungroj C, Maswanna T, Sussadee M, Kanbutra P. Comparison of conventional polymerase chain reaction and routine blood smear for the detection of Babesia canis, Hepatozoon canis, Ehrlichia canis, and Anaplasma platys in Buriram Province, Thailand. Vet World. 2019;12(5):700–5.

9. Batiha GE, Beshbishy AM, Tayebwa DS, Adeyemi OS, Yokoyama N, Igarashi I. Evaluation of the inhibitory effect of ivermectin on the growth of Babesia and Theileria parasites in vitro and in vivo. Trop Med Health. 2019;47:42.

10. Gocko X, Lenormand C, Lemogne C, Bouiller K, Gehanno JF, Rabaud C, Perrot S, Eldin C, de Broucker T, Roblot F, Toubiana J, Sellal F, Vuillemet F, Sordet C, Fantin B, Lina G, Sobas C, Jaulhac B, Figoni J, Chirouze C, Hansmann Y, Hentgen V, Caumes E, Dieudonné M, Bodaghi B, Gangneux JP, Degeilh B, Partouche H, Saunier A, Sotto A, Raffetin A, Monsuez JJ, Michel C, Boulanger N, Cathebras P, Tattevin P. Endorsed by the following scientific societies. Lyme borreliosis and other tick-borne diseases. Guidelines from the French scientific societies. Med Mal Infect. 2019;49(5):296–317.

11. Parveen N, Bhanot P. Babesia microti-Borrelia Burgdorferi coinfection. Pathogens. 2019;8:3.

12. Bogovič P, Lusa L, Korva M, Pavletič M, Rus KR, Lotrič-Furlan S, Avšič-Županc T, Strle K, Strle F. Inflammatory immune responses in the pathogenesis of tick-borne encephalitis. J Clin Med. 2019;8(5)

13. Won YJ, Kang LH, Lee SG, Park SW, Han JI, Paik SY. Molecular genomic characterization of severe fever with thrombocytopenia syndrome virus isolates from South Korea. J Microbiol. 2019;57:927. https://doi.org/10.1007/s12275-019-9174-8.

14. Kim J, Bae JM. Epidemiological and clinical characteristics of confirmed cases of severe fever with thrombocytopenia syndrome in Jeju Province, Korea, 2014-2018. J Prev Med Public Health. 2019;52(3):195–9.

15. Nguyen QD, Vu MN, Hebert AA. Insect repellents: an updated review for the clinician. J Am Acad Dermatol. 2018. pii: S0190-9622(18)32824-X. https://doi.org/10.1016/j.jaad.2018.10.053

16. Saleem F, Iqbal HMN. Environmentally responsive and anti-bugs textile finishes - recent trends, challenges, and future perspectives. Sci Total Environ. 2019;690:667–82. https://doi.org/10.1016/j.scitotenv.2019.06.520. [Epub ahead of print] Review

17. Beard CB, White A, Balanay JA, Richards S, Dyer M, Mather TN, Meshnick S. Bioabsorption and effectiveness of long-lasting permethrin-treated uniforms over three months among North Carolina outdoor workers. Parasit Vectors. 2019;12(1):52. https://doi.org/10.1186/s13071-019-3314-1.

18. Gliniewicz A, Borecka A, Przygodzka M, Mikulak E. Susceptibility of Dermacentor reticulatus tick to repellents containing different active ingredients. Przegl Epidemiol. 2019;73(1):117–25.

19. Tavares EM, Judge BS, Jones JS. Bug off! Severe toxicity following inhalational exposure to N, N-diethyl-meta-toluamide (DEET). Am J Emerg Med. 2019;37(7):1395.e3–4.

20. Swale DR, Bloomquist JR. Is DEET a dangerous neurotoxicant? Pest Manag Sci. 2019;75(8):2068–70. https://doi.org/10.1002/ps.5476.

21. Linske MA, Stafford KC 3rd, Williams SC, Lubelczyk CB, Welch M, Henderson EF. Impacts of deciduous leaf litter and snow presence on Nymphal Ixodes scapularis (Acari: Ixodidae) overwintering survival in coastal New England, USA. Insects. 2019;10(8)

22. Gleim ER, Zemtsova GE, Berghaus RD, Levin ML, Conner M, Yabsley MJ. Frequent prescribed fires can reduce risk of tick-borne diseases. Sci Rep. 2019;9(1):9974.

Spiders and Scorpions

Allison Weiffenbach, Geraldine Ranasinghe,
and Kenneth J. Tomecki

Key Points

- Spiders and scorpions are arachnids, belonging to the same class as ticks and mites.
- In general, spiders are benign Arachnida with few species of clinical significance.
- Envenomation with specific toxins after a spider bite can lead to various clinical syndromes. Diagnosis is based on identification of the spider and the patient's clinical presentation.
- Scorpion envenomation leads to activation of the autonomic nervous system. The clinical severity dictates the treatment and prognosis.

Spiders

Although arachnophobia is a well-known and prevalent fear of spiders, spiders are generally benign Arachnida with few species of clinical significance. They belong to the order Aranea and are related to scorpions, ticks, and mites [1]. Spiders most often have eight legs and lack antennae or wings, differentiating them from six-legged insects [1]. They use sharp fangs to inject venom into their prey, most often insects or other arthropods. This section will focus on the few spiders of medical importance. Emphasis will be placed on spiders from the following five genera/families: *Latrodectus, Loxosceles, Atracinae, Phoneutria,* and *Theraphosidae.* Latrodectism and loxoscelism are the two most important syndromes related to spider bites that occur worldwide. Envenomation with specific toxins leads to these clinical syndromes; the degree of envenomation, location of the spider bite, and age/sex of the spider all contribute to the severity of the clinical syndrome. Australian funnel web spiders are often considered the most dangerous spiders (Table 1) [2].

In general, spider bites occur after a spider's environment has been disrupted. Diagnosis of a spider bite is based on the clinical presentation as there is no laboratory test available to detect spider venom. Identification of the spider is possible if the spider is collected after the bite and it is imperative that physicians are knowledgeable about the spiders endemic to where they practice. A broad differential is important when considering a spider bite; vasculitis, vasculopathy, inflammatory etiologies, infections, and other infestations must be ruled out [3]. Prevention is based on decreasing exposure between medically important spiders and humans. There has been variable success with chemical repellents. Treatment of spider bites with antivenom is usually limited to moderate to severe envenomation syndromes, when local wound care and pain control are insufficient. Antivenoms for spider bites

A. Weiffenbach (✉) · G. Ranasinghe · K. J. Tomecki
Cleveland Clinic, Cleveland, OH, USA
e-mail: weiffea@ccf.org;
ranasig@ccf.org; tomeckk@ccf.org

W. Robles (ed.), *Skin Disease in Travelers*, Updates in Clinical Dermatology,
https://doi.org/10.1007/978-3-031-57836-6_20

Table 1 Selected medically significant Spider species

Spider species		
Family/genus	Selected species and locations	Toxins (clinical disease)
Latrodectus	*Latrodectus mactans*—United States, Caribbean *Latrodectus hasseltii*—Australia, New Zealand *Latrodectus tredecimguttatus*—Mediterranean region	Latrotoxin (Latrodectism)
Loxosceles	*Loxosceles laeta, Loxosceles intermedia, Loxosceles gaucho*—South America *Loxosceles reclusa, Loxosceles deserta*—United States, Mexico	Sphingomyelinase D, Hyaluronidase (Loxoscelism)
Atracinae	*Atrax robustus, Hadronyche formidabilis, Hadronyche cerberea*—Australia	Atracotoxins
Phoneutria	*Phoneutria nigriventer*—Brazil	
Theraphosidae	United States, Mexico, South America, Africa, Asia, Europe	

have proven less effective than those for snake or scorpion bites and few clinical studies exist to support their use.

Latrodectus

The genus *Latrodectus* includes the 30 species of widow spiders whose bites produce a clinical spectrum of disease termed latrodectism. The spiders are found worldwide, classically in warmer climates, hidden under woodpiles, shoes, or other outdoor spots. Females are largely responsible for bites of medical significance as males are not capable of envenomation. Rare reports of male spider bites have been reported in Australia. Bites typically occur when the spider's environment has been disrupted, but rarely lead to significant morbidity or mortality. Risk of envenomation increases when a female spider is protecting an egg sack.

Latrodectus mactans, commonly referred to as the black widow spider, can be found in the southern United States to Caribbean islands. Female spiders are black and classically have a red hourglass-shaped marking on the ventral surface of their abdomen. Additional species include the Australian Redback Black Widow, European black widow, and the South American black widow spider. *Latrodectus tredecimguttatus* is associated with myocardial injury and is most commonly found in the Mediterranean (Fig. 1).

Latrodectism occurs after envenomation with latrotoxin, a neurotoxin that results in depolariza-

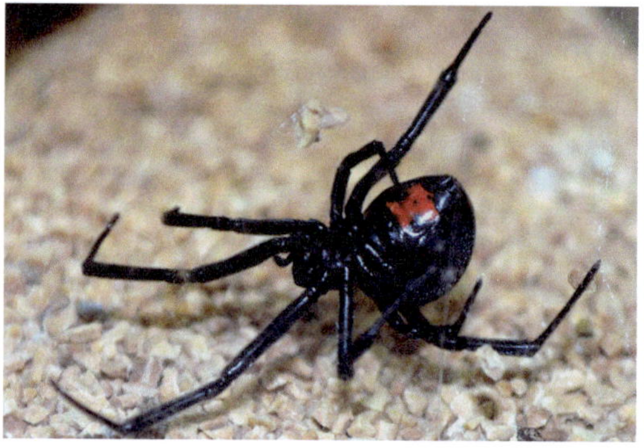

Fig. 1 Black widow spider with hourglass-shaped marking on the ventral surface of the abdomen

tion of neurons. After binding to presynaptic cation channels there is a release of neurotransmitters from motor and adrenergic nerve endings. Symptoms vary depending on the species of widow spider, location, and degree of envenomation. Pain can be localized to the bite site, expand to involve the entire region, or present as radiating pain. Tissue necrosis does not occur. Systemic symptoms include muscle pain and rigidity, vomiting, chills, and symptoms mimicking acute abdomen. Symptoms can very rarely progress to tachycardia, hypertension, shock, and rhabdomyolysis. Diaphoresis localized or radiating from the bite site is a unique presentation that can help distinguish latrodectism from other bite reactions. Latrodectism can be divided into mild, moderate, and major presentations—65% falling into the mild category, with only local symptoms, and 1% falling into the severe category, with life threatening presentations. Symptoms can persist for hours to days [4].

Diagnosis is based on the clinical presentation and history of a spider bite. Mild bite reactions can be treated with gentle wound care and pain control. More severe reactions may require benzodiazepines and calcium gluconate for tetany, and opiates for pain. Antivenom is occasionally used for severe reactions, depending on the geographic location of the bite and perceived efficacy in that region. The risk of allergic reactions, including anaphylaxis, and serum sickness must be taken into consideration, as data regarding efficacy of antivenom are lacking. These reactions are less likely with Fab fragment-based antivenom. For moderate and severe reactions monitoring of potential complications is essential. Tetanus prophylaxis should be considered in the appropriate circumstance [5].

Loxosceles

Loxosceles spiders, known as recluse spiders, violin spiders, and fiddleback spiders are found worldwide and can be best identified by their unique eye arrangement. They have six eyes arranged in three pairs (dyads), in contrast to eight eyes in two rows of four found on other spiders. There are 100 species total, with the majority found in South America. *Loxosceles laeta, Loxosceles intermedia,* and *Loxosceles gaucho* contribute to the majority of recluse bites in South America. *Loxosceles reclusa* and *Loxosceles deserta* are the brown recluse spiders found in the United States and Mexico. Species have also been reported in Europe, South Africa, and Australia. Recluse spiders are typically found inside homes, including hidden in basements, attics, and cupboards. Bites typically only occur when the spider's environment has been disturbed. *Loxosceles recluse* is famous for having a violin-shaped mark on their abdomen, however this feature has led to misidentification [6].

Recluse spiders release two toxins that are responsible for the majority of the clinical symptoms, referred to as loxoscelism. Sphingomyelinase D is a phospholipase that results in cell lysis and death, ultimately leading to skin necrosis. Hyaluronidase is also released contributing to the spread of necrosis. Because the bite is initially painless, it is rare for patients to recognize that the bite occurred and thus identification of the spider rarely occurs. Localized pain and erythema may develop over several hours, often progressing to dermonecrois and ulceration. Occasionally the bite site may take on the appearance of a bull's eye appearance, with a central cyanotic and pre necrotic center, surrounded by a rim of blanching vasoconstriction and finally outer erythematous vasodilation. Within 1 week, an eschar forms that can ultimately heal with or without scar formation. Recluse spider bites can be mistaken for other infections, including cellulitis, anthrax, and erythema migrans. Systemic symptoms are seen in approximately 10% of patients with cutaneous loxoscelism. Symptoms can be nonspecific and include headaches, fever, nausea, and vomiting. Patients should be monitored for signs and symptoms of acute hemolytic anemia, acute renal failure, and disseminated intravascular coagulation. Fatality, though rare in the United States, is more common after the South American recluse spider bite [7, 8].

Diagnosis of loxoscelism is dependent on the classic bite reaction with associated systemic symptoms in the appropriate setting. Treatment of recluse spider bites includes gentle wound care, application of ice, elevation of the affected area, and pain control. Antivenom can be considered when there are signs of impending necrosis or systemic complications, such as acute hemolytic anemia and acute renal failure [9]. Clinical and animal studies demonstrating efficacy and safety of antivenom are lacking, and as a result recluse antivenom is not available in many countries. Monitoring and treatment of any secondary bacterial infections are essential. Additional treatment options, such as systemic corticosteroids, dapsone, and hyperbaric oxygen therapy have not been sufficiently studied to warrant their use [10].

Atrax, Hadronyche, Illawarra

Atrax, Hadronyche, and *Illawarra* are three genera within the *Atracidae* family of Australian funnel-web spiders. The Australian funnel web spiders are some of the most deadly spiders as they inject a potent neurotoxin that leads to catecholamine and cholinergic excess. *Atrax robustus, Hadronyche formidabilis,* and *Hadronyche cerberea* contribute to most cases of severe envenomation. They often form burrows in cool sheltered areas, decreasing the chance that humans will come into contact with these spiders. Most funnel web spider bites have been attributed to the male spiders after they have left the burrow.

Australian funnel web spiders inject various toxins that are collectively called atracotoxins. These toxins bind to presynaptic sodium channels and lead to catecholamine and cholinergic excess with risk of myocardial injury and shock. The venom of female and young spiders is considered less potent than the venom of males. In contrast to many other spider bites, the bite of a funnel-web spider is painful. Severe envenomation is therefore uncommon as the spider is often pushed off soon after the bite occurs. Cutaneous findings can be subtle with erythema, induration, or paresthesia at the bite site. With severe envenomation there is a rapid onset of life threatening systemic symptoms involving neuromuscular and autonomic excitation. Early systemic symptoms include diaphoresis, paresthesias, tachycardia, and hypertension. Symptoms can progress to include nausea, vomiting, shortness of breath, and muscle spasms. Severe envenomation, when untreated, can progress to hypotension, coma, multiorgan failure, and death. Treatment includes urgent application of a pressure bandage along with immobilization of the affected limb, followed by administration of antivenom as soon as possible. Funnel web spider antivenom has proven to be an effective and safe treatment option for patients. No deaths have been attributed to funnel web spider bites since the introduction of antivenom [11–14].

Phoneutria

This genus of spiders, referred to as both Brazilian wandering spiders and armed spiders, is localized to South and Central America. Systemic symptoms only occur in 10% of patients. *Phoneutria nigriventer,* which is localized to Brazil, is the most likely species to cause a human bite. These spiders are nocturnal and bites most frequently occur when they are encountered inside homes during their mating season. Occasionally, *Phoneutria* are transported with bananas. Bite symptoms are typically mild and include localized pain and diaphoresis. Parasympathetic stimulation can present as priapism, bradycardia, and hypotension. Antivenom is the treatment of choice for systemic symptoms, but it is rarely used [15].

Theraphosidae

The theraphosidae family includes various genera of tarantulas that are found worldwide as a result of travel, trade, and "domestication." The largest tarantulas are capable of killing and eating small vertebrates. Although their bites are of little clinical significance, many tarantulas have unique urticaria inducing hairs that are associated with localized reactions. These urticating hairs are largely absent on those species found in Africa and Asia. Cutaneous reactions include urticaria at the site of contact with associated pruritus. Ophthalmia nodosa can occur when tarantulas come into contact with the eye, which can lead to loss of vision. Systemic toxicity amongst tarantulas is rare [16].

Scorpions

Scorpions are arachnids, belonging to the same class as spiders, ticks, and mites. These insects are feared by many due to both their appearance and notoriously painful sting which can have dire consequences. In this section, we will discuss clinically significant scorpions, cutaneous, and systemic manifestations caused by scorpion envenomation, as well as management and prevention.

It is important to understand the anatomy of scorpions as certain characteristics may be useful to differentiate species. All scorpions have seven

Table 2 Scorpion species based on geographic location

Scorpion species		
Geographic location	Species	Comments
Africa	*Parabuthus granulatus, P. capensis, P. transvaalicus, Uroplectes lineatus, and Leiurus quinquestriatus*	Fat tails Highly toxic
Asia and N. Africa	*Androctonus australis* *Buthus occitanus tunetanus*	
Asia	*Androctonus crassicauda* *Hottentotta tamulus*	*H. tamulus* is red
Brazil	*Tityus serrulatus*	Deadly to children
Southwest US (AZ)	*Centruroides exilicauda*	Tubercle found at base of stinger
Central US (TX)	*Centruroides vittatus*	Painful sting
US/Mexico/Central America	*Centruroides noxius* *C. limpidus* *C. suffusus*	Toxic

Adapted from Bolognia J, Schaffer J, Cerroni L. *Dermatology,* 4th ed. Elsevier Saunders, Philadelphia, PA. 2017

sets of appendages: the chelicerae, the pedipalps (claws), four sets of legs, and the pectines. Their unique tail is segmented and curls upward with the telson, the terminal bulbous segment, containing their venom glands and the stinger. During the scorpion's envenomation process, their pedipalps are used to grasp their prey while they curve their tail overhead to sting. Although scorpions can sting many times, their first sting is the most potent and nearly depletes the stored venom in the telson [17]. The majority of scorpions prefer undisturbed areas, such as under table tops, in wood piles, or even in shoes.

There are approximately 2000 species of scorpion, all of which are venomous. These species are divided into roughly nine families. The most notorious scorpion family of clinical importance is the Buthidae family, which contains several species that secrete poisonous venom which is potentially fatal to humans. Notable species within this family include Centruroides, Tityus, Androctonus, Buthus, Buthotus, Leirus, and Parabuthus (Table 2) [18].

Centruroides

Centruroides exilicauda (also called *C. sculpturatus* or Arizona bark scorpion) is found predominantly in the Southwestern United States and Northern Mexico. These scorpions can be yellow

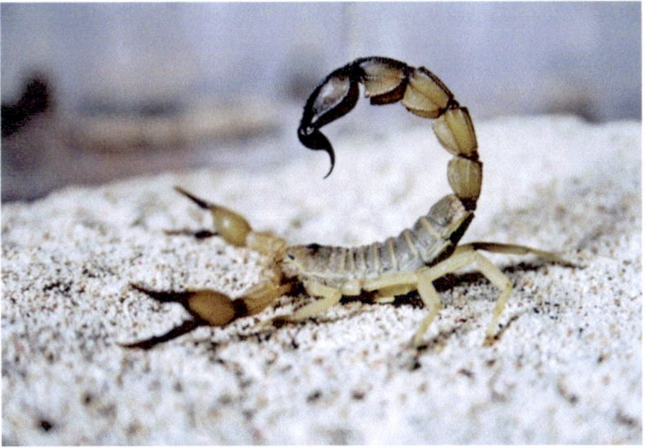

Fig. 2 *Centruroides* can be identified by their tan to yellow color. This family of scorpions is found throughout the Southwestern United States and Northern Mexico

or tan in color and range from 4 to 7 cm in length. These scorpions prefer residing in or near shade trees. Their unique stinger which contains a distinct tubercle at its base serves as a particularly useful clue to identifying this species [19].

Another notable species in the Centruroides family is *Centruroides vittatus* which has a striking appearance with a black interocular triangle and black stripes on the thorax. These scorpions prefer to hide in undisturbed areas in natural habitats, such as crevices in rocky terrain and even attics and basements in man-made buildings. These too are found in Southwest United States, as well as Southern Indiana and Illinois (Fig. 2) [20].

Parabuthus

The Parabuthus family of scorpions is one of the largest in size, ranging from 6 to 15 cm in length. *Parabuthus granulatus* (also called granulated thick-tailed scorpion) is dark yellow to brown in color and possesses thin pincers and with a thick tail. They prefer to dwell beneath grass, shrubs, or sandy soil [5]. *Parabuthus transvaalicus* is a nocturnal thick-tailed scorpion that can be dark brown or black. Its tail is capable of injecting or spraying its kurtoxin venom, which selectively inhibits calcium channels. This type of scorpion prefers thatched roofs as well as burrowing in sandy, dry soil [21, 22].

Androctonus

Androctonus astralis (also called the "yellow fat tailed scorpion") is typically yellow with darker pincers and found in arid desert regions in the Middle East, India, as well as mountains of North America [23]. *Androctonus crassicauda* (Arabian fat-tailed scorpion) is black and slightly larger than *A. astralis,* measuring around 12 cm in length. This species is also found in desert climates in North America and Middle East [24].

Tityus

Tityus serrulatus is found in the warm, tropical climates of Brazil. These scorpions have yellow pincers with dark brown tips, a dark body and typically grow to about 6–7 cm in size. Interestingly, cases of envenomation by this scorpion tend to rise during the rainy season as the scorpions flee their underground burrows for shelter in or near human dwellings. These scorpions secrete a toxin which can cause acute pancreatitis [24, 25].

Buthus

Buthus occitanus is yellow-brown scorpion up to 8 cm in length that lives in deserts of North Africa. There are reports of this scorpion found in southwestern Europe as well. The cases of scorpion envenomation in Europe are not associated with fatal systemic symptoms [26].

Leiurus

Leiurus quinquestriatus (also called "death stalker") is a desert scorpion that grows 8–11 cm in length. This species prefers to burrow into sandy deserts in North Africa and the Middle East. These scorpions are commonly imported from Egypt and sold in Europe or United States as an exotic species. Similarly to *T. serrulatus,* these scorpions secrete a toxin which can cause acute pancreatitis [27].

Hottentotta

Hottentotta tamulus (also called the red scorpion) is the most dangerous scorpion indigenous to the tropical Asian climates found in India, Pakistan, Sri Lanka, and Nepal. This scorpion grows 9 cm in size and is red in color. Envenomations by this scorpion are more commonly reported in rural regions along the southern coast of India during the months of April through June [28–31].

Venom

The scorpion's venom contains a mixture of enzymes and toxins, including acetylcholinesterase, hyaluronidase, mucopolysaccharides, phospholipase, histamine, serotonin, protease inhibitors, histamine releasers, and neurotoxins. Once injected into their victim, these molecules inhibit vital sodium, potassium, and calcium channels. The scorpion α-toxin is the most lethal, as it inhibits voltage-gated sodium channels leading to prolonged depolarization and neuronal excitation. The prolonged and unregulated depolarization stimulates the autonomic centers and the sympathetic system releases excess catecholamines, causing fatal systemic effects such as pulmonary edema, cardiogenic shock, and myocardial dysfunction [32].

Cutaneous and Systemic Manifestations

Scorpions primarily sting as a mode of defense when they feel threatened or endangered. Human envenomations most often occur on the lower extremities when an individual unknowingly encounters a scorpion dwelling under wood, rocks, or sand while walking. Individuals living in endemic regions of the world may encounter scorpions on a frequent basis, as they may hide in crevices of roofs, stone houses, in bedding, or footwear [33].

Depending on the species, scorpion stings often result in a local inflammatory response which can include pain, edema, erythema, muscle fasciculations, and/or numbness at the site of envenomation. While fatal systemic symptoms are typically only seen in approximately 10% of all scorpion stings, envenomation by scorpions in either the *Centruroides* or *Parabuthus* species are associated with significantly increased risk of life-threatening symptoms which can present immediately or up to 5 h later [28, 32, 34].

As the neurotoxins stimulate the autonomic nervous system, both parasympathetic and sympathetic responses are activated, resulting in profuse diaphoresis, lacrimation, miosis, diarrhea, vomiting, bradycardia, hypotension, increased respiratory secretion, hypersalivation, and priapism due to hyperactive parasympathetic system and tachycardia, hyperthermia, hyperglycemia, agitation, mydriasis, and restlessness due to overdrive of the sympathetic system. Acute pancreatitis is a unique symptom seen in patients stung by a *Leiurus quinquestriatus and Tityus species.* Adverse toxin effects on the cardiac conduction result in atrial tachycardia, T-wave inversion, ventricular extrasystoles, and rarely bundle-branch block [32]. An adverse consequence of this cardiac dysfunction could lead to cardiogenic shock and/or pulmonary edema. Neurological symptoms include: uncoordinated neuromuscular activity which may present as respiratory compromise, alarming thrashing of the limbs, abnormal oculomotor movements, visual changes and muscle fasciculations of face, tongue, and extremities [32, 35, 36].

It may be difficult to identify the site of the sting, but pain out of proportion is a common finding. An interesting phenomenon occurs with stings from the *H. lepturus* species. Initially stings are asymptomatic and later develop purpuric, erythematous, and bullous lesions that resolve. However, in 20% of cases there is a delayed tissue necrosis that develops over hours to days. Patients may also experience systemic symptoms described above, such as fever, nausea, and vomiting, as well as acute kidney injury that may require dialysis. In some cases, this presentation may resemble one after loxosceles spider bite [32].

Management

The clinical management of symptoms is directed by a grading system based on severity of symptoms [37]. This grading system is divided into four categories: local, minor, major, and lethal. Grade 1 envenomation describes local pain and paresthesias at the sting site with minimal inflammation. Although not widely recognized, the "tap test" has been used to confirm a *C. exilicauda* sting. With the patient looking away, one can gently tap the sting site, and if symptoms are significantly exacerbated, then this is deemed as a positive result—which is not seen with other scorpion stings [3]. Grade 2 envenomations produce local symptoms plus systemic autonomic effects as described above. Grade 3 envenomations show evidence of cardiotoxicity with acute pulmonary edema or cardiogenic shock. Grade 4 envenomations have features of Grade 3 plus coma, seizures, and/or other signs of multisystem organ failure [32]. Depending on the clinical situation, additional laboratory workup may be warranted, such as serum electrolytes, liver enzymes, serum creatinine, urine analysis, ECG, and cardiac markers if there is suspicion for cardiac involvement.

It is imperative for clinicians in endemic areas to be aware of these symptoms, especially in the pediatric population, as infants and children tend to be the most vulnerable to such injuries and can present with bizarre constellations of symptoms.

Other entities to consider in the differential diagnosis include: bites from other arthropods such as spiders, tetanus, botulism, organophosphate exposure, seizure disorder, neuroblastoma, and meningitis to name a few.

Symptom resolution varies by age and degree of envenomation. Without antivenom treatment, improvement can be seen between 9 and 30 h however, persistent symptoms such as pain and paresthesias can last for up to 2 weeks [19]. For the majority of scorpion stings, which tend to be classified as Grade 1 and 2 envenomation, treatment consists of pain management with ice, oral nonsteroidal antiinflammatory agents, oral or short acting intravenous opioids as suitable for severe pain. As for wound care, gently cleansing the site and providing tetanus prophylaxis if the patient is not up to date on vaccinations is recommended. Patients should be observed for at least 4 h to ensure there is no progression of clinical symptoms [19, 37].

For patients presenting with Grade 3 or 4 envenomation, administration of antivenom should be considered in addition to targeted treatment for specific symptoms such as prazosin for autonomic cascade and dobutamine to restore myocardial function. Antivenom after *Centruroides, Hottentotta, Tityus, Leiurus,* and *Parabuthus* stings is recommended, although there is some evidence that this is not always effective. The specific dosing and administration is dependent on the type of species the patient was stung by [32, 38].

Prazosin is a medication that modulates excessive catecholamine release and subsequent adverse events. In some cases, the use of prazosin in addition to scorpion-specific antivenom is preferred as there have been promising results. In a randomized open-label study [39] of 70 patients in India stung by *Hottentotta* species, the patients with Grade II or higher envenomation who received antivenom and prazosin recovered more rapidly than patients who received prazosin alone. There are several reports and retrospective analyses suggestive of lower mortality rates and better recovery outcomes in patients given prazosin compared to those who were not given the medication. Future studies and further evidence is necessary to make a definite judgement [39]. This medication is also easy to store and can be given orally, which are useful factors to consider in rural or resource depleted areas [40, 41].

Although literature regarding management of scorpion envenomation is limited, the small number of published studies show that with prompt administration of prazosin, supportive care, and addition of scorpion specific antivenom, most patients fully recover from scorpion envenomation within 24–48 h with mortality rates of less than 1% [32, 42].

Prevention

In endemic areas, education on prevention could potentially decrease the incidence of scorpion envenomation. Filling in cracks in homes and placing a bed net below thatched roofs prevents scorpions from entering human dwellings. Clothing, shoes, or undisturbed areas should be carefully searched for scorpions. Another preventative measure is spraying an insecticide around the perimeter of the house, this works by killing other insects and decreasing available food supply for scorpions [39].

References

1. Madsen W, Elfar J. Spider bites. J Hand Surg Am. 2010;35(10):1698–9. https://doi.org/10.1016/j.jhsa.2010.07.004.
2. Isbister GK, Fan HW. Spider bite. Lancet. 2011;378(9808):2039–47. https://doi.org/10.1016/S0140-6736(10)62230-1.
3. Vetter RS, Isbister GK. Medical aspects of spider bites. Annu Rev Entomol. 2008;53:409–29. https://doi.org/10.1146/annurev.ento.53.103106.093503.
4. Prongay R, Kelsberg G, Safranek S. Clinical inquiry: which treatments relieve painful muscle spasms from a black widow spider bite? J Fam Pract. 2012;61(11):694–5.
5. Jelinek GA. Widow spider envenomation (latrodectism): a worldwide problem. Wilderness Environ Med. 1997;8(4):226–31. https://doi.org/10.1580/1080-6032(1997)008[0226:wselaw]2.3.co;2.
6. Forks TP. Brown recluse spider bites. J Am Board Fam Pract. 2000;13(6):415–23. https://doi.org/10.3122/15572625-13-6-415.

7. Malaque CM, Santoro ML, Cardoso JL, et al. Clinical picture and laboratorial evaluation in human loxoscelism. Toxicon. 2011;58(8):664–71. https://doi.org/10.1016/j.toxicon.2011.09.011.

8. Barbaro KC, Knysak I, Martins R, Hogan C, Winkel K. Enzymatic characterization, antigenic cross-reactivity and neutralization of dermonecrotic activity of five Loxosceles spider venoms of medical importance in the Americas. Toxicon. 2005;45(4):489–99. https://doi.org/10.1016/j.toxicon.2004.12.009.

9. McDade J, Aygun B, Ware RE. Brown recluse spider (Loxosceles reclusa) envenomation leading to acute hemolytic anemia in six adolescents. J Pediatr. 2010;156(1):155–7. https://doi.org/10.1016/j.jpeds.2009.07.021.

10. Parekh KP, Seger D. Systemic loxoscelism. Clin Toxicol (Phila). 2009;47(5):430–1. https://doi.org/10.1080/15563650802555515.

11. Oranges T, Janowska A, Tonini A, Romanelli M, Dini V. Necrotoxic spider bite: a successful non-invasive wound management. Int J Dermatol. 2019;58(7):e128–30. https://doi.org/10.1111/ijd.14323.

12. Suchard JR. Spider bite. Ann Emerg Med. 2009;54(1):8–11. https://doi.org/10.1016/j.annemergmed.2008.11.022.

13. Isbister GK, Gray MR, Balit CR, et al. Funnel-web spider bite: a systematic review of recorded clinical cases. Med J Aust. 2005;182(8):407–11.

14. Nentwig W, Gnädinger M, Fuchs J, Ceschi A. A two year study of verified spider bites in Switzerland and a review of the European spider bite literature. Toxicon. 2013;73:104–10. https://doi.org/10.1016/j.toxicon.2013.07.010.

15. Isbister GK, Graudins A, White J, Warrell D. Antivenom treatment in arachnidism. J Toxicol Clin Toxicol. 2003;41(3):291–300. https://doi.org/10.1081/clt 12002111.

16. Isbister GK, Seymour JE, Gray MR, Raven RJ. Bites by spiders of the family Theraphosidae. Toxicon. 2003;41(4):519–24.

17. Campbell NA, Reece JB, Mitchell LG. Biology. 5th ed. Menlo Park, CA: Addison Wesley Longman, Inc.; 1999.

18. Hutt M, Houghton P. A survey from the literature of plants used to treat scorpion stings. J Ethnopharmacol. 1998;60:97–110.

19. LoVecchio F, McBride C. Scorpion envenomations in young children in central Arizona. J Toxicol Clin Toxicol. 2003;41(7):937–40.

20. Stipetic ME, Lugo A, Brown B, et al. A prospective analysis of 558 common striped scorpion (Centruroides vittatus) envenomations in Texas during 1997 (meeting abstract). J Toxicol Clin Toxicol. 1998;36:46.

21. Müller GJ, Modler H, Wium CA, Veale DJH. Scorpion sting in southern Africa: diagnosis and management.

22. Sidach SS, Mintz IM. Kurtoxin, a gating modifier of neuronal high- and low threshold Ca channels. J Neurosci. 2002;22(6):2023–34.

23. Androctonus australis. The Scorpion Files. Available at: http://www.ntnu.no/ub/scorpion-files/a_australis.php

24. Sucard JR. Scorpion envenomation. In: Auerback PS, Cushing TA, Harris NS, editors. Auerbach's Wilderness Medicine, vol. 1. 7th ed. Philadelphia: Elsevier; 2017. p. 1017.

25. Cupo P. Clinical update on scorpion envenoming. Rev Soc Bras Med Trop. 2015;48(6):642.

26. Rein JO. A review of the scorpion fauna of Europe. The Scorpion Files. Available at: http://www.ntnu.no/ub/scorpion-files/european_scorp.php. Accessed on September 18, 2017.

27. Ross LK. Leiurus quinquestriatus. The Scorpion Files. Available at: http://www.ntnu.no/ub/scorpion-files/l_quinquestriatus_info.pdf

28. Bergman NJ. Clinical description of Parabuthus transvaalicus scorpionism in Zimbabwe. Toxicon. 1997;35(5):759–71.

29. Veronika K, Akilan K, Murugananthan A, Eswaramohan T. Diversity and identification key to the species of scorpions (Scorpiones: Arachnida) from Jaffna Peninsula, Sri Lanka. J Entomol Zool Stud. 2013;1:70.

30. Nagaraj SK, Dattatreya P, Boramuthi TN. Indian scorpions collected in Karnataka: maintenance in captivity, venom extraction and toxicity studies. J Venom Anim Toxins Incl Trop Dis. 2015;21:51.

31. Das S, Nalini P, Ananthakrishnan S, Ananthanarayanan PH, Balachander J, Sethuraman KR, Srinivasan S. Scorpion envenomation in children in southern India. J Trop Med Hyg. 1995;98(5):306.

32. Geoffrey KI, Himmatrao SB. Scorpion envenomation. N Engl J Med. 2014;371(5):457 63.

33. Santos MS, Silva CG, Neto BS, Grangeiro Júnior CR, Lopes VH, Teixeira Júnior AG, Bezerra DA, Luna JV, Cordeiro JB, Júnior JG, Lima MA. Clinical and epidemiological aspects of scorpionism in the world: a systematic review. Wilderness Environ Med. 2016;27(4):504.

34. O'Connor AD, Padilla-Jones A, Ruha AM. Severe bark scorpion envenomation in adults. Clin Toxicol (Phila). 2018;56(3):170.

35. Clark RF, Selden BS, Kunkel DB, Frost MD. Abnormal eye movements encountered following severe envenomations by Centruroides sculpturatus. Neurology. 1991;41(4):604.

36. Berg RA, Tarantino MD. Envenomation by the scorpion Centruroides exilicauda (C sculpturatus): severe and unusual manifestations. Pediatrics. 1991;87(6):930.

37. Bergman NJ. Scorpion sting in Zimbabwe. S Afr Med J. 1997;87(2):163–7.

38. LoVecchio F, Welch S, Klemens J, Curry SC, Thomas R. Incidence of immediate and delayed hypersensitivity to Centruroides antivenom. Ann Emerg Med. 1999;34(5):615.
39. Bawaskar HS, Bawaskar PH. Scorpion sting: update. J Assoc Physicians India. 2012;60:46.
40. Al-Asmari AK, Al-Seif AA, Hassen MA, Abdulmaksood NA. Role of prazosin on cardiovascular manifestations and pulmonary edema following severe scorpion stings in Saudi Arabia. Saudi Med J. 2008;29(2):299.
41. Gupta V. Prazosin: a pharmacological antidote for scorpion envenomation. J Trop Pediatr. 2006;52(2):150. Epub 2006 Mar 14
42. Chippaux JP. Emerging options for the management of scorpion stings. Drug Des Devel Ther. 2012;6:165–73.

Part VII

Dermatoses Caused by Parasites

Cutaneous Larva Migrans

Ricardo L. Galimberti

Key Points
- Cutaneous larva migrans
- Nematode parasites of the hookworm family
- Serpiginous lesions
- Pruritic erythematous papules
- Spontaneous relief
- Albendazole
- Ivermectin

Introduction

Cutaneous larva migrans—colloquially called *creeping eruption*—was first described in 1874 [1]. It is considered one of the most common skin diseases in tourists' visits to tropical countries. It is caused by the *larvae* of various nematode parasites of the hookworm family (*Ancylostomatidae*). These parasites live in the intestines of dogs, cats, and wild animals. The disease is characterized by serpiginous lesions with intense itching [2].

Etiology and Distribution

Cutaneous larva migrans is the most frequent helminthic infection in tropical and subtropical dermatosis including Southeast Asia, Africa,

R. L. Galimberti (✉)
Department of Dermatology, Italian Hospital in
Buenos Aires, Buenos Aires, Argentina

Southeastern USA, Central and South America, although lately its frequency has increased in other geographical areas where high temperatures, humidity, and healthcare deficits favor its development [3]. The disease has been reported more frequently during rainy and hot seasons.

The species most frequently involved in this pathology are *Ancylostoma braziliense* (which usually infest dogs and cats), *Ancylostoma caninum* (dogs), *Uncinaria stenocephala* (dogs), among others [4].

Nematode eggs are excreted through feces, usually from dogs and/or cats. They mature into the noninfectious rhabditiform *larvae* in 1–2 days. Then where heat and humidity are appropriate, they develop for approximately 5 days, growing into infective hookworm *larvae*. As such, they remain in the soil until they come into contact with the skin of the primary host (dogs and cats), in which they penetrate [5].

Within the host, they are transported via the lymphatic system and the veins into the lungs. Passing into the alveoli and the trachea they are then regurgitated. They mature in the intestine of the host and produce eggs that are excreted in the feces, thus completing their life cycle.

Occasionally, the infective filariform *larvae* penetrate human skin and remain there without completing their life cycle, since they cannot cross the basement membrane due to their lack of enzymes to do so.

W. Robles (ed.), *Skin Disease in Travelers*, Updates in Clinical Dermatology,
https://doi.org/10.1007/978-3-031-57836-6_21

Exceptionally, the filariform *larvae* do cross the basement membrane and produce a *Visceral larva migrans* condition. Experimental studies show that the larvae penetrate through hair follicles and sweat gland openings [6].

Clinical Features

Clinically, 24–48 hours after making contact with the parasite, the patient presents pruritic erythematous papules at the site of access [7].

During the next 1–2 weeks, below the epidermis, papules grow 2–5 cm per day, thus forming a tunnel or snakelike track, which manifests itself with a linear, erythematous, and pruritic lesion—a clinical sign present in 98% of cases (Figs. 1 and 2).

The most affected areas of the body are those which are in contact with the ground: feet, buttocks, and trunk. Mucosal, scalp, or genital involvement is rare.

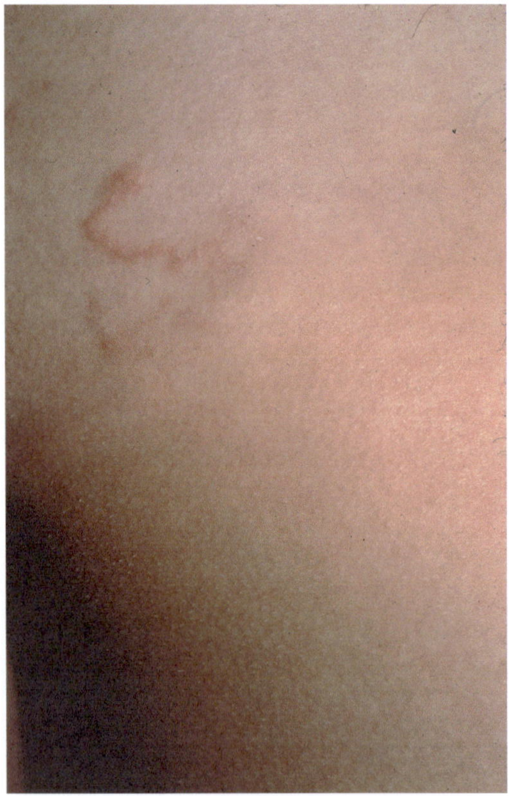

Fig. 1 Cutaneous larva migrans. Indurated worm track. Image Courtesy: Courtesy of Prof Roberto Arenas MD

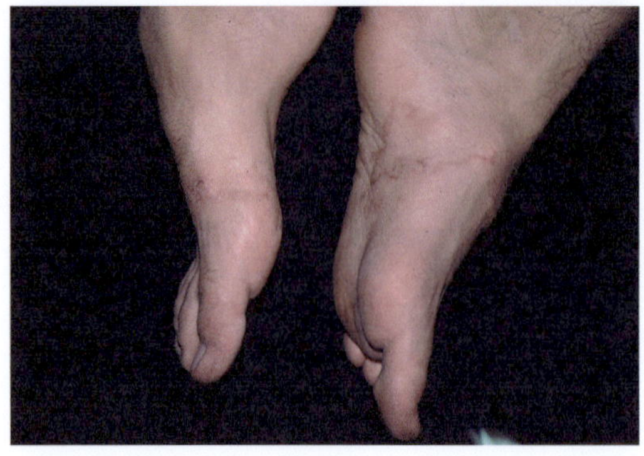

Fig. 2 Cutaneous larva migrans. Creeping eruption with snakelike tracks. Image Courtesy: Courtesy of Prof Roberto Arenas MD

The original lesion becomes dry, scaly, and crusty and may leave transient dyschromia after healing. It is not uncommon to find multiple lesions due to the penetration of more than one *larva*.

In addition to itching, we can find overlapping bacterial infections induced by scratching and, less frequently, blistering lesions associated with edema. The evolution is usually benign and the process is self-limited by the death of the larva in a period that ranges from 1 to 2 months in most cases.

Nevertheless, 10–30% of patients with this disease manifest inflammatory tissue response, intense pruritus, eosinophilia of 9–12%, and increased serum IgE levels as well as increase in IL-5, IL-10 and TNF [8]. Sometimes, Löffler's syndrome may develop along with changing pulmonary infiltrates and eosinophilic pneumonitis [9].

Diagnosis

The diagnosis is clinical and based, first, on the appearance of the lesion and, second, on questions directed towards the possibility of recent travel to an endemic area.

A less common variety has been recognized, called *Larva Currens*, which usually manifests with perianal lesions of *Strongyloides stercoralis*. Its migration is surprisingly fast (10 cm/day) and the eruption is urticarial or linear.

Cases of wandering disease caused by *Gnathostoma larvae*, a parasite acquired by eating raw freshwater fish ceviche, have been described in Mexico, Ecuador, and Thailand [10].

Preventive measures consist in the use of footwear and clothing that prevent direct contact with the ground.

Differential diagnosis of *Cutaneous Larva migrans* should be done with *Larva currens*, *Visceral larva migrans*, Myiasis, Scabies, *Phytophotodermatitis,* and *Chronic erythema migrans.*

Treatment

Although *Cutaneous larva migrans* is a dermatosis of spontaneous relief, where the resolution of the infection ranges from 2 to 8 weeks, itching and bacterial complications should signal the beginning of antiparasitic treatment in order to shorten the natural evolution of the disease and in order to relieve patient's discomfort. Treatment will depend on the degree of morbidity caused by the infection [11].

The most used oral treatments are Albendazole and Ivermectin, the latter being better tolerated with a low rate of adverse events.

There are studies that establish the superiority of treatment with an Ivermectin 12 mg dose when compared to Albendazole 400 mg/12 h. The former has reached approximately 100% success in healing the condition [12].

Topical treatment is used when there is one or only a few lesions. The use of cryotherapy or thiabendazole ointment has been previously described.

Cryotherapy is used on the distal edge of the lesion to prevent further migration of the *larvae.*

Although cryotherapy is an accessible treatment, its response is not entirely effective.

Thiabendazole ointment is the most widely used therapeutic option in the world due to its low cost and easy usage, with an efficacy close to 100% after 4 weeks of treatment (Figs. 1 and 2).

References

1. Lee RJ. Case of creeping eruption. Trans Clin Soc Lond. 1874;8:44–5.
2. Heukelbach J, Feldmeier H. Epidemiological and clinical characteristics of hookworm-related cutaneous larva migrans. Lancet Infect Dis. 2008;8(5):302–9.
3. Klose C, Mravak S, Geb M, Bienzle U, Meyer C. Autochthonous cutaneous larva migrans in Germany. Trop Med Int Health. 1996;1(4):503–4.
4. Davies H, Sakuls P, Keystone J. Creeping eruption. A review of clinical presentation and management of 60 cases presenting to a tropical disease unit. Arch Dermatol. 1993;129(5):588–91.
5. Hochedez P, Caumes E. Hookworm-related cutaneous larva migrans. J Travel Med. 2007;14(5):326–33.
6. Maxfield L, Crane JS. Cutaneous larva migrans. Treasure Island, FL: StatPearls Publishing; 2019.
7. Patel S, Aboutalebi S, Vindhya P, Smith J. What's eating you? Extensive cutaneous larva migrans (Ancylstoma braziliense). Cutis. 2008;82(4):239–40.
8. Gaze S, Bethony J, Periago M. Immunology of experimental and natural human hookworm infection. Parasite Immunol. 2014;36(8):358–66.
9. Hotez P, Narasimhan S, Haggerty J, et al. Hyaluronidase from infective ancylostoma hookworm larvae and its possible function as a virulence factor in tissue invasion and in cutaneous larva migrans. Infect Immunity. 1992;60(3):1018–23.
10. Centers for Disease Control and Prevention. Outbreak of cutaneous larva migrans at a children's camp—Miami, Florida, 2006. Morb Mortal Wkly Rep. 2007;56(3):1285–7.
11. Caumes E. Treatment of cutaneous larva migrans. Clin Infect Dis. 2000;30(5):811–4.
12. Naquira C, Jimenez G, Guerra J, et al. Ivermectin for human strongyloidiasis and other intestinal helminths. Am J Trop Med Hygiene. 1989;40(3):304–9.

African–Asian–European Cutaneous Leishmaniasis

David J. Chandler and Stephen L. Walker

Abbreviations

AAECL	African-Asian-European CL
ACL	American CL
CL	Cutaneous leishmaniasis
DCL	Diffuse cutaneous leishmaniasis
LCL	Localised cutaneous leishmaniasis
MA	Meglumine antimoniate
MCL	Mucocutaneous leishmaniasis
NTD	Neglected tropical disease
NWCL	New World CL
OWCL	Old World CL
PCR	Polymerase chain reaction
PKDL	Post-kala-azar dermal leishmaniasis
SSG	Sodium stibogluconate
VL	Visceral leishmaniasis
WHO	World Health Organisation

D. J. Chandler (✉)
Department of Global Health & Infection, Brighton and Sussex Medical School, Brighton, UK

University Hospitals Sussex NHS Foundation Trust, Brighton, UK
e-mail: d.chandler@bsms.ac.uk

S. L. Walker
London School of Hygiene and Tropical Medicine, London, UK

Hospital for Tropical Diseases and Department of Dermatology, University College London Hospitals NHS Foundation Trust, London, UK
e-mail: Steve.Walker@LSHTM.ac.uk

Key Points
- CL is a neglected tropical disease (NTD).
- CL results in permanent scarring and can be highly disfiguring.
- A wide range of treatment options are available but few have been properly evaluated.
- CL should be considered in anyone with an ulcer or nodule who has recently travelled to an endemic country.
- Species identification is important to understand the risk of developing severe forms of CL or visceral disease and guide management decisions.
- Research is needed to better understand this disease and to develop safe and more effective treatments.

Introduction

Cutaneous leishmaniasis (CL) is a vector-borne parasitic disease caused by a heterogeneous group of parasites belonging to the genus *Leishmania*. CL encompasses a range of clinical forms, from localised self-healing skin lesions, to severe forms which include mucosal and disseminated cutaneous disease. Unlike visceral leishmaniasis (kala-azar), the cutaneous forms of leishmaniasis are not fatal; however, they can be highly disfiguring and result in chronic disability and stigmatisation.

W. Robles (ed.), *Skin Disease in Travelers*, Updates in Clinical Dermatology, https://doi.org/10.1007/978-3-031-57836-6_22

CL is a complex disease. The epidemiology, clinical features and response to treatment vary widely and are influenced by a range of factors which are often specific to the geographic region. Worldwide up to 1.2 million new cases of CL are estimated to occur each year [1].

Post-kala-azar dermal leishmaniasis (PKDL) is a late complication of visceral leishmaniasis. Despite having potentially significant cutaneous manifestations, it is distinct from cutaneous leishmaniasis and is not considered in detail in this chapter.

Leishmania Parasite: An Overview

The life cycle of the *Leishmania* parasite involves a sandfly host and a vertebrate mammalian host.

Flagellated promastigote forms are inoculated into the dermis of the vertebrate host, when the sandfly takes a bloodmeal. The promastigotes are ingested by local skin-resident macrophages where they differentiate into rounded amastigotes (Leishman-Donovan bodies). Amastigotes multiply by simple binary fission within the phagolysosome which leads to rupture of the cell. The released parasites are engulfed by other local macrophages. In most cases the reproductive cycle will continue in the skin and superficial tissues; however, for some parasite species the reproductive cycle can involve mucosal tissue (*L. aethiopica*, *L. braziliensis*, *L. guyanensis*, *L. panamensis*) or deep organs of the reticuloendothelial system such as lymph nodes, bone marrow, liver and spleen (*L. donovani* and *L. infantum*) [2].

When another sandfly takes a bloodmeal, parasitised macrophages from the skin or peripheral circulation are ingested. In the sandfly, parasites return to the promastigote form, completing the reproductive cycle. The taxonomic classification of *Leishmania* parasites into the subgenera *Leishmania* and *Viannia* is based on different anatomical sites in the sandfly gut to which the parasites attach.

Leishmania species may parasite one or many mammalian hosts, which constitute the reservoir of infection. In most cases of CL, humans are accidental hosts. Female sandflies of the genus *Phlebotomus* (Africa, Asia, Europe) and *Lutzomyia* (Americas) are responsible for transmitting the *Leishmania* parasite. Transmission therefore shows seasonal variation according to sandfly levels.

Immunopathogenesis

The host immune response plays a major role in determining disease progression. Most individuals will mount a protective immune response, and the infection will remain subclinical. In cases where the infection is not cleared, a skin lesion will appear at the site of parasite inoculation. Clinical progression from this point is determined largely by the immune response of the host. Mucocutaneous leishmaniasis (MCL) and diffuse CL (DCL) are severe forms of CL which sit at opposite ends of this immunological spectrum. Individuals with MCL demonstrate an exaggerated delayed-type hypersensitivity reaction with high levels of pro-inflammatory cytokines, whilst those with DCL develop a strong humoral response with little cell-mediated immunity [3, 4]. In between these two extremes are patients with localised cutaneous disease, which varies considerably in clinical severity and time to spontaneous healing.

Impaired cell-mediated immunity will limit the ability of the host to both achieve and maintain control of *Leishmania* infection. HIV co-infection and immunosuppressive medications, such as corticosteroids and biologic agents, may influence susceptibility to *Leishmania* infection. These patients are at risk of severe primary infection, atypical presentations and reactivation of previously treated infection. Disseminated cutaneous disease may occur with parasite species that are not normally associated with this form of disease, for example *L. major* [5]. Visceralisation of dermotropic *Leishmania* species has been observed in cases of HIV co-infection. Cases of cutaneous, mucocutaneous and mucosal leishmaniasis have been reported in association with anti-TNF treatment, especially anti-TNF monoclonal antibodies such as adalimumab [6, 7].

Imported CL: Approach to the Patient

CL is commonly divided into "Old World" and "New World" (American) forms, according to the geographic region in which the infection was acquired. In the context of CL, the Old World encompasses the Mediterranean, the Middle East, Central Asia, Africa and the Indian subcontinent, all of which belong to the land mass Afro-Eurasia (Africa, Europe and Asia). The New World includes Central and South America.

This terminology of Old World and New World is outdated and bears historical reference to the European arrival in the Americas in the fifteenth century. We propose the term African-Asian-European CL (AAECL) to replace Old World CL and favour American CL (ACL), a term which is already established in the literature, instead of New World CL.

The distinction between CL acquired in American vs. non-American settings is important. American CL is mostly caused by parasites belonging to *Viannia* subgenus, which tends to manifest a more severe clinical phenotype, with a higher risk of chronic mucosal disease.

The epidemiology of CL in a non-endemic setting is determined by the destinations from which people commonly migrate or return from travel, and patients may therefore present a broad spectrum of clinical disease according to the infection (parasite) acquired. A detailed travel history is a key part of the assessment of any person with suspected CL and has important implications for prognosis and treatment. A history of travel to an endemic area in the preceding weeks to months is important, particularly if this involves high-risk behaviours such as desert or jungle trekking, and sleeping outdoors. Any non-healing ulcer or nodule should be considered suspicious.

Boggild et al. provide the most recent and comprehensive analysis of travel-associated CL, using data collected over a period of 20 years (1997–2017) across the GeoSentinel Surveillance Network, which comprises 72 tropical/travel medicine clinics in 6 continents [8]. This study reported 955 cases of travel-associated CL. Non-migrant travellers accounted for 90% of cases and predominantly comprised of young tourists who had travelled to Central and South America. Migrants accounted for 10% of cases, most of whom were from Syria and Afghanistan. CL was acquired by 10% of all travellers (1 in 6 tourists) while travelling to an endemic areas for less than 2 weeks.

Similar findings were reported in an earlier case series of CL in travellers presenting over a period of 11 years (1998–2009) to the Hospital for Tropical Diseases in London, UK [9]. CL was diagnosed in 223 patients—African-Asian-European CL in 40%, and American CL in 60%. In this study, AAECL cases were comprised of tourists to the Mediterranean region (32%), persons visiting friends or relatives (37%), and military personnel returning from Iraq or Afghanistan (17%). Most cases of ACL occurred in backpackers (44%) and soldiers (29%).

African–Asian–European Cutaneous Leishmaniasis (AAECL)

Epidemiology

Endemic countries with the highest burden of CL include Afghanistan, Algeria, Iran, Syria, Ethiopia and North Sudan. Together, these six countries account for approximately 80% of all new CL cases that occur in Africa, Asia and Europe each year [1]. The epidemiology of CL in these countries is complex and is affected by a number of variables including parasite species, reservoir hosts, vector biology and geography.

All *Leishmania* species responsible for AAECL belong to the subgenus *Leishmania* (Table 1). These include the dermotropic species *L. major*, *L. tropica*, *L. aethiopica* and members of *L. donovani* species complex (*L. donovani* and *L. infantum*), which predominantly cause VL but can also cause cutaneous disease. Globally *L. major* and *L. tropica* account for the majority of CL cases, and these species have a wide geographic distribution (Fig. 1). *L. aethiopica* is restricted to Ethiopia and Kenya, and *L. infantum* is an important cause of CL in Southern Europe, where it also causes visceral disease.

Table 1 Epidemiology and clinical features of Leishmania species (Euleishmania) causing cutaneous leishmaniasis

Geographical classification	African-Asian-European CL				American CL		
Subgenus	Leishmania				Leishmania	Viannia	
Species complex	L. donovani	L. tropica	L. major	L. aethiopica	L. mexicana	L. braziliensis	L. guyanensis
Species	L. donovani, L. infantum	L. tropica, L. killicki	L. major	L. aethiopica	L. mexicana, L. amazonensis, L. venezualensis	L. braziliensis, L. peruviana	L. guyanensis, L. panamensis, L. shawi
Global incidence (cases per year)	Unknown	200,000–400,000	230,000–430,000	20,000–50,000	Unknown (few)	Majority of the 187,200–300,000 cases of NWCL (L. braziliensis)	Unknown (few)
Endemic regions	**L. donovani**: Africa, Indian subcontinent **L. infantum**: Mediterranean basin, Middle East, Central Asia	Mediterranean, Middle East, Central Asia, Northeast Africa (urban)	North and Sub-Saharan Africa, Middle East, Asia	Ethiopia, Kenya (highlands)	South and Central America (tropical forests)	South and Central America (tropical forests, periurban) **L. peruviana**: highlands of Peru and Argentina	South and Central America
Clinical forms	LCL	LCL, Leishmaniasis recidivans	LCL	LCL, MCL, DCL	LCL, DCL	LCL, MCL, DCL	LCL, MCL, DCL
Characteristic clinical features	Localised nodular or ulcerating lesions	Ulcerating lesions (dry), often multiple	Ulcerating lesions (wet)	Complex localised disease affecting face, non-ulcerating lesions MCL and DCL occur commonly	Localised disease often on face/ears, Chiclero ulcer	Lesions often on the limbs, lymphatic involvement	Localised disease with lymphatic involvement
Median healing time	Self-healing in 12 months	Self-healing in 10-14 months Leishmaniasis recidivans: chronic	Self-healing in 2-6 months	Self-healing in 2-5 years MCL and DCL: chronic, progressive	Self-healing in 3-8 months Chiclero ulcer: chronic DCL: chronic, progressive	Self-healing? MCL and DCL: chronic, progressive	Self-healing in 3-8 months MCL and DCL: chronic, progressive

L. naiffi and *L. lainsoni* (*Viannia* species) and *L. colombiensis* (*Paraleishmania*) are not shown in this table

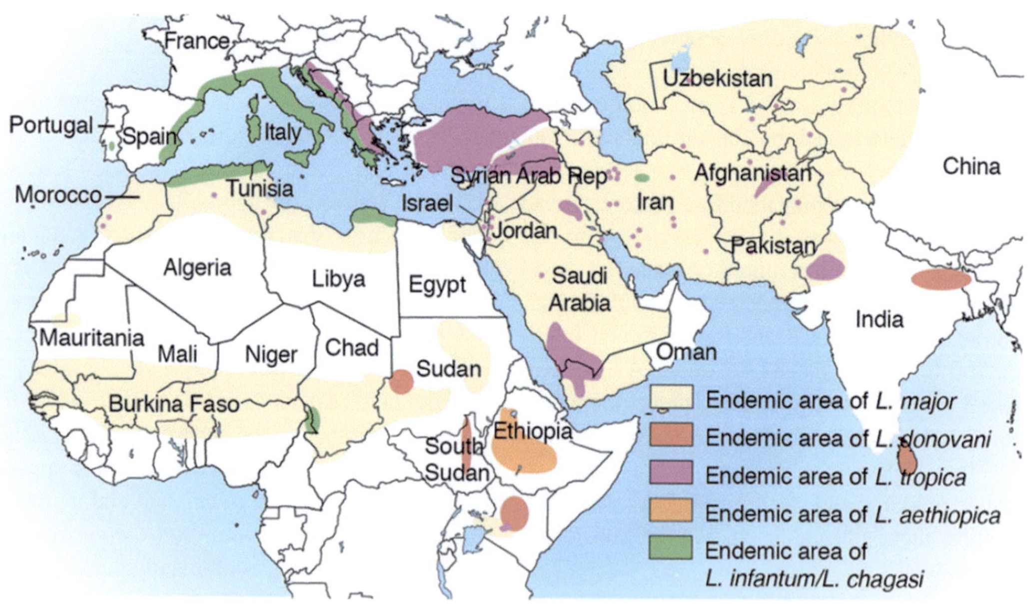

Fig. 1 Distribution of the *Leishmania* species responsible for African-Asian-European CL [10]. *L. major* and *L. tropica* are distributed throughout many countries, in contrast to *L. aethiopica* and *L. donovani* which are geographically restricted [Credit: Aronson S et al. Diagnosis and Treatment of Leishmaniasis: Clinical Practice Guidelines by the Infectious Diseases Society of America (IDSA) and the American Society of Tropical Medicine and Hygiene (ASTMH). *Am J Trop Med Hyg*, 96 (1), 2017]

Most cases of AAECL in travellers, where the causative species has been identified, are caused by *L. donovani* complex; molecular testing is often not available to distinguish *L. donovani* from *L. infantum*. The vast majority of these cases are tourists who have visited the Mediterranean, particularly Spain and the Balearic islands [8, 9]. Significant numbers of cases are also caused by *L. major* (acquired in the Middle East and Mediterranean) and *L. tropica* (Middle East, Pakistan, Africa). Very few cases of travel-associated AECL are caused by *L. aethiopica*.

AAECL is predominantly zoonotic. Infection with *L. major* is acquired in rural areas where humans live in proximity to the animal reservoir—rodents in Sub-Saharan Africa, and gerbils in North Africa, the Middle East and Central Asia. In Ethiopia, rock hyraxes constitute the animal reservoir, and transmission of *L. aethiopica* occurs in highland areas where these animals are found. The exception to this is *L. tropica*, for which humans are the main reservoir, and transmission occurs through anthroponotic cycles. This is particularly the case in urban areas in the Mediterranean basin, Middle East and Central Asia (Turkmenistan, Uzbekistan) and in the highlands and urban areas of Pakistan. Humans serve as a reservoir for *L. donovani* in North-East India, Bangladesh, Burma and Sri Lanka, and possibly in parts of Africa.

Clinical Features

Skin lesions of CL commonly occur on exposed body sites, such as the face and limbs. Clinical manifestations particular to each of the *Leishmania* species are recognised, however clinical presentation is highly variable and significant overlap exists. After a variable incubation period, a skin lesion develops at the site of inoculation. This is typically 2–8 weeks for *L. major*, but as long as 8–9 months for *L. tropica*, *L. aethiopica* and *L. donovani* spp. The initial lesion often appears as a papule or nodule and subsequently ulcerates centrally giving rise to a raised inflamed edge. The lesion may grow to several centimetres in diameter. Some lesions do not ulcerate but persist as nodules or plaques.

AAECL in travellers almost always presents as localised CL (LCL), with few cases of mucocutaneous leishmaniasis (MCL). Multiple skin lesions usually result from different bites although lymphatic spread can occur. Lesions may be clustered together or follow a sporotrichoid (lymphangitic) distribution [11, 12]. Most lesions self-heal resulting in permanent scarring, although some follow a chronic course. Diffuse or disseminated cutaneous forms are very rarely seen in travellers with normal immune systems.

The epidemiology and clinical features of the *Leishmania* species causing AAECL and American CL are summarised in Table 1.

CL Caused by *L. donovani* Species

Leishmania L. donovani and *L. L. infantum* are closely related species belonging to the *L. L. donovani* complex. Infection with *L. donovani/infantum* results predominantly in visceral disease; however some cases will manifest as cutaneous leishmaniasis. This process is influenced by host and parasite factors, although certain subspecies (zymodemes) are recognised for causing cutaneous disease only [13]. Intraspecies variation in *L. donovani* has also been linked to differences in virulence and response to antimonial therapy in Sri Lanka [14, 15]. This form of CL typically displays a mild phenotype. Skin lesions are usually papules or small nodules, which may be multiple, and self-healing occurs in 1–3 years [16]. Mucosal involvement is rare but can occur (Fig. 2).

CL Caused by *L. major*

Infection with *L. major* is frequently referred to as wet, rural or zoonotic CL, reflecting its clinical appearance and epidemiology. After a short incubation period, usually 2–8 weeks, a nodule appears at the site of the sandfly bite. Soon after, the lesion will become crusted which signals ulceration. The ulcer or sore typically has a wet appearance and increases in size over the next few months. Small secondary nodules may appear around the lesion resulting from local lymphatic spread. The majority of cases self-heal

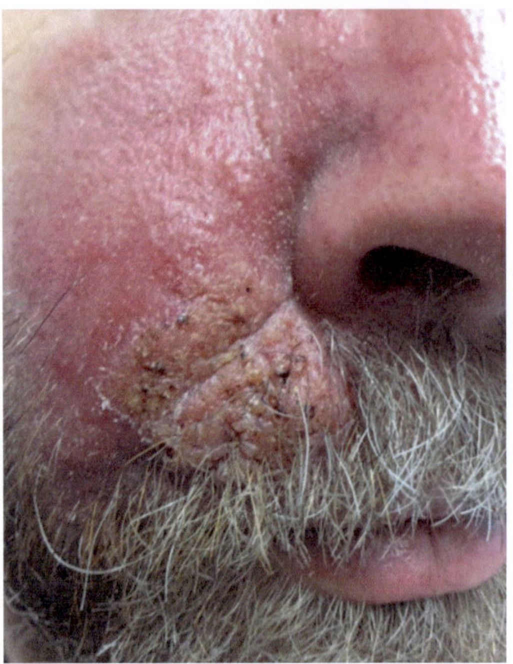

Fig. 2 Clinical image of localised CL. Infection with *L. donovani* (complex) presenting as a nodular and verrucous plaque

in 2–6 months leaving permanent scarring. Variations in clinical appearance of skin lesions have been described which include eczematoid, psoriasiform, verrucous and pseudotumoral lesions [17].

CL Caused by *L. tropica*

This form of CL is often referred to as dry, urban or anthroponotic CL. The incubation period is longer than for *L. major*, and patients often develop multiple ulcerating lesions which are described as dry in appearance, although this is not a reliable distinguishing feature. Lesions begin to heal on average after 12 months.

Lupoid CL and Leishmaniasis Recidivans

These rarer forms of CL share similar clinical features, and the terms have been used interchangeably in the literature to refer to various chronic and relapsing forms of CL; however they are distinct entities and should therefore be distinguished.

Lupoid leishmaniasis is a form of primary CL, characterised by local spread of a cutaneous

lesion to form an indurated plaque. Lesions vary from yellow/red to brown in colour, and may resemble lupus vulgaris (cutaneous tuberculosis). There is often a good response to treatment, without relapse [18].

Leishmaniasis recidivans (LR) is a form of recurrent leishmaniasis, characterised by the appearance of red-brown papules within or adjacent to the scar from a previous healed CL lesion. This commonly occurs as a complication of *L. tropica* CL, in up to 10% of cases, although it can occur in *L. aethiopica* infection. LR can occur months to years after complete healing of the primary lesion and persist for decades following a relapsing-remitting course, with each episode resulting in further scarring. Clinical variants include plaques with annular or psoriasiform appearance, and lesions may worsen and ulcerate during the summer months [19, 20].

CL Caused by *L. aethiopica*

This is rare in travellers. In endemic settings, which are limited geographically to East Africa (particularly Ethiopia), this form of CL presents a broad spectrum of clinical disease. Localised CL is the most common presentation, although this can be complex with multiple non-ulcerated lesions and diffuse skin infiltration. Self-healing occurs in 2–5 years. Severe forms, including DCL and MCL, are common in Ethiopia but are rarely seen in travellers. MCL in Ethiopia typically presents with primary mucosal involvement, early in the course of disease, in contrast to American MCL in which haematogenous spread to mucosal tissue occurs years after primary cutaneous disease. Other clinical presentations reported in the literature include large hypopigmented skin patches mimicking borderline tuberculoid leprosy and lymphoedema (elephantiasis).

Diagnosis

Investigations are useful to confirm a clinical diagnosis of CL and to identify the parasite species.

Direct microscopy of a skin smear allows visualisation of the parasite; with Romanowsky staining (Giemsa or Leishman stain), the nucleus and kinetoplast of the amastigotes are intensely positive. The smear can be prepared as a slit-skin smear or using wound exudate or needle aspirate. Microscopy of H&E stained skin sections, provided by skin biopsy, may reveal macrophages containing amastigotes in the dermis. Part of the biopsy specimen should be reserved for culture on Nicolle-Novy-MacNeal (NNN) medium which allows growth of promastigotes. These investigations confirm the presence of Leishmania parasites but do not permit identification of the parasite species. Using a combination of these techniques is recommended to improve diagnostic accuracy. It has been shown for example, that in the context of a skin biopsy demonstrating granulomata, with or without amastigotes, PCR has a sensitivity of 92–100% [21, 22].

Histopathology may confirm or support the clinical diagnosis, and we recommend performing a skin biopsy for all cases of suspected CL in returning travellers. Early changes consist of a loosely structured mixed dermal infiltrate, including parasitised macrophages, neutrophils, lymphocytes and plasma cells. This is followed by varying degrees of necrosis and granulomatous inflammation. The overlying epidermis becomes hyperkeratotic and frequently ulcerates. In the presence of a strong cell-mediated immune response, parasites may be few or absent. In contrast, histology in DCL often reveals large numbers of heavily-parasitised macrophages with little or no cellular infiltrate. In mucosal leishmaniasis, parasites metastasise to the nasopharyngeal mucosa, and some cases will progress to involve laryngeal mucosa. Histology may demonstrate a perivascular inflammatory infiltrate in the submucosa, with necrosis of cartilage and overlying mucosal tissue; vasculitis and thrombosis can also occur.

Molecular tests using polymerase chain reaction (PCR) to amplify nuclear and kinetoplast DNA can be used for species identification. This is useful to guide management, particularly in regions where multiple *Leishmania* species coexist. PCR amplification coupled with DNA sequencing can be performed, allowing more detailed characterisation of the parasite although this is likely to be available only in specialist centres and research settings.

In AAECL, circulating antibodies are absent or present at low levels so serological tests have very low sensitivity and are not useful in the diagnosis of CL.

Differential Diagnosis

CL has a broad differential diagnosis which varies according to the stage of disease and clinical presentation.

Early nodular lesions might be mistaken for a furuncle or abscess. Cutaneous myiasis should also be considered, as should non-tuberculous mycobacteria and subcutaneous mycoses which can cause nodular lesions in a lymphangitic distribution. The differential diagnosis of an isolated nodular lesion should include cutaneous malignancies, in particular basal cell carcinoma (BCC) and squamous cell carcinoma (SCC). There are several possibilities for ulcerating skin lesions including tropical ulcer, tularaemia, Buruli ulcer, cutaneous anthrax, yaws and neuropathic ulcers of leprosy. Non-infectious causes such as neoplasia, pyoderma gangrenosum and chronic venous disease might also be considered. CL localised to the face, especially involving the nose, may resemble cutaneous sarcoidosis (lupus pernio).

For mucosal leishmaniasis, the differential diagnosis includes rhinoscleroma, paracoccidioidomycosis, granulomatosis with polyangiitis and extranodal NK/T-cell lymphoma, nasal type (previously lethal midline granuloma).

In addition to the clinical considerations outlined above, the differential diagnosis must take into account the geographical context, with attention to the duration of time spent in endemic settings. This will differ considerably for travellers and migrants. For example, in tourists who have recently travelled to the Mediterranean for a short duration, a number of conditions will be irrelevant—Buruli ulcer and yaws are not found in this region, and leprosy has an incubation period of at least 1–2 years. Migrants may have lived for many years in an endemic setting, and conditions such as leprosy and its chronic complications (neuropathic ulcers) may need to be considered. Diffuse CL is rarely seen in travellers, however it might be considered in migrants from endemic settings. In this case, it must be distinguished from lepromatous leprosy; and from PKDL if the patient is from an area where CL and VL are co-endemic.

Treatment

Treatments for CL can be divided broadly into local and systemic therapies. Key factors to take into consideration when deciding on treatment include the clinical presentation, *Leishmania* species, and patient comorbidities.

Clinical guidelines are available to support physicians in the management of imported leishmaniasis. Guidelines produced by Infectious Diseases Society of America (IDSA) and the American Society of Tropical Medicine and Hygiene (ASTMH) are intended to support physicians in the USA and Canada in the management of VL, CL and MCL [23]. Recommendations for treatment of CL and MCL in Europe were published by the expert group "LeishMan" (Leishmaniasis Management) [24].

Systemic treatment should be used for patients with MCL, DCL, leishmaniasis recidivans, complex localised disease, and those at risk of developing MCL (*L. aethiopica* infection) or visceral disease (*L. donovani* spp. infection). Complex localised disease is indicated by a large number (>3) or size (>3 cm diameter) of skin lesions, lymphatic spread, location of skin lesions close to a joint or free margin (nose, lips, eyelid, ears), chronic/progressive course, failure to respond to treatment and an immunocompromised host. For simple localised disease, it is reasonable to begin with local treatment.

In some cases, it may be appropriate to simply observe and allow the lesion(s) to self-heal. This option applies particularly to immunocompetent patients with simple localised disease caused by *L. major* or *L. tropica*, although self-healing may take many months (Table 1). In endemic settings where transmission is anthroponotic, it is important to treat patients in order to reduce the reservoir of infection.

The evidence base for the treatment of CL is limited, and especially so in travellers. Most research is conducted in endemic settings, using a variety of interventions and outcome measures, which limits comparison of studies. Due to the lack of strong evidence, treatment is often influenced by clinician preferences and drug availability.

Local Treatment

Local treatment options for CL include intralesional antimony, physical therapies (cryotherapy, thermotherapy and curettage), topical treatments and photodynamic therapy.

Intralesional injection of pentavalent antimony, either sodium stibogluconate (SSG) or meglumine antimoniate (MA), is used in many countries as first-line treatment. Studies of AAECL report cure rates of 56–75% for intralesional antimony, when given alone [25–27]. Treatment regimens vary although treatment every 3–7 days for a total of 5–8 sessions is common practice. Pain at the injection site and scarring are the main side effects.

Cryotherapy, another commonly used treatment, is ideally suited to treating skin lesions which are small in number and size. Cure rates of 57–81% are reported for cryotherapy alone [25–27]. Adverse effects of cryotherapy in the days after the procedure include pain, localised erythema/oedema and blistering. Long-term sequelae include dyspigmentation and scarring.

Combining intralesional antimony and cryotherapy can be effective, and is the preferred approach in many centres. Combination treatment every 3–7 days for up to 5 sessions has been recommended; however, fewer treatments with a longer interval can be effective. Asilian et al. achieved a 91% cure rate after 1–3 sessions of combined treatment at 2 week intervals [25].

The available data suggest that thermotherapy is an effective treatment for AAECL. Localised heat therapy (50 °C for 30 s) was superior to intralesional antimony in two studies; in Kabul, Afghanistan (83 vs. 74%) [28] and Iran (81 vs. 55%) [29]. It is important to note that in many studies, these two included, *Leishmania* species are not identified and treatment protocols vary.

A large number of topical treatments have been trialled including paromomycin (aminosidine), amphotericin B, azole antifungals, dapsone, miltefosine, trichloroacetic acid, imiquimod and herbal preparations. Paromomycin, an aminoglycoside antibiotic, is the most widely used of these and could be a suitable alternative to other local treatments for treatment of AAECL. A randomised controlled trial in 375 patients with *L. major* CL in Tunisia, showed cure rates of 82% for paromomycin ointment versus 58% using a vehicle control [30]. Paromomycin ointment containing 12% methylbenzethonium chloride (MBCL), applied twice daily for 10–20 days, demonstrated efficacy comparable to intralesional antimony injections against *L. major* CL [31]. However, reports of severe local inflammatory reactions, in some cases resulting in treatment being abandoned, in skin lesions treated with MBCL-containing preparations have led to this treatment being avoided [32, 33]. Paromomycin alone is also recognised as a cause of irritant and allergic contact dermatitis [34].

Topical photodynamic therapy (PDT) was shown to be an effective treatment for CL in Iran [35]. In this randomised trial, topical PDT every week for 4 weeks resulted in complete cure at 2 months in 94% of patients, compared with 41% for topical paromomycin-MBCL and 13% for placebo. Adverse events were mild and tolerable in both active treatment groups.

Systemic Treatment

Systemic treatment is commonly with pentavalent antimony, cither SSG or MA, administered by intravenous or intramuscular injection. Treatment duration varies widely; initial treatment is 20 mg/kg per day for 10–21 days, although this is often extended based on clinical and parasitological response. Despite its widespread use, high quality data on the efficacy and safety of systemic antimony for AAECL are lacking. In a randomised trial of patients with confirmed *L. major* infection, treatment with intravenous SSG (20 mg/kg for 10 days) resulted in cure rates of 54% at 2 months and 90% at 12 months [36]. Other studies have shown similar results. The addition of pentoxyfylline (400 mg three times per day) to intramuscular MA for 20 days increased the cure rate at 3 months to 81%, compared to 52% for intramuscular MA alone [37].

Systemic antimonial therapy is associated with dose-dependent toxic side effects; however these are transient and rarely result in adverse clinical outcomes. Headache, myalgia and arthralgia are reported frequently. Severe adverse events are rare, and it has been shown that low-risk patients (age below 65 years and without comorbidities) can be treated safely with parenteral SSG in an outpatient setting, avoiding the cost and inconvenience of hospital admission [38]. In other studies, cardiotoxicity has been reported in up to 60% of patients, and can result in arrhythmias and QT interval prolongation. Hepatotoxicity, haematological and electrolyte abnormalities, and hyperamylasaemia occur commonly but pancreatitis is rare. Patients require regular blood monitoring and electrocardiogram during treatment.

Miltefosine is an oral alkyl phosphocholine analogue used to treat VL and PKDL. It has also been used to treat AAECL, with two small studies reporting cure rates at 3 months of 93% for miltefosine and 73–83% for systemic antimony [39, 40]. Treatment lasts 28 days and is better tolerated than systemic antimony, however renal impairment and hepatotoxicity can occur and weekly blood monitoring is recommended. Miltefosine is teratogenic and contraindicated in pregnancy.

Liposomal amphotericin B (LAMB) has proved an effective and safe treatment, but evidence is limited to case series. In these studies, in patients with *L. major* and *L. tropica* CL, cure rates were 84–100% following the initial course of treatment [41, 42]. Treatment is by intravenous infusion, 3 mg/kg per day for 7 doses, given on days 1–5, 14 and 21. In one cohort of travel-acquired AAECL, treatment with LAMB was more effective in those with *L. infantum* than *L. major* [43]. Adverse effects include infusion reactions (chest pain, dyspnoea, urticaria), renal impairment and electrolyte disturbance (hypokalaemia).

Pentamidine, an antiprotozoal and antifungal agent, has been used to treat few cases of

AAECL. Data are scarce, although a cure rate of 73% at 3 months was reported in a small series from Southern France which included cases of *L. major*, *L. tropica* and *L. infantum* CL [44]. Many adverse effects have been reported and treatment requires close monitoring. Patients can develop hypoglycaemia, diabetes mellitus and rhabdomyolysis. Cardiotoxicity can occur resulting in arrhythmias, hypotension and cardiac failure.

Limited evidence supports the use of oral imidazoles (ketoconazole and fluconazole) in *L. major* and *L. tropica* infection. Fluconazole 200 mg daily for 6 weeks achieved a cure rate of 79% at 3 months, in patients with *L. major* CL in Saudi Arabia, compared with 34% in the placebo group [45]. Similar results are reported for ketoconazole [46], including a study in Iran which demonstrated superiority over intralesional antimony [47]. These are well tolerated in comparison to other treatments, although mild hepatotoxicity can occur.

The evidence base for the treatment of *L. aethiopica* infection is extremely limited. Cure rates using systemic SSG in two prospective studies were 69–85% [26, 48]. Treatment failure is more likely in patients with MCL and DCL and those with HIV co-infection. Pentamidine appears to be effective in cases that do not respond to antimonials [48]. The treatment of DCL is particularly challenging; treatment with pentamidine or combination antimony and paromomycin has been effective, although experience is limited to a few patients [49, 50]. Miltefosine and LAMB have been used successfully in a small number of cases.

Prevention

There is currently no vaccine or chemoprophylaxis available to prevent infection, although travellers can reduce the risk of acquiring infection by taking steps to avoid sandfly bites.

Pre-travel counselling should emphasise that prolonged travel to "exotic" destinations is not necessary to acquire infection [8]. Travel-associated AAECL is commonly imported by migrants and persons visiting friends or relatives, from the Middle East and North Africa. However, tourists to the Mediterranean region are at risk with many patients acquiring CL from travel lasting less than 2 weeks. Persons visiting friends or relatives are significantly less likely to seek pre-travel medical advice compared with tourists and business travellers.

General advice is to limit outdoor activities as much as possible, especially at night when sandflies are most active. Where possible advice should be tailored to the individual, taking into account local epidemiology and vector biology. Exposed body parts should be kept covered with protective clothing, including long sleeves, trousers and hats, and insect repellents should be applied frequently. The most effective repellents contain DEET. Bednets offer protection against sandflies, although they must be tightly woven to provide an effective barrier; sandflies are small (2–3 mm) and will easily pass through standard bednets. Sleeping in air-conditioned and well-ventilated areas may provide some benefit. Clothing and bednets can be treated with a pyrethroid-containing insecticide, which may be particularly useful if outdoor activities cannot be avoided.

Conclusions

CL is a common dermatological problem in returning travellers. Individuals from non-endemic settings lack protective immunity and are at risk of acquiring AAECL in many countries throughout Africa, Asia and Europe. The diagnosis of CL should be considered in any patient presenting with a new skin lesion, typically a nodule or ulcer on an exposed body site, if there is a relevant travel history. Every effort should be made to identify the *Leishmania* species, as this has important implications for treatment and clinical follow-up. Management decisions are complicated due to the lack of robust evidence on treatment efficacy and toxicity of the available systemic agents. Patients at risk of developing MCL and DCL (*L. aethiopica* infection) or visceral disease (*L. donovani* spp.) should receive systemic treatment.

International travel, particularly for outdoor/ adventure activities, makes it increasingly likely that susceptible individuals will be exposed to the parasite. It is important therefore to be able to recognise and manage this condition in the returning traveller. Additionally, increasing use of novel immunomodulatory therapies will pose diagnostic and therapeutic challenges for clinicians. This group of patients in particular need to be made aware of the risk of acquiring CL in endemic countries which are popular travel destinations.

References

1. Alvar J, Vélez ID, Bern C, et al. Leishmaniasis worldwide and global estimates of its incidence. PLoS One. 2012;7:7. https://doi.org/10.1371/journal.pone.0035671.
2. Nabarro L, Morris-Jones S, Moore DAJ. Arthropod-borne diseases. In: Peter's Atlas of tropical medicine and parasitology. Elsevier, 2020:1–108.
3. Bacellar O, Lessa H, Schriefer A, et al. Up-regulation of Th1-type responses in mucosal leishmaniasis patients. Infect Immun. 2002;70:6734. https://doi.org/10.1128/IAI.70.12.6734-6740.2002.
4. Akuffo HO, Fehniger TE, Britton S. Differential recognition of Leishmania aethiopica antigens by lymphocytes from patients with local and diffuse cutaneous leishmaniasis. Evidence for antigen-induced immune suppression. J Immunol. 1988;141:2461–6.
5. Venencie PY, Bouree P, Hiesse C, et al. Disseminated cutaneous leishmaniasis in an immunodepressed woman. Ann Dermatol Venereol. 1993;
6. Baltà-Cruz S, Alsina-Glbert M, Mozos-Rocafort A, et al. Pseudolymphomatoid cutaneous leishmaniasis in a patient treated with adalimumab for rheumatoid arthritis. Acta Derm Venereol. 2009;89:432–3.
7. Bosch-Nicolau P, Ubals M, Salvador F, et al. Leishmaniasis and tumor necrosis factor alpha antagonists in the Mediterranean basin. A switch in clinical expression. PLoS Negl Trop Dis. 2019;13:e0007708.
8. Boggild AK, Caumes E, Grobusch MP, et al. Cutaneous and mucocutaneous leishmaniasis in travellers and migrants: a 20-year GeoSentinel surveillance network analysis. J Travel Med. 2019;26:1–11.
9. Wall EC, Watson J, Armstrong M, Chiodini PL, Lockwood DN. Epidemiology of imported cutaneous leishmaniasis at the Hospital for Tropical Diseases, London, United Kingdom: use of polymerase chain reaction to identify the species. Am J Trop Med Hyg. 2012;86:115–8.
10. Aronson N, Herwaldt BL, Libman M, et al. Diagnosis and treatment of leishmaniasis: clinical practice guidelines by the infectious diseases society of America (IDSA) and the American Society of tropical medicine and hygiene (ASTMH). Am J Trop Med Hyg. 2017;96:24–45.
11. Kurban AK, Karam PG, Kurban AK. Sporotrichoid leishmaniasis in patients from Saudi Arabia: clinical and histologic features. J Am Acad Dermatol. 1987; https://doi.org/10.1016/S0190-9622(87)70259-X.
12. Iftikhar N, Bari I, Ejaz A. Rare variants of cutaneous leishmaniasis: whitlow, paronychia, and sporotrichoid. Int J Dermatol. 2003;42:807. https://doi.org/10.1046/j.1365-4362.2003.02015.x.
13. Sulahian A, Garin YJF, Pratlong F, Dedet JP, Derouin F. Experimental pathogenicity of viscerotropic and dermotropic isolates of Leishmania infantum from immunocompromised and immunocompetent patients in a murine model. FEMS Immunol Med Microbiol. 1997;17:131–8.
14. Lypaczewski P, Hoshizaki J, Zhang W-W, et al. A complete Leishmania donovani reference genome identifies novel genetic variations associated with virulence. Sci Rep. 2018;8:16549.
15. Kariyawasam UL, Selvapandiyan A, Rai K, et al. Genetic diversity of Leishmania donovani that causes cutaneous leishmaniasis in Sri Lanka: a cross sectional study with regional comparisons. BMC Infect Dis. 2017;17:791.
16. del Giudice P, Marty P, Lacour JP, et al. Cutaneous leishmaniasis due to leishmania infantum. Arch Dermatol. 1998;134:193.
17. Remadi L, Haouas N, Chaara D, et al. Clinical presentation of cutaneous Leishmaniasis caused by leishmania major. Dermatology. 2016;232:752–9.
18. Ul Bari A, Raza N. Lupoid cutaneous leishmaniasis: a report of 16 cases. Indian J Dermatol Venereol Leprol;76:85.
19. Mavilia L, Rossi R, Massi D, Difonzo EM, Campolmi P, Cappugi P. Leishmaniasis recidiva cutis: an unusual two steps recurrence. Int J Dermatol. 2002;41:506–7.
20. PETTIT JH. Chronic (lupoid) leishmaniasis. Br J Dermatol. 1962;74:127–31.
21. Vega-López F. Diagnosis of cutaneous leishmaniasis. Curr Opin Infect Dis. 2003;16:97–101.
22. Safaei A, Motazedian MH, Vasei M. Polymerase chain reaction for diagnosis of cutaneous leishmaniasis in histologically positive, suspicious and negative skin biopsies. Dermatology. 2002;205:18–24.
23. Aronson N, Herwaldt BL, Libman M, et al. Diagnosis and treatment of leishmaniasis: clinical practice guidelines by the Infectious Diseases Society of America (IDSA) and the American Society of Tropical Medicine and Hygiene (ASTMH). Clin Infect Dis. 2016;63:e202–64.
24. Blum J, Buffet P, Visser L, et al. LeishMan recommendations for treatment of cutaneous and mucosal leishmaniasis in travelers, 2014. J Travel Med. 2014;21:116–29.
25. Asilian A, Sadeghinia A, Faghihi G, Momeni A. Comparative study of the efficacy of combined

cryotherapy and intralesional meglumine antimoniate (Glucantime) vs. cryotherapy and intralesional meglumine antimoniate (Glucantime) alone for the treatment of cutaneous leishmaniasis. Int J Dermatol. 2004;43:281–3.

26. Negera E, Gadisa E, Hussein J, et al. Treatment response of cutaneous leishmaniasis due to Leishmania aethiopica to cryotherapy and generic sodium stibogluconate from patients in Silti, Ethiopia. Trans R Soc Trop Med Hyg. 2012;106:496–503.

27. Salmanpour R, Razmavar MR, Abtahi N. Comparison of intralesional meglumine antimoniate, cryotherapy and their combination in the treatment of cutaneous leishmaniasis. Int J Dermatol. 2006;45:1115–6.

28. Safi N, Davis GD, Nadir M, Hamid H, Robert LL, Case AJ. Evaluation of thermotherapy for the treatment of cutaneous leishmaniasis in Kabul, Afghanistan: a randomized controlled trial. Mil Med. 2012;177:345–51.

29. Sadeghian G, Nilfroushzadeh MA, Iraji F. Efficacy of local heat therapy by radiofrequency in the treatment of cutaneous leishmaniasis, compared with intralesional injection of meglumine antimoniate. Clin Exp Dermatol. 2007;32:371–4.

30. Ben Salah A, Ben Messaoud N, Guedri E, et al. Topical paromomycin with or without gentamicin for cutaneous leishmaniasis. N Engl J Med. 2013;368:524–32.

31. Kim DH, Chung HJ, Bleys J, Ghohestani RF. Is paromomycin an effective and safe treatment against cutaneous leishmaniasis? A meta-analysis of 14 randomized controlled trials. PLoS Negl Trop Dis. 2009;3:e381.

32. Bryceson ADM, Moody AH, Murphy A. Treatment of 'old world' cutaneous leishmaniasis with aminosidine ointment: results of an open study in London. Trans R Soc Trop Med Hyg. 1994;88:226–8.

33. El-On J, Halevy S, Grunwald MH, Weinrauch L. Topical treatment of Old World cutaneous leishmaniasis caused by Leishmania major: a double-blind control study. J Am Acad Dermatol. 1992;27:227. https://doi.org/10.1016/0190-9622(92)70175-F.

34. Veraldi S, Benzecry V, Faraci AG, Nazzaro G. Allergic contact dermatitis caused by paromomycin. Contact Derm. 2019;81:393–4.

35. Asilian A, Davami M. Comparison between the efficacy of photodynamic therapy and topical paromomycin in the treatment of Old World cutaneous leishmaniasis: a placebo-controlled, randomized clinical trial. Clin Exp Dermatol. 2006;31:634. https://doi.org/10.1111/j.1365-2230.2006.02182.x.

36. Aronson NE, Wortmann GW, Byrne WR, et al. A randomized controlled trial of local heat therapy versus intravenous sodium stibogluconate for the treatment of cutaneous Leishmania major infection. PLoS Negl Trop Dis. 2010;4:e628.

37. Sadeghian G, Nilforoushzadeh MA. Effect of combination therapy with systemic glucantime and pentoxifylline in the treatment of cutaneous leishmaniasis. Int J Dermatol. 2006;45:819–21.

38. Wise ES, Armstrong MS, Watson J, Lockwood DN. Monitoring toxicity associated with parenteral sodium stibogluconate in the day-case management of returned travellers with New World cutaneous leishmaniasis [corrected]. PLoS Negl Trop Dis. 2012;6:e1688.

39. Rahman SB, ul Bari A, Mumtaz N. Miltefosine in cutaneous leishmaniasis. J Coll Physicians Surg Pak. 2007;17:132–5.

40. Mohebali M, Fotouhi A, Hooshmand B, et al. Comparison of miltefosine and meglumine antimoniate for the treatment of zoonotic cutaneous leishmaniasis (ZCL) by a randomized clinical trial in Iran. Acta Trop. 2007;103:33–40.

41. Solomon M, Pavlotsky F, Leshem E, Ephros M, Trau H, Schwartz E. Liposomal amphotericin B treatment of cutaneous leishmaniasis due to Leishmania tropica. J Eur Acad Dermatol Venereol. 2011;25:973–7.

42. Wortmann G, Zapor M, Ressner R, et al. Lipsosomal amphotericin B for treatment of cutaneous leishmaniasis. Am J Trop Med Hyg. 2010;83:1028–33.

43. Guery R, Henry B, Martin-Blondel G, et al. Liposomal amphotericin B in travelers with cutaneous and mucocutaneous leishmaniasis: not a panacea. PLoS Negl Trop Dis. 2017;11:e0006094.

44. Hellier I, Dereure O, Tournillac I, et al. Treatment of Old World cutaneous leishmaniasis by pentamidine isethionate. An open study of 11 patients. Dermatology. 2000;200:120–3.

45. Alrajhi AA, Ibrahim EA, De Vol EB, Khairat M, Faris RM, Maguire JH. Fluconazole for the treatment of cutaneous leishmaniasis caused by Leishmania major. N Engl J Med. 2002;346:891–5.

46. Weinrauch L, Livshin R, Even-Paz Z, El-On J. Efficacy of ketoconazole in cutaneous leishmaniasis. Arch Dermatol Res. 1983;275:353–4.

47. Salmanpour R, Handjani F, Nouhpisheh MK. Comparative study of the efficacy of oral ketoconazole with intra-lesional meglumine antimoniate (Glucantime) for the treatment of cutaneous leishmaniasis. J Dermatolog Treat. 2001;12:159–62.

48. Padovese V, Terranova M, Toma L, Barnabas GA, Morrone A. Cutaneous and mucocutaneous leishmaniasis in Tigray, northern Ethiopia: clinical aspects and therapeutic concerns. Trans R Soc Trop Med Hyg. 2009;103:707–11.

49. Bryceson ADM. Diffuse cutaneous leishmaniasis in Ethiopia: II treatment. Trans R Soc Trop Med Hyg. 1970;64:369–79.

50. Teklemariam S, Hiwot AG, Frommel D, Miko TL, Ganlov G, Bryceson A. Aminosidine and its combination with sodium stibogluconate in the treatment of diffuse cutaneous leishmaniasis caused by Leishmania aethiopica. Trans R Soc Trop Med Hyg. 1994;88:334–9.

New World Leishmaniasis

Emilia Duarte A. and Wanda Robles

Key Points

- Leishmaniasis is amongst the top 10 neglected tropical diseases with 700,000–1,000,000 new cases annually.
- It is a tropical and subtropical disease caused by an intracellular parasite transmitted to humans by the bite of a female sand-fly.
- In the Americas, there are 15 different species of Leishmaniasis causing disease in humans and in some mammalian hosts which makes it a complex disease with variations within different species, geographical areas, and host factors.
- The diagnosis of Leishmaniasis in non-endemic regions can be delayed since it is not a common disease; this can lead to long term morbidity, scarring, and an increased risk of developing mucocutaneous disease.
- Treatment for this condition in travelers needs to be catered to the type of clinical presentation, the Leishmania species and a very detailed travel history.

E. Duarte A. (✉)
King's College Hospital NHS Trust, London, UK
e-mail: eduartewilliamson@nhs.net

W. Robles
Royal Free Hospitals NHS Trust, London, UK
e-mail: drwrobles@wrobles.com

Introduction

New world cutaneous Leishmaniasis is a tropical disease endemic in most countries in Central and South America. It is transmitted by a female sand fly bite and has a wide range of clinical presentations with localized or disseminated cutaneous skin lesions, Mucocutaneous Leishmaniasis, and more rarely visceral Leishmaniasis.

These wide range of clinical manifestations is directly related to the type and grade of the immune response of the host, as well as on the differences between the infecting Leishmania species.

Due to deforestation, refugee crisis, migrations, tourism, and climate change, Leishmania infections have expanded to unusual populations including developed countries and non-endemic areas.

In this chapter, the main aspects of the disease in the New World will be reviewed, as part of the dermatosis in travelers, given the fact that this is an increasing health problem in patients returning from endemic areas mostly on adventure trips with outdoor activities in forested areas in South and Central America, whilst for OWD it is an increasing issue due to massive migrations from war, civil unrest, and poverty torn areas to Europe and the UK [1, 5].

© The Editor(s) (if applicable) and The Author(s), under exclusive license to Springer Nature Switzerland AG 2024
W. Robles (ed.), *Skin Disease in Travelers*, Updates in Clinical Dermatology,
https://doi.org/10.1007/978-3-031-57836-6_23

Epidemiology

In the Americas, leishmaniasis is caused by parasites of the sub-genera *Leishmania* and *Viannia* with 15 species affecting the skin, mucosal membranes, and more rarely, internal organs as visceral leishmaniasis (VL). Parasites are transmitted to humans and vertebrate animals by the bite of female sand flies of the genus *Lutzomyia*. All the NWCL cycles are predominantly zoonotic, but the reservoir hosts vary by species and location, and in many cases are not completely understood [4]. There is an average of 55,000 cases of CL and MCL, and 3500 cases of VL, per year. It has been recorded in 20 countries of Central and S. America; 84% of the cases are found in Brazil, Peru, Bolivia, Colombia, Nicaragua, and Venezuela. The disease is found in environments with an altitude of 0 to 1500 m above sea level, temperatures higher than 20 °C, and an annual rainfall of 1500–3000 mm (Fig. 1).

The only two South-American countries where the disease has not been reported are Uruguay and Chile. It hasn't been reported in the Caribean Islands either.

In the past, NWCL was predominantly an occupational disease, related to activities such as farming, military operations, road construction, and new agricultural development in forests. Occupational exposure remains important, but widespread deforestation has led to an increase in cases in sub-urban settings and even urban transmission. In the last two decades, there has been an increase in cases presenting in non-endemic areas as tourism to Central and South America develops and becomes more popular [1].

NWCL is caused by numerous *Leishmania* species, belonging to the subgenera *Viannia* and *Leishmania* [7].

L. Viannia species:

L. braziliensis, which is the most frequent causative agent of cutaneous and muco-cutaneous clinical forms.

L. guyanensis, localizes geographically to the north of the Amazon River, Guyana, Venezuela, and Peru and can cause multiple cutaneous lesions.

L. lainsoni is limited almost exclusively to the Brazilian Amazon.

L. shawi, is found in the Brazilian state of Pará.

L. naiffi, distributed in Pará and Amazonas (Brazil) and in the French Guiana causes CL. There is a very similar species reported in soldiers in the forested areas in Belem de Para (North East Brazil) named Leishmania Viana *Lindembergi* in honor of Adolpho Lindemberg, who was the first person to detect Leishmania in cutaneous lesions in Brazil, in patients suffering from "úlcera de Bauru." It causes CL [28].

L. peruviana, which is found mostly in the Peruvian Andes and causes the CL form known locally as "Uta."

L. panamensis, which is the responsible agent of the disease in Panama, Costa Rica, Colombia, Ecuador, and Honduras.

L. colombiensis, which is found in Colombia, Panama, and Venezuela causing CL sporadically.

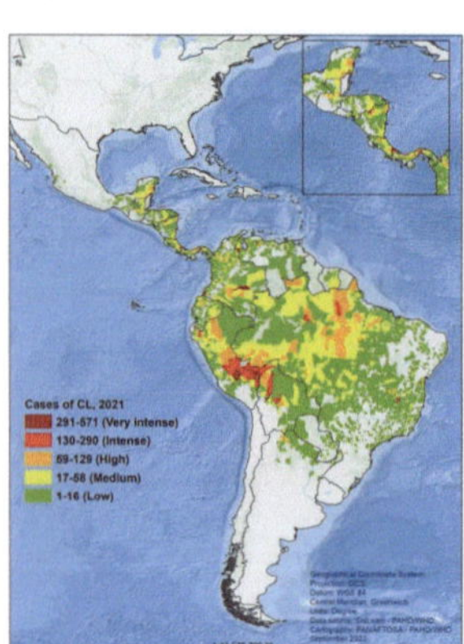

Note: Data reported by countries' leishmaniasis programs and surveillance services. CL: cutaneous leishmaniasis.
Source: Pan American Health Organization. Regional Information System on Leishmaniases in the Americas (SisLeish). Washington, DC: PAHO; 2022 [accessed 2 September 2022]. Limited access.

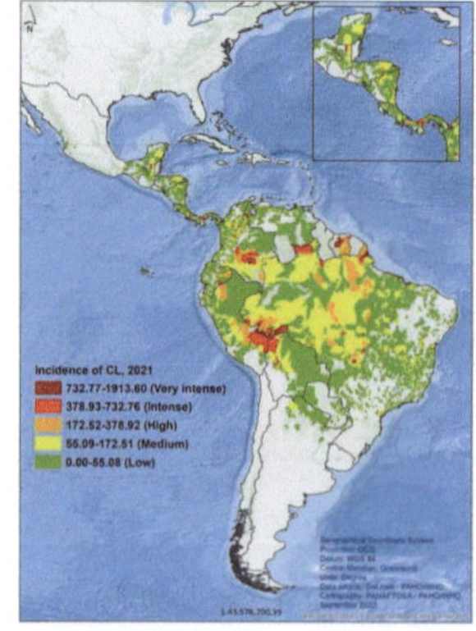

Note: Data reported by countries' leishmaniasis programs and surveillance services. CL: cutaneous leishmaniasis.
Source: Pan American Health Organization. Regional Information System on Leishmaniases in the Americas (SisLeish). Washington, DC: PAHO; 2022 [accessed 2 September 2022]. Limited access.

Fig. 1 PAHO, Pan-American Health Organization, Source: Regional information system for Leishmania in the Americas, Washington DC:OPS,2022, 2nd September

L. Leishmania species:

- *L. amazonensis* is responsible for the anergic diffuse cutaneous form and the cutaneous forms with disseminated lesions.
- *L. mexicana*, which is observed in Mexico, Colombia, the Caribbean Sea region, and Ecuador produces mucocutaneous leishmaniasis (MCL) or "Espundia," and the classic cutaneous form known as Chiclero's ulcer (gum tree harvester's ulcer).
- *L. pifanoi*, is the causal agent of MCL in Venezuela, and *L. venezuelensis* is observed in the Venezuelan Andes.
- *L. chagasi* causes VL and has a wide distribution in Latin America, extending from Mexico to Argentina.

A review article form the Geo-sentinel network, a worldwide communication and data collection network for the surveillance of travel-related diseases, reported in their 20 year analysis that most of the cases of imported NWCL/MCL in non-endemic, developed countries were acquired by travelers to Bolivia and Peru where risk of acquiring L. V. braziliensis and subsequent MCL is high for those visiting these risk areas.

From their reported cases, the risk of MC disease was much higher in patients that didn't get systemic treatment but in all the cases the disease was mild, probably due to the fact that it was diagnosed and treated early [27].

These patients need to be informed of the risk of developing MC disease and need to have careful monitoring for long periods.

Ethiology

Leishmaniasis species is a group of protozoan parasites, with a life cycle that is completed in a mammalian host and an insect vector, with different morphology adapting to either host and vector.

Leishmaniasis species undergo a cycle of development on the gut of female sand-flies of the genera Lutzomya and Psychodopygus in the new world.

All the species share a similar life cycle in which a sand fly transmits a flagellated form of the parasite, called a promastigote, to mammalian hosts, including humans. Once the promastigotes are injected into the skin via the bite of a sand fly, they enter the phagocytic cells. Within the macrophages, promastigotes transform to a round non-flagellated form called an amastigote (2–3 Micras). The life cycle is completed when the sand flies ingest amastigotes while feeding on a host, and the amastigotes subsequently transform to promastigotes (12–20 Micras) and replicate within the sand fly. The amastigotes multiply inside the cell causing its rupture, some continue to infect other macrophages and dendritic cells, some spread to the lymph nodes via lymphatic vessels from where they can disseminate to the mucosae membranes. Mammalians hosts are dogs, horses, mules, foxes, domestic rats, spiny rats, and others [3].

According to the type of immune response, the disease can be localized and have spontaneous healing, or it may become chronic, Progressive, or generalized [3].

Diagnosis

The diagnosis is suspected based on the clinical presentation and epidemiological facts, e.g., history of travel to an endemic area and/or history of an insect bite; to confirm, a smear obtained with a scrapping at the edge of the ulcer, in the wound exudate, or with needle aspiration will demonstrate the parasite by direct light microscopy with Wright, Giemsa, or Leishman stains showing the amastigotes as pale blue structures with deep blue kinetoplasts and nucleus inside the macrophages cytoplasm [7].

The biopsy for histopathology analysis is an useful tool although it can be highly variable depending on the age and type of the lesion, the epidermis can show an ulcer, it can be atrophic or demonstrate pseudo-ephiteliomatous hyperplasia with an inflammatory infiltrate composed by lymphocytes, macrophages, and plasmocytes with focal necrosis. In recent lesions, many parasites can be found inside the histiocytes cytoplasm, in later stages, there will be fewer amastigotes and a lymphocytic infiltrate conforming a tuberculoid granuloma.

Variable profiles of Th1 and Th2 cytokines are found in localized CL lesions and elicited in vitro in response to Leishmania antigens. CD4 and CD8, Interferon Gamma and TNF-Alpha producing T lymphocytes, macrophages and B cells constitute the majority of infiltrating cells [26]. IL-10 and IL-13 have been associated with chronic lesions. IL-4 is rarely detected and if present only in low concentrations. IL-10 is reported to be produced mainly by monocytes and CD4 + CD25 T regulatory cells are found in lesions caused by *L. braziliensis* and *L. guyanensis*. The role of T regulatory cells in human leishmaniasis is not yet clear; however, these cells are more frequently found in chronic lesions [3].

The histopathology for Diffuse CL reflects the absence of cell-mediated immunity, it is characterized by an intense dermal infiltration of vacuolated, macrophages filled with parasite amastigotes, very few lymphocytes and absence of necrosis and ulceration. After treatment, the lesions show features of acquired cellular immunity, including lymphocytic infiltrates and diffuse granulomatous inflammation.

Cell-mediated immune responses to Leishmania antigens in vitro are low or absent in diffuse cutaneous leishmaniasis. An absence of cutaneous delayed hypersensitivity response to leishmanin skin test antigen and low or absent interferon Gamma production by peripheral blood mononuclear cells characterize this disease presentation. Parasites are abundant in histopathological tissue sections. High concentrations of TNF-alpha are found in the serum of patients. The outcome of diffuse cutaneous leishmaniasis is often attributed to host factors but there may be a role for the infecting Leishmania species.

In Mucocutaneous disease, the histology features are similar to those observed in CL. Initially, a nonspecific cellular reaction predominates, with infiltration of lymphocytes, macrophages, and plasmocytes, sometimes associated with minor necrotic and granulomatous reactions. An important aspect of the pathogenesis is acute vasculitis, with coagulation necrosis of the walls of the small blood vessels. At this stage, the lesion can either progress to an epithelioid tuberculoid granuloma or revert to a cellular exudative reaction.

The most severe process is in the deep nasal mucosa, where amastigotes are present in proliferating vascular endothelium, with a heavy perivascular cellular infiltrate and liquefaction of the cartilage. Exuberant lymphocytic proliferation and mixed Th1 and Th2 cytokine responses characterize this disease presentation. Interferon producing CD4 and CD8 T cells abound in mucosal lesion biopsy samples and parasites are scarce in tissue sections [3].

The parasites can also be cultured in a Novy-McNeal-Nicole medium or similar, but some strains don't grow in culture and if they do, it may take up to 4 weeks.

The Leishmania or Montenegro subcutaneous test, consists on an injection of 0.1 ml of phenol killed promastigotes to elicit a cell mediated immune reaction, this determines past and present infections but it is negative in the diffuse or anergic forms of the disease.

PCR using DNA is the most effective and fastest test for diagnosis of Leishmaniasis, it is sensitive 92–98%, specific 100% characterizing the sub species causing the disease. Several target sequences and different PCR protocols have been described for the detection of Leishmania DNA. The most frequently used amplification targets are the Kinetoplast DNA minicircle (kDNA) and the small subunit ribosomal RNA (SSU rRNA). There are various gene targets which are also commonly used such as the ribosomal internal transcribed spacer (ITS), the mini-exon gene (spliced leader), and a repetitive genomic sequence. Real time PCR (or quantitative PCR-qPCR), a molecular technique which has revolutionized the pathogen diagnosis, is considered to be the future reference method for molecular diagnosis. qPCR is highly sensitive especially at the lower parasite loads, specific and reproducible offering the ability to monitor therapy and to prevent relapses. This makes qPCR an attractive alternative to conventional PCR in routine diagnosis.

Differential Diagnosis

Early forms of the disease can mimic an insect bite reaction, folliculitis, bacterial furuncle, and myasis; later on the ulcerated forms of CL can simulate other ulcerative diseases as atypical mycobacterium, tropical ulcer, yaws, neuropathic ulcers of Leprosy, most common skin conditions like venous stasis ulcers, Keratinocytic carcinomas, Pyoderma gangrenosum, although PG ulcers tend to grow more rapidly and become extremely painful. When presenting with verrucous plaques, one needs to consider, sporotrichosis, cutaneous tuberculosis, histoplasmosis, and Blastomycosis.

Facial CL plaques may resemble Lupus vulgaris, lupus pernio, discoid lupus erythematosus; for the mucocutaneous presentations, the differential diagnosis include Rhinoscleroma, Paracoccidiodomycosis, facial lymphomas, and Wegner's granulomatosis.

Diffuse Leishmaniasis must be differentiated form Lepromatous Leprosy and cutaneous lymphomas.

Clinical Features

Cutaneous Leishmaniasis can present as localized, disseminated, diffuse, atypical, and mucocutaneous. There is great variety of clinical presentations and none is species specific. There is a classical presentation affecting the ear; this characteristic chondro-cutaneous form known as the Chiclero's ulcer is seen more commonly in Mexico [2].

All species can cause localized cutaneous disease (LCL) with lesions that originate at the site of inoculation, initially as a papule that spreads centrifugally to form a nodule that ulcerates slowly and presents as a painless oval ulcer with raised indurated edges and sloughy centre; less commonly it can present as non-ulcerating skin nodules or verrucous/vegetating plaques. This process may take weeks, months, or even years after inoculation. Patients don't present any other associated symptoms, occasionally these lesions may be itchy. Primary lesions may be single or multiple; lymphatic involvement manifests as lymphadenitis in a sporotrichoid pattern or lymphadenopathy [3].

Lesions caused by *L. mexicana*, the Viannia subgenus species *L. braziliensis*, *L. panamensis*, *L. guyanensis*, and *L. peruviana* may heal without treatment after 3–6 months, leaving scars. Secondary cutaneous or mucosal lesions can occur.

L. panamensis and *L. brasilensis* can cause mucosal disease which may appear from a few months to many years after the initial skin lesion has healed; the nasal mucosa is almost always affected, causing nasal congestion and obstruction, the inflammation destroys the septum and if not treated with progress to pharynx, larynx, palate, and upper lip causing difficulties with speech and eating. It can progress to cause disfigurement and mutilation. Risk factors are malnourishment, self-healing or partially treated skin lesions, lesions on the upper body, large or multiple lesions. Mucocutaneous leishmaniasis never heals spontaneously. Secondary bacterial infections are frequent [3].

L. mexicana and Amazonensis can cause a NWCL diffuse form, it's been reported in Central America, the Amazonian Basin in Brazil and Venezuela, due to the absence of cellular immunity, the parasite disseminates through the skin, lymphatics, and blood vessels to all over the skin and sometimes mucous membranes, sparing the scalp. It usually starts on exposed areas with erythematous raised nodules, pigmented smooth or verrucous plaques, lymphadenopathy can be found and lymphedema, patients may have fever and constitutional symptoms. This unusual form of the disease if not treated has a chronic protracted course than can last many years. Treatment is difficult with common recurrences.

L. infantum, the species generally associated with visceral leishmaniasis, the skin involvement is often atypical presenting as nodules or plaques.

L. brasiliensis, *L. panamensis*, *L. guyanensis*, and *L. amazonensis* can also present with disseminated cutaneous Leishmaniasis with mixed type (nodules, ulcers, plaques) with more than 10 lesions involving 2 different parts of the body, patients may present with up to a hundred of

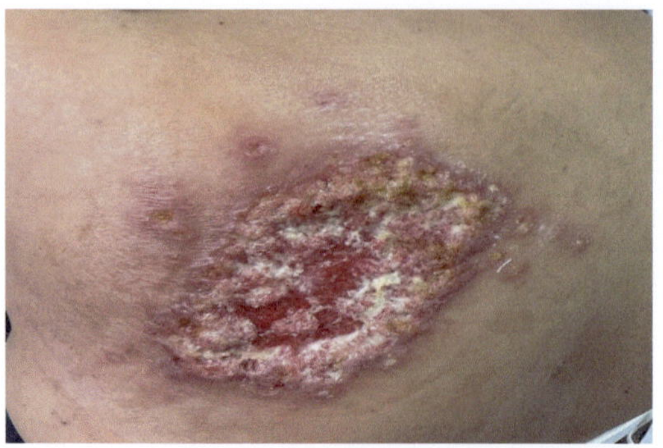

Fig. 2 42-year old female woman living in a farm in Restrepo, Valle del Cauca, she presented in the Federico Lleras Dermatology institute in Bogota, with a history of a 4 weeks insect bite papule that had transformed into an itchy, ulcerated plaque on the back. It was proven Leishmania sp.

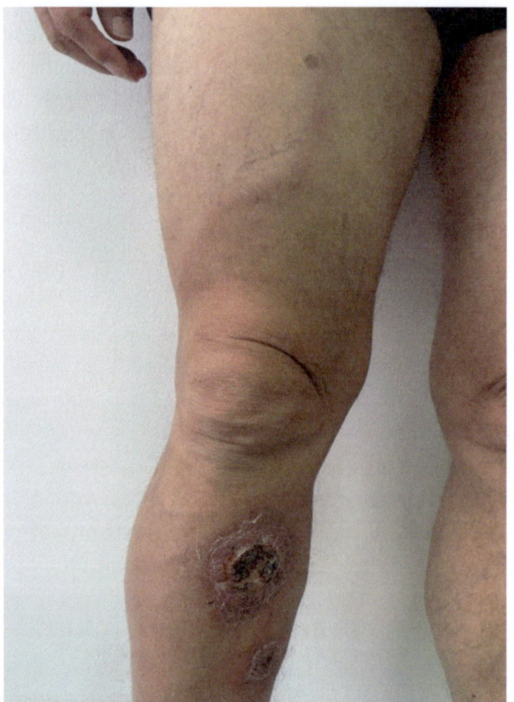

Fig. 3 55-year old man, who went on a holiday to Leticia in the Amazonas department, had a few insect bites but a few weeks later, he developed a few plaques on his right leg that rapidly ulcerated, the photo demonstrates also lymphatic spread. This was a *L. brasiliensis*

these lesions with or without mucosal involvement (Figs. 2 and 3) [3].

The epidemiology and clinical features of New World CL are summarized and contrasted with Old World CL in Table 1, Chap. X.

Clinical photos kindly provided by Dr. Claudia Marcela Arenas, Consultant Dermatologist, Specialist in Medical education at the Military University "Nueva Granada" Bogota-Colombia. Current president for the Colombian Association of Dermatologists (Asocolderma).

Treatment

NWCL in most of the cases requires systemic treatments due the fact that these lesions can disseminate to adjacent skin or mucosa, causing MCL. The risk of developing mucosal lesions varies between in 2 and 30% of untreated cutaneous cases with 2% risk for *L. amazonensis*, 10% for *L. guyanensis* and *L. panamensis* and up to 30% with *L. braziliensis* [6].

Systemic treatments don't guarantee that mucosal lesions will not present a few months to many years later, the high risk of developing side effects to systemic medications, and the high rate of relapses make the treatment for NWCL very challenging.

The lack of a simple drug evaluation system has stopped the development of new drugs for the treatment of leishmaniasis, this is complicated by the various Leishmania species infecting humans and the fact that leishmaniasis is almost exclusively a problem of developing countries where there is little commercial incentives for pharmaceutical companies to develop cheap and effective antileishmanial drugs [3].

Topical Treatments

In general, topical treatment or withholding treatment can be considered in patients with simple CL caused by *L. leishmania* species, unique or few lesions, with lesion size of less than 1 cm, lesions that are showing improvement without treatment and absence of lymphadenopathy.

The topical treatments used in NW cutaneous Leishmaniasis are thermotherapy and paromomycin.

Thermotherapy

It has been demonstrated that several pathogenic Leishmania species are thermo-sensitive from 37 to 39 °C in vitro. Thermo-therapy has been evaluated in a variety of CL species and via a variety of heat-delivery modalities [14]. The Thermo-MedT device, which utilizes radio-frequency (RF) technology remains the most supported by randomized clinical trials and is WHO recommended as an alternative therapy for all American CL species. In some areas, the high cost of this device, healthcare infrastructure limitations, and poverty in endemic areas has restricted its use to research and military settings. One to three applications of localized heat (50 °C for 30 s) were about 70% effective in CL in Colombia and Guatemala 3 months after treatment [6].

Paromomycin

Paromomycin is an aminocyclitol aminoglycoside antibiotic used for the treatment of leishmaniasis. Diverse preparations of topical PR have been tested on CL in animals and humans.

Paromomycin at 15% plus MBCL (methylbenzethonium chloride) 12% ointment, twice daily for 20 days, was 70–90% effective against cutaneous leishmaniasis species in trials in Guatemala and Ecuador. The final clinical response rate at the 12-month follow up examination was 85.7% (31 of 35) in the treatment group and 39.4% (13 of 33) in the placebo group in the RCT in Guatemala. In general, the treatment is well tolerated, the adverse events are mild locally on the treated areas with pruritus and a burning sensation, none of them led to stopping the treatment and all disappeared within 1 week of completing the treatment. However, Paromomycin was ineffective in the treatment of NWCL by *L. mexicana* and *L. chagasi* in Honduras (CR 5.5%) [6]. Paromomycin combinations with short courses of systemic Antimonials have been tried with variable results and can be effective on some serotypes of Leishmaniasis, e.g., *L. panamiensis* in Colombia [6].

Intralesional Injections of Pentavalent Antimonial Compounds

The experience using intra-lesional injections of antimonial compounds is very limited.

In a Brazilian study in 74 patients with NWCL by *L. braziliensis*, meglumine antimoniate was injected intra-lesionally in the four cardinal points of the lesion, until achieving complete blanching, every 3–7 days and for a total of 1–5 sessions with a CR of 80% after 10 years of follow-up [8]. A randomized clinical trial was performed for NWCL caused by *L. braziliensis* in Bolivia where three doses of an intralesional injection of meglumine antimoniate with 70% CR at 6 months follow-up [6].

Systemic Treatments

Pentavalent Antimonials

The pentavalent antimonial compounds remain the main pillar of therapy for leishmaniasis. Sodium stibogluconate (Pentostam) has been the most studied compound and is the only pentavalent antimonial available in the USA. Meglumine antimoniate (Glucantime) is used largely in French-speaking countries and in Latin America. These compounds appear to inhibit bioenergetic pathways such as glycolysis and fatty acid oxidation in Leishmania amastigotes. Its best efficacy is on *L. braziliensis* and *panamensis*, for *L. mexican* and *L. guyanensis*, it may respond well in some areas.

The Pan-American Health Organization (PAHO) guide for the treatment of Leishmaniasis recommends sodium stibogluconate 20 mg Sb/kg/day intramuscularly or intravenously for 20 days as first-line treatment for all Leishmania spp. [4]. This can be repeated 3 months later if needed.

Antimonials are still the first-choice treatment for NWCL in many countries, [10–12] the CRs range from 77% to 90% depending on the species with the exception of *L. guyanensis* infection in French Guinea where pentamidine is the first-choice treatment [9]. Other cases of CL due to *L. guyanensis* in Peru had a response rate to pentavalent antimonials varying from 90% to 73.3%. *L. mexicana* responds in Guatemala only with a 57% CR but got a very good response in Mexico with 100% CR [6, 13].

A combination of oral pentoxifylline with pentavalent antimonials for 30 days reduced the relapse rate and accelerated cure in comparison with pentavalent antimonials alone. Combination therapy has been used in some other studies. Topical administration of imiquimod every other day for 20 days as adjunct therapy to pentavalent antimonials has been tested in Peru (CR 72%). Although no significant difference among CRs was observed, imiquimod accelerated cure in comparison with antimonials alone in patients with relapsing lesions.

The Antimonials are given by intravenous or intramuscular injection and can cause cardiotoxicity, pain at the injection site, chemical evidence of pancreatitis, elevation of transaminase levels, bone marrow suppression, rashes, myalgia, and arthralgia. The higher risk patients for severe side effects are patients under 2 years old and over 45 years old.

Pentamidine

Pentamidine Isethionate is a synthetic amidine derivative, Pentamidine Isethionate is an antiprotozoal and anti-fungal agent that appears to interact with the minor groove of AT-rich DNA regions of the pathogen genome, interfering with DNA replication and function. It is effective in the treatment of trypanosomiasis, leishmaniasis, some fungal infections, and Pneumocystis carinii pneumonia in HIV-infected patients.

In Leishmaniasis, it has been used at a dose of 3–4 mg/Kg intravenously or Intramuscular every 48 h for 3 or 4 doses being effective in *L. panamensis* and *L. guyanensis*, but less effective in *L. brasiliensis*.

Several studies have compared the efficacy of pentamidine isethionate with pentavalent antimonials when treating CL, it is the drug of choice in French Guyana, where over 90% of infections are due to *L. guyanensis* [9, 17].

Similarly, in Brazil with primarily *L. braziliensis*, and in Surinam with *L. guyanensis*, CRs of 73–100% have been reported [16]. Clinical trials have demonstrated a low response in those cases acquired in Brazil caused by *L. guyanensis* (CR 58.1%), with no significant differences in the CR in response to antimonials [15].

In Colombia, where the majority of infections are caused by *L. panamensis*, CRs of up to 95%

have been reached with the standard dose of Pentamidine with a toxicity comparable to that of antimonials [18, 19]. The results obtained in Peru with *L. braziliensis* were less favorable where the efficacy of pentamidine was 35% compared with 78% with antimonials.

The more common side effects for Pentamidine are dizziness, hypoglycemia (can be severe), hypotension (can be severe), local reaction, nausea, rash, altered taste, more rarely patients can have QT interval prolongation, arrhythmia, and cases of acute pancreatitis have been described. Other potential side effects with parenteral use are: acute kidney injury, anaemia, azotemia, electrolyte imbalance, flushing, hematuria, hyperglycemia, local induration, leukopenia, localized pain, myopathy, syncope, thrombocytopenia, vomiting. Patients should be closely monitored for at least 1 h after the injection.

Miltefosine

Miltefosine is an orally and topically active alkylphosphocholine compound with potential antineoplastic activity. It targets cellular membranes, modulating cell membrane permeability, membrane lipid composition, phospholipid metabolism, and mitogenic signal transduction, resulting in cell differentiation and inhibition of cell growth. This agent also inhibits the anti-apoptotic mitogen-activated protein kinase (MAPK) pathway and modulates the balance between the MAPK and pro-apoptotic stress-activated protein kinase (SAPK/JNK) pathways, thereby inducing apoptosis. As an immunomodulator, Miltefosine stimulates T-cells, macrophages and the expression of interleukin 3 (IL-3), granulocyte-macrophage colony stimulating factor (GM-CSF), and interferon gamma (INF-gamma).

It was originally intended for breast cancer and other solid tumors. However, it could not be developed as an oral agent because of dose-limiting gastro-intestinal toxicity and only a topical formulation was approved for skin metastases. Then came the evidence of excellent anti-leishmanial activity from clinical trials and the medication was approved to treat VL and CL.

Miltefosine at 2 mg/Kg day for 28 days can be effective in CL mostly *L. panamensis* but limited effect has been found in *L. brasiliensis* and *L. mexicana*.

Several studies carried out using Miltefosine in Colombia and Guatemala have shown great variability in the CR depending on the Leishmania species isolated. Good results observed in Colombia suggest that Miltefosine may be a good option for MCL [6].

Similarly, a non-randomized clinical trial carried out in Bolivia, using Miltefosine showed a CR of 83% for moderate MCL and 58% for severe cases, versus 50% of patients treated with amphotericin B; the patients were re-evaluated 24 months after the beginning of the trial when it was observed that only 2 of 41 patients relapsed. Prolonging treatment from 4 to 6 weeks increased the CR to 75% [20, 21].

The main and most frequent side effects of Miltefosine are Gastrointestinal side effects with appetite loss, nausea, vomiting and diarrhea which are more prevalent early on the treatment but improve throughout the course of treatment. This is probably related to the oral intake of the drug and the detergent-like properties of Miltefosine affecting the gastrointestinal mucosa. Intake of fatty food together or just before Miltefosine reduces the gastrointestinal side effects and has no effect on bioavailability.

Elevated serum creatinine levels during treatment are frequently observed, possibly related to occasional dehydration by severe vomiting/diarrhea, severe nephrotoxicity caused by Miltefosine is rare. Serum levels of both alanine aminotransferase (ALT) and aspartate aminotransferase (AST) tend to increase mildly in the first week of Miltefosine treatment in VL patients, possibly due to immediate necrosis of pre-damaged hepatocytes. This generally normalizes in the subsequent weeks together with the resolving infection. Ophthalmologic retinotoxic side effects have been reported in pre-clinical studies, but have so far not been observed in any VL or CL patients. Preclinical reproductive toxicity studies in animals showed fetal death and teratogenicity at doses lower than the recommended human dose. Use of Miltefosine during pregnancy is strictly contraindicated, and contraceptive use is mandatory for females of child-bearing age during ther-apy and for 5 months afterwards. Stevens-Johnson syndrome has been reported, therefore therapy should be discontinued if an exfoliative or bullous rash occurs during treatment.

Amphotericin B

Amphotericin B deoxycholate belongs to the polyene class of antifungals. It has been in use for the treatment of invasive fungal infections for more than 50 years. It was first isolated as a natural product of a soil actinomycete. Newer lipid formulations that are less nephrotoxic as compared with conventional Amphotericin B are available [22, 25]. These include: Amphotericin B in a liposomal formulation (LAMB) exhibits increased tolerability and a reduced toxicity profile and Amphotericin B lipid complex in which Amphotericin B is tightly packed in a ribbon-like structure. Amphotericin B cholesteryl sulphate complex-deoxycholate.

Amphotericin B acts by binding to ergosterol in the cell membrane of most fungi, after binding with ergosterol, it causes the formation of ion channels leading to loss of protons and monovalent cations, which results in depolarization and concentration-dependent cell killing. It produces oxidative damage to the cells with the formation of free radicals and increased membrane permeability and has a stimulatory effect on phagocytic cells, which assists with the fungal infection clearance.

It has been used at 0.7/mg/kg/day for 25–30 days for the treatment of MCL by *L. braziliensis*. With liposomal amphotericin B (LAMB), there is more experience with the treatment of mucocutaneous types. The dose usually consists of 3 mg/kg/day up to 10–15 doses (20–45 mg/kg total doses) [23].

Not many controlled clinical trials are able to give a clear response for LAMB in CL. A study in Bolivia for *L. braziliensis*, LAMB proved to be more effective (CR 85%), better tolerated and more cost effective than antimonials [23]. Another clinical trial in Brazil, mainly for infections by *L. braziliensis*, found that low doses of LAMB achieved a high CR (81%), although lower than that obtained by pentavalent antimonials (CR 100%) but with fewer side effects [24].

Side effects of treatment with Amphotericine B 80% of the patients may develop infusion related renal toxicity. Amphotericin B also interacts with cholesterol in human cell membranes, which is responsible for its toxicity. The most common side effects include: hypokalemia, hypomagnesemia, anaphylaxis, fever. Nephrotoxicity: Renal toxicity correlates with conventional amphotericin B use and can lead to renal failure and requirement for dialysis. But the AKI often stabilizes with therapy and renal damage is reversible after discontinuation of Amphotericin.

Avoiding concomitant use of other nephrotoxic agents and appropriate hydration with normal saline before the infusion significantly decreases the likelihood and severity of AKI associated with Amphotericin B.

Other potential uncommon side effect includes demyelinating encephalopathy in patients with bone marrow transplant with total body irradiation or who are receiving cyclosporine. The long-term administration is associated with normochromic, normocytic anaemia due to low erythropoietin levels.

Other systemic medications: Azithromycin, Itraconazole, Ketoconazole, and Allopurinol have been used sporadically in some cases with moderate to good responses but are not supported by good evidence and won't be discussed in this chapter.

References

1. Lawn SD, Whetham J, Chiodini PL, Kanagalingam J, Watson J, Behrens RH, Lockwood DNJ. New world mucosal and cutaneous leishmaniasis: an emerging health problem among British travellers. QJM. 2004;97(12):781–8. https://doi.org/10.1093/qjmed/hch127.
2. Talhari C, Oliviera de Guerra J, Chrusiak-Talhari A, Lima Machado P. Faculty of Medicine, state University of Amazonas, Manaous Brasil. Chapter 15, American tegumentary Lesihmaniasis.
3. WHO Technical report series, Control of the Leishmaniases Report of a meeting of the WHO Expert Committee on The Control of Leishmaniases, Geneva, 22–26 March 2010.
4. Panamerican health organization, World health organization, report Leishmaniases Report # 11 - December, 2022. Epidemiological Report of the Americas on LEISHMANIASES.
5. Pavli A, Maltezou HC. Leishmaniasis, an emerging infection in travelers. Int J Infect Dis. 2010;14(12):e1032–9. https://doi.org/10.1016/j.ijid.2010.06.019.
6. Monge-Maillo B, López-Vélez R. Therapeutic options for old world cutaneous leishmaniasis and new world cutaneous and mucocutaneous leishmaniasis. Drugs. 2013;73(17):1889–920. https://doi.org/10.1007/s40265-013-0132-1. PMID: 24170665
7. Edoardo Torres-Guerrero, Marco Romano Quintanilla-Cedillo, Julieta Ruiz-Esmenjaud, Roberto Leishmaniasis: a review F1000Res 2017 May 26;6:750. doi: https://doi.org/10.12688/f1000research.11120.1.. eCollection.
8. Soto J, Rojas E, Guzman M, et al. Intralesional antimony for single lesions of bolivian cutaneous leishmaniasis. Clin Infect Dis. 2013;56:1255–60.
9. Pradinaud R, Girardeau I, Sainte-Marie D. A pentamidina, excelente terapeutica da leishmaniose cutanea. Esquema de tratamiento idealizado na Guiana Francesa em dose unica. An Bras Dermatol. 1985;60:385–7.
10. Soto J, Valda-Rodriquez L, Toledo J, et al. Comparison of generic to branded pentavalent antimony for treatment of new world cutaneous leishmaniasis. Am J Trop Med Hyg. 2004;71:577–81.
11. Arevalo J, Ramirez L, Adaui V, et al. Influence of leishmania (viannia) species on the response to antimonial treatment in patients with American tegumentary leishmaniasis. J Infect Dis. 2007;195:1846–51.
12. Vargas-Gonzalez A, Canto-Lara SB, Damian-Centeno AG, Andrade-Narvaez FJ. Response of cutaneous leishmaniasis (chiclero's ulcer) to treatment with meglumine antimoniate in Southeast Mexico. Am J Trop Med Hyg. 1999;61:960–3.
13. Romero GA, Guerra MV, Paes MG, Macedo VO. Comparison of cutaneous leishmaniasis due to Leishmania (viannia) braziliensis and L. (V.) guyanensis in Brazil: therapeutic response to meglumine antimoniate. Am J Trop Med Hyg. 2001;65:456–65.
14. Navin TR, Arana BA, Arana FE, de Merida AM, Castillo AL, Pozuelos JL. Placebo-controlled clinical trial of meglumine antimonate (glucantime) vs. localized controlled heat in the treatment of cutaneous leishmaniasis in Guatemala. Am J Trop Med Hyg. 1990;42:43–50.
15. de Paula CD, Sampaio JH, Cardoso DR, Sampaio RN. A comparative study between the efficacy of pentamidine isothionate given in three doses for one week and N-methyl-glucamine in a dose of 20mgSbV/day for 20 days to treat cutaneous leishmaniasis. Rev Soc Bras Med Trop. 2003;36:365–71.
16. Lai A, Fat EJ, Vrede MA, Soetosenojo RM, Lai A, Fat RF. Pentamidine, the drug of choice for the treatment of cutaneous leishmaniasis in Surinam. Int J Dermatol. 2002;41:796–800.
17. Neves LO, Talhari AC, Gadelha EP, et al. A randomized clinical trial comparing meglumine antimoniate,

pentamidine and amphotericin B for the treatment of cutaneous leishmaniasis by Leishmania guyanensis. An Bras Dermatol. 2011;86:1092–101.

18. Soto J, Buffet P, Grogl M, Berman J. Successful treatment of Colombian cutaneous leishmaniasis with four injections of pentamidine. Am J Trop Med Hyg. 1994;50:107–11.

19. Soto-Mancipe J, Grogl M, Berman JD. Evaluation of pentamidine for the treatment of cutaneous leishmaniasis in Colombia. Clin Infect Dis. 1993;16:417–25.

20. Soto J, Toledo J, Valda L, et al. Treatment of Bolivian mucosal leishmaniasis with miltefosine. Clin Infect Dis. 2007;44:350–6.

21. Soto J, Rea J, Valderrama M, et al. Efficacy of extended (six weeks) treatment with miltefosine for mucosal leishmaniasis in Bolivia. Am J Trop Med Hyg. 2009;81:387–9.

22. Wortmann G, Zapor M, Ressner R, et al. Lipsosomal amphotericin B for treatment of cutaneous leishmaniasis. Am J Trop Med Hyg. 2010;83:1028–33.

23. Solomon M, Baum S, Barzilai A, Scope A, Trau H, Schwartz E. Liposomal amphotericin B in comparison to sodium stibogluconate for cutaneous infection due to Leishmania braziliensis. J Am Acad Dermatol. 2007;56:612–6.

24. Solomon M, Pavlotzky F, Barzilai A, Schwartz E. Liposomal amphotericin B in comparison to sodium stibogluconate for Leishmania braziliensis cutaneous leishmaniasis in travelers. J Am Acad Dermatol. 2013;68:284–9.

25. Motta JO, Sampaio RN. A pilot study comparing low-dose liposomal amphotericin B with N-methyl glucamine for the treatment of American cutaneous leishmaniasis. J Eur Acad Dermatol Venereol. 2012;26:331–5.

26. Scott P, Novais F. Cutaneous leishmaniasis: immune responses in protection and pathogenesis. Nat Rev Immunol. 2016;16:581–92. https://doi.org/10.1038/nri.2016.72.

27. Boggild AK, Caumes E, Grobusch MP, Schwartz E, Hynes NA, Libman M, Connor BA, Chakrabarti S, Parola P, Keystone JS, Nash T, Showler AJ, Schunk M, Asgeirsson H, Hamer DH, Kain KC, GeoSentinel Surveillance Network. Cutaneous and mucocutaneous leishmaniasis in travellers and migrants: a 20-year GeoSentinel Surveillance Network analysis. J Travel Med. 2019;26(8) pii: taz055 https://doi.org/10.1093/jtm/taz055.

28. Ishikawa EAY*, De Souza AAA*, Lainson R*. An outbreak of cutaneous Leishmaniasis among soldiers in Belem, Para state, Brazil, CA) caused by Leishmania Viana Lindenberg n. sp a new Leishmanial parasite of man in the Amazon region Silveira F.T Parasite. 2002;9(1):43–50. https://doi.org/10.1051/parasite/200209143.

Myiasis

Omar Lupi and Fabio Franciscone

Introduction

Myiasis is the infestation of live vertebrates with dipterous larvae. Depending on the body's location and the relationship of the larvae with the host, the parasite can cause a broad range of infestations [1]. Myiasis remains a major economic problem in animal production leading to reduced milk production, weight and fertility issues, and also reduced high quality, resulting in economic losses [2]. Human myiasis is distributed worldwide, with more species and greater abundance in poor socioeconomic regions of tropical and subtropical countries. In non-endemic countries, myiasis is an important condition, where it can represent the fourth most common travel-associated skin disease [3].

O. Lupi
Dermatology—Federal University of the State of Rio de Janeiro (UNIRIO), Rio de Janeiro, Brazil

Internal Medicine at the Federal University of Rio de Janeiro (UFRJ), Rio de Janeiro, Brazil

Physician—Immunology Service—HUCFF/UFRJ, Dermatology Department—Policlínica Geral do Rio de Janeiro (PGRJ), Rio de Janeiro, Brazil

F. Franciscone (✉)
Federal University of Amazonas, Manaus, Amazonas, Brazil
e-mail: fabiofrancesconi@ufam.edu.br

Myiasis Classification

There are two main systems for categorizing myiasis:

Anatomical classification—this classification system is based on the one proposed by Bishop [4], later modified by James [5] and by Zumpt [2]:

- *Sanguinivorous or bloodsucking.*
- *Cutaneous myiasis*—subdivided into furuncular, migratory, and wound infestation.
- *Cavitary myiasis*—subdivided into nasopharyngeal myiasis, intestinal myiasis, and urogenital. If an unusual location occurs, the infestation may receive the name of the affected organ—p. ex. cerebral myiasis, aural, ophtalmomyiasis.

Ecological Classification—is the classification based in the relationship between the fly's maggots and the host [2, 4]:

- *Specific/obligatory*—parasite dependent on host for part of its life cycle.
- *Semi-specific/facultative.*
  - *Primary*—normally free-living but may initiate myiasis.
  - *Secondary*—normally free-living and unable to initiate myiasis. May be involved once animal is infested by other species.

W. Robles (ed.), *Skin Disease in Travelers*, Updates in Clinical Dermatology,
https://doi.org/10.1007/978-3-031-57836-6_24

- *Tertiary*—normally free-living and unable to initiate myiasis. May be involved when host is near death.
- *Accidental/pseudomyiasis*—normally free-living larvae. Cause pathological reaction when accidentally in contact with the host.

Diptera (True Flies) Taxonomy

To fully understand the ecological classification and the real impact of myiasis, it is necessary to understand the taxonomic classification of the diptera as shown in graphics 1, 2, and 3.

Myiasis and Travel Medicine

Increasing international travel, both for tourism and business, raises the physicians need to make an accurate and timely diagnosis of myiasis, it is important not only to alleviate the patient's symptoms, but also to prevent the establishment of myiasis causing flies in non-endemic regions.

Epidemiology

Poor hygiene is the most important risk factor for acquiring myiasis, with the exception of *D. hominis* infestation. Other important risk factors are: geographical location, cultural habits, open wounds—especially those with an abundance of suppuration, poor vision, mental illness, and other situations where the maggot cannot be identified or removed.

Clinical Manifestations

Cutaneous myiasis—is the most frequently encountered clinical form [6]. Furuncular, migratory and wound myiases are all included in this group.

Furuncular myiasis (warble)—is due to penetration of the larva into the skin, where an erythematous, furuncle-like nodule develops, with a maggot within it. The typical lesion has a central punctum, which may exude watery, serosanguineous, or purulent fluid. Frequently the patients are aware of movements within the nodule. From the central pore, the presence of the parasite is evidenced by direct visualization of the posterior part of the larva, the respiratory spiracle (usually confused with tiny black eyes), or by bubbles in the discharge. The number of larvae within the lesion varies with the offending species.

D. hominis and *C. anthropophaga* are the most common causative agents of furuncular myiasis. Pruritus, pain, and movement sensation are the most common symptoms, and they usually happen suddenly at night and precede the fluid leak. The difference in the number of lesions and their distribution pattern can be explained by the natural habit of each species. Furuncle-like lesions are the typical manifestation. Clinical variants described are: vesicular, bullous, pustular, erosive, ecchymotic, and ulcerative lesions. Almost always the lesion heals completely without leaving any trace. Sometimes hyperpigmentation and scarring can occur. Clinical variants and severe scarring outcomes are more commonly seen in malnourished children. The most common complication is secondary bacterial infection.

Agents Responsible for Furuncular Myiasis

- *D. hominis (human bot fly)* is the a common cause of furuncular myiasis in the Americas. Human bot flies have a unique and complex life cycle. When the female bot fly is ready to lay eggs, it captures blood-sucking arthropods and attaches the eggs to their abdomen with a quick drying glue—a method of egg delivery called phoresis [7]. After 1 week, when the insect approaches a warm-blooded animal, the heat induces the larvae to hatch. The larvae have 20 days to grab a host with its lid. If it succeeds, the larva leaves the egg and penetrates painlessly through the skin and gains access to the dermis. Within 5–10 weeks, the parasite goes to second instar—stage II and eventually a third instar or stage III, when it leaves the host to pupate in the soil. After a month, the adult flies emerge to mate and begin the life cycle over. Pain is more commonly seen with this species, the presence of larval hooks and the larva's movement of rotation around its axis may explain the pain sensation, typically with sudden paroxysmal episodes of lancinating pain (often nocturnal). The history of an insect bite can be remembered. The infestation favors exposed sites, such as the scalp, face, and extremities, usually a single lesion harboring only one larva [6].

- *Cordylobia anthropophaga (Tumbu fly)* has been endemic to the subtropics of Africa for more than 135 years. Tumbu-fly myiasis has been described in Portugal. Adult flies are more active during the morning and late in the afternoon, when they deposit the eggs on shaded soil, preferably contaminated with urine or feces, or drying clothes (especially improperly washed diapers and damp clothing laid on the ground). Larvae hatch in 1–3 days and remain still until "activated" by host body heat or vibration. People are most commonly parasitized during the rainy season, with a greater number of lesions (compared to other species), distributed more commonly in covered sites, such as the trunk, buttocks, and thighs. After 8–12 days, the mature third instar maggot leaves the host. The infestation of humans is particularly related to the disease of dogs, an important reservoir for the infestation. During rainy season, the rats (*Rattus novergicus*) approach human settlements and may transfer the infestation to house rats and domestic animals—especially dogs. The observation that children are more frequently infested than adults is, probably related to the thinner skin of the infants and the immunity developed by adults living in endemic regions [8].
- Other species reported to cause furuncular myiasis in humans are:
  - *Cordylobia rodhaini* is similar to *C. anthropophaga* infestation, being larger and more painful.
  - *Cuterebra* spp. (rabbit or rodent bot flies) causes facultative myiasis in the summer

months of North America. Most cases occur in children, affecting the face, scalp, neck, shoulders, or chest.
  - *Wohlfahrtia vigil* causes furuncular lesions in children, usually with multiple lesions— with 12–24 maggots in each lesion.
  - *Wohlfahrtia magnifica (Spotted Flesh Fly)* furuncular myiasis develops 24 h after larval infestation. One or few larvae are present in the lesion. Local inflammatory lymph node enlargement with eosinophilia may compose the clinical picture.

Differential diagnoses—furuncle, insect bite, insect prurigo, pyoderma, inflamed cyst, tungiasis. *C. anthropophaga* myiasis can simulate serious soft tissue infection. Some cases can be misdiagnosed as delusion of parasites. Labial cases may be confused with labial cellulitis. Breast myiasis may be confused with periductal mastitis, benign mass with microcalcification, and inflammatory carcinoma. Clinical and radiologic confusion with AV malformation and hemangioma happened in one case of pre-auricular myiasis. Pain, erythema, itchiness, small vesicles, and crusting may pose differential diagnosis with herpes simplex.

Furuncular myiasis (warble) diagnosis is easily done based solely on clinical grounds. Dermoscopy has been used to identify the posterior parts of the maggot. Ultrasound can be very useful to confirm a case of furuncular myiasis and also control the complete removal of the larvae. Color Doppler sonography, which is able to visualize the continuous movement of internal fluids of the larva, has proved to be useful to detect *D. hominis* and *C. anthropophaga* larvae when ultrasound is not able to detect the parasite. Mammography may not be able to exclude malignancy. Magnetic resonance and computed tomography are able to identify a subcutaneous segmented nodule; however, its morphology doesn't aid in the diagnosis.

Laboratory examination is usually normal. In cases of chronic infestation or multiple infestations, laboratory signs of systemic inflammation, peripheral eosinophilia, and elevated Immunoglobulin E may be found.

Molecular diagnosis has been successfully used to identify the offending larva and may be a future method for identifying cutaneous myiasis in hospitals with no expertise in tropical medicine.

Biopsies are not necessary for diagnosing furuncular myiasis and should be restricted for academic purposes.

Treatment

The goal of the treatment of Furuncular myiasis is the complete removal of the larva from the skin with prevention and control of secondary infection. Therapy consists of three general techniques: 1—application of a toxic substance to the larvae and egg; 2—produce localized hypoxia to force the emergence of the larvae; 3—mechanical or surgical removal of the maggots.

C. anthropophaga does not migrate deeper into tissue and is easier to remove. Expression of *C. anthropophaga* may be adequate, preferably with two wooden spatulas—which reduces the chance of rupturing the larva. On the other hand, expression should be avoided when *D. hominis* is the offending agent, because it is usually fruitless and painful with a risk of rupturing the maggot. Reports have noted the successful eradication of *D. hominis* infestation by occluding the punctum (breathing hole in the skin) with a substance to prevent gas exchange [9]. To avoid asphyxiation, the organism emerges far enough to be grasped by the forceps of a vigilant patient or physician. Occluding substances that may be used are: petrolatum, bacon, fingernail, adhesive tape, and others. Occlusion may have to be maintained for 24 h or more to have the desired effect. The risk of attempted occlusion is that the organism may asphyxiate without emerging, and the dead larva may elicit an inflammatory response with formation of a foreign-body granuloma, and eventually progression to calcification. Injection of lidocaine 1% (2 ml per nodule) is sometimes used to paralyze the larva, making the extraction easier [10]. Liquid nitrogen used before extraction stiffens the larva and helps its removal. Topical 1% ivermectin may be used in furuncular lesions caused by *D. hominis*—there is, although, a possibility that the dead larva may be trapped within the skin.

Surgical excision is usually unnecessary for treatment, although it may be needed to remove the larva. Some advocate a cruciate incision to remove *D. hominis*, which prevents damage to the larva and allows easier extraction without leaving remnants in the wound. In some cases, debridement of necrotic tissue surrounding the lesion inside the pocket may be indicated.

Oral treatment is not recommended in furuncular myiasis. Ivermectin may kill the larva inside the lesion with consequent inflammatory reaction. Antibiotics should be exclusively used in the presence of bacterial infection.

Migratory myiasis or creeping myiasis— occurs when a dipteran maggot migrates through burrows within the skin. The deepth of the tunnel and the migration speed are the factors responsible for the clinical manifestations. Larvae of the genera *Gasterophilus* (horse bot fly) and *Hypoderma* (cattle bot fly) cause almost all cases of creeping myiasis. In human skin, unable to complete their life cycle, these larvae start to migrate in the skin, aimlessly, producing the migratory pattern of the lesions. It should be noted that *Hypoderma* spp. could simulate their larval development (although without reaching the fully mature third instars) in human hosts.

Differential Diagnosis

Three clinical features distinguish migratory myiasis from helminthic cutaneous larva migrans. Firstly, larva migrans extends more slowly, and its cutaneous presentation is generally less widespread. Secondly, fly larvae can survive for months in human skin, much longer than helminths. Finally, fly larvae are generally larger than helminths. Cutaneous larva migrans, migratory myiasis, gnathostomiasis, and sparganosis should be remembered in the differential diagnosis of cases with cutaneous migratory lesions with eosinophilia. Hypereosinophilic syndrome can occasionally be caused by creeping myiasis.

Diagnosis

The definitive diagnosis is made with the identification of a dipteran larva in the migratory lesion. The parasite can be visualized with dermoscopy; *Gasterophilus* can be visualized just in advance of the visible line and *Hypoderma* in the furuncle-like lesion. Ultrasound scan can reveal the larva in *Hypoderma* furuncular lesion. *Hypoderma* infestation produces hypodermin C, a circulating antigen that appears to reflect periods of larval activity in cattle. In humans, serology has been useful in confirming the diagnosis of a suspected case of hypodermosis. Polymerase chain reaction-restriction fragment (PCR-RFLP) targeting cytochrome oxidase I (COI) of mitochondrial DNA can be used for parasite molecular identification and differentiating the most common *Hypoderma* species [6].

Treatment

Treatment of the lesion caused by horse bot fly can be made by identification of the position of the larvae and its removal with a needle.

Hypoderma larvae are best removed through a cruciform incision or may be expressed if a furuncle-like lesion is formed. Surgical excision is almost always required for migratory myiasis. When it is migrating deep in tissue, the extraction may not be possible. Use of oral albendazole or ivermectin mobilized the parasites toward the body surface, allowing identification and surgical removal of the maggot in one case caused by *H. sinense* larvae. A case was successfully treated after three rounds of oral ivermectin.

Wound myiasis—occurs when fly larvae infest open wounds in a living host. This kind of infestation may be the result of facultative or obligatory parasites. *Cochliomyia hominivorax, Chrysomya bezziana,* and *W. magnifica* are the most common flies worldwide that cause obligatory human wound myiasis. Numerous species of Muscidae, Calliphoridae, and Sarcophagidae (also known as filth flies) have been implicated in facultative wound myiasis. In one series, 87% of human wound myiasis found in the United States was caused by flies of the Calliphoridae family, which include Lucilia sericata (the green bottle blowfly) and Phormia regina (the black blowfly).

Wound myiasis most often is initiated when flies oviposit in necrotic, hemorrhaging, or pus-filled lesions. Wounds with alkaline discharges (pH 7.1–7.5) have been reported to be especially attractive to blow-flies. In humans, usually there is only one species implicated as the causative agent, although mixed infestation can occur.

Predisposing factors for human wound myiasis include open wounds, cutaneous malignancies, poor social conditions, poor hygiene, elderly, psychiatric illness, alcoholism, diabetes, vascular occlusive disease, leprosy, and other helpless patients, especially those with poor medical care, and inability to discourage flies from depositing eggs or larvae because of a physical handicap. Poor visual acuity may limit the detection of myiasis. Human natural disasters may be another predisposing factor for wound myiasis.

Some dermatological conditions have been described as a predisposing factor for myiasis-causing flies, such as psoriasis, seborrheic keratosis, onychomycosis, vascular insufficiency ulcer, lipedema, herpes zoster, noma, filarial lymphoedema, condyloma acuminatum, and hemorrhoid.

Treatment—The current treatment concept for myiasis comprises mechanical removal of maggots, surgical debridement of the infested wound bed, intensive rinsing with antiseptic solutions, and consistent dressing changes on a daily basis. Irrigation may be particularly useful in lesions with holes and cavities. Oral treatment is not a consensus in the treatment of human myiasis, and studies must be done to consolidate this modality of treatment. Ivermectin is the most commonly used drug in human infestation. Much of the experience came from the veterinary use of this drug.

Cavitary myiasis—this group of myiasis corresponds to the infestation of natural body cavities. The infestation usually receives the name of the anatomic region affected. Internal organs affected by dipteran larvae are also included in this group.

Ophthalmomyiasis—or oculomyiasis is the infestation of any anatomic structure of the eye that is further subclassified into ophthalmomyiasis externa (or superficial) and ophthalmomyiasis interna. Orbital myiasis or "ophtalmomyiase profonde" (French term meaning profound, deep) is used to bring together palpebral or periocular infestation with intraocular myiasis.

Ophthalmomyiasis externa refers to the superficial infestation of ocular tissue. Conjunctival myiasis is the most common form of ophthalmomyiasis, and it is a relatively mild, self-limited, and benign disease. Patients commonly complain of an acute foreign-body sensation with lacrimation, characteristically with an abrupt onset. *O. ovis* is the main causative agent of external ocular myiasis. The majority of the cases were described in the Mediterranean basin and the Middle East. Other agents implicated in this form of the disease are: *Rhinoestrus purpureus, D. hominis, C. bezziana, Lucilia* spp.*, and Cuterebra.* External manifestations are managed by the mechanical removal of larvae.

Opthalmomyiasis internal involves the anterior or posterior segment of the eyeball. This clinical picture may be a complication of ophthalmomyiasis externa. Anterior ophthalmomyiasis interna is less common and appears clinically as anterior uveitis. Posterior ophthalmomyiasis interna is characterized by pigmented and atrophic retinal pigment epithelium (RPE) tracts in a criss-crossing pattern seen in conjunction with hemorrhages, fibrovascular proliferation, exudative detachment of the retina, and even fibrovascular scarring. Red eye, vision loss, floaters, eye pain, and scotomas are the symptoms described in opthalmomyiasis interna. Ophthalmomyiasis interna should be considered in the differential diagnosis of retinal detachment, panuveitis, orbital cellulitis, chorioretinitis, and endopthtalmitis. The reindeer or caribou warble fly *Hypoderma* species are considered the commonest cause, with *Hypoderma tarandi being* the most frequent cause of in northern European countries such as Norway.

Orbital myiasis is a severe clinical picture characterized by intraocular invasion of maggots from eyelid myiasis, a peculiar kind of wound myiasis.

ENT myiasis—is a term used to group myiasis affecting the nose, ears, oral cavity, larynx, and tracheostomy.

Oral myiasis—It is a wound myiasis associated with infestation of the oral cavity. Species reported to cause this clinical picture are: *C. hominivorax, W. magnifica, M. domesticus, C. bezziana, O. ovis, H. bovis, H. tarandi, Musca nebulo.*

Aural Myiasis or Otomyiasis—involves the infestation of the external ear and/or middle ear. Although considered rare, auditory myiasis represented 86.16% of 94 cases of all ENT myiasis in one study [11]. It is usually seen in children younger than 10-y or in debilitated individuals. Chronic otorrhea has been implicated as a risk factor for aural myiasis in healthy, mobile patients. The clinical presentation of aural infestation is variable. Signs and symptoms include: foreign body sensation, otalgia, otorrhea, bleeding, itching, aural malodor, tinnitus, vertigo, restlessness, impaired hearing, and perforation of the tympanic membrane. The most important species causing aural myiasis are: *C. hominivorax, W. magnifica, C. bezziana, C. megacephala, Sarcophaga* [6].

Nasal myiasis—is the infestation of the nasal cavity either by direct ovipositing within the nasal cavity or in the vicinity while the patient is sleeping. In one study, this manifestation represented 70% to 75% of ENT myiasis [12]. In other study, nasal myiasis represented 11.7% of pediatric cases of ENT myiasis [11]. Cases more commonly occur in people who lost the sneezing reflex. Atrophic rhinitis is another important predisposing factor. Leprosy patients are more prone to this kind of infestation. Nasal myiasis signs and symptoms are usually related to the presence and movement of the larvae. The fatality rate may reach up to 8% of the cases [13]. The agents reported to cause nasal myiasis are: *C. hominivorax, C. bezziana, Oestrus ovis, W. magnifica, Lucilia sericata, Drosophila melanogaster, Calliphora erythrocephala.*

Throat myiasis—is mainly caused by *O. ovis,* affecting people in close contact with sheep and goats and should be considered an occupational disease in endemic countries such as Iran and Italy.

Urogenital myiasis—is the infestation of the genitourinary tract of males and females. Depending on the anatomical location, the condition could be sub-classified in external or internal urogenital myiasis.

External urogenital myiasis is, clinically, epidemiologically, and entomologically similar to furuncular myiasis or wound myiasis. Lack of underwear, urethral discharge or a sexually transmitted disease, uterine prolapse, cervix carcinoma, and the presence of a urethral stent are peculiar predisposing factors of the urogenital region.

Internal urogenital myiasis should be, in fact, considered accidental myiasis, since there is no documentation of any species that complete their life cycle within the urinary tract of humans. Dysuria, lumbar pain, ureteric obstruction, microhematuria, albuminuria, and leucocyturia are signs and symptoms related to this kind of infestation, with relief after expelling or removing the maggots. Uncommon myiasis agents are associated with this type of accidental myiasis, for example: *Megaselia scalaris, Psychoda albipennis, Eristalis tenax, Piophila casei, Fannia scalaris, Fannia canicularis, Muscina stabulans.*

Intestinal myiasis—true enteric myiasis does not occur in humans and all cases are classified as pseudomyiasis or accidental myiasis. Intestinal myiasis, in humans, is probably related to ingestion of food or water contaminated with dipteran fly larvae. Water supply is a possible contamination source. The female flies may oviposit the eggs around the mouth; comatose and psychiatric patients, and patients that sleep or keep the mouth open are particularly prone to this infestation.

Clinical presentation is variable and depends on the number of maggots, the species of the parasite, and also their location within the digestive tract. Including asymptomatic cases, abdominal pain, nausea and vomiting, anal pruritus, or rectal bleeding are possible symptoms. Some patients just notice the presence of the larvae in stool or vomitus. The presence of numerous larvae in one or more consecutive stool specimens is diagnostic. Ideally, the sample should be collected in the laboratory so that posterior infestation of the stool can be ruled out. Maggot identification from specimens collect through sigmoidoscopy is more reliable if external contamination is suspected [14]. Myiasis agents associated with this type of accidental myiasis are: *Fannia canicularis, Sarcophaga* spp., *Hermetia illucens, Muscina stabulans, Megaselia scalaris, Eristalis tenax, Musca domestica, Phormia regina, Lucilia cuprina, Stomoxys calcitrans.*

Accidental myiasis or pseudomyiasis—is the presence of any symptom due to the presence of a non-parasitizing dipteran maggot. Pseudomyiasis is mostly a benign event, but the larvae could possibly survive temporarily, causing symptoms. It generally occurs from ingesting fly eggs or larvae on uncooked foods or previously cooked food that have been subsequently infested. Cured meats, dried fruits, cheese, and smoked fish are the most commonly infested foods and the most common sources of accidental myiasis [15]. Accidental myiasis may also occur when the larvae enter the urinary passage.

Nosocomial myiasis—is a term used when the infestation affects subjects in hospital settings. Although this form of infestation is considered rare in rich countries, it may be underreported in developing and poor countries. When considering nosocomial myiasis, the identification of the myiasis-causing species is crucial to recognize the dipteran habits and schedule the pest eradication program. Nosocomial myiasis may complicate other infestations; two cases of nasal myiasis in ICU unity was reported in association with mouse infestation (mouse carcass could have attracted the flies). Comatose and handicapped patients are particularly prone to myiasis with reported cases of nasal myiasis, orothracheal myiasis, myiasis of nasogastric tube. Nets for windows and other ventilation ducts is a simple measure that could help preventing nosocomial myiasis.

Larva Preservation

After removing the larvae from the host, the larvae should be killed in hot water or ethanol to retain their overall shape. The posterior respiratory spiracles are an important means of identification. Larvae should be preserved in 80% alcohol. Identification of accidental or facultative parasites is often difficult, as many species may be involved. In contrast, identification of an obligate parasite is easier. It is even easier to identify the species, or at least the genera, if the larva can develop until the fly stage.

Prevention

Prevention and good sanitation can avert much of the accidental and facultative myiasis. Good sanitation is essential and includes emptying and steam-cleaning dumpsters on a regular schedule. Food should be washed and visually inspected before consumption. Exposed food should not be unattended and should be readily covered to prevent flies from ovipositing. Wounds must be cleaned regularly and dressed, especially on the elderly and helpless. In endemic regions, sleeping nude, sitting outdoors, and on the floor should be avoided. Appropriate precautions will help avoid infestations. The use of screens and mosquito nets is essential to prevent flies from reaching the skin. *D. hominis* infestation may be thwarted by the application of insect repellents containing diethyltoluamide (DEET). Drying clothes in bright sunlight and ironing them is an effective method of destroying occult eggs laid in clothing, especially by the *C. anthropophaga* [16]. Other general precautions include wearing long-sleeved clothing, covering wounds, and avoiding falling asleep outdoors.

A field control of flies is extremely important. All available methods should be used, including aerial sprays, destruction of animal carcasses, elementary sanitary and hygiene practices, and clearing debris and rubbish near houses. Inactivation of females by the release of large numbers of males previously sterilized by ionizing radiation has been highly successful. Reports on the control of *Cochliomyia* infestation in sheep with the use of ivermectin, which has been reported to be 100% effective in controlling existing infestations and as a prophylaxis, suggest that this may be the route of the future.

References

1. Noutsis C, Millikan LE. Myiasis. Dermatol Clin. 1994;12(4):729–36.
2. Zumpt F. Myiasis in man and animals in the old world. London: Butterworths; 1965. p. 267.
3. Caumes E, Carriere J, Guermonprez G, Bricaire F, Danis M, Gentilini M. Dermatoses associated with travel to tropical countries – a prospective study of the diagnosis and management of 269 patients presenting to a tropical disease unit. Clin Infect Dis. 1995;20(3):542–8.
4. Patton WS. Notes on Myiasis producing Diptera of man and animals. Bull Entomol Res. 1922;12:239–61.
5. James MT. The flies that cause myiasis in man. US Depart Agric. 1947;631:1–175.
6. Francesconi F, Lupi O. Myiasis. Clin Microbiol Rev. 2012;25(1):79–105.
7. Guse ST, Tieszen ME. Cutaneous myiasis from Dermatobia hominis. Wilderness Environ Med. 1997;8(3):156–60.
8. Gunther S. Clinical and epidemiological aspects of dermal Tumbu-Fly myiasis in equatorial Africa. Br J Dermatol. 1971;85(3):226–31.
9. Brewer TF, Felsenstein D, Wilson ME. Furuncular myiasis – alternatives to bacon therapy. JAMA J Am Med Assoc. 1994;271(12):901–2.
10. Loong PTL, Lui H, Buck HW. Cutaneous myiasis: a simple and effective technique for extraction of Dermatobia hominis larvae. Int J Dermatol. 1992;31(9):657–9.
11. Singh I, Gathwala G, Yadav SP, Wig U, Jakhar KK. Myiasis in children: the Indian perspective. Int J Pediatr Otorhinolaryngol. 1993;25(1–3):127–31.
12. Arora S, Sharma JK, Pippal SK, Sethi Y, Yadav A. Clinical etiology of myiasis in ENT: a reterograde period – interval study. Braz J Otorhinolaryngol. 2009;75(3):356–61.
13. Sharma H, Dayal D, Agrawal SP. Nasal myiasis: review of 10 years experience. J Laryngol Otol. 1989;103(5):489–91.
14. Sehgal R, Bhatti HPS, Bhasin DK, Sood AK, Nada R, Malla N, et al. Intestinal myiasis due to Musca domestica: a report of two cases. Jpn J Infect Dis. 2002;55(6):191–3.
15. Goddard J. Myiasis (invasion of human tissue by fly larvae). In: Goddard J, editor. Physician's guide to arthropods of medical importance. 4th ed. CRC Press; 2003. p. 61–5.
16. Blacklock B, Thompson MG. A study of the tumbu-fly Cordylobia anthropophaga Gru̇nberg in Sierra Leone. Trop Med Parasitol. 1923;17:443–502.

Human Gnathostomiasis

Marina Romero-Navarrete,
Aureliano Delfino Castillo-Solana,
Roberto Arenas, and M. Elisa Vega-Memije

Key Points

- Parasitic, emergent, neglected zoonosis, transmitted by raw or undercooked food of freshwater fish, eels, snakes, and parasitized birds with advanced third-stage larvae (LA3) of nematodes of the genus *Gnathostoma* sp.
- Of interest to general practitioners, dermatologists, ophthalmologists, neurologists, dentists, otolaryngologists, urologists, internists.
- Thirteen species of *Gnathostoma* sp., six in Asia, seven in the Americas), six related to diseases in humans (*G. spinigerum*, *G. hispidium*, *G. binucleatum*, *G. malaysae*, *G. doloresi*, and *G. nipponicum* have been described).
- The life cycle of *Gnathostoma* sp. requires three guests: (1) a freshwater copepod that ingests eggs that adults throw; (2) a wide range of fish and other intermediate aquatic hosts for larval maturation; and (3) definitive vertebrate hosts for adult development; with the possibility of a paratenic host. The human being is an accidental host, is not compatible with the reproductive life cycle of the nematode.
- Clinical presentations on skin, eyes, visceral organs, nervous system, lung, heart, and tongue have been reported.
- The confirmatory diagnosis is the observation of the larva or by serology by ELISA and Western blot.
- There is no international guide, nor consensus for its management, albendazole 400 mg is used twice daily for 21 days, or ivermectin, 0.2 mg/kg single dose, can be repeated at 7 days, therapeutic efficacy is greater than 90%; Albendazole stimulates larval migration and can make it more accessible for biopsy and subsequent identification.
- In a migrant or traveler returning from an endemic area, or in patients from non-endemic areas with a history of raw or undercooked meat intake of freshwater fish (ceviche, sushi, sashimi), poultry, pork, which present with cutaneous lesions with intermittent and pruritic migration, edema, and peripheral eosinophilia Gnathostomiasis should be suspected.

M. Romero-Navarrete (✉) · A. D. Castillo-Solana
General Hospital of Acapulco,
Colonia Mangos, Guerrero, Mexico

R. Arenas · M. E. Vega-Memije
Dr. Manuel Gea Gonzalez, General Hospital,
México City, Mexico

W. Robles (ed.), *Skin Disease in Travelers*, Updates in Clinical Dermatology,
https://doi.org/10.1007/978-3-031-57836-6_25

Synonymy

Gnathostomosis, Migratory larva syndrome, eosinophilic migratory nodular panniculitis), deep larva-migrans, tuao chid in Japan, Yangtze River edema, and Shanghai rheumatism in China.

Definition

It is an emerging parasitic zoonosis, transmitted by raw or undercooked food of freshwater fish, eels, snakes, and parasitized birds with larvae of the third advanced stage (L3A) of nematodes of the genus *Gnathostoma* sp. It can affect the skin, eyes, visceral, central nervous system, lungs, heart, and tongue.

Etiology

Thirteen species of *Gnathostoma* sp. have been described. Six in Asia and seven in the Americas. Six related to human diseases (*G. spinigerum, G. hispidium, G. malaysae G. doloresi*, and *G. nipponicum* in Asia, and *G. binucleatum* in Latin America).

Biological Cycle

The genus *Gnathostoma* belongs to the Spirurida order, in its passing through the stages of egg life cycle, larva (L1, L2, L3, L4) and adult requires two intermediate hosts (copepods, freshwater fish: snakehead from north (*channa argus*) of China, Russia and Korea, loaches, creole mojarra, guabina, tilapia, trout, bass, eels Asian swamp, and a definitive host (dogs, cats, pigs, wild boars, wild cats, weasels, opossums, raccoons, opossums, otters), with possibility of a paratenic host (snakes, poultry, and wild rats) that feed on fish.

In the definitive hosts adult nematodes, male and female, are in cavitated forms in the stomach or esophagus and their eggs, fertilized, and they are expelled with the stool. When they are eliminated in bodies of freshwater like dams, rivers, lakes, and lagoons, embryogenesis starts, developing the first-stage larvae (L1) that in the food chain are ingested by the first intermediate host, water flea or copepods of the genera *Cyclops, Eucyclops, Mesocyclops, Acantocyclops,* and *Tropocyclops* in which second-stage larvae (L2) develop, these are ingested by a second intermediate host (fish, eels, birds, and reptiles), the larvae are released in their intestine, becoming third stage (L3) larvae, these migrate through their tissues reaching the muscles where they become encysted and develop as L3A larvae, in the definitive hosts, the larvae are released in their gastrointestinal tract, migrate to the liver and abdominal cavity, then return to the stomach where they invade the gastric wall or esophagus, becoming adult worms 13 to 55 mm in length, release eggs that are eliminated with the stool to the environment and the cycle is restarted.

The human being is an accidental host when consuming raw or undercooked food of freshwater fish eels, snakes, and parasitized birds with third-stage larvae, the individual is infected and develops the disease.

Two alternative routes of infection have been suggested: the ingestion of water containing infected copepods (thus replacing a second intermediate host) or by the penetration of the skin of the larvae food handlers of the third stage of infected meat.

It is noteworthy that the larvae resist lemon juice, soy sauce, vinegar, and brine (Fig. 1).

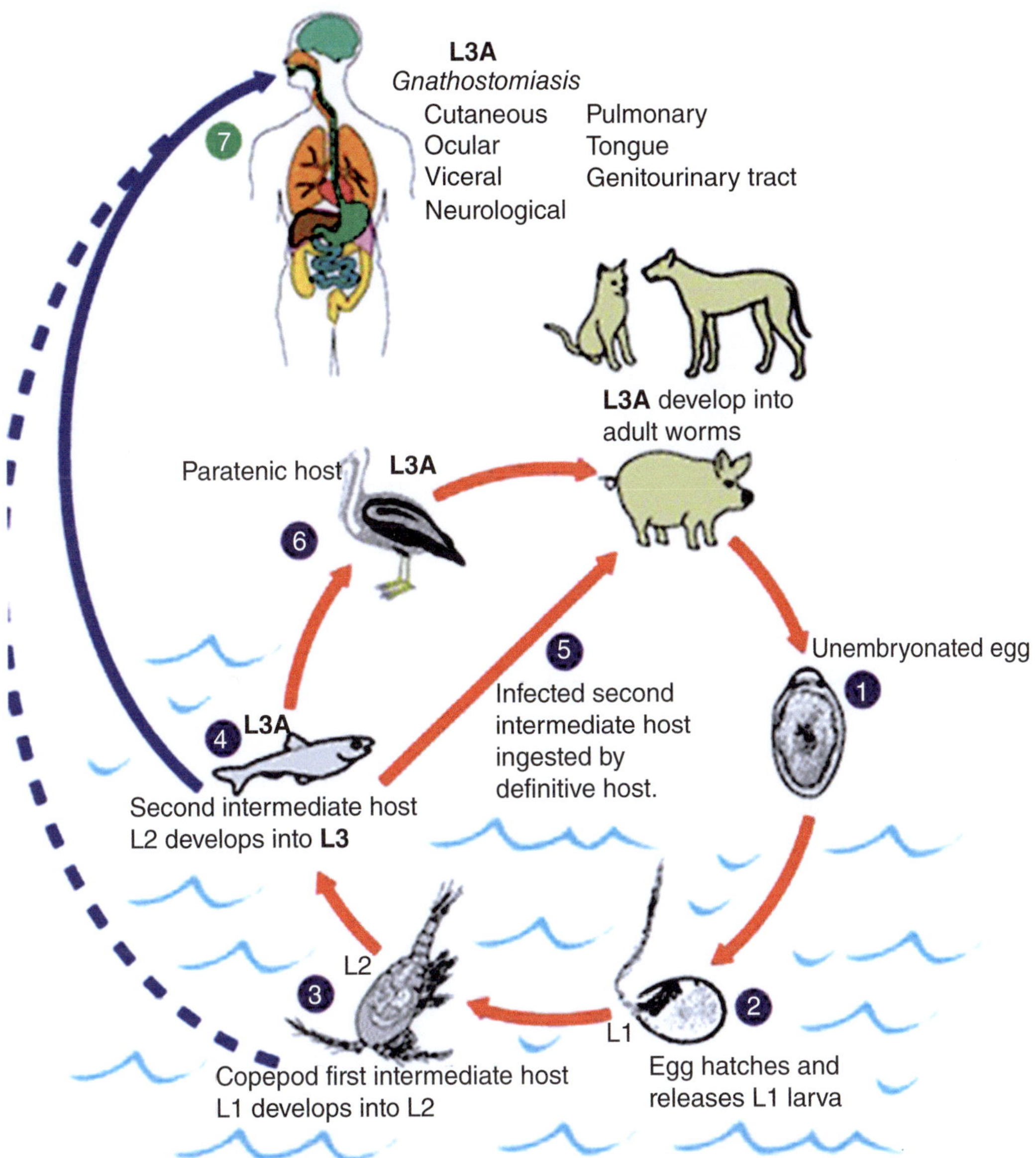

Fig. 1 Life cycle of *Gnathostoma* sp.

Epidemiology

It is a circumstantial parasitosis in humans, not considered by the World Health Organization, foodborne, it is not mandatory notification in the health sector, its incidence is unknown and its prevalence is worldwide. Should be considered within neglected, fish-borne nematodiasis.

The knowledge of this disease is by case reports, endemic in Asia: Bangladesh, Korea, China, India, Japan, Thailand, Cambodia, Laos, Myanmar, Indonesia, Israel, Malaysia, Philippines, Sri Lanka, Vietnam. In North America; in Mexico, and the United States. In Central America Guatemala, in South America Brazil, Ecuador, Peru, and Venezuela. In Oceania

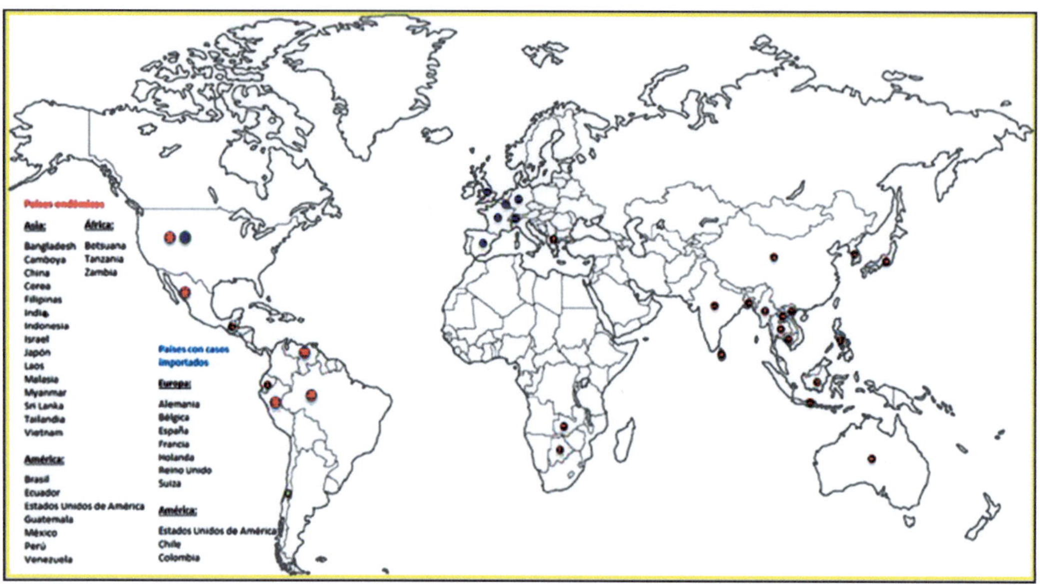

Fig. 2 Endemic countries and imported cases 2020

in New Zealand and southern Africa in Botswana, Tanzania, and Zambia (Fig. 2).

As of 2019, 63 imported cases have been reported, 92% (58 cases) in Europe: France 26, United Kingdom 19, Germany 6, Spain 6, Belgium, Switzerland, South Holland; United States, Chile, and Colombia: 1 in each country. The majority corresponds to immigrants rather than tourists, who traveled to endemic countries with a history of eating raw or undercooked fish, eels, snakes, being considered an emerging disease (Fig. 2).

Most affect the skin, then the central nervous system and brain with 248, most in Thailand with 241 cases, Laos and South Korea with 2 each, Myanmar and Japan 1 case per country. Of the ocular variety, 84 cases have been documented up to 2019, 83% (70 cases) in Asia distributed in Japan 18, India 17, Thailand 16, Bangladesh 5, Malaysia and Myanmar 3 each, China and Cambodia with 2 in each country and with a case in Korea, Israel, the Philippines, and Vietnam. In Mexico 11, Brazil, Ecuador, Venezuela with 1.

The increase in international tourism to endemic countries and an increase in immigrants from Asia and Latin America to the United States have favored exotic ethnic cuisine, especially raw seafood prepared with freshwater species such as trout, tilapia, and eels.

The importation of swamp eels from Asia to the United States resulted in the contamination of local species, in 2014 *Gnathostoma* larvae were detected in 30% of Asian swamp eels of *Monopterus* sp. and in 4.5% of the swamp eels captured in three states, favoring the risk in the increase of native cases.

From 2008 to 2009 in Laos, an endemic country, a seroprevalence study was carried out in 3 provinces, with a total of 29.8% and in the 3 regions of 3.6%, 38.6%, and 47.1%. The seropositivity increased with the age of the participants.

The lethality rate due to cerebral gnathostomiasis reported since 1967 ranges from 7.7% to 25%, identifying *G. spinigerum*.

Pathogeny

Ingested third-stage larvae (L3A) are released into the stomach, pierce the gastric wall, reach the liver, hence migrate to different organs.

The pathogenesis is not well defined, it has been attributed to the combination of several factors, an explosive action in which, *Gnathostoma* feeds on blood cells and hemoglobin, the destruction of tissues due to the penetration and migration of the larva, armed with hooks and cuticle spines, the secretion of substances such as hyaluronidase, proteolytic enzymes, hemolysins, and an enzyme similar to acetylcholine.

During migration through host tissues, *Gnathostoma* induces a Th2-type humoral and cellular immune response, with interleukin release (IL-3, IL-4, IL-5, IL-6, IL-10, IL-13), as well as the stimulator factor of granulocytic and monocytic colonies (GM-CSF), with the production of IgE by plasma cells, generating eosinophil production.

Clinical Manifestations

In the first 24–48 h, there are usually nonspecific signs and symptoms characterized by nausea, vomiting, diarrhea, malaise, hives, pain in the epigastrium and right hypochondrium for 2 to 3 weeks, it is often misdiagnosed as food poisoning, acute appendicitis or adenitis mesenteric. These symptoms are considered to correspond to the penetration of the larva into the intestine and its migration through the portal vein into the liver.

Then there is a latency period from 3 weeks to 5 years with an average of 1 year, then it is expressed in different clinical forms: (1) skin disease, (2) visceral (liver) or gastrointestinal disease (eosinophilic gastritis), (3) neurognathostomiasis (cerebral gnathostomiasis), (4) ocular gnathostomiasis, and less frequently presentations in muscle, lung, and tongue.

Cutaneous Gnathostomiasis

It is the most frequent form, usually, they appear 1 to 12 weeks or months after the ingestion of raw or undercooked meat infected with advanced third-stage larvae (L3A), it is manifested by intermittent migratory erythema, erythematous plaques, edematous with a "serpiginous" border slightly raised and indurated, in trunk, head, or upper limbs, accompanied by pain, pruritus, with intermittent migratory subcutaneous inflammation (Fig. 3).

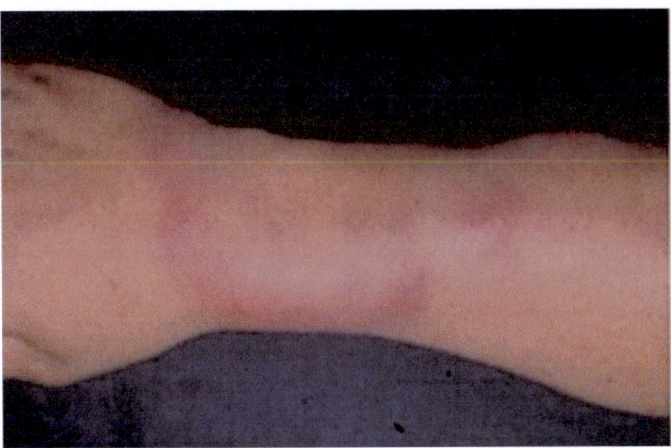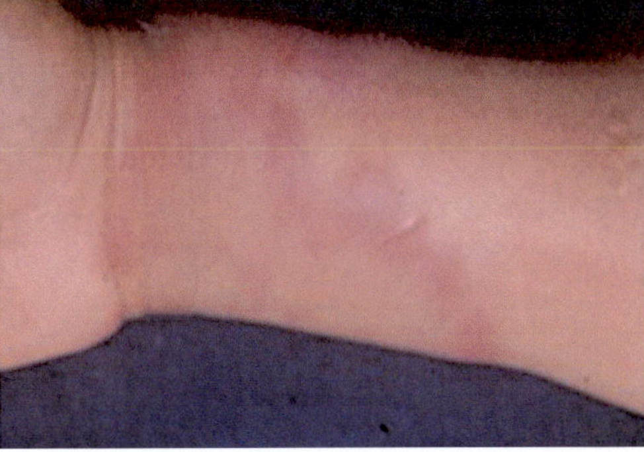

Fig. 3 Plaque with erythema and edema, circular or irregular, serpiginous in internal and external face, in distal forearm

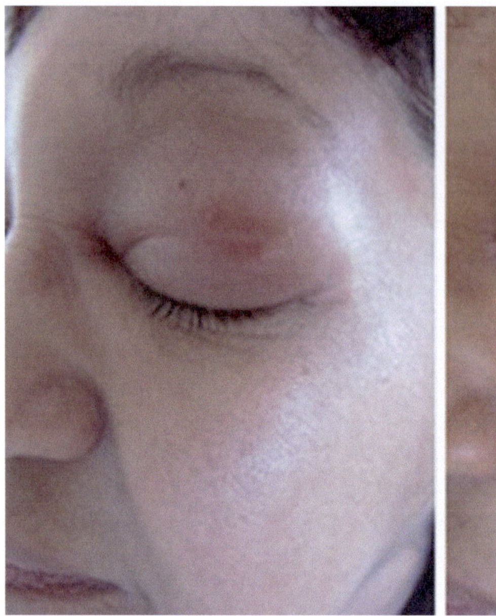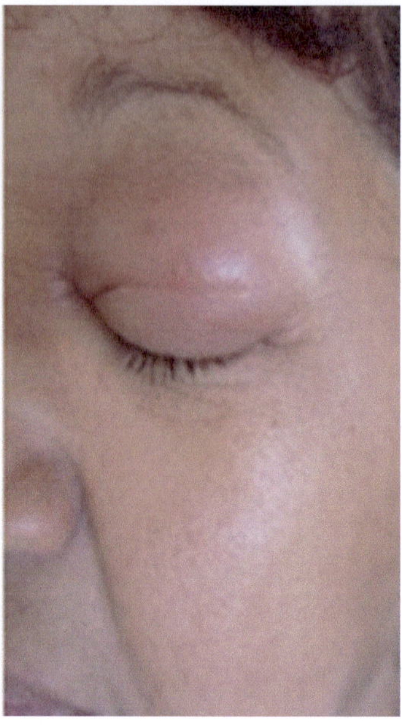

Fig. 4 Edema and erythema of upper left eyelid

Cerebral Gnathostomiasis

Also known as neurognathostomiasis, the main clinical syndromes that occur are radioculomyelitis, radioculomyeloencephalitis, meningitis, meningoencephalitis, subarachnoid, and intracerebral hemorrhage.

In children in Thailand, it has been reported that 15 to 20% of intracranial hemorrhages are caused by this parasite. The damage to the central nervous system is mainly due to a direct mechanical injury: tearing and/or destruction of the nervous tissue and its vascular structures. Migration to the central nervous system has been documented in the first 6 h and up to a month later.

Ocular Gnathostomiasis

Eighty-four cases have been reported in the international literature, the mechanism by which larvae enter this site is unknown, it manifests clinically with severe pain in the eyeball, progressive decrease in visual acuity in up to 40% of cases. The parasite has been located in the vitreous fibers, can cause uveitis, iritis, intraocular hemorrhage, orbital cellulitis, glaucoma, and even scarring and retinal detachment, due to a less frequent invasion of the vitreous. Eye involvement is rarely associated with peripheral eosinophilia (Fig. 4).

Visceral Gnathostomiasis

It can manifest with fever, nausea, vomiting, pain in the epigastrium and right hypochondrium, physical examination may have hepatomegaly and simulate an acute abdomen compatible with appendicitis, acute cholecystitis, or intestinal perforation.

Pulmonary Gnathostomiasis

Migration from larvae to lung can manifest with cough, chest pain, pleural effusions, hemoptysis, pneumothorax, hydropneumothorax, consolidation or pulmonary collapse, and peripheral hypereosinophilia (20%–72%). In some cases, larval expectoration has led to the resolution of symptoms. The triad: eosinophilia, subcutaneous edema, and unexplained eosinophilic pleural effusion with a history of exposure risk should be ruled out gnathostomiasis.

Cases have been reported with the involvement of the genitourinary tract in Thailand, Indonesia, Laos and the back of the tongue in Mexico.

Diagnosis

Until a few years ago the definitive diagnosis was established through the identification and subsequent classification of larvae recovered from lesions by surgical excision, biopsy, or necropsy, which is not frequent in any of the clinical varieties.

In recent years, serological enzyme-linked immunosorbent assays (ELISA) tests have been developed that measure specific antibodies against *Gnathostoma* sp., with acceptable sensitivity values of 59–87% and specificity of 79–96%.

In 2016, a lateral flow immunochromatographic test (ICT) was developed in Taiwan, using a recombinant protein (rGslic18) as an antigen, with a sensitivity of 93.75% and a specificity of 97.01%.

In 2017, a rapid test (DIGFA—dot immune-gold filtration assay) was applied in China using L3A larval antigen, partially purified from *G. spinigerum*, with a sensitivity of 96.7%, a specificity of 100%, and cross-reactivity of 1.6%. This technique can be done in 5 min, it costs $1, its reagents have good stability at 1 year or more, but more types and number of sera are needed to determine its usefulness.

There is another test proposed for the confirmation of the diagnosis and consists of an immunoblot analysis (Western blot) for the detection of IgG antibodies directed against a specific antigenic fraction of 24 kDa, of the L3 larvae of *G. spinigerum*, with specificity of 98.8% at 100% and sensitivity from 83.1% to 100%. This procedure has been considered the gold standard in Asia and Europe and is available in reference laboratories in Thailand, Japan, and Switzerland.

In a 2020 study, the polymerase chain reaction (PCR) was used in Mexico to amplify the ITS (internal transcribed spacer, ITS2) region of the ribosomal RNA, in 2 cases of human gnathosto-

miasis. The L3A extensions of both patients were 321 base pairs. The length and sequence of these fragments were identical to the fragments deposited in GenBank as *G. binucleatum* (accession number JF919679). Therefore, these molecular data confirmed that the etiologic agent of gnathostomiasis was *G. binucleatum*.

Histopathology

In the histological study, irregular epidermis is observed, in the middle and superficial dermis, there is the presence of parasitic structures, surrounded by an inflammatory infiltrate, predominantly of eosinophils, an approximation of the transverse section, inflammatory infiltrate mainly of surrounding eosinophilic is observed (Figs. 5 and 6). Also, the parasitic structure arranged in a channel limited by eosinophils, which have "flame figures" (Fig. 7). In deep dermis and subcutaneous cellular tissue vasodilation and a mixed inflammatory infiltrate, composed of lymphocytes and numerous eosinophils can be observed (Fig. 8). In Mexico, it has been found in 34% and in 66% an eosinophilic panniculitis.

The observation of larvae provides a definitive diagnosis, however, the positivity is low, this can be explained by their small size, their migration

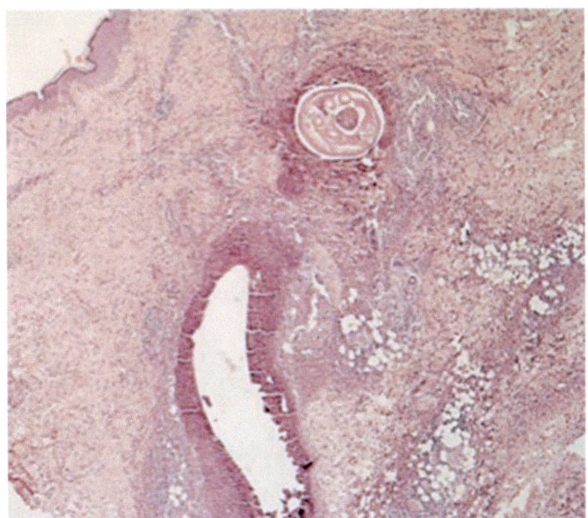

Fig. 5 Irregular epidermis is observed. In the superficial and middle dermis, presence of a parasitic structure surrounded by inflammatory infiltrate, predominantly eosinophils. HE 20×

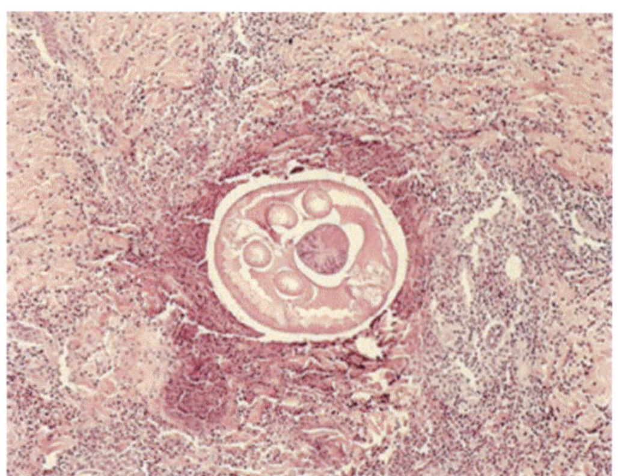

Fig. 6 Structure approach parasitic in a cross section, with an inflammatory infiltrate, mainly eosinophilic surrounding. HE 40×

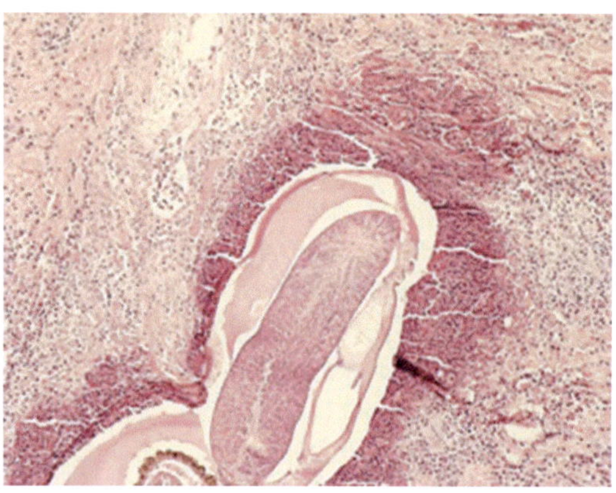

Fig. 7 Detail of the parasitic structure, arranged in a channel limited by eosinophils that form "flaming figures". HE 40×

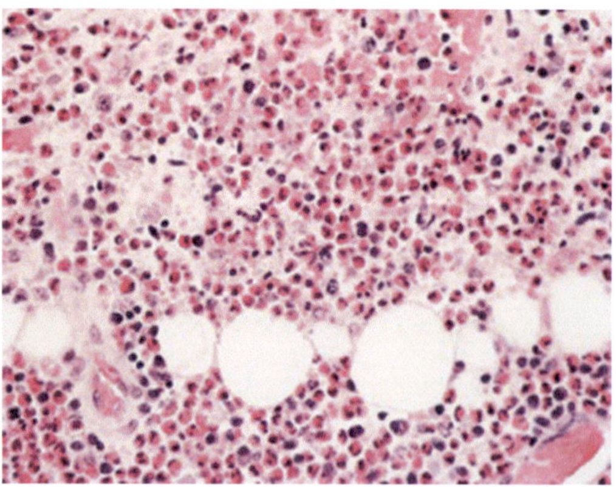

Fig. 8 In deep dermis and subcutaneous tissue, it is observed vasodilation and mixed inflammatory infiltrate, composed of lymphocytes and numerous eosinophils. HE 60×

speed (1 cm/h), the depth of tissue migration and the propagation of the lesions that can reach several centimeters.

Dermoscopy

In 2015, a case of mixed gnathostomiasis with dermatoscopic visualization was reported in Ecuador in 2015, showing an elongated, curved, 1.5 mm brown structure with two ends, one of which was sharp and well defined and another tubular, colored brownish that corresponded to the pigmented intestine of the parasite. Dermatoscopy allows a non-invasive approach to the parasite and facilitates its extraction, especially when it occurs in the form of pseudofurunculosis.

Differential Diagnosis

Mainly with other parasites that cause cutaneous larval migrans syndrome such as trichinosis, myiasis, angioedema, strongyloidiasis, abscesses, sparganosis, cutaneous paragonimiasis, with parasitosis that affect the central nervous system: cysticercosis, toxocariasis, schistosomiasis, baylisascariasis or paragonimiasis, or presentations of ophthalmia uveitis.

Treatment

For many years, there was no effective treatment, only surgical excision, which is not always indicated by the difficulty of knowing the exact location of the larva. Currently, there is no international guide, nor consensus for its management, as of 1992, albendazole 400 mg is used twice a day for 21 days, thus, 7–14 days after initiation of treatment stimulates larval migration, being more accessible for surgical removal or biopsy, its mechanism of action is an inhibitory effect of tubulin polymerization, with loss of cytoplasmic microtubules, affecting glucose absorption, decreasing the body's glycogen stores and immobilization, and as a result death of the parasite. Its side effects may be nausea, dizziness, headache and, occasionally, abnormal liver function tests, and transient leukopenia. In most Latin American countries, ivermectin is used, 0.2 mg/kg as a single dose, it can be repeated after 7 days. In the author's experience, twice the dose can be used to improve effectiveness. It selectively binds to the chloride ion channels activated by glutamate, which occur in the nerve and muscle cells of invertebrates, increasing the permeability of the cell membrane to chloride ions with hyperpolarization of the nerve or muscle cell, generating paralysis and death of the parasite. The therapeutic efficacy is greater than 90% for both. In relapses, both medications can be used individually or simultaneously.

There have been no randomized trials of anthelmintic therapy in neurognathostomiasis, there are reports of management with albendazole, corticosteroids must first be used for cerebral edema that is generated as an inflammatory response due to the presence of larvae, (prednisolone, 60 mg/day) for 7 days).

Prevention

The preventive actions that are being carried out in high-risk regions (Japan and Thailand) are: (a) freezing cooling, by any means, for long periods; (b) cooking, at the boiling point, for more than 15 min; (c) use of latex gloves, who for a long time handle raw fish meat (in fishmongers or at home) because they are vulnerable to larval skin penetration, (d) avoid (not only in endemic areas) the consumption of meat raw or undercooked (in ceviche, marinade, or brine) of any vertebrate (not only freshwater, estuarine, or marine fish), because lemon, vinegar does not kill the larvae present in the musculature of their hosts.

Bibliography

1. Díaz CSP, Parra UJR, Ríos SJ, Delgado VF. Molecular identification of the etiological agent of human gnathostomiasis in an endemic area of Mexico. Jpn J Infect Dis. 2020;73(1):44–50.

2. Sapp SGH, Kaminski M, Abdallah M, Bishop HS, Fox M, Ndubuisi M, Bradbury RS. Percutaneous emergence of *Gnathostoma spinigerum* following praziquantel treatment. Trop Med Infect Dis. 2019;4(4):145.

3. Ma A, Wang Y, Liu XL, Zhang HM, Eamsobhana P, Yong HS, Gan XX. A filtration-based rapid test using a partially purified third-stage larval antigen to detect specific antibodies for the diagnosis of gnathostomiasis. J Helminthol. 2019;93(1):26–32.

4. Sen P, Dutta MP, Biswas J, Rao C, Das K. Role of ultra-wide-field imaging in the diagnosis of intravitreal gnathostomiasis: a case-report. Ocular Immunol Inflamm. 2019;27(3):380–2.

5. Arenas R. Dermatología Atlas, diagnóstico y tratamiento. 7th ed. México: McGraw-Hill; 2019. p. 481–2.

6. Korekawa A, Nakajima K, Makita E, Aizu T, Hara K, Maruyama H, Morishima Y, Nakano H, Sawamura D. Two cases of cutaneous gnathostomiasis after eating raw *Salangichthys* microdon (icefish, *shirauo*). J Dermatol. 2019;46(9):791–3.

7. Bravo F, Gontijo B. Gnathostomiasis: an emerging infectious disease relevant to all dermatologists. An Bras Dermatol. 2018;93(2):172–80.

8. Benavides MA, Baldo MB, Tauber S, Figueiras SF, Incani RN, Nawa Y. Case report: ocular gnathostomiasis in Venezuela most likely acquired in Texas. Am J Trop Med Hyg. 2018;99(4):1028–32.

9. Hamilton WL, Agranoff D. Imported gnathostomiasis manifesting as cutaneous larva migrans and Löffer's Sindrome. BMJ Case Rep. 2018; https://doi.org/10.1136/bcr-2017-223132.

10. Roach REJ, van Doorn R, Arend SM, Visser LG. A recurrent migratory swelling. Lancet Infect Dis. 2018;18(9):1045.

11. Grau PM, Vilar AJ, de la Rosa-del Rey MDP, Hernández FM, AJL P. Migratory, recurrent skin eruption in a returning traveller. Australas J Dermatol. 2018;59(4):e307–8.

12. Nawa Y, Yoshikawa M, Sawanyawisuth K, Chotmongkol V, Fernández FS, Maria Benavides M, Díaz CSP. Ocular gnathostomiasis—update of earlier survey. Am J Trop Med Hyg. 2017;97(4):1232–4.

13. Leroy J, Cornu M, Deleplancque AS, Loridant S, Dutoit E, Sendib B. Sushi ceviche and gnathostomiasis. A Case report and review of imported infections. Travel Med Infect Dis. 2017;20:26–30.

14. Janwan P, Intapan PM, Yamasaki H, Rodpai R, Laummaunwai P, Thanchomnang T, et al. Development and usefulness of an immunochromatographic device to detect antibodies for rapid diagnosis of human gnathostomiasis. Parasit Vectors. 2016;9:14.

15. Martínez LE, Caballero HSE, Toussaint CS, Vega MME, Martínez OJA. Quiz/Serpentine shoulder path. Dermatología Cosmética, Médica y Quirúrgica. 2016;14(4):356–8.

16. Diaz JH. Gnathostomiasis: an emerging infection of raw fish consumers in gnathostoma nematode-endemic and nonendemic countries. J Travel Med. 2015;22:318–24.

17. Úraga PE, Garcés S, Üraga MV, Reyes A, Garcés JC. Dermoscopic features of cutaneous gnathostomiasis. Int J Dermatol. 2015;54:985–8.
18. Jurado LF, Palacios DM, López R, Baldión M, Matijasevic E. Cutaneous gnathostomiasis, first confirmed case in Colombia. Biomedica. 2015;35(4):462–70.
19. World Health Organization. Who estimates of the global burden of foodborne diseases foodborne burden epidemiology reference group 2007–2015.
20. Álvarez GC, Castañeda MA, Benítez VC, Castañeda MJE, Becerro VEM. A case report of lingual gnathostomiasis. Oral. 2014;15(47):1086–8.
21. Vargas TJ, Kahler S, Dib C, Barroso CM, Jeunon SMA. Autochthonous gnathostomiasis, Brazil. Emerg Infect Dis. 2012;18(12):2087–9.
22. Katchanov J, Sawanyawisuth K, Chotmongkoi V, Nawa Y. Neurognathostomiasis, a Neglected Parasitosis of the Central Nervous System. Emerg Infect Dis. 2011;17(7):1174–80.
23. Jarell AD, Dans MJ, Elston DM, Mathison BA, Ruben BS. Gnathostomiasis in a patient who frequently consumes sushi. Am J Dermatopathol. 2011;33(8):e91–3.
24. Nawa Y, Katchanov J, Yoshikawa M, Rojekittikhun B, Dekumyoy P, Kusolusuk T, Wattanakulpanich D. Ocular gnathostomiasis: a comprehensive review. J Trop Med Parasitol. 2010;33:77–86.

Scabies in Travellers

Vijay Zawar and Madhur Kelkar

Key Points
- Travelling has become extremely common in recent times due to a variety of reasons.
- Skin infections and infestations are one of the most frequent diseases acquired in travellers.
- Scabies is an ectopasitic infestation due to a mite, *Sarcopties scabiei var hominis,* affecting humans all over the world.
- Longer travel periods, especially to low income countries often predisposes to scabies.
- Extremely pruritic erythematous papules and vesicles are the most common presentation.
- Returning travellers complaining of pruritus should be carefully investigated for possible scabies and treated early to prevent outbreak in the community.

military service and medical tourism are different reasons for travelling.

Skin infections are common in the returning traveller from tropical or subtropical countries.

Skin complaints are the third most common reason for consultation and request for treatment among returning travellers. This accounts for approximately 10% of all patients. A few of these may have serious infections leading to hospitalization and in-patient management [1–4].

Scabies is the most common ectoparasitic transmissible disease. It has long been associated with humans as this variant infects humans only. It is a global disease and over 200 million people are affected worldwide. It is one of the top 10 dermatological diseases observed in the returned travellers [5–9].

Introduction

Travelling has greatly increased in the last few decades. Immigration, tourism, business, missionary and volunteer work, research work, visiting friends or relatives, and also for the education,

Epidemiology

Scabies has worldwide distribution and affects all races, ages, genders and socioeconomic groups. It is found more predominantly in places of overcrowding, with lack of public awareness and delayed treatment. There is definite variation in the prevalence of scabies with rates in low income countries ranging from 4%–100% [6, 9]. Incidences are high in overcrowding related to natural disasters, war, economic depression and refugee camps [7]. Scabies is most commonly transmitted by close personal contact or by com-

V. Zawar (✉)
Consultant Dermatologist, Skin Diseases Centre, Nashik, India

M. Kelkar
Consultant Dermatologist, Sanjivan Hospital, Nashik, India

W. Robles (ed.), *Skin Disease in Travelers*, Updates in Clinical Dermatology,
https://doi.org/10.1007/978-3-031-57836-6_26

ing in contact with objects used by the infected individual. Transmission via sexual contact is also known.

Predisposition

Children, close contacts at home or work place and sexually active individuals are commonly affected.

Crusted scabies, previously known as Norwegian scabies is more prevalent in immunocompromised individuals such as the elderly, people infected with Human immunodeficiency virus (HIV) or human T-cell lymphotropic virus type 1(HTLV-1), solid organ transplant recipients. It can also be seen in patients with decreased sensory functions or ability to scratch, e.g. patients with leprosy or paraplegic individuals where despite a large number of infested mites, the pruritus is minimal.

For patients who have just returned from travel, we have to consider the following points.

Duration of the Travel

Scabies is more prevalent in patients who have travelled for longer periods of time, weeks, instead of days [10, 11].

Reason for Travel

People who travel for fun and luxury are less exposed and affected than the people who are backpackers and travel for adventure, sports, camping.

Trips for missionary and voluntary work may show higher number of people affected [10, 11].

Location of the Travel

In general, travelling to the tropics or countries with low socio economic income and overcrowding are higher risk factors for infestation with scabies since the incidence is also higher [6].

Etiopathogenesis [7–10]

Scabies in humans is caused by a mite known as *Sarcoptes scabiei* var. *hominis* of family Sarcoptidae, class Arachnida. The one responsible for scabies in animals is called *Sarcoptes scabiei* var. *canis* (in dogs). It does not cause scabies in humans but may cause bite reactions.

Scabies mite found in humans is species-specific, eight legged which lives its entire 30 day life cycle in the epidermis. The mite is a translucent, pearl-like, white, eyeless and oval in shape with four pairs of short stubby legs. The size of an adult female mite its approximately 0.4 × 0.3 mm and the male is slightly smaller, just too small to be seen by naked eye. In a sterile test tube it can survive for 3 days and in a mineral oil mount up to 7 days. Mites cannot fly or jump.

Copulation occurs in a burrow excavated by the female, when the adult male mite goes in. Fifteen minutes copulation occurs once per female lifetime. In 1 to 2 days, the female burrows and lays eggs in the tunnel. Each day a female mite lays three eggs. They mature in a matter of 2–3 days into larvae. This larva has three pair of eggs instead of four. These larvae spend 1 day on skin and then go back into the burrow. After 3–4 days, it matures into protonymph and then 3 days later into tritonymph. After 2–3 days, this tritonymph finally transforms into adult mites. In an infested host the average number of mites living can vary, though they are usually 10–15, and not more than a hundred. However in patients with crusted scabies large number of mites are present. The scabies mite usually survives up to 3 days off human host, but in crusted scabies it may live off, feeding on sloughed skin, for about 7 days.

The incubation period of the mite may vary from days to months, but on first exposure the usual incubation period is 2–6 weeks, after which the host immune system kicks in and becomes sensitized to the mite and its by-products, resulting in the most common symptoms of pruritus and cutaneous lesions. In case of a subsequent infestation, the patient may become symptomatic with 1–2 days. Asymptomatic scabies carriers have also been known.

Clinical Features

Intense pruritus, which is generally worse at night or may be aggravated by a hot bath is the most common complain. This severe desire to scratch may be felt immediately before or after the appearance of the new lesions, generally the papules or early tiny vesication.

Typically, the pathognomic lesions of scabies are burrows. These consist of a serpiginous tract formed by the advancing movement of mites in the superficially epidermis. The commonly affected areas may show typical papular or vesicular excoriated lesions. These include the interdigital spaces (Figs. 1 and 2), inner aspect of wrists, elbows, axillae, post auricular area, waist(including the umbilicus), ankles, feet and buttocks. In men, penile and scrotal lesions are common (Fig. 3). In females, the areola, nipples and vulva are commonly affected. In elderly and immune-compromised individuals, all skin surfaces are susceptible including the face and the scalp, so do the infants [2, 7]. The latter may show plantar and palmar lesions (Fig. 4).

Other than the burrow, small erythematous papulo-vesicular lesions can also be present with varying degrees of associated pruritus and excoriation. Intensely pruritic erythematous nodules especially on male genitalia and in the groins and axillae in either sexes is a common feature in hosts with good immune response against the mite (Fig. 5).

In many patients, especially in warm climates or after long periods of infestation, it is difficult to observe burrows because they might have been distorted due to scratching.

In immunocompromised patients, elderly, unkempt homeless people there is often a widespread scaly, crusted eruption (crusted scabies) (Figs. 6 and 7). Instead of the regular signs and symptoms, it presents with marked hyperkeratosis and maybe no or minimal itching (Norwegian scabies). Large number of mites could be seen in skin scrapings (Fig. 8).

It's common to see patients with pruritus in the absence of typical recognizable lesions after

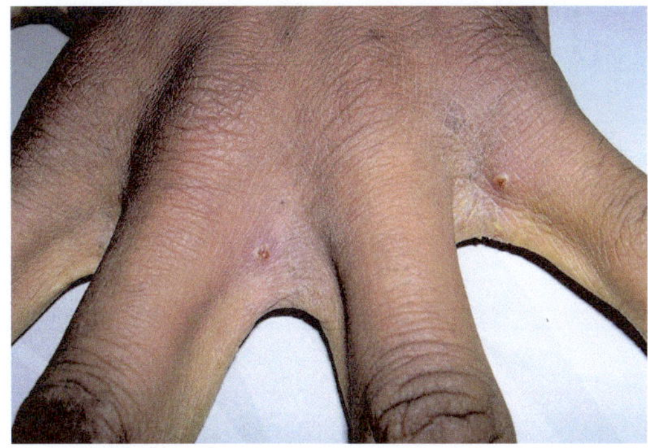

Fig. 2 Early lesions of scabies often show itchy papules and vesicles on closer look

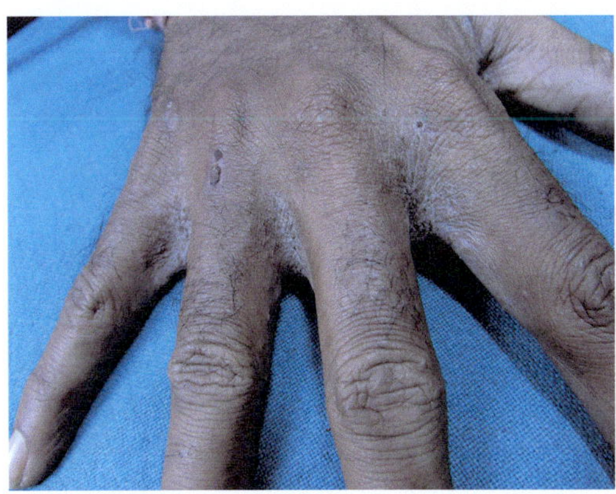

Fig. 1 Typical involvement of finger webs in a man with untreated scabies

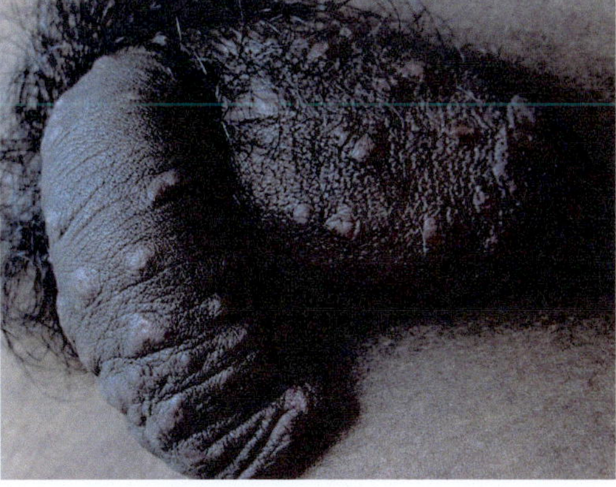

Fig. 3 Classic presentation of intensely pruritic nodular lesions in a sexually active man

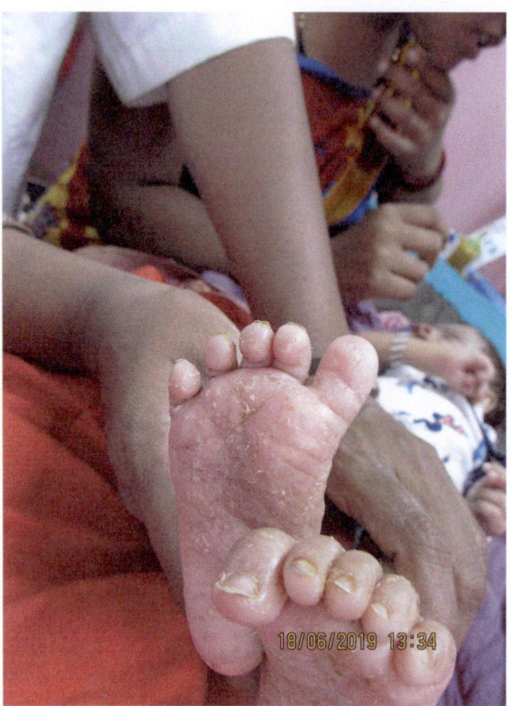

Fig. 4 Irritable infant with plantar vesicular eruptions whose mother was suffering from scabies

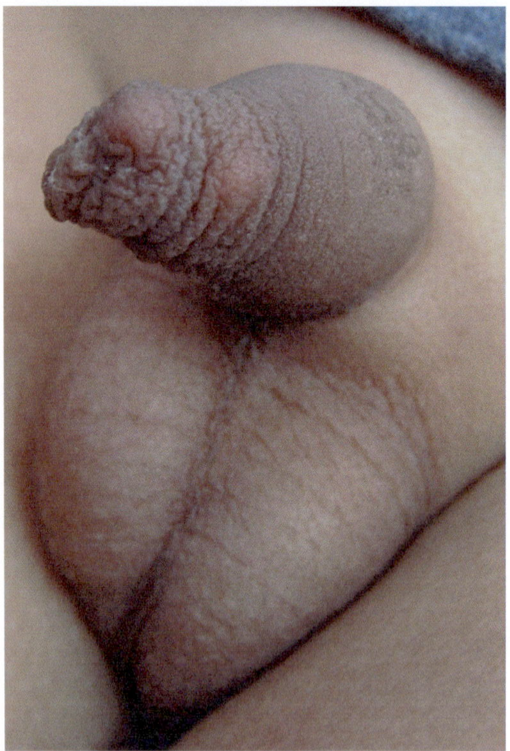

Fig. 5 Persistent penile erythematous pruritic lesions on penis in a child, as the only presentation of scabies

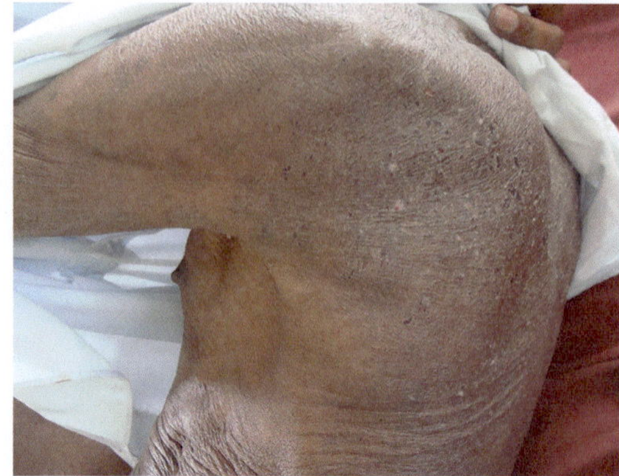

Fig. 6 Widespread crusting and scaling in an elderly man: Crusted scabies

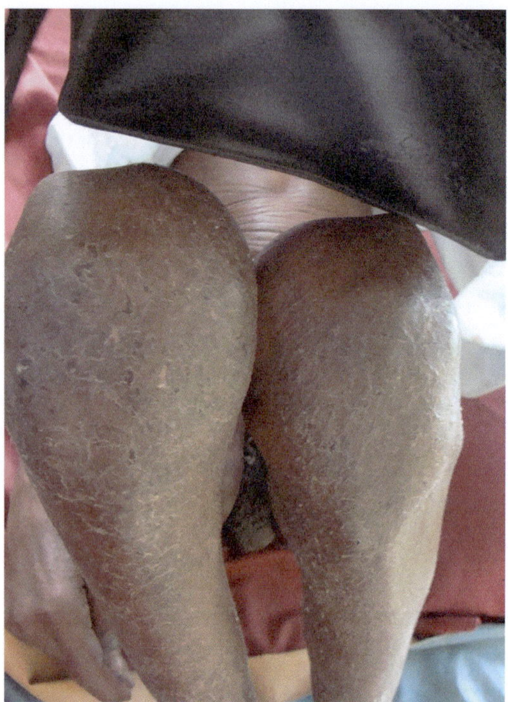

Fig. 7 Widespread crusting and scaling in an elderly man: Crusted scabies

application of over the counter potent topical steroid preparations. These are referred to as Scabies incognito (Fig. 9). Scabies acquired from pet animals (frequently cats or dogs) presents with highly pruritic excoriated papules (Fig. 10).

Senile population is more affected. Immunocompromised elderly patients may exhibit bullous eruptions (Fig. 11).

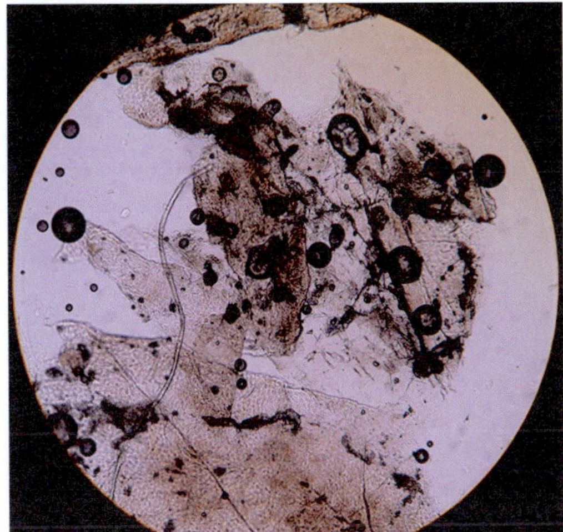

Fig. 8 Skin scraping showed dead mites and with its parts and eggs with faeces

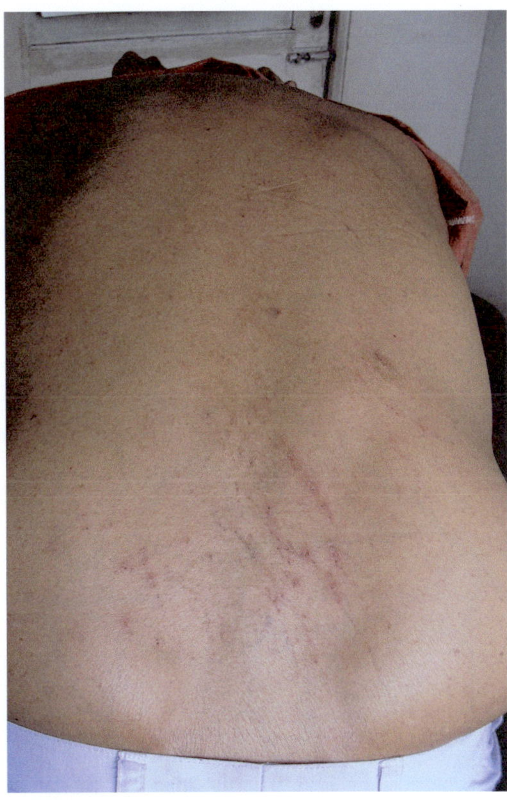

Fig. 10 Intense pruritus on trunk of a man, whose pet dog suffered from scabies (Animal scabies)

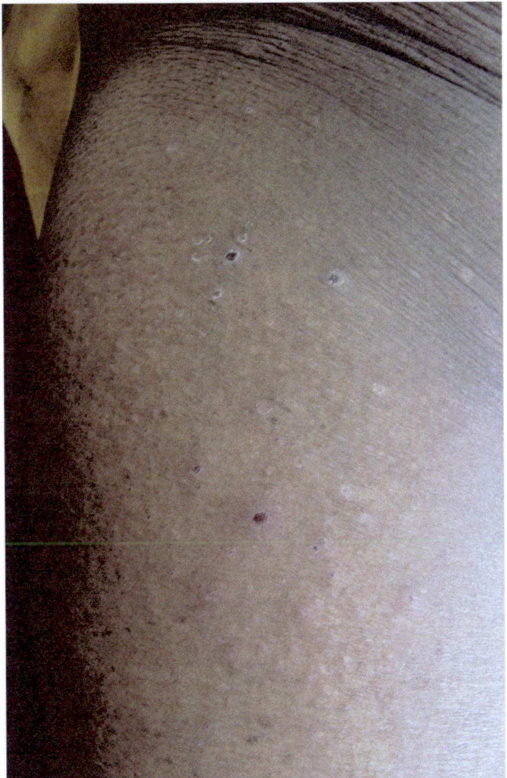

Fig. 9 Potent steroid topical application masks the classic symptoms and signs of scabies (Scabies incognito)

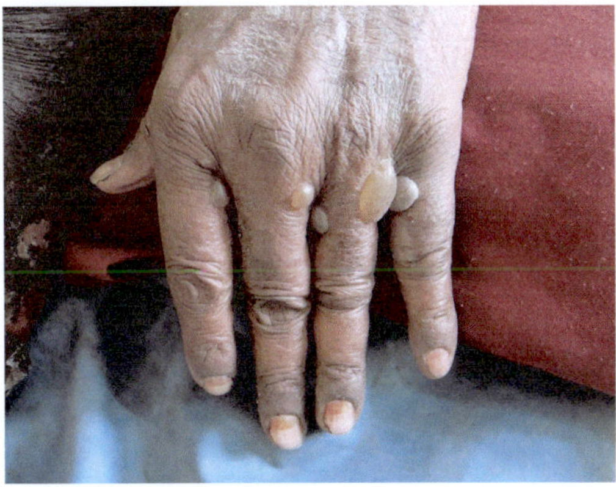

Fig. 11 Bullous eruptions in the finger webs of an immunocompromised homeless man, who was confirmed having Scabies (Bullous scabies)

HIV seropositive patients may present with thickened hyperkeratotic pruritic papules on buttocks and lower extremities (Keratotic scabies) (Fig. 12).

The presentation of patients who have travelled and have been infested with scabies can be different than the usual manifestations. Patchy areas affected with confined itching are commonly seen. Sometimes there can be erythema-

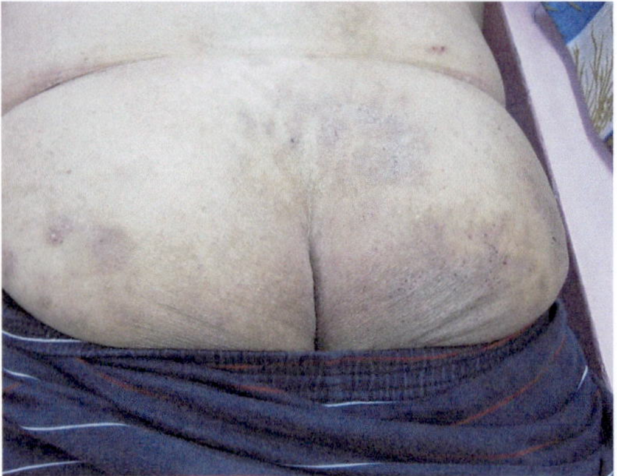

Fig. 12 Excoriations and keratotic papules on lower back and gluteal areas in HIV seropositive man (Keratotic scabies)

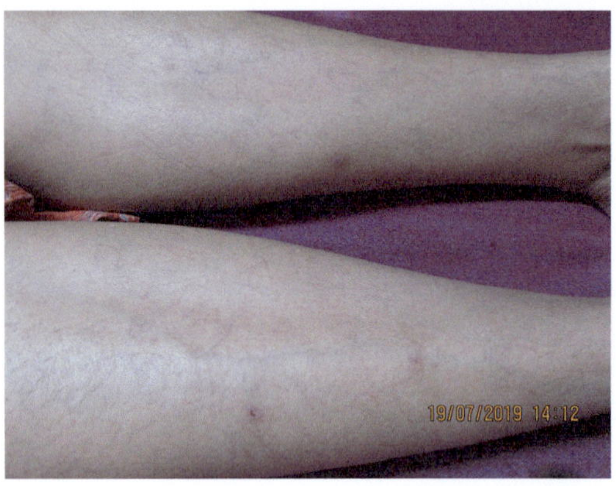

Fig. 13 Sparse excoriations on legs of very hygienic lady (clean man's scabies)

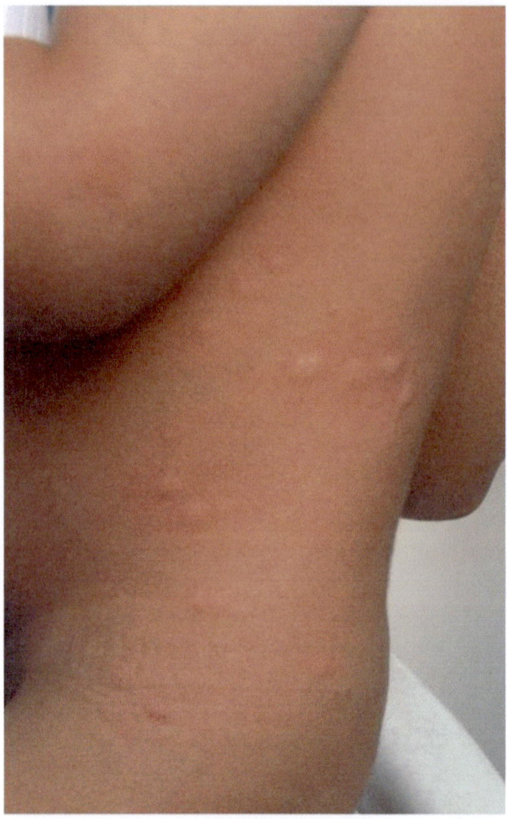

Fig. 14 Urticaria as presenting manifestation of scabies

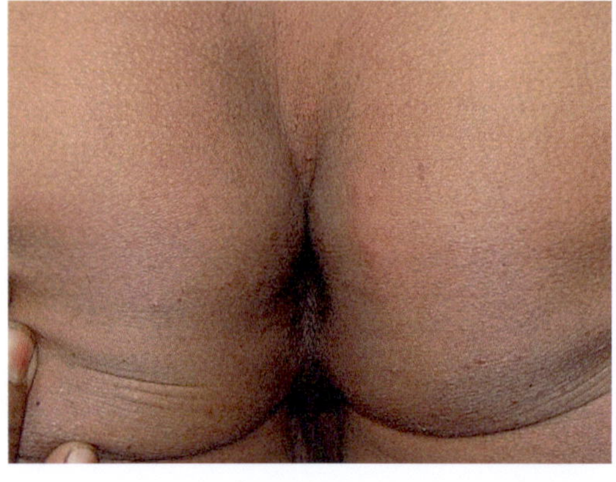

Fig. 15 Urticaria as presenting manifestation of scabies

tous, pruritic nodules in the axillae and groin and commonly over genitalia. In a family, or group of travellers who have travelled to the same place, some may be asymptomatic and hence the presentations may be confusing.

Mild itching with very few lesions or only excoriations on extremities or trunk may be seen in certain healthy hygienic individuals may sometimes referred to as "Clean man's scabies" (Fig. 13).

Infants and young children may present with facial, scalp or palmar lesions, often with severe nocturnal pruritus.

Unusual variants of urticarial lesions (Figs. 14 and 15) or symptomatic dermographism (Fig. 16) as presenting manifestations of scabies is known, especially in the Indian patients [12].

Diagnosis The diagnosis of scabies is based on typical clinical manifestations and history. In cases of doubt various bed-side and laboratory tests can be performed.

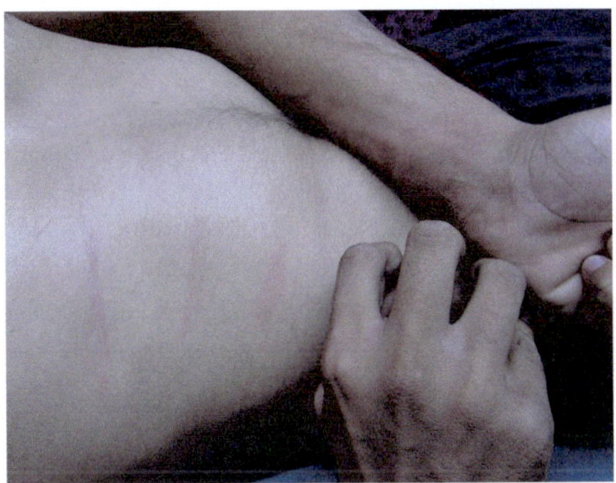

Fig. 16 Symptomatic dermographism as a presenting manifestation of scabies

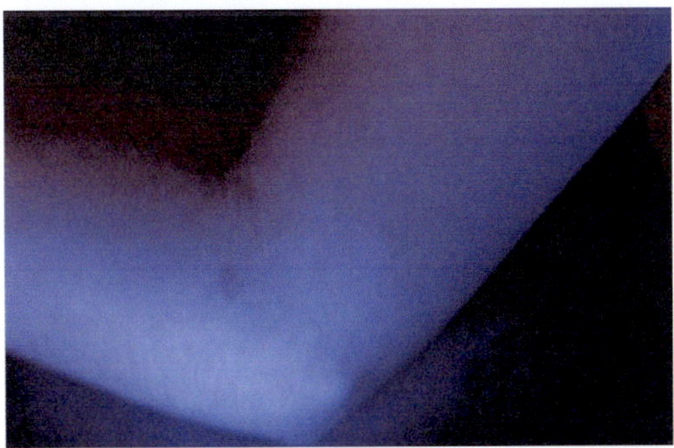

Fig. 17 Wood's lamp helps detection of scabeitic burrow, a pathognomonic sign of scabies

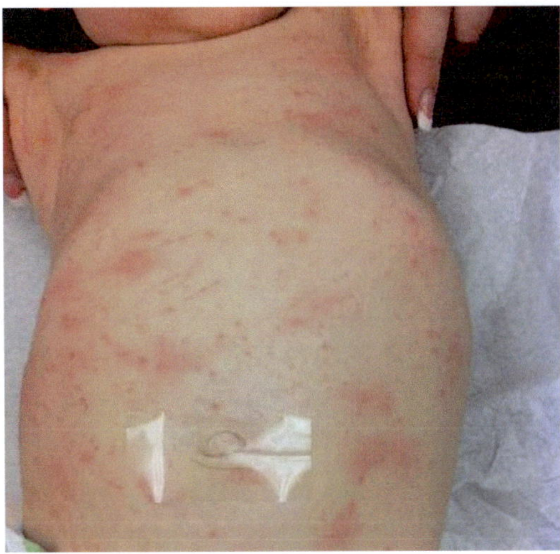

Fig. 18 Tape stripping of suspected scabies lesions is a rapid method of diagnosis

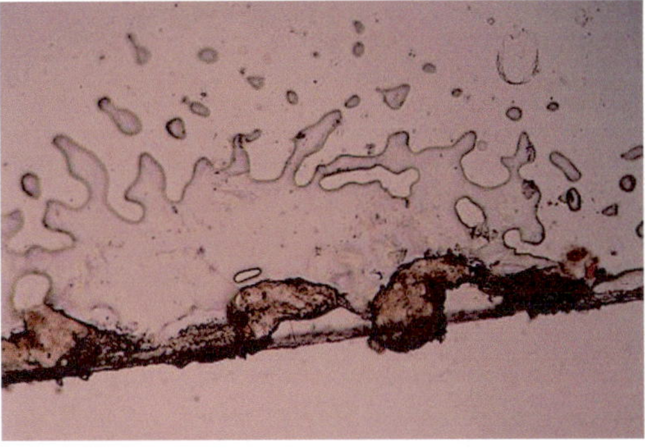

Fig. 19 Tape stripping of suspected scabies lesions is a rapid method of diagnosis

1. **Observation of Burrows with the Help of–** India ink preparation, crystal violet stain, is smeared on it and removed after sometime by wiping with cotton alcohol swab. The burrows take up the ink and retain it and are seen more clearly. Wood's lamp may come handy in improving visualization of scabies mite burrow, with or without smearing of tetracycline powder (Fig. 17).

2. **Skin scrapings under light microscope–** scrapings from commonly affected areas observed under a mineral oil preparation with the help of a light microscope. Adult mites, eggs and faecal pellets (scybala) may be seen.

   Adhesive tape can be applied to scabietic lesions, which is then transferred onto a clean glass slide and observed under light microscope to visualize mite or its parts (Figs. 18 and 19). This may be useful in very busy out-patient clinics and time saving for quick diagnosis especially in doubtful patients.

3. Confocal microscopy and dermoscopy can be used for direct visualization of mites and eggs in vivo.

4. Skin biopsy—this will clinch the diagnosis if it reveals mite or its mouth parts or faces in the stratum corneum of the affected skin (Fig. 20).

   It shows patchy or diffuse eosinophilic infiltrate, with lymphocytes and histiocytes in the reticular dermis. Attached to the stratum corneum can be pink pig-tail like structure that represent adult mite exoskeleton and can add to the clue.

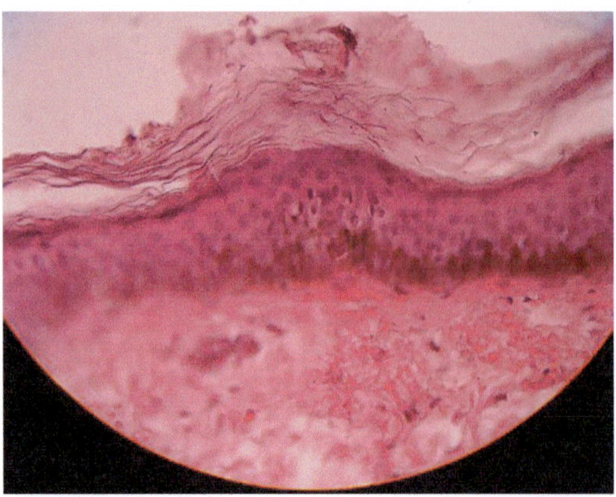

Fig. 20 Skin biopsy of a doubtful lesion reveals mite in the stratum corneum on histopathology

5. Serological tests—for detection of IgE specific for a recombinant *S.scabiei* antigen are under investigation [13].

Differential Diagnosis

In context of travellers, the most common differential to think about in case of scabies are:
   Most likely

1. Atopic dermatitis
2. Allergic contact dermatitis
3. Auto sensitization (id eruption)
4. Dyshidrotic eczema
5. Nummular eczema
6. Insect bite reaction
7. Pyoderma in case of infected scabies
   Also consider
1. Dermatitis herpetiformis
2. Psoriasis
3. Bullous pemphigoid
4. Drug eruption

5. Systemic causes of pruritus
6. Delusions of parasitosis
7. Langerhans cell histiocyosis, clinically and hisopathologically
8. In infants—inflammatory stage of incontinentia pigmenti, acropustulosis of infancy in case of second day infection

Treatment [9–11]

To treat scabies, various scabicides are available and choice depends on the availability, the age group, pregnancy and extent of the disease.

There are topical as well as oral scabicidal drugs. A second application after a week of starting the therapy is a must to treat all the adult mites and eggs.

Topical agents are to be applied overnight, all over the body except for head in adults. In infants, the application should involve the head area. The hands and feet are to be covered so as to avoid contact with mouth. During topical application, special care must be taken to apply it in the creases, interdigital spaces, clefts of buttocks, belly button, and under finger and toenails.

Most patients will experience reduction in symptoms by third day. However, the rash and pruritus may persist for another 4–6 weeks, and that is because of the body's reaction to the dead mite and debris. This is known as "post-scabitic itch" and patients should be informed that this is not due to treatment failure and the itching will reduce. Oral anti-histaminic and emollients considerably reduce this itch. Patients should also be informed that excessive washing of skin with harsh soaps and detergents may dry the skin and further aggravates the itching.

The following are a few scabicidal drugs:

Drug	Mode of action	Dose	Comment
1. Permethrine 5% cream	Synthetic pyrethroid inhibits sodium transport in neurons and thus paralyses the mite and death due to respiratory paralysis to the mite	Topically overnight, all over body on days 1 and 8	Most common treatment used recently, pregnancy category B, tolerance seems to be developing
2. Lindane 1% lotion or cream	Gamma-hexacholocyclohexane, an organochlorine agent. Neurotoxic to mite. Thus, acaricidal	Topically overnight, all over body on days 1 and 8	US FDA "black box" approved. Banned in California. Potential CNS toxicity. Pregnancy category C

Drug	Mode of action	Dose	Comment
3. Crotomiton 10% cream	Antiparasitic and antipruritic	Topically overnight, all over body on days 1, 2, 3 and 8	Has antipruritic properties, effectiveness is limited. Pregnancy category C
4. Precipitated sulphur 5–10%	Weak antiparasitic, antipruritic	Topically overnight for 3 consecutive days	Pregnancy and infants. Low efficacy
5. Benzyl benzoate 10% lotion	Neurotoxic to mite (acaricidal)	Topically apply for 24 h	Cheap but may have a potential for causing irritant dermatitis
6. Ivermectin	Macrocyclic lactone produced by streptomyces avermitilis. Blocks neural transmission nerve synapses that utilize (GABA) glutamate or gamma aminobutaric acid and cause paralysis of peripheral motor function [2]	Oral dose, 0.2 mg per kilogram of body weight, repeat after 8 days and more times in cases of crusted scabies [2]	Not recommended in infants with weight below 15 kg, pregnant women and breast-feeding mothers because of lack of safety data in these groups [2] Pregnancy category C

In case of a clean man's scabies, the mainstay of treatment is managing intense pruritus due to severe hypersensitivity to scabietic mite from dogs or cats. Escalated doses of antihistamines or a short course of corticoids or topical application of mid potency topical steroids often helps in resolution.

In case of crusted scabies, emollients and keratolytic agents play important role to make it easier for the scabietic agents to penetrate. Some patients may require Methotrexate therapy [14].

Nodular scabies occurs with persistent intensely pruritic nodules due to hypersensitivity reaction to retained antigenic parts of the mite. The scrotum and the shaft of the penis are frequently affected anatomic locations. Common effective treatments include potent topical steroid creams, intralesional injection of triamcinolone, short course of systemic corticoids or topical Tacrolimus. However, it could be challenging at times to manage the unresponsive persistent or recurrent nodules. Cryotherapy has been tried with success by the authors [15].

Treatment of fomites and contact avoidance forms an important part of treatment of scabies. Appropriate community health education is a must. Clothing should be changed daily and clothes and bed linen should be washed in hot water 60 °C. If hot water is not available, all clothing should be wrapped together in a plastic bag and stored away for 5–7 days because scabies mite does not survive for more than 4 days outside human body.

Prophylactic anti scabies therapy is to be organised for all family members and close contacts, irrespective of symptoms.

Appropriate systemic antibiotics in case of secondary infection, antihistamines and/or a short course of corticoids may be recommended in case of eczematous complication of scabies.

Complications

Scabies lesions and the subsequent excoriation may become secondarily infected with *Saphylococcus aureus* or *Streptococcus pyogenes leading to pustulation folliculitis or cellulitis* (Figs. 21 and 22). **Recurrent ecthyma especially over gluteal areas is known in Indian patients** (Fig. 23).

In countries with endemic scabies, post streptococcal glomerulonephritis is a noteworthy issue. Lymphangitis and septicemia are also known to happen in crusted scabies.

In patients with disorders of keratinization, peripheral eosinophilia can rarely be a primary sign.

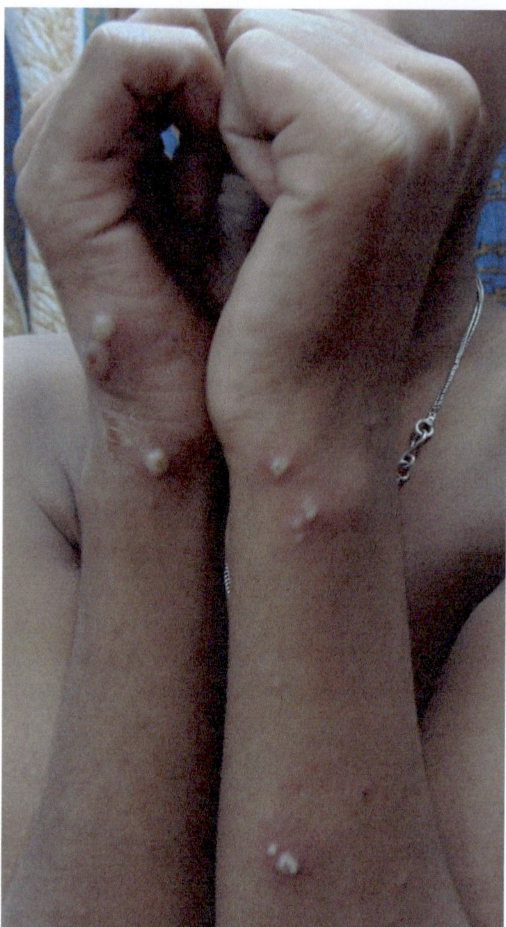

Fig. 21 Pustulation of scabies lesions on forearm of a man. Bacterial folliculitis is a frequent complication of untreated scabies

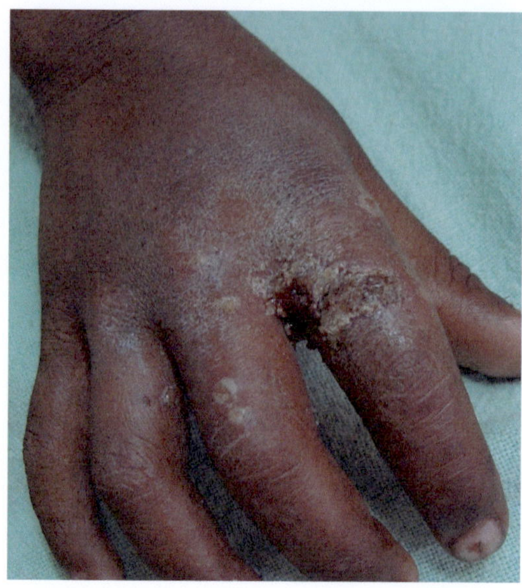

Fig. 22 Cellulitis of hand as a complication of untreated scabies

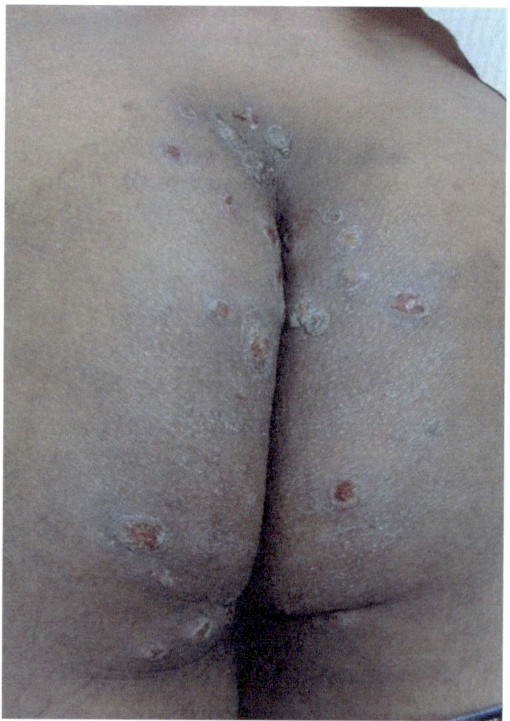

Fig. 23 Recurrent ecthyma of gluteal areas is often seen as a complication in children

Summary

Scabies is one of the most common dermatological diseases found in travellers. It is common in those individuals from low socioeconomic background, who have been travelling for more than 2 weeks, especially who are travelling for social causes. Any complaints of pruritus following travelling could be scabies. Such patients and their contacts and family members should be carefully examined and screened for scabies even if they have small nonspecific lesions. Appropriate treatment at the earliest may help to avert epidemic of this important public health problem.

References

1. Caumes E. Skin diseases. In: Keystone J, Kozarsky P, Freedman D, Nothdurft H, Connor B, editors. Travel medicine. Spain: Mosby; 2004. p. 491e502.
2. Harvey K, Esposito DH, Han P, Kozarsky P, Freedman DO, Plier DA, et al. Centers for Disease Control and Prevention. Surveillance for travel-related disease—GeoSentinel Surveillance System, United States, 1997–2011. MMWR Surveill Summ. 2013;62(3):1–23.
3. Korzenlewski K, Juszczak D, Jerzemowski J. Skin lesions in the returning travellers. Int Marit Health. 2015;66:173–80.
4. Freedman DO, Weld LH, Kozarsky PE, et al. Spectrum of disease and relation to place of exposure among ill returned travelers. N Engl J Med. 2006;354:119–30.
5. Herbinger KH, Siess C, Nothdurft HD, von Sonnenburg F, Löscher T. Skin disorders among travellers returning from tropical and non -tropical countries consulting a travel medicine clinic. Trop Med Int Health. 2011;16:1457–64.
6. O'Brien MB. A practical approach to common skin problems in returning travellers. Travel Med Infect Dis. 2009;7:125–46.
7. Meinking TL, Burkhart CG, Burkhart CN. Ectoparasitic diseases in dermatology: reassessment of scabies and pediculosis. Advances in Dermatology -Chicago Then St Louis MO- 2000:67–108.
8. From the URL: wwwnc. cdc. gov, accessed 15 Jun 2020. Traveler's health, Skin and soft tissue infections, chapter 11 authors Karolyn Wanat and Scott Norton travelers health, skin and soft tissue.
9. Lederman ER, Weld LH, Elyazar IR, von Sonnenburg F, Loutan L, Schwartz E, Keystone JS. Dermatologic conditions of the ill returned traveler: an analysis from the GeoSentinel Surveillance Network. Int J Infect Dis. 2008;12(6):593–602.
10. Hicks MI, Elston DM. Scabies. Dermatol Ther. 2009 Jul;22(4):279–92.
11. Jacks SK, Lewis EA, Witman PM. The curette prep: a modification of the traditional scabies preparation. Pediatr Dermatol. 2012;29(4):544–5.
12. Zawar V, Godse K. Acute urticaria presenting manifestation of scabies in children. Asian J Ped Pract. 2009;
13. Jayaraj R, Hales B, Viberg L, Pizzuto S, Holt D, Rolland JM, O'Hehir RE, Currie BJ, Walton SF. A diagnostic test for scabies: IgE specificity for a recombinant allergen of Sarcoptes scabiei. Diagn Microbiol Infect Dis. 2011;71(4):403–7.
14. Ward WH. Scabies norvegica. Treatment with methotrexate. Aust J Dermatol. 1971;12:44–51.
15. Zawar V, Pawar M. Liquid nitrogen cryotherapy in the treatment of chronic unresponsive nodular scabies. J Am Acad Dermatol. 2017;77:e 43–4.

Tungiasis

Carlos D. Sánchez-Cárdenas, Cristhian Moreno-Leiva,
M. Elisa Vega-Memije, Eder R. Juarez-Duran,
and Roberto Arenas

Key Points

- Tungiasis is a parasitic skin disease caused by *Tunga penetrans*.
- Risk factors: lack of footwear, living with domestic reservoir animals.
- It affects mainly the periungual region, toes, the soles and heels.
- Clinical features: intense inflammation and a bacterial superinfection.
- Macroscopic findings: dark spot, black nodule and body-like structure.
- Dermoscopic findings: epidermal and superficial parasitic structures.
- Best treatment: sterile surgical extraction.
- Affects the quality of life and household economy.

C. D. Sánchez-Cárdenas · E. R. Juarez-Duran ·
R. Arenas (✉)
Mycology Section, "Dr. Manuel Gea Gonzalez"
General Hospital, Mexico City, Mexico

C. Moreno-Leiva
Facultad de Ciencias de la salud, Bioquimica—
Quimica y Farmacia, USCA San Francisco,
Coaguazu, Paraguay

M. E. Vega-Memije
Dermatopathology Department "Dr. Manuel Gea
Gonzalez" General Hospital, Mexico City, Mexico

Introduction and History [1, 2]

Tungiasis is a parasitic skin disease caused by penetration of the gravid female sand flea *Tunga* spp. (Insecta, Siphonaptera, Tungidae).

Medical entomology claims that South American region was the original site of Tungiasis, mainly restricted to tropical and sub-tropical areas. Since mid-nineteenth century, it has been observed also in countries with template climates due to transatlantic voyages.

The first reports goes back to the pre-Incan period, Peru has been an endemic area of tungiasis for at least fourteen centuries, artists of the Moringa and Chimu cultures depicted morphological features of *Tunga* on ceramic jars. Multiple names have been given to the sand flea in endemic areas, such as nigua, pique, jigger, chigoe, puce-chique and tchique. The first contact of Europeans with this entity was when Christopher Columbus's sailors landed in Haiti. Then, tungiasis became a critical problem for the colonizing troops, who had no previous experience with this parasite. For instance, the Spanish military expedition in Colombia (1538), leaded by Gonzalo Ximenez de Quesada, had to stop for an extended period in Sororoca town, where infestation made soldiers suffer so severe that walking was a challenge. Native women had compassion and showed them how to remove the embedded fleas. This ancient extraction method of the fleas are still used in some areas in South America and Africa.

The British ship "Thomas Mitchell", during its 1872–1873 voyage brought the flea from Brazil to Angola inside bags of sand used as ballast. *Tunga penetrans* spreaded rapidly along the African West Coasts and sub-Saharan regions following the trading caravans. Indeed, towns and villages were so infested that inhabitants were often forced to migrate, since it caused painful lesions on the feet, unable to work and eventually starve.

Tunga penetrans is one of the few parasites that spread from the Western to the Eastern hemisphere.

Aleixo de Abreu provided the first scientific description of *T. penetrans* and tungiasis in 1623. The first specie, *Tunga penetrans*, was described by Linnaeus in the eighteenth century (*Pulex penetrans*, Linnaeus 1758), and a second Tunga specie, which infects humans (*T. trimamillata*), was taxonomically described by Pampiglione et al. in 2002.

Epidemiology [3, 4]

This disease belongs to the ever-growing group of neglected tropical diseases (NTDs); present in poor communities of the tropical and subtropical parts of the world, like South America, Caribbean, and sub-Saharan Africa, and sporadically affects travellers who become infected in endemic areas and acquired from walking barefoot or with open-toed shoes. This disease is more frequent in dry seasons but also can be found in the rain forest as well as in banana plantations located on laterite soil.

Infestation is more prevalent in children than in adults, mainly among 5–10 year-old and also in elderly (85%). In Africa, the prevalence of tungiasis among children within 5–14 years old as in Ethiopia is 58.7% (95% CI: 53.7%–63.8%), but in some areas can be between 1.2%–34.7%. In Cameroon, the prevalence range has been reported from 60.5% to 70.2%, in Northern

Tanzania is about 97%, in Kenya is 25% (95% CI 22.4–27.5%). In some parts of African households, prevalence is 42.5%, meaning that at least one individual has tungiasis. In America, it can be found from Mexico to northern Argentina, the prevalence is between 16%–54%. It is endemic in Peru but, as in other countries, there's not sufficient information about the prevalence and geographical distribution. The top exposure countries are Brazil, Madagascar, Uganda and Ethiopia.

Regardless of gender, prevalence depends on the region; in Ethiopia and Kenya, the prevalence among males and females do not have significant difference. However, in Cameroon, tungiasis is more prevalent among males.

Prevalence is more frequent in farmers (46.1%), also in houses with mud or sand/dust as floor material (58.4% and 30% respectively), in walls made with mud (84.5%), in persons who use traditional latrine or bushes for their defecation (32.6%, 56.7% respectively).

In endemic areas, the walking time between the community and any health center increases the prevalence. A period of 30–39 min increases 30%.

Tungiasis is more frequent in low social economical resources.

Risk Factors [3]

Living with domestic reservoir animals such as cats (4.95 times higher odds), dogs and pigs, poor personal hygiene, poor sanitation of the housing and residential environment, and lack of footwear (7.42 times higher odds) are risk factors to get tungiasis. In Northeast Brazil, street dogs and cats are essential reservoirs in urban areas, whereas in rural areas pigs are the most important. Pigs were also identified as the primary reservoir of *T. penetrans* in Nigeria and Uganda.

Being Muslim was identified as a significant protective factor, this can be explained because they wash their feet several times a day before entering the mosque for prayer.

Children under 15 years, living in a house with a sandy floor, mud walls, using traditional latrine or bushes as toilet, disposing waste on a pile, using mud puddles as a water source, sleeping together with many others persons in a room, sleeping on the floor are also risk factors.

Other risk factors are low maternal educational status, like children of illiterate mothers (3.62 times higher odds) and mothers with primary education (2.72 times higher odds).

Walls of stone or concrete would reduce the prevalence of tungiasis by 64%.

Etiology

T. penetrans and *T. trimamillata*

Physiopathology [4–6]

Tunga penetrans is the smallest known flea, adult being less than 1 mm length. Once embedded in the epidermis of the host within 6–8 h, the female sand flea leaves the rear abdominal segments protruding, and within 2–5 weeks reaches the size of a pea. Then the parasite makes a skin hole of about 250 μm, which remains in contact with the environment, through which it is fertilized, breaths, defecates, producing and releasing hundreds of eggs (Fig. 1). Once fertilized, the female sand flea undergoes extraordinary hypertrophy, growing by 2000 times within 1 week. The female lays 100–200 eggs throughout 2 weeks; after all eggs have been expelled, the involution of the lesion begins and, 3 to 4 weeks after penetration, it finally dies and eventually is sloughed from the epidermis by tissue repair mechanisms (Fig. 2).

If the floor in the rooms consists of sand, dried mud or rugged cement with holes and cracks, eggs that have been expelled by embedded female sand fleas overnight and which have fallen on to the floor are swept into crevices or cracks. Eggs can develop into larvae after 3–4 days, pupae after 5–7 days in such cracks, and adults emerge ready to infect the next host after another 9–15 days.

Female sand fleas are fertilized by males exploring the skin only after females are embedded in the epidermis. There is circumstantial evidence that males are attracted by odour emitted from the faecal material released by females. The faecal material spreads into dermal papillae around the lesion, and since it is very sticky, it needs soap to be washed off. Hence, when soap is not used, or unavailability of water exists, more male sand fleas are attracted to the skin and this will lead to a higher intensity of infection.

Embedded sand fleas cause an intense inflammatory response.

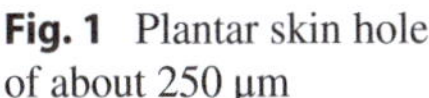

Fig. 1 Plantar skin hole of about 250 μm

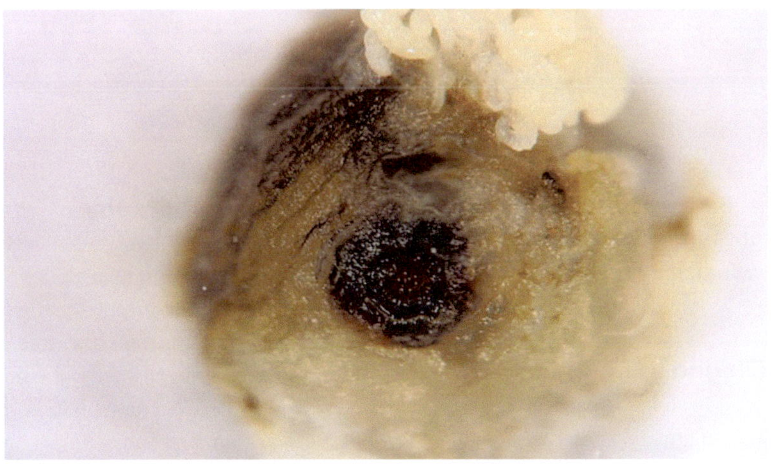

Fig. 2 Female sand flea of *Tunga penetrans*

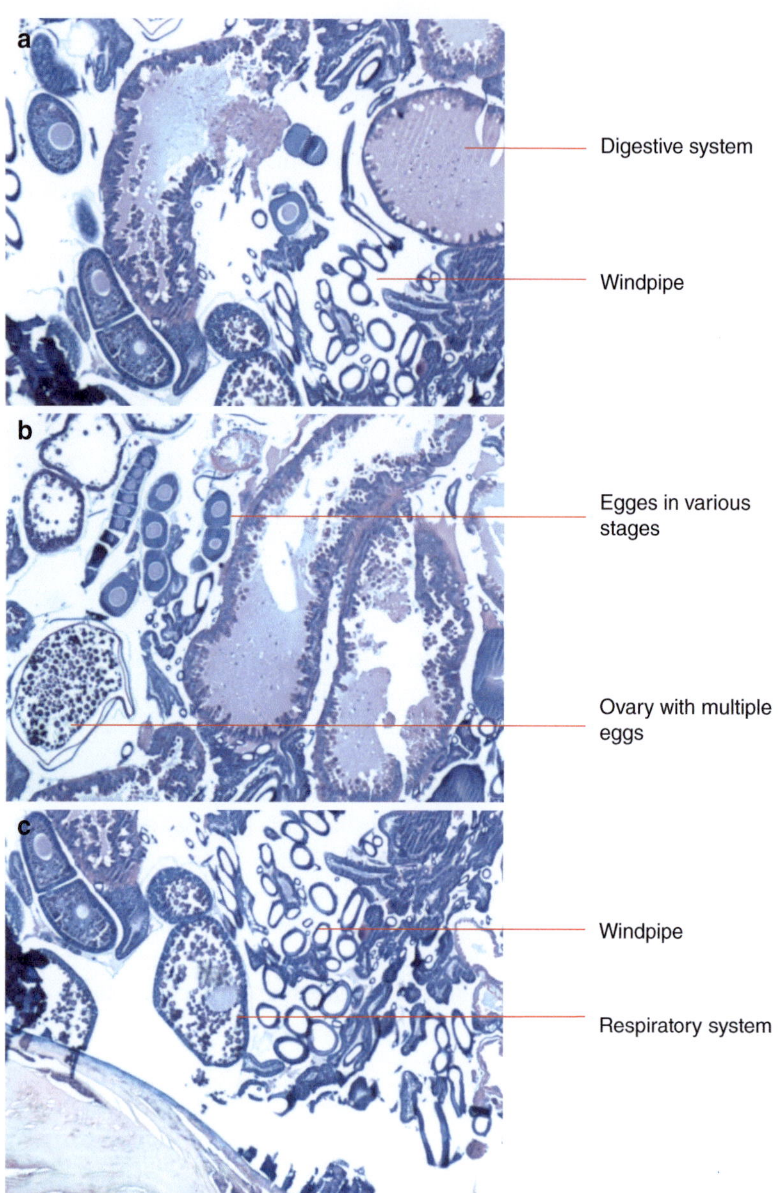

Bacterial superinfection is common and intensifies the inflammation, including cellulitis and necrotizing fasciitis, gangrene and sepsis.

Diagnosis [3, 6]

The diagnosis is made clinically.

Topography

In endemic areas, 95 to 98% of all tungiasis lesions affect the feet (Fig. 3). The periungual region, toes, the sole and the heel are the most preferred site by the flea, although infestation can also occur in hands, elbows, neck, genital and anal region.

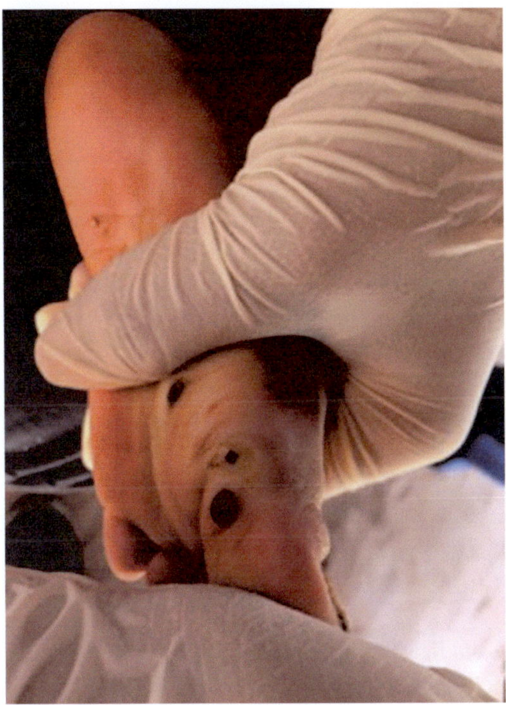

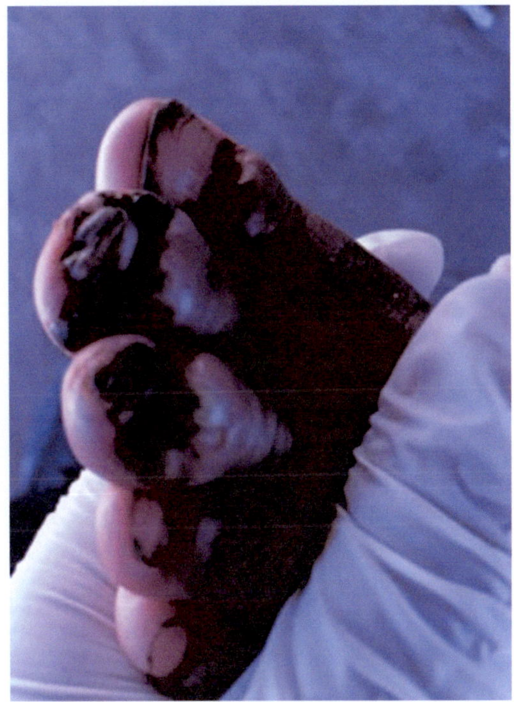

Fig. 3 Tungiasis affecting the plantar surface of the foot

Fig. 4 Acute symptoms of periungual tungiasis

Morphology

The natural history of tungiasis can be divided into five stages. In stage I (30 min to several hours) a tiny reddish spot of about 1 mm appears. In stage II (beginning of hypertrophy, 1 to 2 days after penetration), the parasite becomes more evident as a growing whitish or nacre-like nodule develops. In the protruding rear cone of the flea, the anal-genital opening appears as a black central dot, which is surrounded by increasing erythema. In stage III (maximal hypertrophy, 2 days to 3 weeks after penetration), a watch-glass-like white patch with well-defined borders and a central black dot appears, often in association with hyperkeratosis and desquamation of the surrounding skin. Expulsion of eggs and faeces are typical in this stage. In stage IV (3 to 5 weeks after penetration), a black crust covers this lesion containing a dead parasite. A residual scar in the stratum corneum is characteristic for stage V (6 weeks to several months after penetration).

We can observe the parasite intensity in mild (presence of one to five lesions), moderate (presence of six to thirty lesions) and heavy/ severe (presence of 30 or more lesions). The parasite intensity in children can be 6.8 jiggers per child. In general, the intensity prevalence in children is about 74% with a mild infestation, 23.3% moderate and 2.8% heavy/severe infestation.

Signs and Symptoms

When there is an infestation, signs are an ulcer, loss of nails, deformation of toes, and suppuration. Intense pain and itching are almost constant.

The acute symptoms are erythema, edema, pain and itching. Chronic manifestations include desquamation, hyperkeratosis, a formation of deep fissures, ulcers and hypertrophy of nail rims (Fig. 4).

Macroscopically suggestive of tungiasis: particular central dark spot, black nodule, or intraepidermic foreign body-like structure.

The observation of eggs being expelled, around the skin or the release of brownish threads of faeces are pathognomonic signs. Faeces threads are helical structures and often spread into the dermal papillae. Expulsion of eggs can be provoked by massaging the hypertrophy zone slightly.

Classification

The lesions can be classified by Fortaleza scale (described by Eisele and others in 2003); it permits the staging of the cycle of infection of Tunga spp. in the host:

- Stage I: penetrating sand flea (3–7 h).
- Stage II: Beginning of hypertrophy with a brownish/black dot with a diameter of 1–2 mm surrounded or not by an erythema (1–2 days after penetration).
- Stage III: circular yellow-white watch-glass-like patch with a diameter of 3–10 mm and with a central black dot, with two sub-stages.
  - First (3a): lasts for 2–3 days.
  - Second (3b): lasts for 2 weeks.
- Stage IV: brownish-black crust with or without surrounding necrosis. It is the involution of the lesion and has two sub-stages:
  - First (4a): live flea, 3–4 weeks after penetration.
  - Second (4b): 4–6 weeks, dead flea.
- Stage V: Residues.

Stage I to III are viable sand fleas; in stage IV–V, the parasite is dying or already dead.

Dermoscopic Findings [7, 8]

Dermoscopic examination allow us the visualization of the epidermal and superficial dermal structures (dark central pores, whitish oval structures, silver dendritic fibres, and blue-black blotches); it can be a valuable diagnostic tool in non-endemic areas and atypical cases.

We observe a brown pigmented ring with a dark central pore (corresponding to the genital opening of the flea or posterior end of the exoskeleton), a peripheral pigmented ring (corresponds to the posterior abdomen), also a radiated crown have been described between the pore and the peripheral ring, which is a zone of parakeratosis with hemorrhagic zones in a radiated arrangement, blue-blackish blotches (presumed to be the eggs or hematin in the gastrointestinal tract) and whitish oval structures linked together forming chain-like structures (corresponding to the eggs in the flea's abdomen) (Fig. 1).

Anatomical and Histopathologic Characteristics [9–11]

Sand fleas of the genus *Tunga* is the smallest flea species known with 1 mm length. Two species parasitize human: *Tunga penetrans* and (recently discovered) *T. trimamillata*.

Tunga eggs have an average length of 604 µm and a width of 327 µm. The larvae have a length of 1500 µm; the 6-day-old larvae grow up to 2900 µm.

Mature sand fleas have (in contrast to other flea specimens) a well-developed laciniae and an epipharynx, which are essential for females, concerning their invasive way of living. The head is flattened and has no ctenidial combs. Female adults are smaller than males, but their mouthparts have nearly the same size. The difference between the two sexes, is the shape of the abdominal end; because the posterior end of the female shows a depression. Size measurements of an adult *Tunga* shows that females are smaller than males in all extremities except for the epipharynx. The maxillary palp of females is only a little bit smaller than males.

Between species of *Tunga* that affect humans, *T. trimamillata* shows three protrusions surrounding, the presence of three anterior abdominal humps observed by the naked eye, a greater length of the first maxillary palps, and the presence of spines in the tibia of the third legs and thus hiding the head. *T. penetrans*, in contrast, has a chitin clasp, which shows a cloverleaf structure. Midgut diverticula is another presumed anatomical difference present in gravid *T. trimamillata*, but not in *T. penetrans*.

General Parts of *Tunga*:

Male

Aedeagus, accessory glands, abdominal spiracle, blood ingested, brain, claspers, epididymis, fat body, muscles, midgut, nerve chord, oesophagus, *proventriculus*, pleural arch, pharynx, resilin pad, rectal pad, specialized cells, trachea and testes.

Non-gravid Female

Area cribriformis, abdominal spiracles, *bulga*, brain, eye, hindgut, *hilla,* lens, muscles, midgut, malpighian tubules, nerve chord, oesophagus, optic nerve, *proventriculus,* pigmented layer, rectal *ampulla,* rectal pad, *spermatheca,* trachea.

Gravid Female

Area cribriformis, bulga, cuticula, *diverticulum,* eggs, head, hypodermal cells, muscles, midgut, midgut epithelium, mouth parts, oviduct, oocites, oral parts, pharynx, *spermatheca,* spermathecal glands.

There are different findings in histopathology, we can divide this into two parts, the Tunga histologic findings and the particular findings of the host.

Tunga findings: Eosinophilic cuticle, eggs in different stages of development, tracheal rings, a brown-yellowish intracuticular chitin (representing the last abdominal segment of the embedded flea), oviducts, midgut and intraparasitic red blood cells, hypodermis, hypertrophied striated muscle.

Host histopathological changes: Basal hyperplasia, acanthosis, hyperkeratosis, parakeratosis, hypergranulosis, papillomatosis, spongiosis, and microabscesses, with an infiltrate of lympho-cytes, neutrophils, eosinophils and histiocytes in the epidermis and dermis

Complications [3, 6]

Tungiasis is associated with acute and chronic inflammation and pain of toes, fissures, lymphoedema and deformation, loss of toe nails and auto-amputation of digits. Severe inflammation, ulceration and fibrosis, and though rarely, death might occur in case of profound infestation. The lesion may also be complicated by bacterial superinfection by aerobe and anaerobe bacteria, lead to formation of pustules, suppuration and ulcers; even tetanus may be causally linked to tungiasis in areas with low immunization coverage when the people try to keep out the parasite with dirty material. Constant reinfection is the rule in endemic setting, impairs mobility, eventually leads to tissue necrosis and gangrene and then mutilation of the feet and immobilization of the patient.

Patients with severe infections develop a characteristic walking, as they try to avoid placing pressure on painful lesions and walk with their toes pointing upwards. The risk of transmitting blood-borne pathogens such as hepatitis B and C viruses exist because of the use of inappropriate sharp instruments to remove or kill the embedded fleas used subsequently by several individuals.

Life Impact [5, 6]

Tungiasis harms the quality of life and household economy, limiting their productivity. Associated morbidity in endemic areas can cause severe foot pain, foot mutilation and nail dystrophy, complicating walking and contributing to stigmatization. It also affects school attendance and performance of children, mainly due to high absenteeism; also, children are bullied. It is reasonable to assume that tungiasis causes mental strain and distress. In communities where people rarely wear closed shoes, the disease cannot be hidden in public and, since it is associated with poverty, it stigmatizes its victims.

Table 1 DLQI score in Tungiasis

Score	Impact on patient's life quality
I	None
II–III	Light
IV–VII	Moderate
IX–XIII	High
XIV–XVIII	Very high

The quality of life can be measured by the Dermatology Life Quality Index (DLQI). It has 6 categories and a score ranging from 0 to 18 points including: feeling of shame, impairment of leisure activities, difficulty in walking, impairment of concentration during classes, social exclusion and sleeping problems. The first 2 categories are evaluated verbally in this order: Not at all = 0 points, Only a little = 1 point, Quite a lot = 2 points, Very much = 3 points. The last 4 are examined and evaluated visually. In Table 1, there is the interpretation of the tungiasis-related DLQI scores.

According to Wiese S, Elson L, Feldmeier H (2018) Tungiasis-related life quality impairment in children living in rural Kenya. PLoS Negl Trop Dis 12 (1):1–13.

Treatment [3, 6, 12–14]

Because the sandflies typically die within 6 weeks after penetration, tungiasis is self-limited. The aim of treatment is to reduce symptoms and prevent secondary bacterial infection with appropriate antibiotics. Also, tetanus vaccination must be implemented to prevent secondary tetanus.

Surgical removal of the organism is crucial. Sterile surgical extraction can be performed in a medical setting. Local people extract the mature flea using sterile needle; in poor areas, people are forced to try to get rid of the flea from the body using thorn or other sharp materials. After extraction, the wound should be flushed thoroughly with sterile saline and dressed with antibiotic ointment. Tetanus prophylaxis is indicated.

Various attempts have been made to use topical anthelminthic including metrifonate, thiabendazole and ivermectin, none of which proved useful. Oral ivermectin showed no efficacy in a RCT.

Likewise, oral ivermectin did not affect embedded fleas. Successful topical treatments include cryotherapy.

Home Remedies and Myths [15, 16]

In some countries, including Kenya, the government recommends soaking the feet in potassium permanganate (at a concentration of 0.05%) for 15 min followed by applying Vaseline to counteract the dehydrating effect of the permanganate. However, a recent trial demonstrated that this treatment has only marginal efficacy.

In Brazil, several communities use coconut oil for prevention. This was tested in a trial with a coconut-based insect repellent, Zanzarin. Its efficacy varied from 86% to 100% when applied twice daily, and morbidity was reduced after 3–4 weeks.

In Kenya, a remedy based on Neem seed oil (*Azadirachta indica*) and coconut oil (*Cocos nucifera*) are used, but the efficacy of the mixture has yet to be determined.

Recently, a mixture of two dimethicones with a low viscosity and the propensity to cover microscopic surfaces (NYDA®) has been tested in a randomized proof-of-principle study. When the whole foot was covered with NYDA®, it killed 78% of the embedded fleas within 7 days. A subsequent trial with a targeted application to the flea's abdominal tip four times over 20 min showed an efficacy of 98%.

Topical dimethicone has been shown to reduce inflammation and hasten parasite death in 1 RCT,165 with targeted application to areas of parasite protrusion being more effective than to the entire foot [16, 17].

Prevention [4, 6, 18, 19]

Widespread control has never been attempted, only isolated efforts to treat infected individuals, often by non-governmental organizations.

Tungiasis can be controlled with simple housing improvements, improved access to water and hygiene practices; such as: using closed shoes and socks (complete protection cannot be achieved by these means), making a daily inspection of the feet and immediate extraction of embedded fleas, sealing house floors with concrete, treating domestic animals with an appropriate insecticide, and keeping animals away from the houses.

For travellers planning to enter endemic villages, it is highly recommended that they use insect repellent and wear closed shoes.

For travellers to endemic areas, improving education and footwear is essential as one of the best preventive measure.

But people living in endemic areas are usually re-infested unless proper footwear and improving housing changes.

Finally, increasing tetanus vaccination coverage in tungiasis-endemic regions will help prevent secondary tetanus.

References

1. Vaira F, Nazzaro G, Veraldi S. Tungiasis "The greatest curse that has ever afflicted Africa". JAMA Dermatol. 2014;150(7):708.
2. Maco V, Tantaleán M, Gotuzzo E. Evidence of tungiasis in pre-Hispanic America. Emerg Infect Dis. 2011;17(5):855–62.
3. Girma M, Astatkie A, Asnake S. Prevalence and risk factors of tungiasis among children of Wensho district, southern Ethiopia. BMC Infect Dis. 2018;18(1):456.
4. Wiese S, Elson L, Reichert F, Mambo B, Feldmeier H. Prevalence, intensity and risk factors of tungiasis in Kilifi County, Kenya: I. Results from a community-based study. PLoS Negl Trop Dis. 2017;11(10):1–19.
5. Wiese S, Elson L, Feldmeier H. Tungiasis-related life quality impairment in children living in rural Kenya. PLoS Negl Trop Dis. 2018;12(1):1–13.
6. Elson L, Fillinger U, Feldmeier H. Tungiasis. In: Tyring S, Lupi O, Hengge U, editors. Tropical dermatology. 2nd ed. Edinburg: Elsevier; 2017. p. 401–4.
7. Abarzua A, Cataldo K, Alvarez S. Dermoscopy in tungiasis. Indian J Dermatol Venereol Leprol. 2014;80(4):371–3.
8. Criado PR, Landman G, dos Reis VMS, Belda WJ. Tungiasis under dermoscopy: in vivo and ex vivo examination of the cutaneous infestation due to Tunga penetrans. An Bras Dermatol. 2013;88(4):649–51.
9. Nagy N, Abari E, D'Haese J, Calheiros C, Heukelbach J, Mencke N, et al. Investigations on the life cycle and morphology of Tunga penetrans in Brazil. Parasitol Res. 2007;101(Suppl 2):233–42.
10. Maco V, Maco VP, Tantalean ME, Gotuzzo E. Case report: histopathological features of tungiasis in Peru. Am J Trop Med Hyg. 2013;88(6):1212–6.
11. Pampiglione S, Fioravanti M, Gustinelli A, Onore G, Rivasi F, Trentini M. Anatomy of Tunga trimamillata Pampiglione et al., 2002 (Insecta, Siphonaptera, Tungidae) and developmental phases of the gravid female. Parasite. 2005;12(3):241–50.
12. Karmouta R, Mikailov A, Johnson R. Young woman with black spot on foot. Ann Emerg Med. 2018;71(1):151–6.
13. Joseph JK, Bazile J, Mutter J, et al. Tungiasis in rural Haiti: a community-based response. Trans R Soc Trop Med Hyg. 2006;100:970–4.
14. Heukelbach J, Franck S, Feldmeier H. Therapy of tungiasis: a double-blinded randomized controlled trial with oral ivermectin. Mem Inst Oswaldo Cruz. 2004;99:873–6.
15. Buckendahl J, Heukelbach J, Ariza L, Kehr JD, Seidenschwang M, Feldmeier H. Control of tungiasis through intermittent application of a plant-based repellent: an intervention study in a resource-poor community in Brazil. PLoS Negl Trop Dis. 2010;4(11):e879.
16. Thielecke M, Nordin P, Ngomi N, Feldmeier H. Treatment of tungiasis with dimeticone: a proof-of-principle study in rural Kenya. PLoS Negl Trop Dis. 2014;8(7):1–10.
17. Nordin P, Thielecke M, Ngomi N, Mudanga GM, Krantz I, Feldmeier H. Treatment of tungiasis with a two-component dimeticone: a comparison between moistening the whole foot and directly targeting the embedded sand fleas. Trop Med Health. 2017;45:1–7.
18. Leung A, Woo T, Robson W, Trotter M. A tourist with tungiasis. CMAJ. 2007;177:343–4.
19. Elson L, Wright K, Swift J, Feldmeier H. Control of tungiasis in absence of a roadmap: grassroots and global approaches. Trop Med Infect Dis. 2017;2:1–13.

Onchocerciasis

Michele E. Murdoch

Key Points

- Onchocerciasis should be considered a diagnosis in travelers or migrants presenting with pruritus and skin lesions.
- Such patients should have a detailed travel history taken. There can be a long latency period between the time of infection and the onset of symptoms. Hence, patients may forget to mention a relevant visit to an endemic country. Latency periods of 3 months to 3 years have been reported with a mean period of 18 months.
- A peripheral eosinophilia may or may not be present.
- The diagnosis is confirmed by the finding of *O. volvulus* microfilariae in skin snips.
- A combination of doxycycline for 4–6 weeks in addition to a single dose of ivermectin is advised for imported cases of onchocerciasis.
- Loiasis should be excluded before using ivermectin in patients who have traveled from co-endemic areas.

M. E. Murdoch (✉)
Department of Dermatology, West Herts Teaching Hospitals NHS Trust, Watford General Hospital, Watford, Herts, UK
e-mail: michele.murdoch@nhs.net

Introduction

Onchocerciasis is a parasitic infection caused by the nematode worm *Onchocerca volvulus*. It is transmitted to humans by bites of *Simulium* blackflies that breed alongside fast-flowing rivers. There are an estimated 19.6 million infected people worldwide [1] most of whom live in tropical Africa. Short-term travelers are at risk of infection whenever they visit endemic areas, especially if they spend time in or near rivers. Cases of imported onchocerciasis present differently in travelers compared with migrants from endemic areas. Onchocerciasis in travelers has subtle and non-specific features that may lead to misdiagnosis or under-reporting by physicians in non-endemic areas who are unfamiliar with the disease. Onchocerciasis should be considered a diagnosis in travelers or migrants presenting with pruritus and skin lesions, with or without eosinophilia.

Epidemiology

Notably, 99% of cases are seen in 31 countries across tropical Africa. Previously, there were also 13 small foci of infection within six countries of Latin America, but the Onchocerciasis Elimination Program for the Americas (OEPA) succeeded in eliminating transmission of

W. Robles (ed.), *Skin Disease in Travelers*, Updates in Clinical Dermatology,
https://doi.org/10.1007/978-3-031-57836-6_28

infection in Colombia in 2013 [2], followed by Ecuador, Mexico, and Guatemala in 2014, 2015, and 2016, respectively [3] (Fig. 1). The two remaining foci with ongoing transmission in Brazil and Venezuela together form a single large transmission zone along the border of these two countries. It is difficult for the control program to reach the Yanomani tribes within this remote region. Foci of infection are also seen in Yemen.

Cases of imported onchocerciasis to non-endemic areas are relatively rare. The Geosentinel Surveillance Network is a global network of medicine/travel clinics established in 1995 to detect morbidity trends in travelers. Their data published in 2007 revealed that 271 (0.62%) of 43,722 cases were filarial infections, of which 37% were infected with *O. volvulus.* Migrants and migrants visiting friends and family in endemic areas formed the majority of cases of diagnosed onchocerciais (48%) compared with

non-endemic visitors (20%). The majority of patients with *O. volvulus* infections had trip durations of up to 1 month [4]. A retrospective study of a cohort of immigrants and travelers with one of the 13 core neglected tropical diseases (NTD) at a Tropical Medical Referral Unit in Spain from 1989 to 2007 found that onchocerciasis was the most frequent NTD in immigrants with 240/2634 (9.1%) cases, mainly acquired in sub-Saharan Africa and was the second most frequent NTD in travelers with 17/3277 (0.5%) cases. Of these, 16 had had stays of >3 months (range 3–336 months), and one patient had traveled for 1 month. All had visited sub-Saharan Africa, and some patients had visited more than one country. Onchocerciasis was also the most commonly diagnosed NTD in any traveler who had traveled back to their country of origin to visit family and friends (VFR) with 14/257 (5.4%) cases [5]. The study also noted a reduction in the number of new cases of

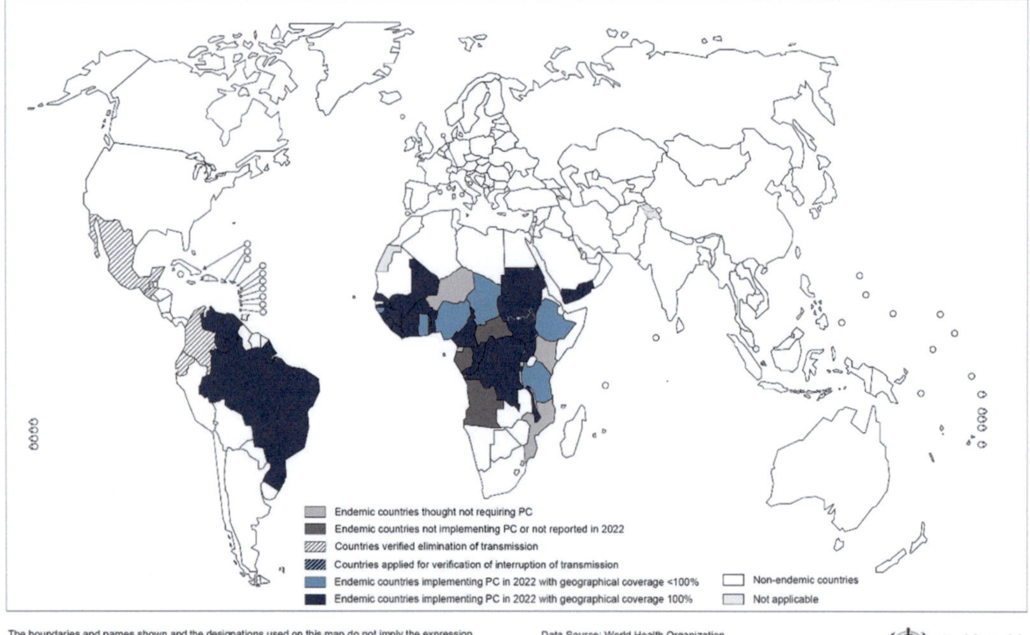

Fig. 1 Distribution of onchocerciasis and status of preventive chemotherapy in endemic countries, 2022. Data source: World Health Organization. Map Production: Control of Neglected Tropical Diseases (NTD), World Health Organization. Reproduced from WHO Preventive Chemotherapy Joint Reporting Form. Annual country reports, 2022. https://www.who.int/images/default-source/maps/onchocerciasis_2022.png?sfvrsn=407395cf_1 (accessed 12 July 2024). With permission from the World Health Organization

onchocerciasis per new African immigrants each year over the period of the study. A medical literature review of English and French articles from 1994 to 2014 identified 29 cases of imported onchocerciasis (migrants 18 (60%), returned travelers 3 (10%), and expatriates 9 (30%) [6]. A review of 31 cases of filariasis in Paris between 2002 and 2011 found four cases of onchocerciasis (3 immigrants from Cameroon, Sierra Leone, and Senegal and one traveler from Central Africa with arm swelling) [7]. A review of 289 NTD cases in 283 patients from 2000 to 2015 at the Infectious and Tropical Diseases Unit in Florence found two (0.7%) cases of onchocerciasis [8]. The largest case series of imported onchocerciasis to date from a reference clinical unit in Spain over a 17-year period identified 400 imported cases in migrants, all from sub-Saharan Africa and their most common symptom was pruritus [9].

The incidence of imported cases of onchocerciasis appears to be decreasing, no doubt a reflection of the success of global control and elimination programs, but at present, both migrants and travelers remain at risk for onchocerciasis [10].

Mode of Infection

The life cycle of onchocerciasis is shown in Fig. 2. Humans become infected whenever they are in the vicinity of rivers, as the pupae of the vector blackfly develop attached to stems of vegetation which trail in the water. Once the pupae have developed into adult flies, the female fly has to take a human blood meal to ensure the maturation of her eggs. Humans therefore become bitten whenever they are in contact with the water (such as swimming, fishing, collecting water, or washing) or in close proximity to the rivers. The infective L$_3$ larvae of *O. volvulus* are transmitted to the dermis of the human at the same time as the fly takes its blood meal and enters the subcutaneous tissue. Over a period of 6–12 months, the nematode larvae develop into adult worms within the human, but at this stage, the infection is essentially asymptomatic. The adult worms subsequently mate, and then the female worm starts to produce thousands of microfilariae each day which concentrate in the dermis of the skin and eyes and start to produce symptoms. This long latency period before microfilariae are produced and cause symptoms means that is very important

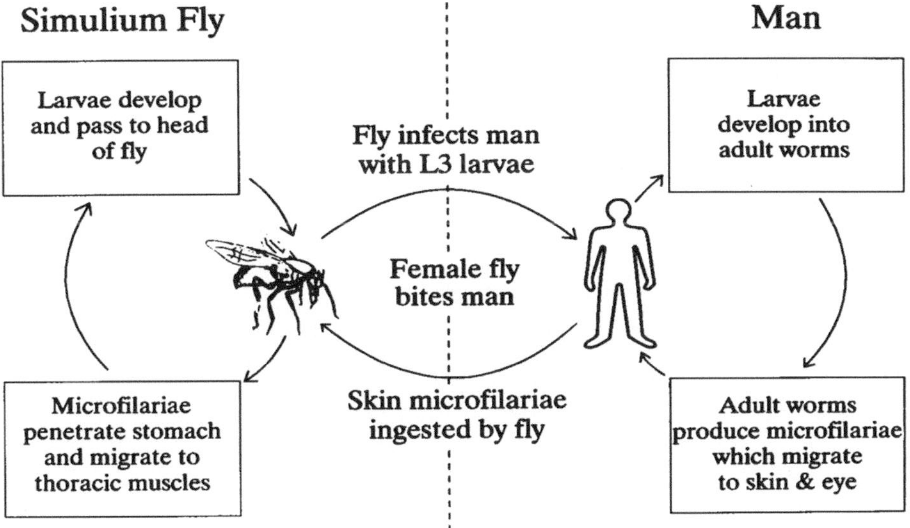

Fig. 2 The life cycle of *Onchocerca* volvulus (courtesy of the International Centre for Eye Health, London)

to take a full travel history in anyone presenting with fever +/− a non-specific itchy rash as the patient may have forgotten to mention travel which had occurred so many months previously. Latency periods of 3 months to 3 years have been reported with a mean period of 18 months [11].

Clinical Features

Travelers

Travelers who only remain within endemic areas for short periods of time (less than 3 months) are generally at low risk of infection because many bites are needed before becoming infected. In contrast, travelers such as long-term missionaries, long-term volunteers, field researchers, and servicemen who remain in endemic areas for longer periods are at higher risk of infection. In most case series, infected travelers had a minimum stay of 3 months with a median of approximately 2 years.

However, a cluster of cases was reported in one group of young people who went on a short-term Operation Raleigh expedition to a highly endemic region of Cameroon during the transmission season. A total of 143 people went to the area with a mean duration of stay of 3 months (range 27 days to 15 months). Onchocerciasis was diagnosed in 22 (26%) of the 85 respondents to a follow-up questionnaire after the initial case was diagnosed 15 months after leaving the endemic area [12]. The correct diagnosis of onchocercal infection may be delayed as physicians in non-endemic areas are unfamiliar with onchocerciasis. The most common presenting features are changes in the skin including itching and/or an itchy nonspecific urticated papular eruption, often limited to one limb or to one particular area of the body such as the shoulder or waist [13] (Fig. 3). Limb edema may also occur either in association with the rash [14–17] or on its own [18] and affected 43.3% of travelers/expatriates in one review [6]. Other early manifestations include arthralgia and fever. Onchocercal nodules, or onchocercomata, are rare in travelers.

Eye lacrimation, itching, burning, and conjunctival congestion may also occur, but, in general, serious eye pathology is not common in infected travelers.

Travelers have been noted to be symptomatic for 6 months before onchocerciasis was considered a diagnosis but had a shorter time to diagnosis compared with migrants [10]. Asymptomatic infection is a common finding with imported onchocerciasis with cases only detected when referred for unexplained eosinophilia, a raised IgE, or as a result of a similar exposure history to another known case.

Long-Term Residents and Migrants

Long-term residents in endemic areas have different clinical manifestations with itching in addition to a variety of skin and ocular clinical findings. If long-term residents migrate to a developed country then they may present with these more florid

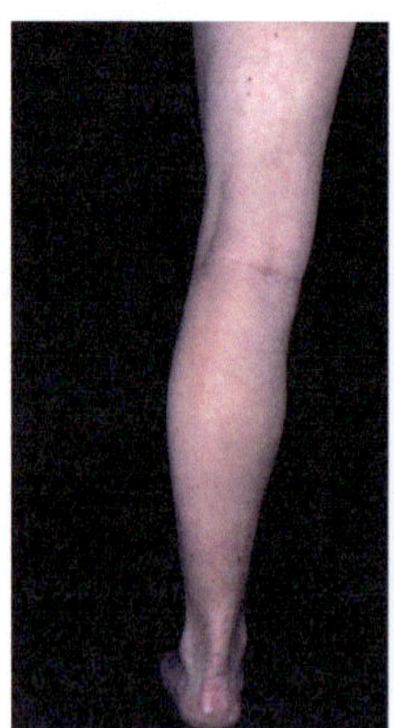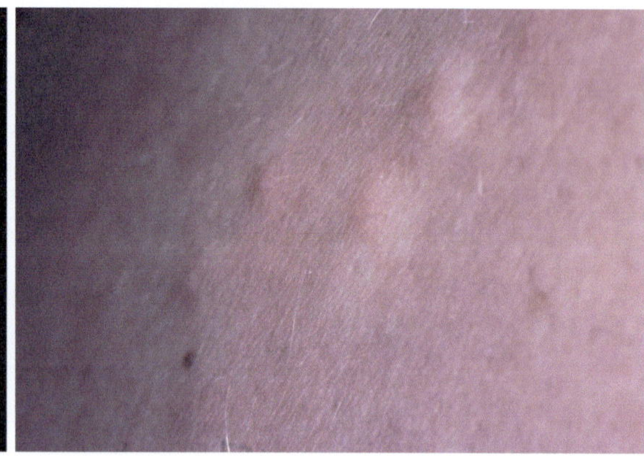

Fig. 3 Subtle urticated papular rash on one leg in a young female traveler who presented 15 months after leaving Cameroon (inset—close up of urticated papules)

clinical signs. The various forms of onchocercal skin disease in long-term residents of endemic areas have been classified into acute papular onchodermatitis, chronic papular onchodermatitis, lichenified onchodermatitis, atrophy, and depigmentation [19]. Migrants from the highly endemic Kuwara province of Ethiopia were found to have these typical onchocercal skin manifestations, as well as eye disease, when they immigrated to Israel [20]. A later study of 27 Ethiopian migrants from this endemic area to Israel also found that the most common presentation was skin changes typical of long-term residents of endemic areas with lichenifed onchodermatitis in combination with atrophy and depigmentation [21]. (These cases had all been missed during a general health screening on arrival in Israel and were later identified by active referral and screening of patients with a rash or pruritus.)

Approximately two-thirds of migrants report ocular symptoms and 20–80% have ocular involvement on slit-lamp examination [6, 11, 20]. Old corneal scarring, subepthelial infiltrates, corneal haze, active anterior segment inflammation, and ocular microfilariae have been reported [20]. Most ocular involvement in imported cases is mild, and posterior segment eye disease is rarely observed.

Onchocercal Nodules (Onchocercomata)

Residents of endemic areas often have firm, smooth, asymptomatic subcutaneous nodules overlying bony prominences which can often be palpated overlying the iliac crests of the pelvic girdle in adults and on the head in children. The nodules consist of adult female *Onchocerca* worms coiled up and surrounded by fibrous tissue. Nodules are more common on the scalp in Central and Southern America. Subcutaneous nodules were present in 29% of immigrants in the large Spanish case series [9].

Diagnosis

FBC

A peripheral eosinophilia may be present in two-thirds of travelers [11].

Serum IgE

Between 50% and 90% of patients have elevated IgE levels [9, 11].

Skin Snips

The finding of *O. volvulus* microfilariae in skin snips is the most reliable form of diagnosis. However, travelers are likely to be only lightly infected, and therefore skin snips may well prove negative. The higher the number of skin snips taken, the greater the sensitivity of the test. Usually, six skin snips are taken in travelers, one from each side of the iliac crests, scapulae, and calves. If there is a rash affecting one side of the body, it is worth taking a skin snip from the affected site.

Other Parasitological Forms of Diagnosis

Microfilariae may be detected in the cornea and anterior chamber of the eye on slit lamp examination. Patients are asked to keep their heads down for 2 min prior to the examination.

If an onchcoercal nodule is present, this may be surgically excised and adult *Onchcoerca* visualized, but nodules are uncommon in travelers and nodulectomy is not a standard diagnostic procedure.

PCR Diagnosis

A highly sensitive and specific technique available in research laboratories is the detection of onchocercal DNA in skin snips by targeting the repetitive DNA sequence known as O-150 (found only in *O. volvulus*) [22]. PCR can also detect parasite DNA in skin scrapings.

Serology

Although IgG anti-filarial tests are positive in onchocerciasis, they lack specificity as they have cross-reactivity with other filarial infections. A commercially available IgG$_4$ rapid diagnostic test (RDT) using a recombinant antigen OV-16, SD Bioline Onchocerciaisis RDT, (Standard Diagnostics, now Abbott, Gyeonggi-do, South Korea) has a high specificity and sensitivity) [23, 24]. Although primarily used as a field tool for confirmation of elimination of transmission, it may be useful diagnostically in patients with suspected onchocerciasis.

Prevention

The mainstay of prevention of infection is to avoid endemic areas if possible, but if travel to such areas cannot be prevented, then expert advice on regional and seasonal health risks for the areas should be sought prior to travel. Onchocerciasis may be acquired during a relatively short visit to a highly endemic region during the transmission season [12]. The best advice is to limit time near any known river breeding sites and to take active measures against insect bites. Blackflies are daytime biters, i.e., when most humans are active. Travelers in endemic areas should wear loose-fitting clothing, long sleeves, long trousers, and socks if out of doors from dawn to dusk to minimize accessibility for bites from *Simulium* blackflies. Garments may be sprayed or impregnated with an insect repellent, such as N,N-diethyl-3-methylbenzamide (DEET) and an insect repellent should also be applied to any exposed skin. The efficacy of various DEET concentrations and NO MAS (active component: para-menthane-3,8-diol and lemon grass oil) skin repellents studied in an endemic area in Ghana found that the highest protection provided was 80.8% by NO MAS and the least at 42.5% by the 13% DEET product. The period of absolute protection was 5 h by NO MAS and 1 h by 50% DEET product. No significant increase in protection was offered beyond 25% active DEET [25]. There is no treatment routinely given to prevent onchocerciasis at present, and no preventive vaccine is available.

Treatment

Ivermectin

The standard treatment is a single dose of ivermectin 150 µg/kg orally, which is repeated at intervals depending on the recurrence of symptoms and eosinophilia [26]. Ivermectin is primarily microfilaricidal and theoretically cure would require long-term annual or 6-monthly treatment throughout the approximate 10 year life span of the adult *O. volvulus* worms. In practice, though, short courses do seem to be sufficient in this group of lightly infected travelers and a group reassessed 10 years after treatment had stopped appeared to be free of infection despite having stopped ivermectin when symptoms resolved after an average of 3.9 doses over a median length of treatment of 1.75 years [27].

N.B. Prior to any treatment with ivermectin, it is important to check whether or not the patient has visited an onchocerciasis area which is also co-endemic for loiasis because if the patient has high numbers of *Loa loa* microfilariae in the bloodstream ivermectin can cause neurological side effects, including even fatal encephalopathy. Onchocerciasis and loiasis are co-endemic in parts of many central African countries including Angola, Cameroon, Central African Republic, Chad, Congo, Democratic Republic of Congo, Equatorial Guinea, Ethiopia, Gabon, Nigeria, and Sudan.

Doxycycline

Doxycycline is macrofilaricidal as it kills the endosymbiotic *Wolbachia* bacteria which reside within *O. volvulus* and are essential for is fertility. Various treatment regimens have been tried but the macrofilaricidal effect is strongest with 200 mg/day for 6 weeks. Doxycycline is macrofilaricidal on its own, but ivermectin may also be given 1 week before doxycycline for faster symptom relief, as microfilariae are not affected by *Wolbachia* depletion and otherwise would only reduce by natural decay [28]. Doxycycline is contra-indicated in children less than 9 years of age and in pregnancy.

Future Treatments

Moxidectin has been shown to be a more effective microfilaricidal drug than ivermectin in a randomized, controlled, double-blind phase 3 trial in endemic communities [29], but it is not in routine use yet to treat individual travelers. A single dose or short-course macrofilaricidal drug is much needed. There is no vaccine available yet for onchocerciasis.

References

1. GBD 2021 Diseases and Injuries Collaborators. Global incidence, prevalence, years lived with disability (YLDs), disabilityadjusted life-years (DALYs), and healthy life expectancy (HALE) for 371 diseases and injuries for 204 countries and territories and 811 subnational locations, 1990-2021: a systematic analysis for the Global Burden of Disease Study 2021. Lancet. 2024;403(10440):2133–61.
2. Nicholls RS, Duque S, Olaya LA, López MC, Sánchez SB, Morales AL, et al. Elimination of onchocerciasis from Colombia: first proof of concept of river blindness elimination in the world. Parasit Vectors. 2018;11:237.
3. World Health Organization. Progress towards eliminating onchocerciasis in the WHO Region of the Americas: elimination of transmission in the northeast focus of the Bolivarian Republic of Venezuela. Wkly Epidemiol Rec. 2017;92:617–23.
4. Lipner EM, Law MA, Barnett E, Keystone JS, von Sonnenburg F, Loutan L, et al. Filariasis in travelers presenting to the GeoSentinel Surveillance Network. PLoS Negl Trop Dis. 2007;1(3):e88.
5. Norman FF, de Ayala AP, Pérez-Molina JA, Monge-Maillo B, Zamarrón P, López-Vélez R. Neglected tropical diseases outside the tropics. PLoS Negl Trop Dis. 2010;4(7):e762.
6. Antinori S, Parravicini C, Galimberti L, Tosoni A, Giunta P, Galli M, et al. Is imported onchocerciasis a truly rare entity? Case report and review of the literature. Travel Med Infect Dis. 2017;16:11–7.
7. Develoux M, Hennequin C, Le Loup G, Paris L, Magne D, Belkadi G, et al. Imported filariasis in Europe: a series of 31 cases from Metropolitan France. Eur J Intern Med. 2017;37:e37–9.
8. Zammarchi L, Vellere I, Stella L, Bartalesi F, Strohmeyer M, Bartoloni A. Spectrum and burden of neglected tropical diseases observed in an infectious and tropical diseases unit in Florence, Italy (2000–2015). Intern Emerg Med. 2017;12:467–77.
9. Puente S, Ramirez-Olivencia G, Lago M, Subirats M, Perez-Blazquez E, Bru F, et al. Dermatological manifestations in onchocerciasis: a retrospective study of 400 imported cases. Enferm Infecc Microbiol Clin. 2018;36(10):633–9.
10. Showler AJ, Nutman TB. Imported onchocerciasis in migrants and travelers. Curr Opin Infect Dis. 2018;31(5):393–8.
11. Mc Carthy JS, Ottesen EA, Nutman TB. Onchocerciasis in endemic and nonendemic populations: differences in clinical presentation and immunologic findings. J Infect Dis. 1994;170:736–41.
12. Pryce D, Behrens R, Davidson R, Chiodini P, Bryceson A, McLeod J. Onchocerciasis in members of an expedition to Cameroon: role of advice before travel and long term follow up. BMJ. 1992;304:1285–6.
13. Glover M, Murdoch M, Leigh I. Subtle early features of onchocerciasis in a European. J R Soc Med. 1991;84(7):435.
14. Harvey RJ. The early diagnosis and treatment of onchocerciasis. Cent Afr J Med. 1967;13:242–5.
15. Nguyen JC, Murphy ME, Nutman TB, Neafie RC, Maturo S, Burke DS, et al. Cutaneous onchocerciasis in an American traveler. Int J Dermatol. 2005;44:125–8.
16. Ezzedine K, Malvy D, Dhaussy I, Steels E, Castelein C, De Dobbeler G, et al. Onchocerciasis-associated limb swelling in a traveler returning from Cameroon. J Travel Med. 2006;13(1):50–3.
17. Wolfe MS, Petersen JL, Neafie RC, Connor DH, Purtilo DT. Onchocerciasis presenting with swelling of limb. Am J Trop Med Hyg. 1974;23(3):361–8.
18. Jopling WH. Onchocerciasis Presenting Without Dermatitis. BMJ. 1960;1(5176):861. https://doi.org/10.1136/bmj.1.5176.861.
19. Murdoch ME, Hay RJ, MacKenzie CD, Williams JF, Ghalib HW, Cousens S, et al. A clinical classification and grading system of the cutaneous changes in onchocerciasis. Br J Dermatol. 1993;129(3):260–9.
20. Enk CD, Anteby I, Abramson N, Amer R, Amit Y, Bergshtein-Kronhaus T, et al. Onchocerciasis among Ethiopian immigrants in Israel. Isr Med Assoc J. 2003;5:485–8.

21. Baum S, Greenberger S, Pavlotsky F, Solomon M, Enk CD, Schwartz E, et al. Late-onset onchocercal skin disease among Ethiopian immigrants. Br J Dermatol. 2014;171:1078–83.
22. Zimmerman PA, Guderian RH, Aruajo E, Elson L, Phadke P, Kubofcik J, et al. Polymerase chain reaction-based diagnosis of Onchocerca volvulus infection: improved detection of patients with onchocerciasis. J Infect Dis. 1994;169:686–9.
23. Weil GJ, Steel C, Liftis F, Li B-W, Mearns G, Lobos E, et al. A rapid-format antibody card test for diagnosis of onchocerciasis. J Infect Dis. 2000;182:1796–9.
24. Dieye Y, Storey HL, Barrett KL, Gerth-Guyette E, Di Giorgio L, Golden A, et al. Feasibility of utilizing the SD BIOLINE Onchocerciasis IgG4 rapid test in onchocerciasis surveillance in Senegal. PLoS Negl Trop Dis. 2017;11(10):e0005884.
25. Wilson MD, Osei-Atweneboana M, Boakye DA, Osei-Akoto I, Obuobi E, Wiafe C, et al. Efficacy of DEET and non-DEETbased insect repellents against bites of Simulium damnosum vectors of onchocerciasis. Med Vet Entomol. 2013;27:226–31.
26. Godfrey-Faussett P, Dow C, Black ME, Bryceson AD. Ivermectin in the treatment of onchocerciasis in Britain. Trop Med Parasitol. 1991;42:82–4.
27. Henry NL, Law M, Nutman TB, Klion AD. Onchocerciasis in a nonendemic population: clinical and immunologic assessment before treatment and at the time of presumed cure. J Infect Dis. 2001;183:512–6.
28. Hoerauf A. Filariasis: new drugs and new opportunities for lymphatic filariasis and onchocerciasis. Curr Opin Infect Dis. 2008;21:673–81.
29. Opoku NO, Bakajika DK, Kanza EM, Howard H, Mambandu GL, Nyathirombo A, et al. Single dose moxidectin versus ivermectin for Onchocerca volvulus infection in Ghana, Liberia, and the Democratic Republic of the Congo: a randomised, controlled, double-blind phase 3 trial. Lancet. 2018;392:1207–16.

Part VIII

Dermatoses Caused by Injury

Cold Injuries

Markus Starink

Key Points

- Low temperatures can cause direct injuries to the skin or trigger or worsen underlying skin diseases.
- Cold injuries and cold-related skin diseases are not strictly confined to cold/freezing conditions, but can also be induced by wind and humidity.
- Vasoconstriction plays a pivotal role in cold injuries and cold-induced skin diseases.
- Frostbite and trench foot are medical emergencies and rewarming should be started as soon as possible.
- Pernio and Raynaud phenomenon are relatively common and harmless conditions. However, they can also be a manifestation of an underlying systemic condition.
- Prevention of cold injuries consists of keeping the area (hands, feet, face) warm and dry.

Introduction

Low temperatures can have several effects on the skin. It can cause direct injuries to the skin, as in frostbite. Low temperatures can also trigger or worsen underlying skin diseases, such as pernio/

M. Starink (✉)
Department of Dermatology, Amsterdam University Medical Centre, Huid Medical Centre,
Amsterdam, The Netherlands

chilblains, Raynaud, and cold urticaria. Travelers to cold areas such as mountains (climbers, winter sports) or arctic environments can be affected. However, travelers do not necessarily have to be in these environments. Humidity, rain, and wind can produce hypothermia with temperatures around 10 °C (50 °F). Of note, wet skin loses heat 25 times faster compared with dry skin [1]. For example, pernio and Raynaud can also occur in summertime when there is rain and wind. Exact numbers on how often travelers present with cold-related injuries are lacking. This chapter starts with the injuries directly caused by coldness, followed by more or less common diseases that are triggered or worsened by low temperatures and that can affect travelers. Rare diseases such as cold urticaria, cold panniculitis, cryoglobulinemia, and cold agglutinins are beyond the scope of this book.

Frostbite

Clinical Manifestations

Frostbite can occur when exposure to low temperatures (usually below −2 °C/28 °F) causes freezing of skin and/or other tissues. It is most often seen in exposed areas such as face (ears, nose), fingers, and toes. The first symptom is numbness, followed by clumsiness with swelling

W. Robles (ed.), *Skin Disease in Travelers*, Updates in Clinical Dermatology,
https://doi.org/10.1007/978-3-031-57836-6_29

and white or blue-purple coloration of the skin. These symptoms (called "frostnip") still resolve with rewarming, without permanent tissue damage. The symptoms progress to frostbite with prolonged exposure to cold [2].

There are several classifications, each with advantages and disadvantages. Classification similar to burns is still widely used and divides frostbite into superficial (first- and second-degree injury) and deep (third- and fourth-degree injury) [2, 3]. These symptoms are only recognizable upon rewarming. *First-degree* frostbite is very superficial and characterized by redness with a central area of pallor and anesthesia of the skin, surrounded by edema ("frostnip"). Usually, full recovery is expected. In *second-degree* frostbite, large blisters containing clear fluid develop, usually within 24 h. The blisters are surrounded by edema and erythema. Healing occurs, often with long-term sensory neuropathy with significant cold sensitivity. In *third-degree* frostbite, there is full-thickness dermal involvement, with hemorrhagic bulla formation or development of waxy, dry, mummified skin. The tissue loss is permanent. In *fourth-degree* frostbite, there is full-thickness involvement and loss of skin, muscle, tendon, and sometimes even bone. Usually, this results in amputation. A more recent classification uses four grades for frostbite of hand and foot, based on the appearance of the lesion after rapid rewarming. This classification better predicts sequelae. In this classification, *first-degree* frostbite is characterized by no cyanosis on the extremity. This predicts no amputation and no sequelae. *Second-degree* involves cyanosis isolated to the distal phalanx. This predicts only soft tissue amputation and fingernail or toenail sequelae. *Third-degree* frostbite is characterized by intermediate and proximal phalangeal cyanosis. This predicts bone amputation of the digit and functional sequelae. *Fourth-degree* frostbite involves cyanosis over the carpal or tarsal bones. This predicts large bone amputation of the limb with systemic effects [4].

Epidemiology

Frostbite is most frequently seen in winter sporters, mountaineers [3], other cold weather sporters, soldiers, people working in the cold, and the homeless. Modern equipment and clothing are available to protect adventure tourists from frostbite. The condition now occurs mainly as the result of accidents, severe unexpected weather, or failure to plan appropriately [1].

Pathogenesis

Frostbite is the consequence of a combination of formation of extracellular and (in case of rapid freezing) intracellular ice crystals, vasoconstriction (alternated by vasodilatation, known as "hunting reaction"), vascular occlusion, and damage due to inflammatory mediators. This leads to both immediate cold-induced cell death and development of reperfusion-related localized inflammatory processes and tissue ischemia [3].

Diagnosis

Frostbite is a clinical diagnosis. It is not possible to reliably judge the extent of damage shortly after the frostbite. Determining the depth of the injury requires clinical tests (like the cold-water immersion test) and imaging studies [3].

Management

Rapid rewarming in a warm (37–39 °C, 98.6–102.2 °F) water bad is the cornerstone of the therapy [2]. If not available, body heat can be used (placing frostbitten fingers in the axillae). Rubbing areas in an attempt to rewarm them is not advised, this can make the tissue damage worse. The same goes for walking after rewarming. For that reason, rewarming should only start as soon as a patient is "safe" in a warm area where he/she can stay. For example, if a hiker must walk to obtain help, do not start the warming process. Refreezing the injured area causes damage that is worse than the original frostbite. Usually, rewarming takes 15–30 min, until the tissue is red or purple and soft to touch. It is usually painful, so adequate analgesia (NSAID/Ibuprofen 12 mg/kg/day divided twice daily to a maximum of 2400 mg/day divided four times daily, opiates) should be given. Ibuprofen also works as an anti-inflammatory drug and should be continued until wounds are healed or amputation occurs. Blisters should be kept intact or drained; deroofing is not recommended. Removal of dead tissue should be delayed till there is a clear division between vital and dead tissue (often several weeks to months) [1–3]. In general, patients should be admitted for supportive care, in an attempt to prevent secondary infection and amputation. In extensive cases, thrombolytic therapy (rTPA) and/or vasodilatation (Iloprost) is given [3]. If systemic hypothermia is present, this should, of course, be given priority.

Trench Foot

Clinical Manifestations

Trench foot is also known as "immersion foot" and "nonfreezing cold injury". Trench foot is the consequence of prolonged exposure of the feet to cold, humid/wet, occluded, and/or often unhygienic conditions. It usually occurs at temperatures above freezing, unlike frostbite. Initial symptoms are tingling or itching, which progresses to numbness or pain. Later, when the patient is removed from the cold environment and rewarming is performed, the feet become red or purple and start to swell. There is a smell of decay as skin and underlying tissue become macerated. Often blisters and open sores are seen, usually due to pressure injury or mechanical damage. The affected feet are prone to gangrene and secondary infection. Because of hypoxic injury to nerves, often neuropathy persists indefinitely.

Epidemiology

Military people are most commonly affected. It was seen frequently in the trenches during World War I – it was estimated that trench foot contributed to the deaths of approximately 75,000 British soldiers. Travelers, hikers, and survivors of plane or ship accidents in wet environments are other known victims, due to exposure to cold and wet conditions for days, without removing wet boots and socks. Recently, it was described by visitors of festivals where there were cold, wet, and muddy conditions [5]. It is also seen in homeless. The frequency is unknown.

Pathogenesis

Trench foot can occur in temperatures up to 15 °C/59 °F. It can commence within 10–13 h. Cold alone does not cause trench foot; there is always a moisture component and often infection. The exact pathogenesis is unknown. It is probably the consequence of vasoconstriction, vascular damage, and destruction of nerves [5]. Risk factors are immobility, malnutrition, fatigue, tight boots, and poor hygiene.

Diagnosis

Trench foot is a clinical diagnosis. Typically, there is a history of prolonged exposure to cold (0–15 °C) and wet conditions. It can sometimes be difficult to distinguish trench foot from frostbite. They can even coexist. If there was no exposure to below-freezing temperatures, frostbite can be ruled out [6].

Management

Keeping the feet dry, warm, and clean are the first steps in the prevention. Changing socks regularly, applying emollient and/or talcum powder, regular inspection, bathing followed by patting dry, and letting the air dry the feet further are effective measures to prevent trench foot. For treatment of trench foot, see "Management" in the Frostbite paragraph. The major difference in the treatment of trench foot is that rewarming should be performed gradually by air drying at room temperature instead of warm water (unless frostbite co-exists). The affected extremity should be elevated [6].

Pernio

Clinical Manifestations

Pernio is one of the most prevalent cold-induced skin disorders. Pernio, also known as chilblains, perniosis, and chill burns, is an abnormal reaction of the microvasculature of the skin to coldness. It is characterized by red to purple, painful, burning, and often itchy macules, papules, plaques, or nodules on the acral parts of the body—the dorsal side of the fingers, hands, toes, feet, and heels. Sometimes the tip of the nose, helix, hips, and lower legs are affected. In severe cases blistering, wounds, ulcers, and secondary infection can occur. On examination, the affected skin feels cold. The lesions develop 12–14 h after exposure to coldness. They subside over the next couple of weeks [7]. One has to be aware that pernio is not strictly confined to cold conditions, but also to temperature changes, wind, and humidity. For example, cycling outside in summertime when it is raining and windy can cause significant temperature drops and induce pernio.

Epidemiology

Pernio can affect every gender and age group, but it is mostly seen in young and middle-aged women. Low body mass index, genetic predisposition, smoking, and vasoconstrictive medications are predisposing factors. Usually, patients have poor peripheral circulation (acrocyanosis), characterized by cold, blue-red-white mottled acral skin after exposure to coldness. Pernio is most common in cold climates and has a seasonal presentation, usually beginning in early winter and resolving by spring [7].

Pathogenesis

The exact pathogenesis is unclear. It is thought that pernio is caused by constriction of the small arteries and veins in the (acral) skin as a response to cold exposure. This results in hypoxemia, which in turn stimulates an inflammatory response [8]. Some people consider it as a kind of localized lymphocytic vasculitis.

Pernio can be associated with connective tissue diseases, especially with systemic lupus erythematosus (chilblain lupus) [9]. It can also be seen in association with amongst others Raynaud phenomenon, systemic sclerosis, rheumatic arthritis, anti-phospholipid syndrome, myelodysplastic disease, leukemia, and viral infections. Of note, pernio and pernio-like lesions are well-known skin manifestations of COVID-19 [10]. Especially if pernio persists beyond the cold season, one has to be wary of underlying disease.

Diagnosis

Pernio can be diagnosed based on clinical features and history taking.

A biopsy can be taken in atypical cases or if concomitant (systemic) disease is suspected. There are no strictly pathognomonic histopathological features, but the combination of papillary edema and superficial and deep, moderate to dense perivascular and peri-eccrine lymphocytic infiltrate, sometimes with lymphocytic vasculitis, is suggestive of the diagnosis. In addition to these features, chilblain lupus erythematosus shows interface changes.

Laboratory investigations can be performed for the evaluation of concomitant medical disorders.

Management

Patients should be aware that it is not a disease of just coldness, but that rapid temperature drops, wind, and humidity can also trigger pernio. It can usually be prevented by keeping hands and feet warm and dry, by wearing gloves, warm socks, and footwear. These days, battery-operated heated gloves and socks are available, in case normal gloves and socks/footwear are not sufficient. Some patients benefit from soaking hands in warm water for several minutes before exposure to cold. Others can benefit from Capsicum cream. Smokers have to be encouraged to stop smoking, as nicotine causes vasoconstriction. In severe cases, vasodilating drugs can be prescribed (Nifedipine) during colder periods. If patients present with pernio, topical corticosteroid cream can partly relieve itch and swelling [9, 10].

Raynaud Phenomenon

Clinical Features

Raynaud phenomenon is an episodic spasm of small arteries as an exaggerated response to low temperature or emotional stress. It is characterized by well-demarcated "tricolore" (white, blue, red) discoloration of the distal parts of the digits/toes. Rarely, the nose, ears, or lips are affected. Usually, it starts with a single finger turning cold, with a sharply demarcated white color. It then spreads to other digits, symmetrically on both hands. Digits II, III, and IV are most frequently involved, while the thumb is usually spared. Involvement of the thumb can even indicate a secondary cause. The white phase is followed by a blue phase, indicating cyanotic skin. Often numbness, pain, a burning sensation, and clumsiness of the hand occur. With rewarming, the ischemic phase (white/ blue) usually fades away after 15–20 min, resulting in the erythema of reperfusion. In total, attacks last minutes to several hours [11].

There are two variants. *Primary Raynaud phenomenon* (or "Raynaud disease") is not associated with underlying medical problems. Usually, there are symmetric attacks, <5 per day. Ischemic injury is absent, and lab investigations show no abnormalities. Nowadays, there is evidence that the primary Raynaud phenomenon may comprise several entities that include a functional vasospastic disorder, a physiologically appropriate thermoregulatory response, subclinical atherosclerosis, and "cold intolerance" [12]. *Secondary Raynaud phenomenon* (or "Raynaud syndrome") is uncommon and is associated with an underlying medical problem, for example, systemic sclerosis, systemic lupus erythematosus, thoracic outlet syndrome, thromboangiitis obliterans, cryoglobulinemia, myeloproliferative disorders, drug-induced, carpal tunnel syndrome. Depending on the cause, there can be among others asymmetric/single-digit attacks, absent pulses, asymmetric blood pressure, tissue necrosis, (intense) pain, abnormalities like sclerodactyly, digital pits, ulcers, nail-fold capillary abnormalities, and lab abnormalities [12].

Epidemiology

Primary Raynaud phenomenon is common. The prevalence is estimated at 3–20% in women and 3–14% in men. These percentages depend on the populations that are studied, for example, in colder climates, the prevalence is much higher. It is more common among young women, younger age groups, and family members of patients with Raynaud phenomenon [13]. The secondary Raynaud phenomenon is rare. The exact prevalence is not known.

Pathogenesis

When exposed to low temperatures, the blood flow to the skin is reduced, thereby reducing the loss of body heat and preserving normal core temperature. Raynaud phenomenon is an exaggerated vascular response to cold temperatures or emotional stress. As a consequence, the blood supply to fingers or toes is markedly reduced and the skin turns white, later blue, and finally red. The primary Raynaud phenomenon is thought to be caused by a possible local defect in normal vascular responses. In the secondary Raynaud phenomenon, the pathogenesis depends on the underlying disorder [11].

Diagnosis

Raynaud phenomenon is a clinical diagnosis with typical symptoms: the fingers are sensitive to cold temperatures and change color (white, blue, red) when exposed to cold. Differentiating primary from secondary Raynaud phenomenon can be difficult and requires careful history taking and physical examination. History taking includes signs and symptoms of underlying systemic disease, age of onset, involved digits, degree of symmetry and severity of the attacks, the presence of digital ulcerations, medication, and intoxication. Nailfold capillary microscopy is the method most commonly used to help distinguish primary from secondary variants. Enlarged or distorted capillary loops and/or dropout or loss of loops suggest an underlying autoimmune disease. When nailfold capillary microscopy is not available, serological testing (antinuclear antibody) can be performed [12].

Management

Usually, the symptoms of primary Raynaud phenomenon are completely reversible on rewarming or reduction of stress. In severe secondary Raynaud phenomenon, pain or ulceration of the tips of the fingers/toes may result from critical tissue ischemia.

The primary prevention is avoiding the cold and relative shifts from warmer to cooler temperatures. If people smoke or use stimulants, they should be encouraged to discontinue. In severe cases, medical treatment can be given: calcium channel blockers (Nifedipine) and/or Iloprost.

The primary Raynaud phenomenon can go into remission in the majority of patients. In up to 37% of patients with primary Raynaud phenomenon, eventually, a systemic disease can develop [11]. And thus, there can be a transition from presumed primary to secondary Raynaud phenomenon. Raynaud phenomenon can precede scleroderma for many years. Especially patients with primary Raynaud phenomenon and abnormal nailfold capillary patterns and serological abnormalities have to be followed up.

References

1. Travelers' Health, Centers for Disease Control and Prevention 2024, Section 4 (https://wwwnc.cdc.gov/travel/yellowbook/2020/noninfectious-health-risks/extremes-of-temperature).
2. McIntosh SE, et al. Wilderness Medical Society Clinical Practice Guidelines for the Prevention and Treatment of Frostbite: 2019 Update. Wilderness Environ Med. 2019;30(4S):S19–32.
3. Handford C, et al. Frostbite. Emerg Med Clin North Am. 2017;35(2):281–99.
4. Cauchy E, et al. Retrospective study of 70 cases of severe frostbite lesions: a proposed new classification scheme. Wilderness Environ Med. 2001 Winter;12(4):248–55.
5. Mistry K, et al. A review of trench foot: a disease of the past in the present. Clin Exp Dermatol. 2020;45(1):10–4.
6. Zafren K, et al. Nonfreezing cold water (trench foot) and warm water immersion injuries. Uptodate.com. Jun 02, 2020.
7. Whitman PA, Crane JS. Pernio. 2020 Aug 10. In: StatPearls [Internet]. Treasure Island, FL: StatPearls Publishing; 2020.
8. Shahi V, et al. Vasospasm Is a Consistent Finding in Pernio (Chilblains) and a Possible Clue to Pathogenesis. Dermatology. 2015;231(3):274–9.
9. Cappel JA, et al. Clinical characteristics, etiologic associations, laboratory findings, treatment, and proposal of diagnostic criteria of pernio (chilblains) in a series of 104 patients at Mayo Clinic, 2000 to 2011. Mayo Clin Proc. 2014;89(2):207–15.
10. Freeman EE, et al. American Academy of Dermatology Ad Hoc Task Force on COVID-19. Pernio-like skin lesions associated with COVID-19: A case series of 318 patients from 8 countries. J Am Acad Dermatol. 2020;83(2):486–92.
11. Wigley FM, et al. Raynaud's Phenomenon. N Engl J Med. 2016;375(6):556–65.
12. Pauling JD, et al. Raynaud's phenomenon-an update on diagnosis, classification and management. Clin Rheumatol. 2019;38(12):3317–30.
13. Wigley FM. Clinical manifestations and diagnosis of Raynaud phenomenon. Uptodate, July 2023.

Sunburn

Nisha Rishi Arujuna and Ljubomir B. Novaković

Key Points

- Sunburn is an acute inflammatory reaction of the skin induced by over-exposure to ultraviolet (UV) radiation.
- Primary prevention of sunburn is critical.
- The key to the prevention and treatment of sunburn is good sun protection behavior including the use of sunscreens.
- Sunburn is a self-limiting condition and typically requires only supportive care.
- Cellular damage caused by sunburn is irreversible and increases the risk of skin cancer.

Introduction

The Sun is a powerful center of attention for Earth and other planets that revolve around it. It holds the solar system together; provides life-giving light, heat, and energy to Earth; and generates space weather [1]. The sun is essential to sustain life on Earth, providing energy that organisms like plants use to form the basis of many food chains. The connection and interactions between the Sun and Earth drive the seasons, ocean currents, weather, climate, radiation belts, and auroras. The volume of the sun (radius of 432,168.6 miles or 695,508 kilometers) would need 1.3 million Earths to fill it [2]. The Sun is 93 million miles (150 million kilometers) from Earth, a distance defined as one astronomical unit (AU) [2]. The Sun has many names in different cultures. The Latin word for Sun is "sol," which is the main adjective for all things Sun-related: solar.

Deep in the sun's core, nuclear fusion converts hydrogen to helium, which generates energy. Photons which are particles of light, carry this energy through a spherical shell called the radiative zone to the top layer of the solar interior, the convection zone. Here, hot plasmas rise and fall, which transfers energy to the sun's surface, called the photosphere. It can take 170,000 years for a photon to complete its journey out of the sun, but once it exits, it zips through space at more than 186,000 miles a second. Solar photons reach Earth about eight minutes after being freed from the sun's interior, crossing an AU.

The sun emits substantial amounts of ultraviolet (UV) radiation, visible light (VL), and infrared radiation (IR), each of which carries photons of varying energies. The electromagnetic (EM) spectrum's classification is based on wave fre-

N. R. Arujuna (✉)
St John's Institute of Dermatology, Guy's and St Thomas' Hospitals NHS Foundation Trust, Kingston Hospital NHS Foundation Trust, London, UK
e-mail: nisha.arujuna3@nhs.net

L. B. Novaković
St John's Institute of Dermatology, Guy's & St Thomas' Hospitals NHS Foundation Trust and Lewisham & Greenwich NHS Trust, London, UK
e-mail: novakovic@doctors.org.uk

W. Robles (ed.), *Skin Disease in Travelers*, Updates in Clinical Dermatology,
https://doi.org/10.1007/978-3-031-57836-6_30

Table 1 Differences between UVA and UVB summarized

Characteristics	UVA	UVB
Wavelength	320–400 nm	290–320 nm
Percent of UV radiation	~95%	~5%
Depth of penetration	Dermis and hypodermis	Epidermis, top dermis layers
Erythema potential	Low	High
Pigment darkening potential	Immediate (IPD) Persistent (PPD)	Delayed (DT-delayed tanning)
Mechanism of tanning	Oxidation of melanin precursors in basal cell layers	Increased synthesis of melanin and increased melanocyte density
Mechanism of DNA damage	Indirect DNA damage via the formation of reactive oxygen species resulting in oxidative stress	Direct DNA damage via the formation of cyclobutane pyrimidine dimers and 6–4 photoproducts
Role in vitamin D	Breaks down vitamin D bound to vitamin D receptors	Directly involved in vitamin D production
Impact on skin	"Aging rays"; causes wrinkling, loss of elasticity, and pigmentation	"Burning rays"; causes sunburn and tanning, increasing the risk of skin cancer

quency. It includes, starting with the lowest frequency/energy and longest wavelengths, radio waves, microwaves, IR, VL, UV light, X-rays, and gamma rays.

The human body is exposed to terrestrial sunlight that contains UVB (290–320 nm), UVA (320–400 nm), VL (400–700 nm), and IR (700–1000 nm).

The depth of penetration of UV light depends on wavelength; longer wavelengths are with deeper penetration, so UVA would penetrate deeper into the skin in comparison with UVB. Practically, all of UVC (100–290 nm) is absorbed by the ozone layer.

UVA is 95% of UV radiation that reaches Earth with the remainder being UVB. UVA penetrates deeper into the skin layers including into the dermis and hypodermis. UVA has a low erythema potential. UVA causes tanning via oxidation of melanin precursors in basal cell layers not through an increase in melanin content, resulting in immediate pigment darkening (IPD) and persistent pigment darkening (PPD). In comparison, UVB induces a delayed tanning 3–7 days postexposure that lasts for weeks via increased synthesis of melanin and increased melanocyte density (Table 1).

UV radiation in small amounts is essential in the production of vitamin D. In the medical setting, controlled levels of UV radiation are used to treat skin diseases such as psoriasis, eczema, and vitiligo. Excessive UV radiation exposure acutely can result in tanning and sunburn and, in the longer term, UV radiation-induced degenerative changes leading to premature skin aging. Two significant public health problems as a result of chronic UV exposure are skin cancers and cataracts. Human behavior in the sun is considered to be a major cause of the rise in skin cancers; between two and three million non-melanoma skin cancers and approximately 132,000 melanoma skin cancers occur worldwide annually [3].

Factors Influencing UV Radiation Levels (Fig. 1)

Sun Elevation

The UV radiation path length through the Earth's atmosphere is determined by the elevation of the sun. The higher the sun is in the sky, the higher the UV radiation level. Hence, UV radiation varies with time of day and time of year.

Latitude

The closer the UV is in proximity to the equator, the higher the UV radiation level.

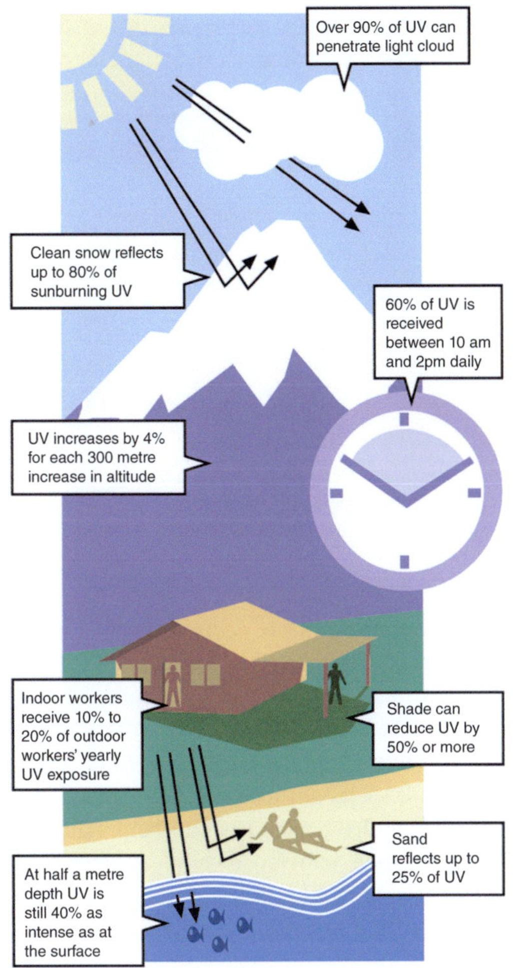

Fig. 1 Factors influencing UV radiation levels [3]. Reproduced with permission from the World Health Organization (WHO), accessed from https://www.who.int/uv/publications/en/UVIGuide.pdf

Cloud Cover

Cloudless skies result in the highest UV radiation levels. Over 90% of UV can penetrate through light cloud [3]. Dense cloud can reduce UV levels by a factor of six. Scattering can have the same effect as reflectance by various surfaces thus increasing total UV radiation levels.

Altitude

Less UV radiation is absorbed through thinner atmospheres at higher altitudes. With every 300 m increase in altitude, UV radiation levels increase by 4%. With every 1000 m increase in altitude, UV radiation levels increase by 10–12% [3].

Ozone

Ozone levels vary over the year and even across the day. Ozone absorbs some of the UV radiation that would otherwise reach the Earth's surface.

Reflection

UV radiation is scattered to varying degrees by different surfaces. Fresh clean snow can reflect as much as 80% of sun-burning UV radiation, sea foam about 25%, and dry beach sand about 15% [3]. Water transmits UV radiation to the extent that at half a meter in its depth, the UV radiation is still 40% as intense as it is at the surface [4].

Shade

Shade can reduce UV radiation by at least 50% [3]. However, it is important to appreciate that 2 h in the shade is equivalent to 1 h in the sunlight.

Windows

UV radiation transmission is approximately 0.2% for 4 mm window thickness and 0.004% for thickness with double glazing [4]. In particular, UVA is transmitted through windows effectively and can be a marker of abnormal sensitivity to

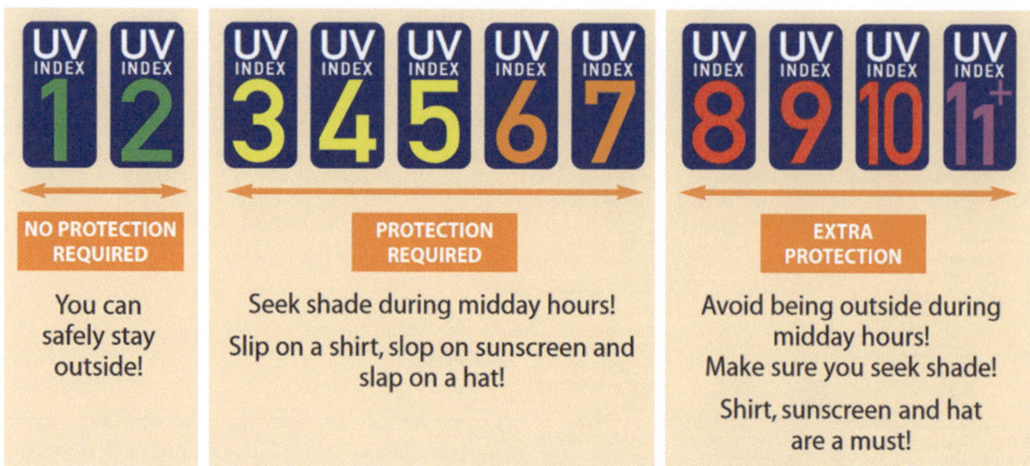

Fig. 2 Recommended sun protection scheme with simple "sound bite" messages [3]. Reproduced with permission from the World Health Organization (WHO), accessed from https://www.who.int/uv/publications/en/UVIGuide.pdf

UVA in patients who have photosensitivity responses through window glass. Plastic blinds can provide UV radiation and VL protection below 470 nm which is helpful in managing severe photodermatoses patients [4]. Indoor workers receive 10–20% of outdoor workers' yearly UV exposure [3].

Pollution

Haze in the atmosphere can increase UV radiation exposure.

The Global Solar UV Index

The Global Solar UV Index (UVI) should be an essential component in having an integrated and longer-term public health approach to sun protection. UVI is a measure of the intensity of UV radiation on the Earth's surface that is relevant to its effects on the human skin. It is an important vehicle to raise public awareness of the risks of excessive exposure to UV radiation. Both sunburn and cumulative UV radiation exposure play roles in the development of skin cancer.

The UVI range runs from 1 to 11+ and has UV radiation exposure categorized as follows: low is <2, moderate is 3–5, high is 6 and 7, very high is 8–10, and extreme is 11 and above. Basic sun protection measures are advised for UVI 3 to 7 and extra care is to be taken for UVI 8 and above. As more than 90% of non-melanoma skin cancers have been observed to occur in skin types I and II, basic sun protective messages associated with the UVI should focus on fair-skinned individuals who have a tendency to burn. Although darker-skinned individuals have a lower incidence of skin cancer, they are nevertheless susceptible to the harmful effects of UV radiation, especially on the immune system and the eye (Fig. 2).

Effects of UV Radiation on the Skin

UV has many effects on skin physiology, with some consequences occurring acutely and others in a delayed manner. The skin is the organ exposed to the vast majority of UV radiation the body encounters, and as a result of potentially uniquely damaging properties of UV, the biological protective response of the skin to UV is necessarily complex.

Skin chromophores, which are conjugated multiple bonded (unsaturated) atoms, absorb solar UV or visible radiation to cause a complex series of photochemical and photobiological events resulting in clinical features of cutaneous solar exposure. A chromophore may itself be a target biomolecule, for example, urocanic acid or DNA whereby its direct structural alteration by UV or visible radiation absorption initiates a biological response. Alternatively, a chromophore could also be a normal endogenous molecule, for example, porphyrin causing indirect photosensitized damage to adjacent biomolecules.

The acute clinical effects of solar UV radiation on the skin include inflammation resulting in sunburn, epidermal thickening, melanogenesis causing tanning, and immunosuppression for which the smaller UVB component is mainly responsible. Solar UVB radiation is also responsible for the synthesis of vitamin D. Skin type determines sensitivity to both the acute and chronic effects of UV radiation on the skin. Molecular and cellular effects underpin both the acute and chronic clinical effects.

Inflammation and Sunburn

UVB radiation induces a cascade of cytokines, vasoactive and neuroactive mediators in the skin that together result in an inflammatory response resulting in "sunburn." When the dose of UV exceeds a threshold damage response, keratinocytes activate apoptotic pathways that result in cell death. Such apoptotic epidermal keratinocyte cells can be identified by their characteristic eosinophilic cells with shrunken cytoplasm and pyknotic nuclei; these are known as "sunburn cells" (SBCs) [4].

Epidermal Hyperplasia

Following UV radiation exposure, cell injury induces damage signals such as p53 activation, which markedly alters keratinocyte physiology, mediating cell cycle arrest, activating DNA repair, and causing apoptosis if the damage is sufficiently great. However, after several hours of UV exposure, the damage response signals abate and the profound increased cellular DNA, RNA, protein synthesis, and mitosis mediated by a variety of epidermal growth factors result in cutane-

ous hyperplasia that lasts for several weeks [5]. This several-fold hyperplasia, particularly in the stratum corneum layer may then give some protection against later photodamage, in association with that provided by melanogenesis.

Melanization

Adaptive melanization, also known as tanning, is likely a complex physiological response involving multiple skin cell types interacting in a variety of ways. UV radiation enhances epidermal production and accumulation of melanin pigment. UV-mediated skin darkening is biphasic; the initial UVA-mediated skin darkening occurs from redistribution and/or molecular changes to existing epidermal melanin (through oxidation of melanin precursors in basal cell layers) and the delayed UVB-mediated skin darkening occurs from upregulation in melanin synthesis, increased melanocyte density, and subsequent transfer to keratinocytes that begins several hours to days after UV exposure [6]. Epidemiological data indicate that constitutive pigmentation protects against skin cancer as defects in the adaptive melanization pathway are linked with increased malignant neoplasm susceptibility [5].

Immunosuppression

Mechanisms involved in the induction of immunosuppression involve absorption of UVR by chromophores, damage/loss of resident Langerhans cells, local production of inflammatory mediators, infiltration of the skin by macrophages, and the generation of regulatory T-lymphocytes. Cytokine induction may be mediated through DNA photodamage; however, the precise chromophore initiating the actual immunosuppression itself remains controversial, with both DNA and urocanic acid being considered as candidate molecules. Exposure of keratinocytes to UV radiation results in the release of cytokines, such as tumor necrosis factor-alpha (TNF-α) and interleukin-10 (IL-10), and of adhesion molecules, some of which play a role in UV radiation-induced inflammation and immunosuppression [5]. UV radiation-induced inhibition of intercellular adhesion molecule-1 (ICAM-1) gene expression in fibroblasts appears to be mediated through DNA photodamage [5].

Vitamin D Production

Important factors affecting vitamin D status include extrinsic factors such as the amount of UVB exposure at a particular time of day, latitude and season, weather, pollution, and intrinsic factors such as genetic polymorphisms, degree of skin melanization, age, health, nutrition, and the practice of sun avoidance or protection. UV radiation is involved in the production of vitamin D in the stratum basale by direct conversion of 7-dehydrocholesterol (7-DHC) into pre-vitamin D_3 (cholecalciferol) [7]. Thermally converted into vitamin D3, it then binds to vitamin D binding protein in the blood to be activated sequentially by the liver and kidney. Cytochrome P 450 enzymes are crucial for the synthesis of biologically active vitamin D3 (calcitriol), which binds to intracellular vitamin D receptor (VDR) in most cells in the body. UVA tends to break down vitamin D bound to VDRs, whereas UVB is directly involved in vitamin D production. Feedback mechanisms and catabolism of pre-vitamin D3 to inactive metabolites (inactive tachysterol and inactive suprasterol) determine that vitamin D3 achieves plateau levels below the erythema threshold dose, so excessive UVB exposure cannot lead to vitamin D toxicity. The main function of vitamin D is the maintenance of calcium and phosphorus levels in the blood to support metabolic functions, bone mineralization, and neuromuscular transmission.

A high UVA-protection factor sunscreen enables significantly higher vitamin D synthesis than a low UVA-protection factor sunscreen because the former, by default, transmits more UVB than the latter [8]. Judicious use of daily broad-spectrum sunscreens with high UVA protection will not compromise vitamin D status in healthy individuals [9]. However, photoprotec-

tion strategies for patients with photosensitivity disorders that include high sun protection factor (SPF) sunscreens, along with protective clothing and encouraging shade-seeking behavior, are likely to compromise vitamin D status. Screening for vitamin D and supplementation are recommended in patients with photosensitivity disorders, for individuals with deeply pigmented skins, those wearing clothing that covers most of the body surface area, especially during pregnancy, in the elderly or in persons living at institutions. The concentration of serum 25(OH)D is a good indicator of vitamin D status and the target serum 25(OH)D should be at least 50 nmol/L (20 ng/mL) [9].

Skin Phototypes and Sunburn Staging

Fitzpatrick Skin Phototypes

The Fitzpatrick skin phototype classification is dependent upon the amount of melanin pigment in the skin (Table 2). This is determined by the individual's constitutional color (white, brown, or black skin) and the result of exposure to UV radiation (burning and tanning). Fairer skin burns easily and tans slowly, needing more protection against sun exposure. Darker skin burns less and tans more easily, needing less protection against sun exposure; however, it is more prone to developing post-inflammatory hyperpigmentation after injury. The amount of UV radiation, measured in energy per unit area, to produce erythema at an exposed site is referred to as the minimal erythema dose (MED), and this is significantly lower in individuals with a lower Fitzpatrick skin phototype grading.

Stages of Sunburn

Sunburn is an acute inflammatory reaction of the skin induced by over-exposure to UV radiation. The presentation of sunburn will vary based on the Fitzpatrick skin phototype and length of

Table 2 Fitzpatrick skin phototypes I–VI

Fitzpatrick skin phototype	Phenotype	Geographical origin	Epidermal eumelanin	Tanning ability	MED (mJ/cm^2)
I	**Unexposed skin is bright white** Blue/green eyes typical Freckling frequent	Northern European/British	+/−	Always burn, does not tan	15–30
II	**Unexposed skin is white** Blue, hazel, or brown eyes Red, blonde, or brown hair	European/Scandinavian	+	Burns easily, tans poorly	25–40
III	**Unexposed skin is fair** Brown eyes Dark hair	Southern/Central European	++	Tans after the initial burn	30–50
IV	**Unexposed skin is light brown** Dark eyes Dark hair	Mediterranean, Latino, Asian	+++	Burns minimally, tans easily	40–60
V	**Unexposed skin is brown** Dark eyes Dark hair	East Indian, Native American, Latino, African	++++	Rarely burns, tans darkly easily	60–90
VI	**Unexposed skin is black** Dark eyes Dark hair	African, Aboriginal ancestry	+++++	Never burns, always tans darkly	90–150

exposure to UV radiation. Fifteen minutes of midday, sun exposure may cause sunburn in a white skin individual, while a darker-skinned individual may tolerate sun exposure for several hours. Signs of sunburn include erythema and edema, with or without vesiculation, followed by desquamation. Symptoms include pain and/or pruritus.

1. *Erythema*

Erythema is a direct result of vasodilatation of cutaneous blood vessels causing visible redness. UVB is much more potent at causing erythema in comparison with UVA, being up to 1000 times more erythemogenic, and is the most significant causative factor of sunburn [10]. UV induces p53 tumor suppressor proteins within keratinocytes, leading to a transient cell cycle arrest during which either DNA is repaired or an apoptotic pathway is initiated. These apoptotic keratinocytes known as "sunburn cells" typically have a shrunken dark (blue) pyknotic nucleus with dense eosinophilic (red) cytoplasm seen histologically (Fig. 3). SBCs appear as early as 30 min after irradiation, are maximal at 24 h when they are distributed throughout the epidermis, and by 72 h are mainly confined to the superficial layers [4]. SBCs seen at 72 h have sustained significant DNA damage, have retained a basal-cell level of differentiation immunohistochemically, and are being eliminated by apoptosis. Redness of the skin following first-degree burns/sunburn can be visible from about 2 h after UV radiation exposure with peak levels at about 24 h.

2. *Edema*

Vasodilatation and increased vascular permeability of blood vessels in the upper dermis layer to nourish damage occurring in the epi-

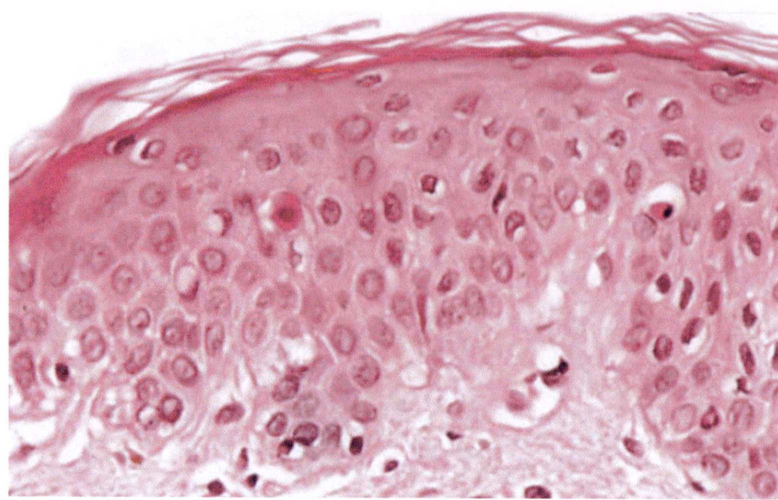

Fig. 3 Sunburn cells; typical apoptotic SBC at different stages of evolution [4]. Reproduced with permission from Dr. Graham Lowe, Consultant Dermatologist, Dundee

dermal layer may contribute to swelling visible during the early stages of sunburn. Within an hour of UVR exposure, mast cells release preformed mediators including histamine, serotonin, and TNF, resulting in prostaglandin and leukotriene synthesis [10]. Cytokine release additionally contributes to the inflammatory reaction, leading to an infiltrate of neutrophils and T lymphocytes. Within 2 h after UV exposure, damage to epidermal skin cells is seen and Langerhans cells undergo apoptotic changes, become depleted within 24 h, and take 2–3 weeks to return to baseline [4]. Other features seen include spongiosis, mast cell depletion/degranulation, early neutrophil infiltration, and endothelial cell enlargement within the superficial vascular plexus.

3. ***Pain and/or Pruritus***

Redness, swelling, and inflammation eventually result in pain. The pain may be noticeable from around 6 h following UV radiation exposure. Histamine release can cause itch symptoms.

4. ***Blistering***

The formation of vesicles or bullae arising from the skin can begin anywhere between 6 and 24 h after the initial UV radiation exposure. In more extreme sunburn episodes, in addition to cell damage in the epidermal layer, there is also damage to cells in the dermal layer, resulting in a second-degree burn. Plasma fluid starts to leak outside of cells and collects between two skin layers separating the epidermal from the dermal layer. The creation of this soft, liquid, protective bubble has the purpose of enabling the wounded dermal tissue underneath to heal.

5. ***Peeling and Healing***

The usual keratinocyte 28-day cell turnover is accelerated with sunburn episodes resulting in cells that stick together like a sheet of tissue rather than having their usual time to mature and separate. Once peeling starts from about 2 days following the initial UV radiation exposure, it can last for several days.

In very severe cases of sunburn, the burn of the skin may result in third-degree burns, dehydration, electrolyte imbalance, secondary infection, shock, and even death.

Sunburn Treatment and Prevention (Sun Protection)

Primary prevention of sunburn is critical as although acute sunburn is a self-limiting condition and typically requires only supportive care, cellular damage caused by UV radiation is irreversible and increases the risk of skin cancer with time.

Sunburn Treatment

The first thing to do is to get out of the sun and preferably stay indoors. The following advice should be given to those affected to help relieve the discomfort:

1. **Take frequent cool showers or baths to help relieve the pain.** As soon as you get out of the shower or bathtub, gently pat yourself dry, but leave a little water on your skin. Then apply a moisturizer to help trap the water in your skin. This can help ease the dryness.
2. **Use a moisturizer that contains aloe vera or soy to help soothe sunburned skin.** If a particular area feels especially uncomfortable, you may want to apply a hydrocortisone cream that you can buy without a doctor's prescription. Do not treat sunburn with "-caine" products (such as benzocaine), as these may irritate the skin or cause an allergic reaction.
3. **Consider taking aspirin or ibuprofen to help reduce any swelling, redness, and discomfort.** Aspirin or ibuprofen which can be bought without a doctor's prescription can help in this regard.
4. **Drink extra water.** A sunburn draws fluid to the skin's surface and away from the rest of the body. Drinking extra water when you are sunburned helps prevent dehydration.
5. **If your skin blisters, allow the blisters to heal.** Blistering skin means you have a second-degree sunburn. You should not pop the blisters, as blisters form to help your skin heal and protect you from infection.
6. **Take extra care to protect sunburned skin while it heals.** Wear clothing that covers your skin when outdoors. Tightly-woven fabrics work best.

Sun Protection with Clothing

1. *Ultraviolet Protection Factor (UPF)*

   The degree of sun protection by clothing is determined by the UPF, which is analogous to the SPF used for sunscreens. UPF indicates how much UV radiation (both UVB and UVA) a fabric allows to reach the skin. For example, a UPF 50 fabric blocks 98% of the sunlight rays and allows 2% (1/50th) to penetrate, thus reducing the sun exposure risk significantly [11]. UPF is generally measured *in vitro* by recording the UV transmittance. The UV transmittance is then applied to the sunlight spectrum and erythema action spectrum which enables computation of the level of protection afforded by the fabric. A fabric must have a UPF of 30 to qualify for The Skin Cancer Foundation's Seal of Recommendation [11]. A UPF of 30–49 offers very good protection, while a UPF of 50+ rates as excellent [11].

   The level of UPF provided by clothing depends on several factors outlined below (Table 3).

2. *Weave*

   The weave of clothing is the most important element affecting the transmission of UV radiation. The majority of UV penetration through fabrics occurs via the spaces between yarns; hence, the more closely woven a fabric is, the less UV radiation is transmitted [4]. Woven textiles such as denim, canvas, wool, or synthetic fibers will have smaller spaces between yarns affording more protection against UV radiation in comparison with knit

Table 3 Factors influencing clothing UPF summarized

Characteristics	Impact
Weave	Woven; denim, canvas, wool or synthetic fibers—high UPF Knit; sheer, thin, loosely woven cloth—low UPF
Composition	Polyester—high UPF Nylon, wool, lightweight satiny silk—moderate UPF Cotton, viscose, rayon—low UPF
Stretch and transparency	Low stretch ability and less transparency affords higher UPF
Weight	Heavier fabrics afford higher UPF
Color	Darker shades afford higher UPF
Washing	Repeated washing affords higher UPF (especially with cotton)
Water and wetness	Dryness affords higher UPF (especially with cotton)
UV absorbers	Laundry detergents and rinse cycle affords higher UPF

fabric or sheer, thin, loosely woven cloth with larger spaces between yarns. One of the simplest means of checking a fabric's sun safety is to hold it up to the light; if it is an easily see-through material, UV radiation will more easily penetrate the fabric to reach the skin.

3. *Composition*

Unbleached cotton contains natural lignins that act as UV absorbers. Shiny polyesters and even lightweight satiny silks can be highly protective due to their ability to reflect UV radiation. High-tech fabrics treated with chemical UV absorbers or dyes prevent some penetration from UV rays [11].

4. *Stretch*

The amount of UV transmission is highly dependent on the degree of stretch of the fabric type. For example, the UPF of elastane is lessened by about 50% when stretched by 10% [4]. Fifteen denier stockings provide a UPF of <2 which is further lessened when stretched [4]. Tight clothing can stretch and reduce the level of protection offered, as the fibers pull away from each other and allow more UV light to pass through. For this reason, loose-fitting apparel is preferable to have better sun protection.

5. *Weight*

Heavier fabrics afford higher levels of UPF in the setting of identical weave and color as UV radiation would have to penetrate through more material of the fabric to reach the skin.

6. *Color*

Fabrics darker in color absorb UV radiation better affording higher levels of UPF. This is mainly a result of the absorption band of dyes often extending into the UV region.

7. *Washing*

Most fabrics can undergo a mixture of relaxation and shrinkage when washed which reduces spaces between yarns thus increasing the UPF over time. UPF of cotton or polyester/cotton garments rises significantly after the first wash. For example, one study reported that a mean UPF of 20.2 ± 2.5 when new, increased to 38.3 ± 4.2 after one wash and was finally 39.9 ± 3.1 after 36 washes [4].

8. *Water*

The presence of water in the spaces of fabric depending on the type of fabric can reduce optical scattering. For example, in cotton T-shirts, when wet, can lessen the UPF to about half the dry value which becomes an important consideration if worn at the beach during high UVI hours [4].

9. *UV absorbers*

Application of UV absorbers in the form of laundry detergents and rinse cycle significantly increased the UPF of a garment. This will be particularly useful for intrinsically low UPF clothing, for example, non-dyed lightweight summer fabrics.

Sun Protection with Sunscreens

1) *Active ingredients*

TOPICAL PHOTOPROTECTORS

Topical sunscreens usually contain either chemical or physical compounds as active ingredients.

i) *Chemical sunscreens*

Chemical sunscreens absorb over relatively narrow wavebands, mainly in the UVB range but of more recent also extend into the UVA range affording better sun protection overall. Chemical sunscreens typically include a combination of two to six of the following active ingredients: oxybenzone, avobenzone, octisalate, octocrylene, homosalate, and octinoxate. In chemical sunscreens, UV radiation is traditionally absorbed by alternating single and double bonds in heterocyclic rings, and these structures have the capacity to undergo further photochemical transformation resulting in phototoxic and photoallergic reactions.

ii) *Physical sunscreens*

In contrast, titanium dioxide (TiO_2) and zinc oxide (ZnO) are physical sunscreens. These inorganic or mineral filters absorb, reflect, and refract UV photons but function in photoprotection primarily by absorbing UV radiation. TiO_2 and ZnO generally provide good broad-spectrum protection when used together and have no photosensitizing properties. For this reason, sunscreens for sensitive skin usually contain physical substances and exclude chemical absorbers, preservatives and fragrances. Nanoparticles (<100 nm in diameter) of TiO_2 and ZnO have the advantages of a non-greasy formulation that is transparent, inexpensive and does not degrade with UV radiation exposure.

ORAL PHOTOPROTECTORS

Oral photoprotectors can complement topical photoprotectors. These include lycopene, beta (β)-carotene, xanthophylls, nicotinamide, vitamins (C, D, and E), dietary non-botanicals (omega-3 polyunsaturated fatty acids, probiotics, and idebenone), and dietary botanicals (*Polypodium leucotomos* extract, green tea polyphenols, and isoflavones) [12]. These will function to minimize erythema (through increasing MED), reduce oxidative stress (by decreasing lipoperoxide levels), reduce DNA damage (inhibiting cyclobutane pyrimidine dimers (CPD)), and minimize inflammation (by decreasing edema and epidermal vesiculation). It will also reduce photocarcinogenesis by inhibiting tumor skin formation via the increase of p53 expression [12].

2) **Sun protection factor**

The SPF is the ratio of the dose of UV radiation that causes a minimal erythema in unprotected skin to that which causes a minimal erythema in sunscreen protected skin (Table 4). For this reason, SPF is more accurately the sunburn protection factor, as it primarily shows the level of protection against UVB, not the protection against UVA. If a sunscreen has SPF 15, it implies that the application of the sunscreen has caused an increase by a factor of 15 in the dose required to induce erythema. SPFs are rated on a scale of 6–50+ based on the level of protection offered, with ratings between 6 and 14 forming the least protected end of the spectrum and ratings of 50+ offering the strongest forms of UVB protection. The British Association of Dermatologists recommend a sunscreen with an SPF of 30 as a satisfactory form of sun protection in addition to protective shade and clothing [13].

3) **UVA star system**

It is important to choose a high SPF as well as a high UVA protection within sunscreens to ensure that the latter provides a defense against photoaging and potentially skin cancer. Sunscreens that offer both UVA and UVB protection are often referred to as "broad spectrum." A sunscreen with an SPF of 30 and a UVA rating of 4 or 5 stars is generally considered as a good standard of sun protection in addition to shade and clothing.

4) **Thickness of application**

There is a significant difference between the highly controlled conditions in the sunscreen laboratory and the outdoor real-life sunscreen product use. For example, SPF is determined based on a uniform application thickness of 2 mg/cm^2 of the product. In practice, however, there is uneven spreading, loss of product due to wash-off or rub-off, and a high-cost factor to take into account; all which may contribute to only between 0.5 and 1.5 mg/cm^2 of the product being used.

A sunscreen labeled SPF 16 is reduced to an SPF 2 when the consumer applies only 0.5 mg/cm^2 [4]. For this reason, it is recommended to re-apply sunscreens at regular intervals, of at least every 2 h while remaining outdoors in sunny weather, and immediately after swimming, perspiring, towel drying or if it has rubbed off and with any other vigorous or abrasive activity.

Table 4 Levels of protection afforded by SPF

New Label	SPF
Low protection	6–14 (i.e., SPF 6 and 10)
Medium protection	15–29 (i.e., SPF 15, 20 and 25)
High protection	30–50 (i.e., SPF 30 and 50)
Very high protection	50+ (i.e., SPF 50+)

5) *Impact on the environment*

On May 1, 2018, the Hawaiian state legislature passed a bill banning the sale of organic filter sunscreens such as oxybenzone and octinoxate. This is due to environmental effects of these filters including an impact on coral reefs, prevalence in water supply and in aquatic animals, as well as a negative hormonal effect in animal models of which the effect in humans is continued to be examined. Studies have had conflicting results regarding the risk of nanoparticles in the environment as TiO_2 and ZnO are minerals found in the environment, so it has been difficult to differentiate the effect of the nanoparticles from naturally occurring particles. At this time, the overall risk to the environment is considered extremely low [14].

Sun Protection with Behavior

As Outlined Above in the "Factors Influencing UV Radiation Levels" Section.

Individuals with Extra Needs for Sun Protection

All individuals with photodermatoses will need diligent sun protection. Photodermatoses with a sensitivity to predominantly UVA include solar urticaria and polymorphic light eruption. Chronic actinic dermatitis patients very sensitive to both UVA and UVB may benefit from UV protective window films. Porphyria patients will need sunscreens that provide protection in the VL range. The importance of epidermal DNA photodamage and nucleotide excision repair in skin cancer is evident from xeroderma pigmentosum (XP) individuals who have an extremely high incidence of all types of skin cancer with an onset in childhood as a result of a hereditary deficiency in DNA nucleotide excision repair. XP patients will need protective clothing including gloves, hoods or hats, and visors with UV blocking face shields.

Patients taking oral photosensitizing medication (e.g., tetracyclines, non-steroidal anti-inflammatory drugs, amiodarone, and retinoids) may develop phototoxic or photoallergic reactions. They require high level broad-spectrum photoprotection.

Long-Term Consequences (Photoaging and Photocarcinogenesis)

Photoaging

Photoaging is the premature aging of skin as a result of repeated exposure to UV radiation, primarily from the sun but also from artificial UV sources, for example, artificial tanning sources. An individual's lifetime exposure to sunlight is a key risk factor.

Hypertrophic Versus Atrophic

The gross appearance of photodamaged skin of individuals with skin types I and II often differs from that of individuals with skin types III and IV. Fairer skin types generally show atrophic skin changes with fewer wrinkles, focal depigmentation (guttate hypomelanosis), dysplastic changes (actinic keratosis (AK)), and epidermal malignancies. Darker skin types generally reveal hypertrophic skin changes including deep wrinkling, coarseness, and leathery textures [15] (Table 5).

Photocarcinogenesis

1. *DNA photo-induced lesions (CPDs and 6,4 photoproducts)*

There are three stages to photocarcinogenesis: initiation, promotion, and progression. In the first stage of initiation, DNA damage results in pyrimidine dimers within keratinocytes. The key mutagenic types of lesions induced by UV acutely, especially UVB, result in binding together of adjacent pyrimi-

Table 5 Characteristics of atrophic versus hypertrophic photoaging summarized

Characteristics	Atrophic	Hypertrophic
Skin types	I–II	III–IV
Appearance	Shiny	Sallow
Texture	Smooth, thin	Rough, leathery
Wrinkling	Minimal, fine surface lines	Coarse, deep
Pigmentation	Focal depigmentation (guttate hypomelanosis), freckles	Dyspigmentation, lentigines
Vasculature	Telangiectasia, senile purpura	Minimal/absent vascular changes
Dysplastic changes (AK) and epidermal malignancies (basal cell carcinomas and squamous cell carcinoma)	Common	Uncommon
Other	Associated with Poikiloderma of Civatte	Associated with Favre-Racouchot syndrome

dine bases in DNA; the two crucial DNA photo-induced lesions are CPD (C-C or T-T) and the 6,4 photoproducts. The nucleotide excision pathway of repair mends these DNA photo-induced lesions.

The second stage is when there is promotion of photocarcinogenesis through biochemical changes resulting in increased cellular stimulation and inflammation, activation of the ornithine decarboxylase, and increased cellular proliferation. UVA may cause indirect DNA damage by reactive oxygen species. If these DNA photo-induced lesions transit into the next cycle of cell division and DNA replication before being restored, it can be misrecognized by the DNA replication mechanism resulting in a mutation; the characteristic mutation is the CC → TT or C → T "UVB signature mutations" which are found in all types of skin cancer. These mutations are seen in the tumor suppressor p53 gene and other key genes in non-melanoma skin cancers. There may also be activation of protooncogenes.

The final stage in photocarcinogenesis is progression which occurs through COX2 synthesis and PGE2 production, whereby there is a loss of normal cell regulation resulting in abnormal epidermal proliferation, enabling AK to become squamous cell carcinomas (SCC) with the potential to metastasize.

2. *Basal cell carcinomas*

The development of basal cell carcinomas is dependent on previous sun exposure and repeated sunburn episodes.

3. *AK→ Bowen's disease→ SCC*

The development of SCC is the consequence of accumulated sun exposure over an individual's lifespan.

4. *Malignant melanoma*

The development of malignant melanomas is more dependent on patterns of sun exposure such as childhood sun exposure and intermittent high dose sun exposure, for example, during sunny holidays [3].

5. *Drug-induced immunosuppression*

The development of skin cancers in organ transplant recipients due to immunosuppressive therapy is widely recognized. Abnormally proliferative epidermal cells that are usually highly antigenic escape immunosurveillance and rejection with immunosuppression, becoming skin tumors.

The key to prevention and treatment of sunburn is good sun protection behavior including the use of sunscreens. Topical retinoids such as tretinoin may antagonize the UV signaling pathways that result in photoaging which provides a major step forward in preventing and reversing photoaging. Advances in UV protective mechanisms in the future will not only enable the improved appearance of the skin in older age groups but also greatly reduce the accompanying burden of the rise in skin cancer.

Acknowledgments We are very grateful to the World Health Organization for their permission to reproduce Figs. 1 and 2, and to Dr. Graham Lowe, Consultant Dermatologist, Dundee, for his permission to reproduce Fig. 3.

References

1. Greshko M et al. 2018. The sun, explained. *National Geographic*, 15 September, accessed August 2019. https://www.nationalgeographic.com/science/space/solar-system/the-sun/
2. 'Our Sun In Depth', *NASA Science Solar System Exploration*, 25 April 2019, accessed August 2019. https://solarsystem.nasa.gov/solar-system/sun/in-depth/
3. 'Global Solar UV Index: A Practical Guide', A Joint Recommendation of the World Health Organization, World Meteorological Organization, United Nations Environment Programme, International Commission on Non-Ionizing Radiation Protection, 2002, accessed September 2019, https://www.who.int/uv/publications/en/UVIGuide.pdf
4. Ferguson J, Dover JS. Photodermatology. 4th ed. London: Manson; 2010.
5. Young AR. The molecular and genetic effects of ultraviolet radiation exposure on skin cells. In: Hawk JLM, editor. Photodermatology. London: Chapman & Hall; 1998. p. 25–42.
6. D'Orazio J, Jarrett S, Amaro-Ortiz A, Scott T. UV radiation and the skin. Int J Mol Sci. 2013;14(6):12222–48.
7. Vanchinathan V, Lim HW. A dermatologist's perspective on vitamin D. Mayo Clin Proc. 2012;87(4):372–80.
8. Passeron T, et al. Sunscreen photoprotection and vitamin D status. Br J Dermatol. 2019;181(5):916–31.
9. Young AR, et al. Optimal sunscreen use, during a sun holiday with a very high ultraviolet index, allows vitamin D synthesis without sunburn. Br J Dermatol. 2019;181(5):1052–62.
10. Payne AS 2018. 'Sunburn', BMJ Best Practice, March 2018, accessed October 2019. https://bestpractice.bmj.com/topics/en-gb/613/pdf/613.pdf
11. Richard EG 2019. 'Sun-protective clothing'. Skin Cancer Foundation, June 2019. accessed December 2019. https://www.skincancer.org/skin-cancer-prevention/sun-protection/sun-protective-clothing/
12. Parrado C, Philips N, Gilaberte Y, Juarranz A, González S. Oral photoprotection: effective agents and potential candidates. Front Med (Lausanne). 2018;5:188.
13. 'Sunscreen and sun safety factsheet'. British Association of Dermatologists, 2013, accessed December 2019. http://www.bad.org.uk/shared/getfile.ashx?id=3917&itemtype=document
14. Schneider SL, Lim HW. A review of inorganic UV filters zinc oxide and titanium oxide. Photodermatol Photoimmunol Photomed. 2019;35(6):442–6.
15. Sachs DL, et al. Atrophic and hypertrophic photoaging: Clinical, histologic and molecular features of two distinct phenotypes of photoaged skin. J Am Acad Dermatol. 2019;81(2):480–8.

Part IX

Marine Dermatosis

Aquatic Dermatoses

Reynaldo Arosemena S. and Alex Jeffrey Kew

Key Points

- It comprises a group of diseases associated with aquatic activities, caused primarily by marine invertebrates, marine vertebrates, and agents that produce secondary infection in open wounds. It also encapsulates miscellaneous dermatoses such as swimmer's xerosis, aquagenic acne, contact dermatitis, surfer's nodules, swimmer's shoulder, and green hair.
- Clinical manifestations can range from a simple dermatitis to severe morbidity and death, as can be seen in cases where toxins are absorbed and cause systemic effects.
- Treatment varies depending on the type of clinical manifestation; it may include, but is not limited to, extraction of encrusted structures, thorough rinsing of the affected area, use of antibiotics, antihistamines, and/or steroids, and extensive preventative measures when engaging in risky activities.

R. Arosemena S. (✉)
Hospital Santo Tomás, Panama City, Panamá
e-mail: dr@arosemena.com.pa

A. J. Kew
University College London Hospitals NHS
Foundation Trust, London, England
e-mail: a.kew@nhs.net

Introduction

Fishing, scuba diving, surfing, swimming, and water skiing form an integral part of many individuals' lives, spanning across different continents and cultures. For some, these activities are hobbies; for others, they are competitive sports activities. Finally, for an essential few, these water activities dominate and are simply a way of life, especially for those who wish to develop a more intimate relationship with nature. Unfortunately and consequently, engaging in such water sports may result in cutaneous dermatoses that need to be accurately recognized, diagnosed, and treated. Contact with nature can give rise to a large variety of cutaneous diseases. For example, the development of contact dermatitis can be the result of a great variety of marine animals such as jellyfish, stingrays, or starfish.

The multiple creatures of the sea, rivers, lakes, aquariums, and pools have different physiologic characteristics that confer distinct levels of protection for adequate survival. As such, varied cutaneous manifestations may result. Dermatologists must be able to recognize the varied cutaneous manifestations and be able to both prevent and treat these dermatoses.

Lesions may be divided as follows:

I. Dermatitis by marine invertebrates
II. Dermatitis by marine vertebrates

W. Robles (ed.), *Skin Disease in Travelers*, Updates in Clinical Dermatology,
https://doi.org/10.1007/978-3-031-57836-6_31

III. Wound infections
IV. Miscellaneous dermatoses, including but not limited to:

Swimmer's xerosis, aquagenic acne, contact dermatitis secondary to sports equipment, surfer's nodules, swimmer's shoulder, and green hair.

Dermatitis by Marine Invertebrates

The most common marine invertebrates to produce cutaneous lesions are those that belong to the phylum Cnidaria (e.g., corals, jellyfish, and sea anemones). These organisms contain nematocysts which are small, elongated capsules found on their surface. These specialized capsules are capable of penetrating the epidermis of aggressors or prey. After penetration, they subsequently release toxins. Toxins released include 5-hydroxytryptamine, catecholamines, quinine, quaternary ammonium compounds, proteases, and substances that stimulate histamine release. The clinical response to these toxins may vary from a simple dermatitis to significant morbidity or even death. The response is dose-, potency-, and exposure-dependent. Host susceptibility is also an influencing factor in determining clinical manifestations of dermatitis secondary to exposure to marine invertebrates [1].

The two most frequent localized cutaneous reactions include [2] linear urticarial eruptions at the site of contact and [3] white-colored papules that may evolve quickly into erythematous papules, hemorrhagic lesions, vesicles, ulcers, or necrotic lesions. It is also possible to observe fat atrophy, necrosis, localized hyperhidrosis, lymphadenopathy, and/or gangrene. Persistent pruritus may also be observed, which may produce lichenification of the affected area [3].

Jellyfish Dermatitis

Toxins produced by jellyfish may cause cutaneous, mucosal, and even corneal lesions. These toxins produce immediate pain or burning sensation at the side of contact. One can observe localized erythema and edema almost immediately. Within a few hours, the rash fades and may progress to bullae and vesicles, possibly with necrosis and gangrene of the affected area.

Exaggerated local reactions can manifest as recurrent episodes of rashes, usually every 4 days, sometimes with associated angioedema. These lesions are usually pruritic rather than painful. With every successive exacerbation, the duration of the episode is shortened, as is the symptom-free period between each of them. Delayed apparition of lesions occurs with the nodular and granulomatous forms.

Linuche and *Physalia* stings have been known to induce inflammatory skin reactions distal to the place of contact by the tentacle. Additionally, local lymphadenopathies have been reported to accompany the cutaneous rash. While rare, the primary cutaneous eruption may resolve as a hypo or hyperpigmented scar or keloid with associated fat atrophy, muscular contractions, gangrene, and/or local cutaneous thrombophlebitis. Some of these nodular or granulomatous lesions may heal appropriately, especially if treated with systemic or intralesional corticosteroids [1].

Physalia Physalis (Portuguese Man o' War)

The Portuguese Man o' War is a large violet-blue colored animal with multiple long tentacles that descend from the center of its body. These tentacles are capable of inoculating the skin, leaving a typical mark that immediately produces sharp pain that can persist for hours. A linear erythematous rash develops with localized sweating, followed by piloerection. Muscle spasms are frequent. Inoculation around the eyes can produce small corneal ulcerations and vision problems. Systemic symptoms may include nausea, vomiting, painful lymphadenopathies, syncope, seizures, and muscle spasms. Cases of recurrent rashes have been reported after a single sting. Serious complications may include multiple mononeuritis, acute renal failure, and macroscopic hematuria.

The venom of *Physalia physalis* is characteristically hemolytic and dermonecrotic and may be a potentially deadly antigen in humans and small animals. Cross-reactions with other jellyfish venoms have been observed. In the event of systemic collapse, resuscitation and support measures should be initiated immediately.

Sea Bather's Eruption

Sea bather's eruption is characterized by its unique cutaneous distribution. It affects areas covered by a bathing suit after an individual has been swimming in infected waters. Sea bather's eruption is a hypersensitivity reaction to the larval form of jellyfish or sea anemones. The condition tends to be observed more frequently in the dry season as the wind encourages the migration of jellyfish to shallower waters. Larval forms get contained under the bathing suit or hair of the sea bather, and the slightest stimulation of larval nematocysts results in toxins being injected into the adjacent skin. Keeping bathing suits on for prolonged periods after swimming, bathing in freshwater, and/or rubbing the affected area may worsen the associated dermatitis [1].

Seaweed Dermatitis

Similarly, to sea bathers' eruption discussed above, seaweed dermatitis is the name given to a skin condition, mainly a rash, caused by direct skin exposure to certain species of cyanobacteria and algae, commonly known as seaweed. The most common species involved in causing this condition is a filamentous cyanobacterium called *Lyngbya majuscula* or "fireweed," a green/black, worldwide distributed colonial organism that tends to grow in clumps and is often described as looking like matted hair on the sea floor.

Much like sea bathers' eruption small parts of the seaweed can end up getting caught underneath swim or footwear during water activities. The trapped seaweed produces toxins, such as lyngbyatoxin A, which, on continued exposure to the skin, can lead to skin itching and burning sensations as well as in some cases a blistering, red rash. Often the tell-tale sign of seaweed dermatitis is that of a red itchy rash in a swimwear distribution on the body, which is why it can often be mistaken for sea bathers' eruption or contact dermatitis second to swimwear.

Prevention is the key to avoiding the seaweed but other than never swimming in the sea, avoiding seaweed blooms as well as thoroughly washing skin and swimwear after exiting the water can help. If a rash occurs treatment is mainly symptomatic with sunburn remedies such as after-sun creams and wet towels often employed. Occasionally, hydrocortisone cream can be used for severe rashes and oral steroids for extreme reactions.

Dermatitis and Wounds by Anthozoa

Anthozoa is the largest class of phylum cnidaria. It contains organisms of diverse shapes and colors, such as sea anemones and coral polyps. Sea anemones are usually harmless. However, they can produce erythema and pain in areas of direct contact, especially if it occurs on the face or axilla. Corals have nematocysts that upon contact with skin may cause edema and erythema of the affected area [4].

Additionally, corals contain a calcium carbonate skeleton that may easily wound the skin. Wounds by coral are very common, and generally, they heal very well. Abrasions or lacerations by coral may be complicated by one of the following:

- Direct physical damage
- Bleeding from an affected blood vessel
- Deposit of coral polyp material and other foreign bodies in the wound
- Introduction of coral venom into the wound
- Contamination of the wound by microorganisms
- Production of a local or systemic antigen–antibody reaction

Patients with an underlying systemic disease such as diabetes mellitus, peripheral vascular disease, chronic liver disease, or immunosuppression due to treatment with corticosteroids tend to present with a delayed response to cutaneous symptoms.

The lesion becomes edematous, pruritic, and very painful. Initially, a clear discharge emerges that later may become purulent. Regional lymphatics enlarge and become painful. Secondary infection of the wound may result in chills, headache, and local edema [4].

Red Coral Contact Dermatitis

Contact with fire coral immediately produces a highly pruriginous, urticarial rash. This causes the affected person to leave the sea immediately. Within minutes, the area becomes erythematous and edematous, with subsequent formation of blisters that resolve as violet papular lesions and plaques. From a clinical and histopathological point of view, it is indistinguishable from lichen planus. This dermatitis should be considered one of the causes of lichenoid eruptions.

Individuals with a greater risk of manifesting dermatological symptoms after contact with red coral are those that are allergic to shellfish and those suffering from atopic dermatitis [3].

General Recommendations and Treatment for Dermatitis by Coelenterates

- Always use gloves.
- Avoid contact with fresh water as it activates the nematocysts.
- Avoid ingestion of meat with softeners because they contain proteolytic enzymes.
- Submerge the area in hot salted water, as the toxin is thermolabile.
- If a secondary infection is suspected, a blood culture should be ordered and antibiotic treatment initiated.
- Administer a tetanus shot.

- Systemic analgesics reduce acute pain.
- Application of sodium bicarbonate is recommended in dermatitis by *P. physalis*.
- Topical antihistamines, local anesthetics, topical corticosteroids, and aluminum preparations may be applied on the affected area.
- X-rays may be helpful in some cases.

Treatment of Cercarial Dermatitis

- It can be prevented with molluscicides and avoiding contact with marine vegetation.
- Prevention using a 20% copper solution is effective.
- It is a self-limited condition, as the cercaria does not reside in the skin.
- Symptomatic antipruritic treatment is indicated.
- The affected area may be rubbed and dried with a towel to remove the drops containing cercaria.

Dermatitis Caused by Poisonous Aquatic Animals

Echinoderms (Sea urchin)

These animals belong to the phylum echinodermata, class echinoidea. They can be circular, ovoid, or flat and without arms and are covered by mobile spines of variable length. These animals are found in all oceans, especially in rocky areas and coral reefs. The most poisonous are found in the tropics and subtropics (Indo-Pacific region). They cause traumatic injuries to surfers, fishermen, and divers.

The spines of some species are poisonous and contain a neurotoxin. The most poisonous echinoderms contain venom in their spines and pedicles. These spines produce physical damage when they get lodged in the skin. They break easily and may dissolve. Those that are not easily removable must be surgically treated [3].

Poisoning may also occur by ingesting certain organs of these animals. Ingestion of their ovaries has been reported in the literature to have resulted in death. The poison is a thermolabile protein that can produce acute toxicity and allergic reactions [4].

Lesions and Poisoning by Spines

Immediate local reactions include erythema, edema, and profuse bleeding. Initially, the pain is intense and decreases several hours later, followed by a sensation of direct pressure. If a spine gets into a joint, it can result in synovitis. Some Panamanian sea urchins produce very serious injuries. Secondary infections are very common, as are painless ulcerations. The systemic effects vary depending on the degree of entry into the layers of the skin [4].

Nausea, local numbness, muscle weakness, and respiratory depression are the main systemic effects produced by sea urchin stings. In the case of multiple stings, patients may experience delirium. At the tip of the spine, there are glands with an epithelial covering that contain vasopressors such as adrenaline. This has been related to cases of cardiac arrhythmia [3].

Foreign-body granulomas or skin-colored, spine-like nodules can form 3–4 months after inoculation. Delayed hypersensitivity reactions may occur, especially on fingers and toes. These include vesicular eruptions or edema that can produce a fusiform type of deformation [3].

Treatment

- First, stabilize the patient and see if cardiovascular resuscitation maneuvers are necessary.
- Clean the affected area with hot water.
- Acidic acid (vinegar) can be helpful because it dissolves thin spines.
- To continue removing everything that protrudes from the affected area, remember that the spines break easily [1].
- Compressive bandages should not be placed, unless there are signs of anaphylaxis.

- To identify fragments of spines that remain inside the wound, xeroradiography may performed with a skin tag marker, as to facilitate its surgical removal.
- If necessary, surgically remove the spine or fragment. Anesthesia is applied, and pain medication, antibiotics, and tetanus immunization should administered [1].
- The risk of secondary infection is significant. Treatment with antibiotics should be considered.
- The response to corticosteroids is variable.

Lesions and Poisoning by Pedicles

Lesions caused by pedicles can be very serious. The associated pain is very intense and irradiated. The area becomes numb, followed by respiratory distress and paralysis in an average of six hours. Hemorrhage, hypotension, and bronchospasm follow. Some cases of facial paralysis have been reported by some species [4].

Treatment

- Submerge the affected area in hot water.
- Immediate removal of the pedicle with shaving cream and a razor to avoid continuous poisoning by the pedicle.
- Administer antibiotics and tetanus immunization [2].

Starfish: Phylum Echinodermata, Class Asteroid

They are mainly found in the reefs of the Indo-Pacific, East Africa, and Central America. They are not found in the Atlantic reefs. Starfish are shaped like a large disk with 14–18 arms capable of regenerating if injured by a predator.

They come in a great variety of colors and contain four types of thorns which contain sulfated steroid glycosides called saponins that are responsible for their toxic nature. These saponins are bioactive substances, they act as a neurotoxin and a histamine-like substance. Animal research demonstrates hematological and even fatal reactions to crude extracts of the toxin. Myotoxicity, by phospholipase A2 activity, has been observed in experimental studies [4].

Starfish passively deposit venom and bacteria into the wound. Contact with starfish may cause intense local pain, burning sensations, bleeding, erythema, edema, itching, numbness, and swelling of the affected area. Serous exudate may seep from the wound, secondary infection, and enlarged regional lymph nodes may ensue. Localized allergic reactions as well as generalized sensibilization have been observed. Divers should be especially careful as the pain can cause loss of control, disorientation, and panic. The pain may last several hours. Unfortunately, diving suits are unable to completely protect against spines.

If there are multiple injuries, systemic symptoms may ensue such as fever, nausea, and vomiting, which may last several days. The affected area turns blue-violet, which may spread and may be surrounded by a region of erythema that lasts for several days. If swelling or pruritus persist, the patient may be experiencing an allergy to the toxin [1].

Treatment

- Extract protruding fragments of spines that protrude and have no danger of breaking.
- Deep fragments may require an X-ray.
- Apply direct pressure on the bleed.
- The wound should be carefully washed.
- In the absence of a severe allergic reaction, which is unlikely, the patient should be immobilized with bandages.
- The affected area may be submerged in hot water. Very cold water also relieves pain.
- Local anesthetics can be injected and/or potent analgesics may be administered.
- Administer tetanus toxoid [2].

Prophylaxis or Treatment of Secondary Infection

- Bed rest and elevation of the affected limb or area.
- The inability to remove these parts of the spines may lead to serious bacterial infections [3].

Marine Vertebrates

Ray-like fishes are marine vertebrates that cause injuries. They belong to the class Chondrichthyes, subclass Elasmobranchii, order Rajiformes, and are flattened, cartilaginous fish. The venom is found in the fish's tail, in a spine with an integumentary sheath that contains poisonous glands. The latter is known as the stingray and the poison it secretes is thermolabile. There may be more than one spine on the dorsal aspect of the tail [1].

They are fish with great perception and are not aggressive. However, if one is frightened, caught, or stepped on, it can react quickly. They are found in tropical and subtropical waters around the world and they prefer the bottom of the ocean where they can find camouflage in the sand [2].

Signs and Symptoms of Poisoning

The damage can occur in one of two ways: by direct trauma or by the effects of the poison. When trauma by the spine occurs, it tends to be in the lower limbs. However, if it occurs somewhere on the trunk, it is considered a serious medical emergency, because there is necrotizing action in the area where the poison is deposited. The actions of the poison are similar in all types of ray-like fish. They generally affect the cardiovascular system in mammals; at low concentrations, it can cause vasodilation or peripheral vasoconstriction and can induce grade I and II AV blocks [1].

Higher doses of venom can result in the ST segment and the T wave changes, resulting in ischemia or injury to cardiac muscle.

Additionally, it can also depress breathing and produce seizures. The toxin may cause necrosis locally, similar to bacterial cellulitis. When the venom is deposited, intense and persistent pain can ensue, sometimes with resulting paresthesias of the area. Necrosis of tissue may also lead to secondary infection that may subsequently lead to the formation of chronic, difficult-to-treat ulcers [3].

Treatment

- The affected area should be cleaned as soon as possible and any foreign body removed.
- Visible active bleeding should be controlled.
- Compressive or immobilizing bandages should not be applied.
- The affected area can be submerged in hot water.
- If the heat does not relieve the pain, cold compresses may be applied for 30 min, as many times as necessary.

- Nerve blocks are preferred over local anesthetics, as the latter may contribute to the spreading of the affected area.
- An X-ray of the area should be ordered to rule out the presence of foreign bodies.

References

1. Marianne Kolbach R, Cossio ML, Luisa Sáenz M, de Santa MP, Néstor Carreño O, Claudia de la Cruz F, Ximena FW. Dermatosis en los deportistas. Rev Med Chile. 2008;136:249–55.
2. Haddad V Jr, Lupi O, Lonza JP, Tyring SK. Tropical dermatology: marine and aquatic dermatology. J Am Acad Dermatol. 2009;61:733–50.
3. Adams BB. Dermatologic disorders of the athlete. Sports Med. 2002;32(5):309–21.
4. Kennedy CTC, Bruid DAR. Mechanical and thermal injury. Rook's textbook of dermatology. Black Science; 2004. p. 1023–6.

Schistosomiasis

Bernard Naafs

Key Points

- Always ask travelers: Where they have you been and have they come into contact with stagnant or river water?
- Dermatological symptoms of schistosomiasis are rare: Urticaria or volatile erythema is the most common present one (cercarial dermatitis and Swimmer's itch).
- Katayama syndrome may occur 2–14 weeks after non-immune individuals have been exposed. It may also be accompanied by urticaria and transient erythema. A serological test may be helpful here.
- A late symptom that is often overlooked is Bilharziasis cutanea tarda. Clinical papules can turn into wart-like lesions with fistulas. The perineum, genital, perianal mucosa, and skin are most often involved, especially in women.
- It is the eggs that are causing the problem, not the adult worm.
- The gold standard for diagnosis is still the finding of the eggs in urine or stool.
- Eosinophilia may be present.
- The most effective treatment available for both urinary and intestinal schistosomiasis is Praziquantel.

B. Naafs (✉)
Foundation Global Dermatology,
Munnekeburen, Friesland, The Netherlands
e-mail: benaafs@dds.nl

Introduction

A dermatologist interested in "exotic" skin diseases is familiar with swimmer's itch, is aware of the Katayama syndrome, and warns patients not to swim in contaminated water because of the risk of getting bladder and liver problems. However, generally, that is all. This chapter wants to give some background.

Schistosomiasis or Bilharzia is caused by a parasite, a flatworm, or trematode (fluke). It is a water-borne parasitic infection that may result in a debilitating chronic disease with extensive morbidity and organ pathology. It belongs to **Family**: Schistosomatidae, **Order**: Diplostomida, **Class**: Trematoda, **Phylum**: Platyhelminthes, and **Kingdom**: Animalia.

The characteristic feature of these helminths is that the adult worms are truly blood parasites, but their offspring are excreted with stool and urine of the infected host. Only part of the eggs produced manage to reach the intestinal lumen or the bladder cavity. Many die "en route" and are the cause of problems in the subsequent predilection sides or elsewhere [1].

There are four important species to humans: *Schistosoma haematobium*, *Schistosoma mansoni*, *Schistosoma intercalatum*, and *Schistosoma japonicum*. In the early stage of human infection, these organisms may cause similar skin manifestations and generalized symptoms. In the chronic

W. Robles (ed.), *Skin Disease in Travelers*, Updates in Clinical Dermatology,
https://doi.org/10.1007/978-3-031-57836-6_32

phase bladder abnormalities, ureter and kidney problems (*S. haematobium*), and iliac and liver abnormalities (the others). The trematodes are recognized for their suction cups. They are endemic in 76 countries worldwide. The majority (88%) of the people infected with schistosomiasis live on the African continent [2]. A systematic review and meta-analysis published in 2006 estimated that more than 200 million people are infected across Africa, Asia, and South America, 123 million of them are children, and close to 800 million are at risk of infection, particularly the children [3]. Meta-analyses have estimated that the current disease burden may exceed 70 million disability-adjusted life years [4, 5].

Travelers and expatriates are the ones potentially at risk: development aid workers and volunteers, missionaries, soldiers, adventure travelers, and ecotourists. Outbreaks of schistosomiasis have occurred among travelers on river trips particularly in Africa.

Life Cycle

The life cycle of schistosomes includes two hosts: humans as definitive hosts, where the parasite undergoes sexual reproduction, and snails as intermediate hosts, where a series of asexual reproductive takes place (Fig. 1) [1].

Schistosoma eggs leave the host in feces or urine, depending on the species. The cycle starts within 15 min when the egg comes in contact with water. A larva (miracidium) frees itself from

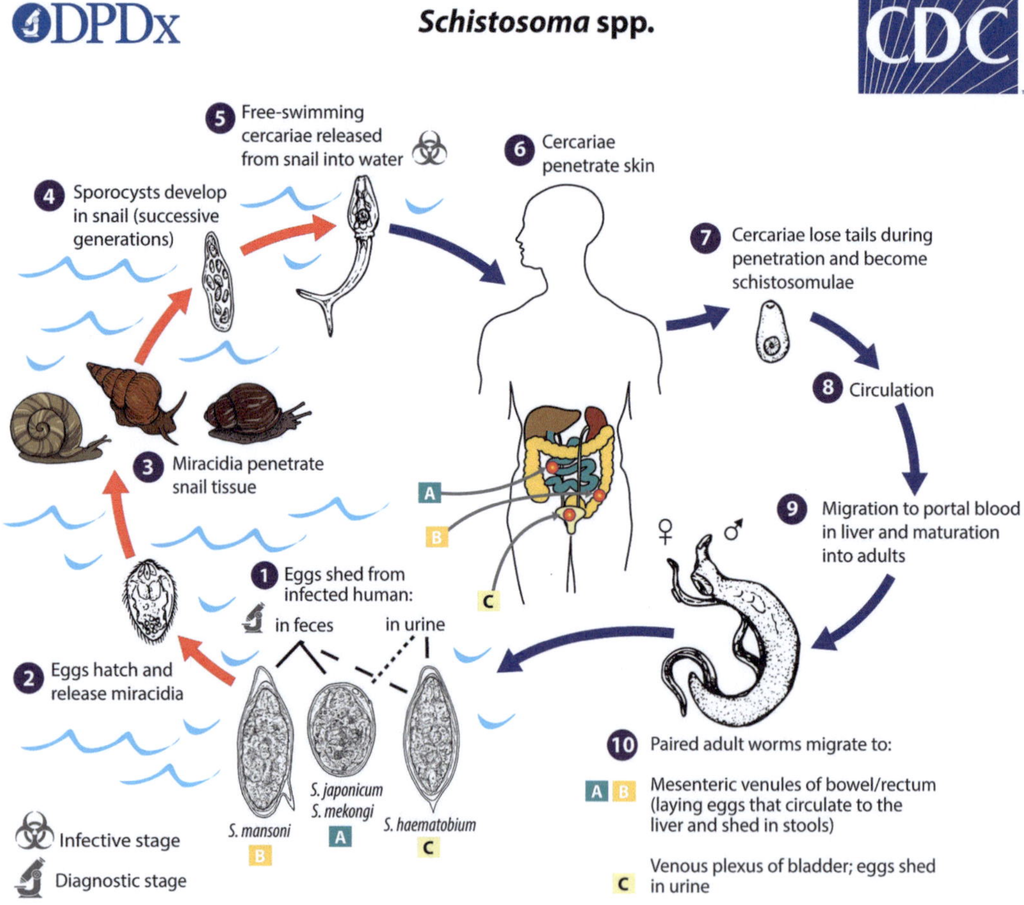

Fig. 1 Life circle of *Schistosoma* species. Thanks to CDC

the egg; each miracidium is either male or female. The miracidium swims around in stagnant freshwater looking for an intermediate host, usually a mollusk. It has to find a host within 24–48 h. In the hepatopancreas of the snail, the miracidium develops into a spherical form, the sporocyst, which develops within 4–8 weeks into the adult larvae or cercariae [6–8]. One "mother" sporocyst produces many "daughter" sporocysts. The daughter sporocyst ruptures and the liberated cercariae leave the snail, having already all the organs of an adult (being male or female), looking for its final host. One sporocyst produces hundreds of thousands of cercariae. The cercariae must find a host within 4–6 days. When the human host comes in contact with infested water, the cercariae attach themselves to the skin using their suckers and penetrate the skin by secreting proteolytic enzymes, losing their biforked swimming tail. They are assisted by the surface tension when the body area is removed from the water and allowed to dry naturally [8]. This process takes about 3–5 min. From here onward, they are called Schistosomulae. They stay in the skin for 2 days, enter the circulation, and reach the heart and lungs and then the liver within 24 h [8]. There they develop into sexual maturity. In pairs, they enter the portal vein, against the bloodstream, and reach different parts of the body [6]. They mate there. After about 50 days, eggs can be found in the urine or feces. The total cycle lasts 2–3 months. They can live for 20–30 years. However, mostly it is much shorter, a few years.

Evading detection by the host's immune system appears to be possible due to several parasite adaptations that occur soon after infection is initiated. Foremost are the processes that result in reduced surface antigenicity and the development of a tegument intrinsically resistant to immune damage. The worms have many tools that help in this evasion, including the tegument, antioxidant proteins, and defenses against the host membrane attack complex [9]. The tegument coats the worm and acts as a physical barrier to host antibodies and complement. Host immune defense produces superoxide, but this is counterattacked by antioxidant proteins produced by the parasite. Schistosomes have four superoxide dismutases,

and levels of these proteins increase as the schistosome grows [10].

The adult worms live in the venulae of the bladder, urinary tract, and pelvic floor (*S. haematobium*), plexus rectalis and vena mesenterica inferior (*S. mansoni* and *S. intercalatum*), and vena mesenterica superior (*S. japonicum*). Individual worms sought out opposite sexes. The male is shorter and wider than the female who is slender and lives in a longitudinal ventral groove of its male. The male permanently carries its female in this gynecophoric canal (schist) (Fig. 2) [6–8]. The body surface of the male is rough and spiny (*S. haematobium* and *S. mansoni*), the female, in all species is smooth, and both have an oral sucker and an acetabulum (a specialized sucker for parasitic adaptation in trematodes by which the worms are able to attach on the host). There is an esophagus with distinct esophageal glands, but no pharynx is present. Paired caeca come together posteriorly, forming a single cecum that extends the remaining length of the schistosome [11, 12]. Adult worms continuously bathed in blood take up nutrients directly across their body surface and also by ingestion of blood into the gut. Their body surface is the principal entry route for glucose, whereas the gut dominates amino acid acquisition, especially in females. Adult worms digest erythrocytes, and although most of their energy is obtained by glucose metabolism, egg production is dependent on fatty acid oxidation. Both glucose and fatty acids are derived from the host. Schistosomes have no anus and cannot excrete waste products, so they regurgitate waste into the bloodstream among which heme, a potentially toxic hemoglobin degradation product [13].

The male has four- or five-pair dorsally situated testes, and the male gynecophoral canal opens ventrally, immediately posterior to the ventral sucker, and a short vas deferens arises from the testes and joins a seminal vesicle which enters in a cirrus (penis), that opens by a gonopore below the acetabulum. The male appears to be essential for the complete maturation of the ovary and passes on, just after joining, "material" which completes the female's development, whereupon they will reproduce sexually [8, 14].

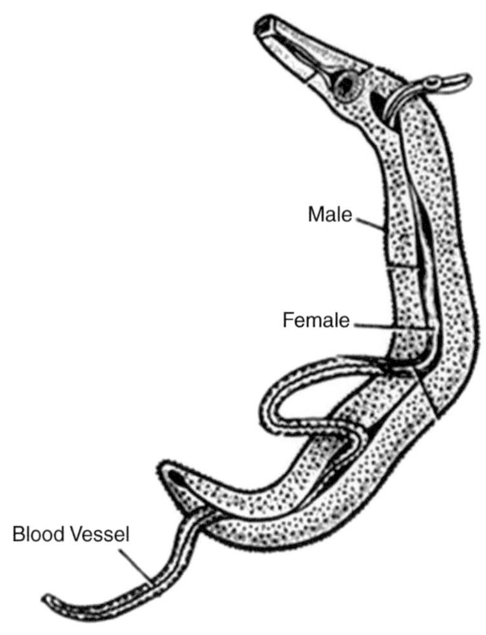

Fig. 2 Paired adult worms (Drawn after fig in Medhekar A in biologicaldiscussion.com)

The spermatozoa passed to a female migrate up the female reproductive tract and are stored in the seminal receptacle located posterior to the ovary.

A single elongated pear-shaped ovary is located in the anterior portion of the body of the female. The uterus can be long or short, depending on the position of the ovary above the point where the caeca join. From the ovary, an oviduct passes in front relative to the female genital pore [12]. From the seminal receptacle, sperm is able to begin the fertilization process as oocytes emerge from the ovary. In the posterior part of the female, are vitelline (yolk) glands from which a vitelline duct joins the oviduct. Oocytes pass through the oviduct that merges with the vitelline duct (now the ovo-vitelline duct). This duct reaches the ootype—the central portion of the ovarian complex—in which fertilization takes place and the vitellarian or eggshell materials are coated over the egg; this occurs in a rapid, stamping-mill sequence, after which eggs pass further into the uterus for tanning of the shell, storage, and passage toward the genital pore, surrounded by the Mehlis gland [15]. A variety of functions have been proposed for the Mehlis gland, including providing lubrication for the reproductive tract, activating sperm, and providing materials for the eggshell biosynthesis gland directly posterior to the ootype [12, 15]. It opens with a female gonopore below the acetabulum [15]. After fertilization, the female leaves the male briefly to lay eggs. She has to because only alone she can enter the small and narrow peripheral venule in the submucosa so that the eggs can be released into the bladder or intestine. Although rare, occasionally mated schistosomes will "divorce," wherein the female will leave the male for another male [16]. The exact reason is not understood, although it is thought that females will leave their partners to mate with more genetically distant males. Such a biological mechanism would serve to decrease inbreeding and may be a factor behind the unusually high genetic diversity of schistosomes [16]. The embryonated eggs penetrate the mucosa using proteolytic enzymes, aided by their spines and by the contraction of the intestines or bladder. The enzyme is a toxin, damaging (necrosis) the tissue. Under normal circumstances, the eggs released into the bladder or intestine do not cause pathological symptoms. The fluke continuously lays eggs throughout her life.

Pathogenesis [1, 7]

The symptoms of infection can be considered reactions to the toxic and sensitizing products produced by the living worms or their eggs. The penetration by the cercariae can by itself cause symptoms but more so in an already sensitized person, leading to a more or less severe dermatitis (cercariae dermatitis, swimmer's itch). During their migration, being in the maturation stage, one may encounter severe illness. These are also mostly allergic by nature (Katayama syndrome). Living worms in general are hardly noticed but the dead ones may give severe reactions. The eggs, however, are the major culprits [6–8]. Not all eggs reach the lumen from the bladder or intestine, some stay behind in the mucosae. After

3–4 weeks, the miracidium dies. A live or dead miracidium elicits a foreign body reaction. Around the egg or a group of eggs, a granulomatous reaction occurs with mononucleotides, eosinophils, epithelioid cells, and giant cells. Small granuloma may "melt" together to the so-called bilharzia-tubercle. The exact nature of this T-cell reaction is not known. Several studies point in the direction of a Th1 response, with the production of TNF-alpha and INF-gamma, with severe morbidity in children infected with *S. mansoni*, while Th2 responses with IL-5 production are associated with mild or absent morbidity [8, 17]. After some time, fibrous tissue replaces the granulation tissue and the eggs calcify. The chronic stimulus may eventually lead to malignancy, particularly in the bladder [6, 18].

Some of the eggs are taken by the bloodstream to the liver and further to the lungs, embolization of the eggs. They get stuck in the fine branches of the vena portae, respectively, the pulmonary arteries where they may cause a granulomatous reaction. These resolve to fibrous tissue, narrowing the blood vessels. The end result after many embolisms could be portal and/or pulmonary hypertension [6, 8].

The eggs may get stuck in other organs as well, even in the CNS.

In a few patients, they may end up in the skin (Bilharziasis cutanea tarda) [19]. There they give first an eosinophilic reaction, which later results in a granulomatous inflammation with epithelioid cells. In a later stadium, fibrous tissue is formed around the granuloma and the eggs calcify.

Clinically, one notices single or multiple grouped papules that may transform into verrucous lesions with fistula. These can be extensive (did tuberculosis or HPV infect). The perineum, genital and peri-anal mucosa, and skin are most often involved, particularly in women [6, 8]. The diagnosis is often missed. Eggs can also be found extragenital. Clinically, itchy papules can converge into irregularly shaped plaques which may ulcerate. Usually, they are located on the trunk, but locations elsewhere have been reported too, face and neck. Peri-umbilical seems to be the preferred localization. The arrangement of the papules is often zosteriform [19].

Symptomatology of Schistosoma Infection

The invading cercariae generally do not produce symptoms; a few of their hosts may have experienced a transient immediate hypersensitivity reaction that occurs within 15 min. However, they can give strong itching, a delayed reaction, within 24 h and then show an atypical spectrum of scratch marks, erythematous, small welts, and papules (Fig. 3); these generally last less than a week [6–8]. The distribution of the lesions is on those parts of the body that were immersed in the water. This cercarial dermatitis does usually not appear after the first contact because the individual must first become sensitized. A cercarial dermatitis may happen after contact with mammalian and avian schistosomes cercariae (swimmer's

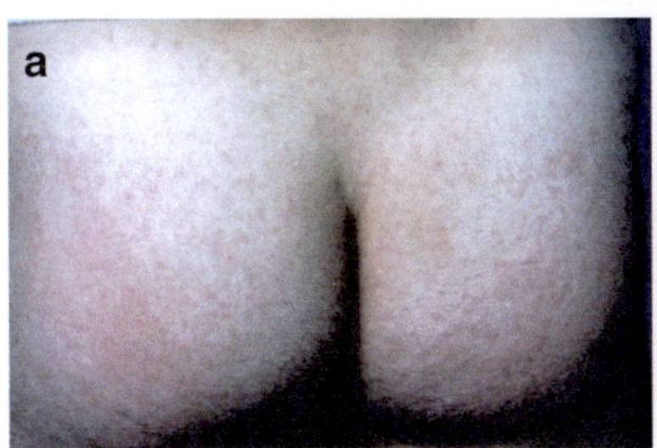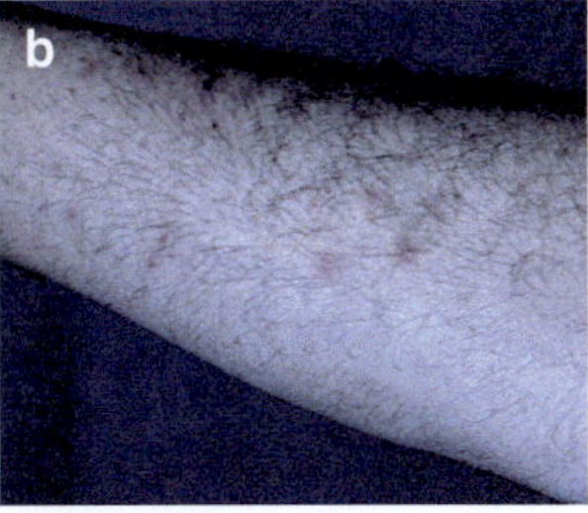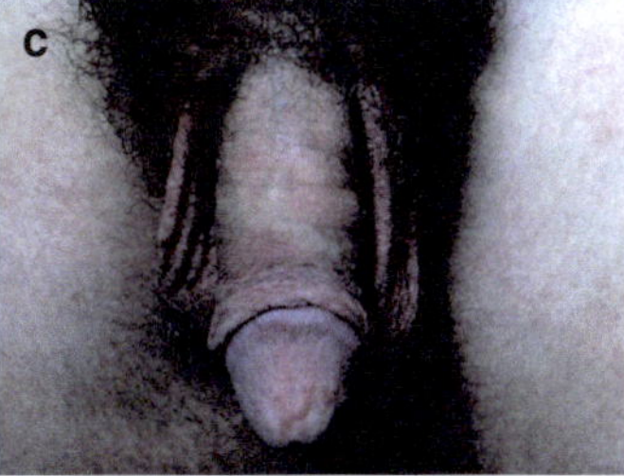

Fig. 3 Swimmer's itch: Non-specific itchy eruption, short-lasting. (**a**) Buttocks, (**b**) arm, and (**c**) genital (penis). (Courtesy: Dep. Dermatology Dijkzigt Hospital, The Netherlands. Photographer: J. Van der Stek)

itch). The acute phase occurs only in a few, more often in the non-immune travelers than in residents from the area. The avian cercariae are responsible for the majority of the reported dermatitis outbreaks around the world. Although these cercariae may penetrate the human skin, they do not mature and usually die in the skin [6, 7].

Occasionally, a part of the group that went for bathing or swimming becomes sick 2 weeks to 3 months after contact with cercariae of schistosomes (Katayama syndrome). This is a more serious event; the cercariae have developed into schistosomula and subsequently into sexual maturity. The most severe are the infections with *S. japonicum* [6, 7]. Important for diagnosis, similar to most worm infections, is eosinophilia. When one consults a patient with fever and eosinophilia and has been bathing in potentially contaminated water, one should think of the acute stage of schistosomiasis.

Katayama syndrome is an early clinical manifestation of schistosomiasis that occurs several weeks post-infection with *Schistosoma* spp. Because of this temporal delay and its non-specific presentation, it is the symptom of schistosomiasis most likely to be misdiagnosed by physicians in non-endemic countries. Katayama syndrome appears 2–14 weeks after non-immune individuals have been exposed to a first schistosome infection or to a heavy reinfection [20].

The constellation of symptoms seen in Katayama syndrome is secondary to an eosinophil-mediated systemic vasculitis [20]. Small vessel thrombosis may accompany this vasculitis. This eosinophilic response is triggered by the migrating schistosomula [21]. Katayama syndrome represents a hypersensitivity response; it resembles classical serum sickness [8]. It may rarely occur in outbreaks [22]. Mini-epidemics have been reported by Loutan et al. [23].

The disease onset is usually acute. The possible symptoms are [6–8] as follows:

1. Important for dermatologists: Urticaria or volatile erythema (This dermatological symptom is certainly not the most common).
2. Fever: The temperature can be recurrent or intermittent, sometimes marginal or mildly increased. The duration may last from a week to some months.
3. Abdominal complaints: vague abdominal pain, nausea, watery diarrhea, and sometimes blood in the stool. The liver usually is enlarged, and sometimes, the spleen is palpable too.
4. Coughing, usually unproductive.
5. Severe headache, great fatigue, severe sweating, and vague muscle and joint pains are occasionally observed.

In general, symptoms and signs involving the respiratory tract tend to occur in the initial phase of the syndrome, while abdominal signs and symptoms tend to occur much later during the course of the syndrome. Neurological manifestations are typically seen during the early phase of Katayama syndrome [24].

Anti-schistosomal antibodies are usually positive in Katayama syndrome and support an early diagnosis of the syndrome. Serological tests have an overall sensitivity of 95.5% in detecting schistosomiasis [25]. The swimmer's itch is an exception, due to the short time from exposure. Egg detection is another way of confirming the diagnosis. It still provides the gold standard (Fig. 4). Peripheral blood examination reveals significant eosinophilia in over 90% of the patients. Eosinophilic counts as high as 3080 cells/mm^3 have been reported [26]. Chest X-rays may reveal diffuse infiltrates within the lung fields. Rocha et al. have also reported micro-nodules in the inferior lung fields in patients with Katayama syndrome [27]. These nodules usually have a beaded appearance [27].

Differential diagnoses include gastroenteritis, hepatitis A, B, and C, HIV, salmonellosis, and urinary tract infections [20].

Even without treatment, the acute stage wains and heals. When a reinfection occurs, the symptoms are less or absent.

Months to years later, the chronic stage may start. This stage is caused by the eggs present in

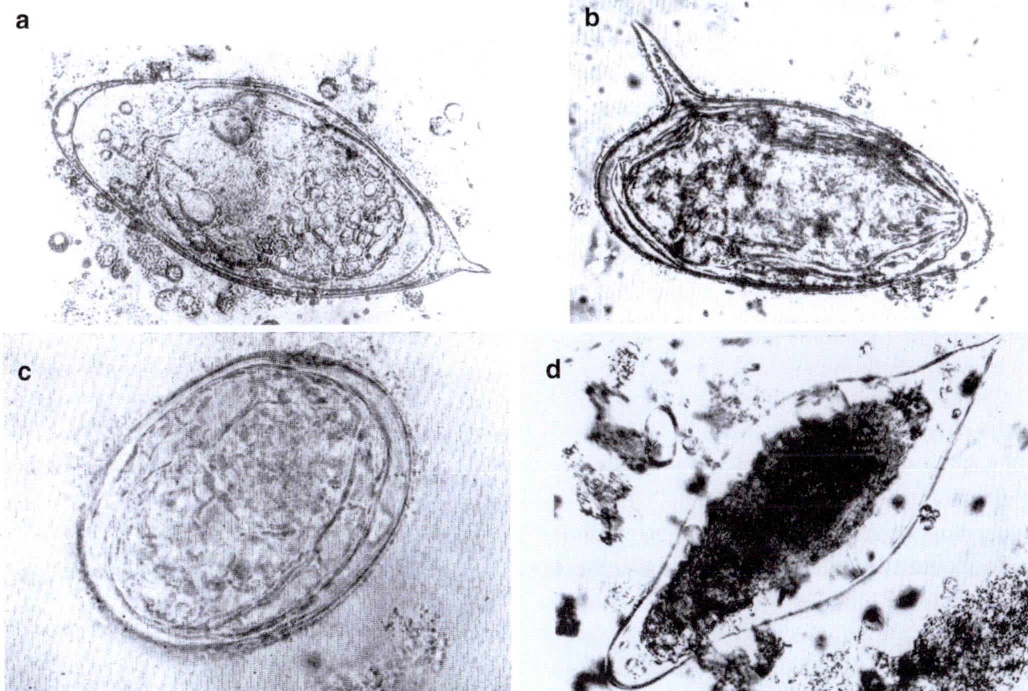

Fig. 4 Eggs of *Schistosoma*. (**a**) *S. haematobium*, end standing spike. (**b**) *S. mansoni*, a lateral spike. (**c**) *S. japonicum*, oval does not have a spike. (**d**) *S. intercalatum*, a terminal spike but a little waisted. (Courtesy: Dr. P.J. Zuidema. University of Amsterdam, the Netherlands)

the tissues. The symptoms for the different schistosomes may differ, and knowing this may assist in establishing the definitive diagnosis.

S. haematobium (Schistosomiasis of the Urinary Tract)

Geographically, it is present in the whole of Africa and the Middle East. It disappeared from the South of Portugal where it was present till the 1950Th. However, the intermediate host is still present in Portugal, Spain, and Corsica, and it may reappear [28]. And indeed, there was a recent (2016) outbreak of urogenital schistosomiasis in Corsica (France) [29].

The male worm is 10–15 mm long, the female is 20 mm, the egg is yellow brown (80–160 × 30–60 μm large), and it has an end-standing spine (Fig. 4a).

The schisotomulae of *S. haematobium* reach the vesical vessels through anastomotic channels between radicles of the inferior mesenteric vein and pelvic veins. After living inside small venules in the submucosa and the wall of the bladder, they migrate to the peri-vesical venous plexus (a group of veins at the lower portion of the bladder) to attain full maturation, which takes about a month. Eggs that reach the lumen of the bladder cause minimal loss of blood. However, more severe are the eggs that remain in the mucosae and are encased by granulation tissue (tubercles). The mucosa may contain thousands of eggs, centers of larger or smaller granulomata. Superficial tubercles may even protrude in the lumen of the bladder and, in later stage, may ulcerate. After some time, the granulomata will fibrose and the eggs calcify. Sometimes, there may be papillomata. In some endemic areas, the process may lead to carcinoma [6–8].

Some worms reside in the venulae of the ureters. There, they may cause similar problems as in the bladder. Fibrosis may obstruct the ureter causing hydro-ureter and hydronephrosis afterwards and even pyelonephritis. The worms may also be present in venous plexi of the salpinx, cervix uteri, prostate, and vesicula seminalis. Occasionally, they are present in the rectum wall, colon, or appendix but cause hardly ever clinical symptoms. The eggs may find their way to the stool [6–8].

Symptomatology

Hematuria is the major symptom. Often some blood can be seen at the end of the urination. Only when ulcerations and/or papilloma are present in the bladder, there may be some anemia. The hematuria often goes together with frequent and painful micturition and a burning feeling along the ureter afterward. The painful micturition might also be caused by secondary bacterial cystitis. The fibrosis of the bladder may also be a reason for the frequent micturition because the bladder capacity is diminished [6–8].

Diagnosis: hematuria and eggs in the sediment. The urine produced between 10.00 and 12.00 o'clock contains most eggs. The sediment also contains leukocytes of which a high percentage are eosinophils. Cystoscopy shows bilharzia tubercles, spelled button large shiny yellow papules surrounded by hyperemia. Fibrosed granuloma shows a sandy aspect. *S. haematobium* eggs are occasionally seen in the stool as well. They can be found in a rectum biopsy. There is some blood hyper-eosinophilia. Radiology shows calcifying but also hydro-ureter and nephrosis. Serology is of great help [6–8].

S. mansoni

It can be found in the whole of Africa and parts of South America and the Caribbean.

The male is 8 mm long and the female is 10 mm. The egg 122–175 μm × 45–75 μm has a lateral spike (Fig. 4b).

The worms live in the venulae of the rectum and sigmoid. The eggs reaching the lumen give no real tissue damage. The eggs that do not reach the lumen but stay in the mucosae are encased. The severe pathology is the result of embolized eggs that end up in the liver where they get stuck in the small portal venulae. Mild infections hardly give any symptoms. When the infestation is more severe, the complaints are those of a proctitis or mild colitis. There may be periods of diarrhea with or without mucous and blood in the feces. Sometimes, the patient may complain of abdominal cramps or painful defecation. A very heavy infection may give a "bilharzia-dysentery". On palpation, the colon is tender. In a late stadium, the colon may become fibrotic resulting in a papilloma, fistulas, and sometimes a rectum prolapse. The diagnosis is confirmed when eggs are found in the stool. There may be mild eosinophilia. Proctoscopy may show smaller or larger tubercles with hyperemia surrounding them. Scraping of the mucosa may show eggs [6–8].

Schistosomiasis of Organs

Liver

S. haematobium infections often cause an embolism from eggs to the liver, but this hardly ever gives clinical symptoms. In contrast, the eggs of *S. mansoni* may, with time, cause many more problems. It may lead to diffuse periportal fibrosis which, at the end, may show as pipe stem fibrosis (Symmers). The liver parenchyma stays intact for a long time. At the beginning, there are only dyspeptic complaints such as no appetite and flatulence. The liver and spleen may be slightly enlarged. Later, it may turn into portal hypertension with a large spleen, collateral circulation, and esophagus varices. Liver function remains intact for a long time. The end results are esophageal bleeding, leg edema, and ascites [6–8].

Lungs

The eggs of both *S. haematobium* and *S. mansoni* may embolize to the lungs and cause obliterative endarteritis in the lung arterioles. At the end, there may be so much obstruction that this may result in pulmonary hypertension and cor pulmonale [6–8].

CNS

Eggs of *S. haematobium* and *S. mansoni* are occasionally found in the spinal cord and the brain. This may happen in early and late infections. Particularly, in early infections, this can easily be missed. The eggs are surrounded by granulation tissue. They may give no symptoms but can lead to spinal cord injury (transverse myelitis) or epileptic insults. Magnetic resonance and computed tomographic images of the brain may show nonspecific, contrast-enhancing infiltrates, which suggest brain tumors. To prevent irreversible damage, early treatment with corticosteroids is essential, after which the adult worms can be eliminated. A high degree of suspicion is therefore needed to avoid treatment delay [24, 30].

Other Schistosomes

S. intercalatum

They are present in the Dem. Rep of Congo, in Gabon and Cameroon. The worms live in the venulae of the rectum and colon. The eggs, 140–240 µm × 50 × 85 µm, are similar to those of *S. haematobium* with a terminal spike but a little waisted or diamond-shaped (Fig. 4d). The spine is a little longer. They give only mild problems, proctitis [6–8].

S. japonica

It is present in the Far East (China, Taiwan, Japan, and Philippines). It also infects many animals (cats, dogs, and cattle). The worms live in the venulae of the small intestine and the proximal part of the colon. There is a large egg production, and the eggs may embolize to the liver, lungs, and brain. The results are periportal fibrosis, portal hypertension, and pulmonary hypertension with cor pulmonale. The eggs are oval (50 × 70 µm) and do not have a spike (Fig. 4c). The initial symptoms are diarrhea with mucous and blood, periods of fever, anorexia, and weight loss. The localization in the brain may lead to epilepsy and even hemiplegia. In general, one may say that the *S. japonica* infection is worse than the others [6, 7].

Diagnosis: The best form of diagnosis is the finding of the eggs in urine or stool. Sometimes, special concentration techniques are needed. However, this requires the adult worms to produce eggs; serological tests can diagnose the less advanced infection [31].

Antibody detection can be useful in specific circumstances, but its application is limited. A positive serological test may be diagnostic in patients who do not excrete eggs, such as those with Katayama syndrome. Serological testing can be useful in field studies for defining regions of low-level endemicity, where individual patients have low egg burdens, and may also be useful in determining whether the infection has re-emerged in a region after an apparently successful control program. It is also important for the diagnosis of travelers or immigrants from endemic areas who have not been treated appropriately for schistosomiasis in the past. For new infections, the serum sample to be tested should be collected at least 6–8 weeks after a likely infection, to allow for the full development of the parasite and antibody to the adult stage. Commercially available immunodiagnostic kits are less sensitive than multiple fecal examinations and less specific, due to antibody cross-reactivity with antigens from other helminths. Most techniques detect IgG, IgM, or IgE against soluble worm antigen or soluble egg antigen by enzyme-linked immunosorbent assay (ELISA), indirect hemagglutination, or immunofluorescence [32]. A cercarial antigen ELISA equivalent to the soluble egg antigen assay has been developed for serodiagnosis of schistosomiasis [32, 33]. The POC-CCA (Point-of-Care Circulating Cathodic Antigen) rapid test offers the best option for the rapid screening of *S. mansoni* infection in communities with a high prevalence of HIV-1 infection [34].

Specific and highly sensitive PCR-based assays have been developed for the detection of schistosome DNA in feces, urine, sera, or plasma [35–37]. This approach has the potential to provide a test for the diagnosis of schistosomiasis in all phases of clinical disease, including the capacity to diagnose Katayama syndrome and active disease, as well as for the evaluation of treatment.

Treatment

A safe and effective medication is available for treatment of both urinary and intestinal schistosomiasis: Praziquantel. It is taken for 1–2 days to treat infections caused by all schistosome species. The currently available formulation of praziquantel presents several problems. First, it is a large tablet, making it difficult for young children and infants to swallow it, and thus it requires breaking/crushing to allow for a safe uptake. Second, it is bitter, so it is often mixed with a sweetener to make it palatable for young children. Third, the current formulation of 600 mg does not permit flexible dose adjustments for this age group. Thus, there is a need to formulate a child-appropriate praziquantel. This should be:

1. Safe and well tolerated with little to no side effects;
2. Small and easy to swallow to avoid chocking;
3. Orally disintegrated and can be taken with or without water (in cases of unsafe water supply);
4. Improved taste for minimization of bitterness, easy dose adjustment by number of tablets to avoid having to break tablets;
5. Stability in hot and humid conditions [2].

Doses of S. haematobium and S. mansoni
≥1 year. Orally, 40 mg/kg/day in one to two doses just 1 day.
S. Japonica and S. mekongi
≥1 year. Orally 60 mg/kg/day in one to three doses. Just 1 day.

Use in pregnancy: Praziquantel is pregnancy category B. There are no adequate and well-controlled studies in pregnant women. However, the available evidence suggests no difference in adverse birth outcomes in the children of women who were accidentally treated with praziquantel during mass prevention campaigns compared with those who were not. There is also no teratogenic effect noticed neither in animal experiments nor during mass campaigns [38].

Lactation: Praziquantel is excreted in low concentrations in human milk. According to WHO guidelines for mass prevention campaigns, the use of praziquantel during lactation is encouraged. For individual patients in clinical settings, praziquantel should be used by breastfeeding women only when the risk to the infant is outweighed by the risk of disease progress in the mother in the absence of treatment [39].

Adverse Effects

These may not only be related to the drug but also to its effects on the worms and eggs. It works by killing; dead worms and eggs have no opportunity to actively evade the immune system any longer.

The administration is usually not associated with significant side effects. However, in those with heavy parasite burdens, abdominal pain, nausea, and vomiting may occur. Other side effects may be tiredness, sleepiness, headache, dizziness, weakness, muscle pain, tachycardia, and epilepsy. Hypersensitivity reactions may occur but are usually not severe. The drug is effective in producing a parasitic cure in approximately 80% of the treated individuals and achieves over 90% reduction in egg count in the remaining 20%. Follow-up urine or stool examination for eggs within 3 months is advised. Treatment of the chronic sequelae may necessitate other therapeutic measures.

As this article is meant for travelers, I will not dwell on the successful mass campaigns of which the success will diminish the risk for the traveler to become infected. However, it is always important to consult the local responsible authorities before coming in contact with stagnant water. However, a local claim that there is no schistosomiasis in a body of freshwater is not always reliable.

References

1. Polderman AM. Schistosomiasis, Chapter 17. In: Faber RW, Hay RJ, Naafs B, editors. Imported skin diseases. 1st ed. Maarsen: Elsevier Gezondheidszorg; 2006. p. 227–32.
2. Mduluza T, Mutapi F. Putting the treatment of paediatric schistosomiasis into context. Infect Dis Poverty. 2017;6:85. https://doi.org/10.1186/s40249-017-0300-8.
3. King CH, Dickman K, Tisch DJ. Reassessment of the cost of chronic helminthic infection: a meta-analysis of disability-related outcomes in endemic schistosomiasis. Lancet. 2005;365:561–9.
4. Steinmann P, Keiser J, Bos R, et al. Schistosomiasis and water resources development: systematic review, meta-analysis, and estimates of people at risk. Lancet Infect Dis. 2006;6:411–25.
5. King CH, Dangerfield-Cha M. The unacknowledged impact of chronic schistosomiasis. Chronic Illn. 2008;4:65–79.
6. Janssens PG, Zuidema PJ. Infecties door treponematoden (Schistosomiasis). In: Importziekten. Stafleu's wetenschappelijke. Leiden: Uitgeversmaatschappij B.V; 1973. p. 69–83.
7. Davis A. Schistosomiasis, Chapter 72. In: Cook GC, editor. Manson's tropical diseases. 20th ed; 1996. p. 1413–57.
8. Butterworth AE, Ouma JH, Vennervald BJ, Dunne DW. Schistosomiasis, Chapter 47. In: Mabey D, Gill G, Parry E, et al., editors. Principles of medicine in Africa. 4th ed. Cambridge: Cambridge University Press; 2013. p. 441–52.
9. Wilson RA, Coulson PS. Immune effector mechanisms against schistosomiasis: looking for a chink in the parasite's armour. Trends Parasitol. 2009;25(9):423–31. https://doi.org/10.1016/j.pt.2009.05.011.
10. Sayed AA, Simeonov A, Thomas CJ, et al. Identification of oxadiazoles as new drug leads for the control of schistosomiasis. Nat Med. 2008;14(4):407–12. https://doi.org/10.1038/nm1737.
11. Medhekar A. Structure and life cycle of trypanosome (with diagram). https://www.biologydiscussion.com/parasites/the-life-cycle-of-schistosoma-with-diagram/2705
12. Bogitsh BJ, Carter CE, Oeltmann TN. Blood flukes, chapter 11. In: Human parasitology. 3rd ed. Academic; 2005. p. 305–32.
13. Skelly PJ, Da'dara AA, Xiao-Hong L, et al. Schistosome feeding and regurgitation. PLoS Pathog. 2014;10(8):e1004246. https://doi.org/10.1371/journal.ppat.1004246.
14. LoVerde PT, Chen L. Schistosome female reproductive development. Trends Parasitol. 1991;7:303–8. https://doi.org/10.1016/0169-4758(91)90263-N.
15. Collins JJ III, King RS, Cogswell A, et al. An Atlas for Schistosoma mansoni. Organs and life-cycle stages using cell type-specific markers and confocal microscopy. PLoS Negl Trop Dis. 2011;5(3):e1009. https://doi.org/10.1371/journal.pntd.0001009.
16. Zimmer C. Even blood flukes get divorced. The Loom October 8, 2008 9:54 PM. https://en.wikipedia.org/wiki/Schistosoma
17. Wilson S, Jones FM, Mwatha JK, et al. Hepatosplenomegaly is associated with low regulatory and Th2 responses to schistosome antigen in childhood schistosomiasis and malaria coinfection. Infect Immun. 2008;76:2212–8.
18. Pearce EJ, MacDonald AS. The immunobiology of schistosomiasis. Nat Rev Immunol. 2002;2(7):499–511. https://doi.org/10.1038/nri843.
19. Faber WR. Schistosomiasis, Chapter 8. In: Faber WR, Naafs B, editors. Import dermatologie. Glaxo Nieuwegein; 1991. p. 125–8.
20. Ross AG, Vickers D, Olds GR, et al. Katayama syndrome. Lancet Infect Dis. 2007;7(3):218–24.
21. Jaureguiberry S, Caumes E. Neurological involvement during Katayama syndrome. Lancet Infect Dis. 2008;8(1):9–10.
22. Zuidema PJ. The Katayama syndrome; an outbreak in Dutch tourists to the Omo National Park, Ethiopia. Trop Geogr Med. 1981;33(1):30–5.
23. Loutan L, Farinelli T, Robert CF. La schistosomiase aiguë ou syndrome de Katayama: á propos de deux mini-épidémies. Schweiz Med Wochenschr. 1996;126(35):1482–6.
24. Clerinx J, van Gompel A, Lynen L, Ceulemans B. Early neuroschistosomiasis complicating Katayama syndrome. Emerg Infect Dis. 2006;12(9):1465–6.
25. Kapoor S. Katayama syndrome in patients with schistosomiasis. Asian Pac J Trop Biomed. 2014;4(3):244. https://doi.org/10.1016/S2221-1691(14)60239-2.
26. Mohamed AE. The Katayama syndrome in Saudis. J Trop Med Hyg. 1985;88(5):319–22.
27. Rocha MO, Rocha RL, Pedroso ER, et al. Pulmonary manifestations in the initial phase of schistosomiasis mansoni. Rev Inst Med Trop Sao Paulo. 1995;37(4):311.
28. Bisoffi Z, Buonfrate D, Beltrame A. Schistosomiasis transmission in Europe. Lancet Infectious Dis.

2016;16(8):878–80. https://doi.org/10.1016/S1473-3099(16)30061-5.

29. Berry A, Moné H, Iriart X, et al. Schistosomiasis Haematobium, Corsica, France. Emerg Infect Dis. 2014;20:1595–159.

30. Silva LCS, Maciel PE, Ribas JGR, et al. Treatment of schistosomal myeloradiculopathy with praziquantel and corticosteroids and evaluation by magnetic resonance imaging: a longitudinal study. Clin Infect Dis. 2004;39:1618–24. https://doi.org/10.1086/425611.

31. Gray DJ, Ross AG, Li Y-S, et al. Diagnosis and management of schistosomiasis. BMJ. 2011;342:d2651.

32. Bergquist R, Johansen MV, Utzinger J. Diagnostic dilemmas in helminthology: what tools to use and when? Trends Parasitol. 2009;25:151–6.

33. Chand MA, Chiodini PL, Doenhoff MJ. Development of a new assay for the diagnosis of schistosomiasis, using cercarial antigens. Trans R Soc Trop Med Hyg. 2010;104:255–8.

34. Mazigo HD, Heukelbach J. Diagnostic performance of Kato Katz technique and point-of-care circulating cathodic antigen rapid test in diagnosing schistosoma mansoni infection in HIV-1 co-infected adults on the shoreline of Lake Victoria, Tanzania. Trop Med Infect Dis. 2018;3(2):54. https://doi.org/10.3390/tropicalmed3020054.

35. Wichmann D, Panning M, Quack T, et al. Diagnosing schistosomiasis by detection of cell-free parasite DNA in human plasma. PLoS Negl Trop Dis. 2009;3:e422.

36. Oliveira LM, Santos HL, Gonçalves MM, et al. Evaluation of polymerase chain reaction as an additional tool for the diagnosis of low-intensity Schistosoma mansoni infection. Diagn Microbiol Infect Dis. 2010;68:416–21.

37. Gomes LI, Dos Santos Marques LH, Enk MJ, et al. Development and evaluation of a sensitive PCR-ELISA system for detection of Schistosoma infection in feces. PLoS Negl Trop Dis. 2010;4:e664.

38. CDC. Parasites-Schistosomiasis. Resources for Health Professionals. https://www.cdc.gov/parasites/schistosomiasis/health_professionals/index.html

39. CDC - Schistosomiasis - Resources for Health Professionals. https://www.cdc.gov/parasites/schistosomiasis/health_professionals/index.html

Part X

Miscellaneous

Insect Repellents

Elizabeth Salazar-Rojas

Key Points

- The most common topical chemical used as an insect repellent (IR) is N, N-diethyl-3-methylbenzamide (DEET); it is very efficient, its toxicity is low, allergic reactions are uncommon, and serious adverse effects are rare.
- Picaridin is also used as an IR in concentrations of 5–20% as effectively as DEET.
- Other compounds that are used as repellents are IR3535 (3 N-butyl-N-acetyl) amino-propionic acid, oil of lemon eucalyptus, 2-undecanone, and citronella oil.

Introduction

Arthropod bites such as mosquitoes and ticks, not only can cause annoying pruritic or painful lesions but can also transmit important vector-borne diseases to humans, including malaria, Zika virus, dengue virus, and Lyme disease, hence the importance of insect repellents (IRs). These are natural or synthetic substances applied to exposed skin or clothing to protect against insect bites (Table 1). Their use is strongly recommended by de Centers for Disease Control and Prevention (CDC) and the Environmental Protection Agency in addition to other protective measures, such as wearing special clothes and avoiding outdoor activities during peak mosquito-biting times [2].

The advice is to apply the repellent on non-irritated skin, mainly on the neck, wrists, and ankles, avoiding areas near the mouth, eyes, or nose. In small children, hands should also be avoided. The effectiveness of repellents usually lasts between 15 min up to 10 h depending on the substance and the presentation (cream, spray, gel, or lotion). Therefore, the ideal IR must have low toxicity, long-lasting and broad action, an esthetic formulation, water and sweat resistance, low cost, and a pleasant scent.

Table 1 Types of repellents [1]

Synthetic	Natural
DEET	Lemon eucalyptus plant
Picaridin	Citronella
IR3535	Neem oil
DEPA	Andiroba
Permethrin	Wild tomato plant

Synthetic

The most common topical chemical used as repellent is N, N-diethyl-3-methylbenzamide (DEET), previously called N, N-diethyl-3-

E. Salazar-Rojas (✉)
Hospital Angeles Pedregal, Mexico City, Mexico

W. Robles (ed.), *Skin Disease in Travelers*, Updates in Clinical Dermatology, https://doi.org/10.1007/978-3-031-57836-6_33

methylbenzamide. This chemical is very efficient in repelling chiggers, fleas, gnats, and some flies as well. DEET formulations contain between 5% and 99%. CDC recommends a concentration of the active ingredient of at least 20% in adults and 10% in children over the age of 6 months. The safety of topical DEET application is acceptable, toxicity is low, and it can be used by pregnant women, but it should be avoided in children under 6 months of age [3].

Allergic reactions are uncommon, and serious adverse effects are rare (local skin reactions). If the concentration is at 50–75%, patients may develop vesiculobullous skin necrosis, scarring, or erythema. DEET works by disturbing mosquito antenna receptors and masking the host's smell [1]. DEET formulations are generally oily and can be sticky as well; it can damage synthetic fiber, clothing, and plastic used in eyeglasses and watches [4]. The effect lasts for as long as 6 h. It is the IR of choice for the CDC to prevent West Nile virus, Lyme disease, and Zika virus infection [1], but it must not be used in children under 2 years of age or in concentrations greater than 33% [5].

Picaridin or icaridin is also used as IR in concentrations of 5–20% as effectively as DEET for 10 h. It is more commonly used in Europe and Australia as an active ingredient; it is more cosmetically acceptable, and, occasionally, can cause skin and eye irritation. It does not feel sticky and is odorless. Its activity against Culicine mosquitoes, flies, and biting midges is very high [4]. Picaridin alters mosquito's odorant receptor proteins [6].

IR3535 repels mosquitoes and other insects for 4 h; its concentration between 10% and 20% is effective. This repellent can cause eye irritation, and it may damage plastic and clothing. It is safe during pregnancy and in children over 6 months of age [1]. Formulations with this compound are colorless and biodegradable and are effective against mosquitoes, deer ticks, body lice, and biting flies [1].

DEPA (N, N diethyl phenylacetamide) at 20% gives an 8-h duration; there are new prolonged releasing formulations for this compound.

Natural

Oil extracted from the lemon eucalyptus plant (*Corymbia citriodora*) (OLE p-menthane-3,8-diol) is efficient like DEET but can cause eye irritation and allergic skin reactions. It should not be used in children under 3 years of age. It is less effective than DEET or picaridin (depending on the concentration) but is the best of the natural repellents [7]. Its mechanism of action is unknown but could act from 6 to 12 h. This compound has better efficacy if used with picaridin compared with DEET [1].

The wild tomato plant (*Lycopersicon hirsutum*) produces a compound called 2-undecanone (methyl nonyl ketone) and its synthetic version, known as BIO-UD-8, is available as a 7.75% concentration spray for use on skin, clothing, and gear. This compound gives protection for 4.5 h for mosquitoes but only 2 h for ticks. It is also used as a pesticide in paths, patios, and containers of ornamental plants.

Citronella (*Cympobogon* sp.) oil is effective only against mosquitoes for a short term (less than 2 h) because of its rapid evaporation. It can cause allergic contact dermatitis. This compound is effective against Anopheline mosquitoes (malaria) and Culicine mosquitoes (arbovirus) [1]. There are new nanoemulsions that increase efficiency with a great aesthetic formulation. Citronella is less effective than DEET products but adding vanillin could prolong the protection time [8]. Despite its popularity, it is not recommended for use in disease endemic areas [9].

Neem oil is obtained from an Indian plant used in Brazil, it is less effective than synthetic repellents, and it has a short action.

Other oils from clove, geraniol, catnip, and patchouli are used but with limited efficiency. Garlic has provided evidence of systemic mosquito repellence but not significantly [10].

Clothing IRs

Permethrin (chrysanthemum flower extract) is considered a drug (to treat scabies and lice), an insecticide, as well as an IR. It is applied on clothing, nets, shoes, tents, and sleeping bags and acts for several weeks against mosquitoes, ticks, and flies [1]. Adverse effects include neurotoxic effects such as tremors, paralysis, skin and eye irritation, reproductive effects, and alteration in the immune system [10].

Wearable devices such as wristbands or collars impregnated with several repellents are not effective.

There are different products with IRs such as coils, vaporizing mats, aerosols, and insecticide-impregnated curtains. World Health Organization recommends the use of aerosol sprays in combination with a coil or bed nets [2].

Topical IRs must be used after sunscreen application. The repellent can reduce the sun protection factor, but applying it before sunscreen may increase DEET absorption [11].

Bug zappers are ineffective, and they may kill beneficial insects.

Reducing vector-borne disease may be possible by suppressing mosquito populations with novel methods like the sterile insect technique with irradiated or chemically treated males, or incompatible insect technique using a bacteria named *Wolbachia* or various genetic modification strategies carrying a transgene that cause larvae death before reaching the pupal stage. These are promising strategies for reducing mosquito infestations [8].

Some fish species like *Gambusia affinis* and nonpathogenic bacteria like *Bacillus thuringiensis* consume mosquito larvae and can be released into the environment to control insects [1].

Conclusion

IRs are chemical or organic substances widely used to prevent vector-borne diseases. However, they could generate concern among people due to the potential adverse effects on health such as endocrine disruption, allergic contact dermatitis, asthma, or migraine as well as environmental changes produced by them [12].

DEET is known to be the best IR, but there are plenty of them approved. Therefore, people must be aware that the ideal IR has low toxicity, long-lasting and broad action, an aesthetic formulation, water and sweat resistance, low cost, and a pleasant scent.

Consumers must know the possible toxicities and should follow the product label indications such as favoring creams, gels, or lotion over sprays to minimize the risk of absorption through mucosae, but they must understand and be aware of the risks of vector-borne diseases as health issue as well. As many cultures have edible insects in their diets, consumers must be aware of the possible contamination with this pesticides to avoid toxicity as well.

References

1. Nguyen QD, Vu MN, Hebert AA. Insect repellents: an updated review for the clinician. J Am Acad Dermatol. 2018: S0190-9622(18)32824-X.
2. World Health Organization. A global brief on vector-borne diseases. WorldHealthOrganization. 2014. https://apps.who.int/iris/handle/10665/111008 (cited 2020 Sept 11).
3. Diaz JH. Chemical and plant-based insect repellents: efficacy, safety, and toxicity. Wilderness Environ Med. 2016;27(1):153–63.
4. Insect repellents. Med Lett Drugs Ther. 2016;58(1498):83–5.
5. Benenson AS. Medical advice for the traveler. Am J Public Health. 1971;61(9):1920.
6. Bohbot JD, Dickens JC. Insect repellents: modulators of mosquito odorant receptor activity. PLoS One. 2010;5(8):e12138.
7. Juckett G. Arthropod bites. Am Fam Physician. 2013;88(12):841–7.
8. Flores HA, O'Neill SL. Controlling vector-borne diseases by releasing modified mosquitoes. Nat Rev Microbiol. 2018;16(8):508–18.
9. Goodyer LI, Croft AM, Frances SP, Hill N, Moore SJ, Onyango SP, Debboun M. Expert review of the evidence base for arthropod bite avoidance. J Travel Med. 2010;17(3):182–92.
10. Katz TM, Miller JH, Hebert AA. Insect repellents: historical perspectives and new developments. J Am Acad Dermatol. 2008;58(5):865–71.
11. Tavares M, da Silva MRM, de Oliveira de Siqueira LB, et al. Trends in insect repellent formulations: a review. Int J Pharm. 2018;539(1–2):190–209.
12. Roy DN, Goswami R, Pal A. The insect repellents: a silent environmental chemical toxicant to the health. Environ Toxicol Pharmacol. 2017;50:91–102.

Sun Protection

Yasaman Mansouri

Key Points

- The sun protection factor (SPF) is a worldwide standard for measuring the effectiveness of sunscreens.
- UV filters are divided into inorganic and organic.
- The inorganic filters titanium dioxide and zinc oxide are preferred for patients with sensitive skin, rosacea, sunscreen allergies and for children.
- Organic UV filters are the most widely used sunscreen agents. There have been recent concerns by the public over their safety, as systemic absorption of some of the organic filters was demonstrated in 2019. Furthermore, the organic UV filters oxybenzone and octinoxate are being banned in some parts of the United States due to possible damage to coral reefs.
- Some organic UV filters, such as oxybenzone and octinoxate may lead to the development of allergic contact dermatitis and photocontact allergy.

Sunscreens are an integral part of protection against UV radiation-induced skin damage. They block, absorb, or reflect ultraviolet radiation (UVR) to protect the skin against the harmful rays of the sun. UVR is absorbed by chromophores in the skin, which leads to photobiologic changes. Chromophores are molecules that absorb energy from the UV and visible spectrum. These chromophores include urocanic acid, melanin, DNA, and RNA. In relation to the biological effects of UV, DNA is the most important of the chromophores [1]. UVR-induced changes can damage DNA directly or indirectly via reactive oxygen species, leading to mutation or cell death by apoptosis or necrosis. Nevertheless, sunlight, mainly UVB, is necessary for the production of vitamin D, which is essential for human health [2].

Sunscreens can prevent the damage caused by UVR. Sunscreens have been shown to reduce the development of pre-cancerous lesions and some skin cancers, [3] they decrease the number of nevi in children [4] and reduce photoaging [5]. Sunscreen agents can be divided into two broad categories: organic and inorganic formulations.

Organic sunscreens absorb specific photons of UVR. Energy is absorbed by the UV filter in the sunscreen, which then leads to the excitation of the molecule that absorbed the energy. The excited molecule then harmlessly dissipates that energy.

Inorganic sunscreens physically block the UV radiation from penetrating the skin. They have been used since the early days of sunscreens, but their large particle size left a visible white film on the skin surface, thus rendering them cosmetically unappealing. Micronized forms have been devel-

Y. Mansouri (✉)
NYC Health + Hospitals/Woodhull Hospital,
Brooklyn, NY, USA

W. Robles (ed.), *Skin Disease in Travelers*, Updates in Clinical Dermatology,
https://doi.org/10.1007/978-3-031-57836-6_34

325

oped, and these have become popular. However, because of their smaller particle size, potential systemic absorption has created concern.

History

The ancient Egyptians were the first to use ingredients such as rice bran, jasmine, and lupine to protect the skin from tanning. Other cultures used other materials, such as olive oil. Sunscreens were used to maintain lighter skin, which was considered more desirable in earlier times. However, the dangers of UV rays were not discovered until much later, in 1889 [6]. In the nineteenth century, the first chemical sunscreens were used, and these early sunscreens contained ingredients such as tannic acid, acidified quinine sulfate, aesculin, 2-naphthol-6,8-disulfonated sodium, para-amino-benzoic acid, cinnamates, and lanolin.

In 1935, the future founder of L'Oreal, Eugene Schueller, used benzyl salicylate in an oily vehicle to create the first major commercial sunscreen, "Ambre Solaire" [7, 8].

After suffering sunburns while climbing the Piz Buin alpine peak in 1938, Franz Greiter, developed "Gletscher Crème" or Glacier cream, a sunscreen developed for mountaineers. The product is still sold today, under the brand Piz Buin [9]. During World War II, the U.S. Army provided troops with red veterinary petrolatum, a heavy and greasy substance that worked as a physical barrier, to prevent sunburns. Sunscreens then became an integral part of photoprotection strategy.

Schulze was the first to introduce a protection factor for sunscreens, later called "Schulze Factor" [10]. He determined the minimal erythema dose (MED), which had already been described in 1934, [10] for human skin, and then, in the same person, exposed skin protected by sunscreen to multiples of the MED, to determine efficacy. The MED is the lowest dose of UVR that produces the first perceptible unambiguous erythema with defined borders appearing over the field of UV exposure, 16–24 h after exposure.

In 1974, Franz Greiter popularized the concept of the "sun protection factor" (SPF), a new name for the "Schulze factor." The SPF has become a worldwide standard for measuring the effectiveness of sunscreens [10]. Greiter also described a method for studying the water resistance of sunscreens. He used a comparison of laboratory tests assessing UV filter adherence to merino wool and pig skin combined with tests in humans undergoing activities such as swimming or exercise to induce sweating [11]. Widespread usage of sunscreens did not occur until the 1970s and 1980s when public health campaigns informed the public of the dangers of UV-induced skin damage. In 1978, the U.S. Food and Drug Administration (FDA) started regulating sunscreen products [10].

Sunscreen products have evolved over the years, from the initial "Glacier cream" to a wide variety of available UV filters. Today, sunscreens are widely used, and products have become more cosmetically appealing. Meanwhile, there are increasing controversies and concerns about the safety of sunscreens as well their impact on the environment. Potential adverse reactions to sunscreens, albeit rare, include irritant, allergic, phototoxic, and photoallergic contact dermatitis [12]. One concern has been that sunscreens may prevent the synthesis of vitamin D [13]. Insufficiency of vitamin D can lead to poor skeletal health, multiple dermatological disorders, systemic infections, [14] as well as an increased risk and poor prognosis of some internal malignancies [2, 15]. However, normal usage of sunscreen by adults has not shown to decrease cutaneous synthesis of vitamin D [16]. Additionally, the current understanding is that UVB-induced vitamin D production in the skin is not superior to dietary vitamin D supplementation.

Ultraviolet Radiation

The electromagnetic radiation reaching the surface of the earth includes infrared, visible, and UV light. There are three categories of UVR, divided based on their wavelength; these are referred to as UV-A (400–320 nm), UV-B (320–290 nm), and UV-C (290–100 nm). UVA is further divided into UVA1 (340–400 nm) and UVA2 (320–340 nm). The shorter wavelength

UVB penetrates the epidermis and causes sunburn, delayed pigmentation, photoaging, and photocarcinogenesis by direct DNA damage. UVA radiation reaches deeper into the dermis. It causes immediate pigment darkening, photoaging, and worsening of photodermatoses, such as lupus erythematosus and polymorphous light eruption. UVA further causes indirect DNA damage through the formation of reactive oxygen species [17]. The Earth has a natural UV filter, the ozone layer, which is very effective in blocking UVC (100% of UVC absorbed) and UVB (95% of UVB is absorbed). However, it is essentially transparent to UVA (only 5% of UVA is absorbed). Thus, most of the UVR reaching the Earth's surface is UVA. Unfortunately, the ozone layer has been depleted over the past decades, and more UV radiation is reaching the Earth's surface [18]. Early sunscreens were produced with the aim of avoiding sunburn and therefore contained only UVB-absorbing agents. Today, broad-spectrum sunscreens protect against both UVB and UVA.

Sun Protection Factor

SPF is a measure of how much UVR is required to develop erythema on sunscreen-protected skin relative to the amount of UVR required to produce erythema on unprotected skin. It represents the fraction of erythema-producing UV light (primarily UVB and some UVA2) that penetrates through the product to reach the skin. To evaluate protection against UVA radiation, the critical wave-length method is recommended by the U.S. Food and Drug Administration.

When properly applied, an SPF 15 sunscreen allows penetration of 1/15th (7%) of erythemogenic UV photons, an SPF 50 sunscreen transmits 1/50th (2%), and an SPF 100 sunscreen transmits 1/100th (1%). Accordingly, SPF 50 and 100 sunscreens are only moderately more protective than SPF 15 sunscreens: 98% or 99% vs. 93%. A sunscreen with SPF 30 is not twice as strong as one with SPF 15, as many people might think. Determination of the SPF value for use on product labels has been standardized for sunscreens at an application level of 2 mg/cm^2 [19].

However, consumers apply only 0.5–1.0 mg/cm^2 [19–21]. This leads to a lower-than-predicted beneficial effect of sunscreens and it may provide the user with a false sense of security regarding the level of protection [22–24]. Consequently, the application of sunscreen prolongs the time needed to develop sunburn.

UVA Protection

There is no unanimity regarding the ideal assay to assess protection against UVA. In the United States, there is no specific rating system for the amount of UVA protection provided by a sunscreen. The FDA allows sunscreens to be labeled "broad-spectrum" if they provide UVA and UVB protection and if the UVA protection is proportional to the UVB protection. Broad-spectrum sunscreens with an SPF ≥15 can claim that they can reduce the risk of skin cancer and early skin aging if used as directed along with other sun protection measures. The FDA mainly regulates three claims for sunscreen labeling: SPF, water resistance, and UV protection spectrum. The FDA and the US Preventive Services Task Force (USPSTF) both recommend the use of a broad-spectrum sunscreen with an SPF ≥15. The American Academy of Dermatology (AAD) recommends that patients use sunscreen with broad-spectrum protection, SPF 30 or higher, and water resistance [25].

In 2011, an *in vivo* method using UVA-derived persistent pigment darkening (PPD) of the skin became an international standard (International Organization for Standardization—ISO) as an endpoint for measuring UVA protection [26]. PPD measures the minimal UVA radiation required to induce visible pigment darkening in sunscreen-protected skin compared with unprotected skin. This method was later combined with an *in vitro* method, thus delivering two endpoints for the labeling of sunscreen products.

The "Critical Wavelength" is an *in vitro* method. It is defined as the wavelength at which 90% of the area under the absorbance curve between 290 and 400 nm is obtained. In 2011, the FDA adopted the Critical Wavelength value to assess UVA or broad-spectrum protection. Only products with a critical wavelength at 370 nm or higher can be labeled as providing broad-spectrum protection [27]. A multicenter comparison of the FDA and ISO methods for assessing UVA protection of sunscreens found that the method adopted by the FDA was weaker compared with the ISO method. Thus, sunscreen products approved in the United States might have insufficient UVA protection to be marketed in the European Union (EU) [28]. Indeed, almost half of the sunscreens tested did not pass standards set in the EU [27].

Substantivity

The term substantivity describes the ability of a sunscreen to maintain efficacy and resist removal by water, including repeated immersion in water and sweating [29]. Highly substantive preparations are preferred, especially in circumstances where they may be washed or rubbed off.

Sunscreen Regulation

Regulation of sunscreens varies widely around the world [30]. While in the United States, sunscreens are regulated as over-the-counter (OTC) drugs by the FDA; they are classified as cosmetics in Europe. In Australia, beach sunscreens are regulated as therapeutic drugs, whereas daily-wear moisturizer sunscreens are regulated as cosmetics. Authorities in Japan regulate sunscreens as "quasi-drugs" with regulations on the types of UV filters and concentrations allowed.

Common UV Filters

Inorganic Filters

Inorganic filters (also known as mineral filters) include titanium dioxide (TiO_2) and zinc oxide (ZnO), which absorb and reflect UV photons. Titanium dioxide is a very efficient UV filter, predominantly blocking UVB radiation [31]. Zinc oxide has been FDA-approved since 1998. It acts as a broad-spectrum sunscreen that is more efficient in UVA absorption than TiO_2. ZnO and TiO_2 can be used together, and this combination provides robust broad-spectrum coverage [32].

Initial inorganic filters contained large particle sizes of around 100–400 µm. While this prevented systemic absorption, the thick formulations left a white film on the skin that was cosmetically unappealing [33]. To improve consumer satisfaction, their particle sizes were decreased to micronized and later, nanosized (<100 nm) preparations. These are more cosmetically pleasing than the older inorganic sunscreens as they are less visible after application. Thus, the micronized and nanosized preparations have popularized the use of inorganic UV filters. However, nanosized UV filters have created concern regarding possible systemic absorption [32, 34] as well as the generation of free radicals [34]. Despite concerns about the potential of systemic absorption, nanosized zinc oxide was not found to penetrate through the stratum corneum or cause toxicity in the skin after repeated applications on human skin [35]. Based on increased internal cancers in rat models, [32, 36] TiO_2 has been classified as a possible carcinogen when inhaled in large doses. Inhalation of TiO_2 is more likely to occur during the manufacturing process rather than during the application of sunscreens.

UVR-induced skin damage includes the formation of free radicals and reactive oxygen species. ZnO and TiO_2, especially their nanosized forms, can induce free radical formation *in vitro*. This has created some concern regarding their use as sunscreens [37, 38]. However, other studies have shown that the risk of free radical formation appears to be very low because these products are not absorbed [31].

Overall, based on current scientific evidence, inorganic UV filters pose no or negligible risk to human health, [31, 39] and they pose a lower risk than most other sunscreen ingredients in the U.S. market [40]. Inorganic filters are preferred for sunscreen-allergic individuals, patients with sensitive skin, persons with rosacea, and children. It should further be noted that TiO2 is used as an additive in food and personal care products, thus attesting to its safety [31].

Organic Filters

Organic filters remain the most widely used sunscreen agents, but the use of inorganic sunscreens is increasing [31]. The latter have a higher spectrum of protection and do not cause skin sensitization [41]. Organic filters absorb UVA, UVB, or both. These chemicals are commonly used ingredients, not just in sunscreens but in many personal care products including cosmetics, fragrances, shampoos, and hair sprays [42]. There are five main types of organic filters: para-aminobenzoic acid (PABA) derivatives, cinnamates, salicylates, benzophenones, and a "miscellaneous" group. The latter include oxybenzone (benzophenone-3), 4-methylbenzylidene camphor (4-MBC), octocrylene, octinoxate (ethylhexyl methoxycinnamate, octyl methoxycinnamate (OMC)), PABA, octyl dimethyl PABA (padimate), and menthyl anthranilate (meradimate). 4-MBC has been approved in the EU but is not listed as an approved filter by the FDA.

Oxybenzone (benzophenone-3) is a broadband organic filter that absorbs UVB and UVA2. It is the most commonly used benzophenone [43]. Oxybenzone is rapidly oxidized under UV radiation, thus reducing its efficacy and generating significant levels of reactive oxygen species. The maximum allowed concentration of oxybenzone in the United States is 6%. In personal care products, concentrations of around 0.5% are used. Approximately 4% of benzophenone-3 applied to the skin is absorbed [44].

Oxybenzone is one of few filters approved in the United States and it is still widely used there. However, there are growing concerns about the use of this chemical.

Octinoxate belongs to the group of cinnamates. Oxybenzone and also octinoxate have been shown to cause hormonal disruptions in humans and wildlife. They also cause coral bleaching, and they are allergenic. Octinoxate is approved as a cosmetic ingredient in the United States and the EU. Oxybenzone can lead to allergic contact dermatitis, photocontact allergy, and contact urticaria [42]. In fact, the American Contact Dermatitis Society listed benzophenone-3 as the 2014 Allergen of the Year, covering both allergy and photoallergy.

Studies have shown that oxybenzone and octinoxate can impact the endocrine systems of humans and other organisms [45]. Oxybenzone has been detected in serum, urine, and breast milk [46, 47] and maternal exposure to this organic filter has been associated with Hirschsprung's disease in the offspring [48]. In recent years, concerns over potential risks to the environment have increased. UV filters have been identified in water sources worldwide [47]. There are various ways in which organic UV filters enter the environment. They are excreted in the urine, which enters plumbing. The majority of the applied chemical UV filters (approximately 96%) remain on the skin and are eventually washed off into bath water. These chemicals are further found in waste from manufacturing facilities, [49] as well as in treated water of wastewater treatment plants, which are used to recycle water. Removal of these organic filters is difficult.

It is estimated that around 14,000 tons of sunscreen enter coral reefs annually [50].

In 2018, the legislature of the State of Hawaii of the United States passed a bill banning the sale and distribution of sunscreens containing oxybenzone and octinoxate without a doctor's prescription. This ban went into effect on January 1, 2021 [51]. California, Key West (Florida), and the Pacific island country of Palau have enacted similar legislation banning oxybenzone and octinoxate [52]. The U.S. Virgin Islands also banned sunscreens containing oxybenzone, octinoxate and octocrylene. This went into effect in March 2020. However, evidence also exists that a major cause of coral reef damage may be climate change leading to ocean warming [53–55]. Similar bans are being considered in Brazil and the EU.

Avobenzone (butyl methoxydibenzoylmethane or Parsol® 1789) is one of the most widely used UVA filters in sunscreens [56]. It has one of the highest protection factors against UVA, and its action spectrum spans from 310 to 400 nm. However, its photolability renders it prone to degradation in the presence of UV radiation [56].

Notably, 60% of avobenzone photodegrades in 1 h and 90% in 4 h after UV radiation exposure [57]. To overcome the photo-instability of avobenzone, various photostabilizers have been added, and these include octocrylene, diethylhexyl 2,6-naphthalate, ethylhexyl methoxycrylene, and antioxidants such as vitamin C, vitamin E, and ubiquinone [56]. These combinations reduce photo-degradation, although they do not completely eliminate it. While there have been reports of photoallergy caused by avobenzone, its potential for inducing allergy is small compared to other sunscreen agents [58].

PABA derivatives are highly effective UVB absorbers and were the first widely used UV filters. Padimate O (octyldimethyl PABA) was the most common of this group. Their use has declined due to sensitivities to PABA, leading to photoallergy and contact allergy. When combined with oxybenzone, they also lead to severe photodegradation.

Salicylates are weak UVB absorbers with a peak absorption of about 300 nm. They are typically used in combination with other organic agents. Octyl salicylate, homomenthyl salicylate (homosalate), and trolamine salicylate are currently approved in the United States. The FDA uses Homosalate as the standard sunscreen in testing procedures to determine the SPF of a product. Trolamine salicylate is water soluble and frequently used in hair products as a photoprotective agent.

Ensulizole (phenylbenzimidazole sulfonic acid) is a pure UVB absorber. It is water-soluble and commonly used in cosmetics for a lighter feel. Ensulizole is used in combination with other organic or inorganic agents to enhance the SPF of the final sunscreen.

Meradimate (menthyl anthralinate) absorbs mainly in the UVA2 range.

Ecamsule (terephthalyidene dicamphor sulfonic acid) is a photostable and water-resistant broad-spectrum UV organic filter.

In 2019, an open-label, randomized, pilot study in 24 adult participants demonstrated systemic absorption of all 4 sunscreen ingredients tested (avobenzone, oxybenzone, octocrylene, and ecamsule) [59]. The resultant plasma concentrations exceeded the 0.5 ng/mL threshold set by the FDA that triggers a requirement for further systemic safety testing [59]. A more recent randomized clinical trial by the same group assessed the systemic absorption of 6 active ingredients (avobenzone, oxybenzone, octocrylene, homosalate, octisalate, and octinoxate) in 48 healthy subjects. All the tested ingredients were found to be systemically absorbed, with plasma concentrations greater than the FDA safety threshold [60]. While the authors concluded that "these results do not indicate that individuals should refrain from the use of sunscreen," this has led to growing concern by the public whether the use of these sunscreens is safe.

It remains unknown whether the systemic absorption of these sunscreen ingredients has any health impacts.

Two questionnaire studies have suggested a possible association between frontal fibrosing alopecia and the use of leave-on facial skincare products and sunscreens [61, 62]. While the results of these studies do not prove any causal role, further research would be beneficial.

Over the past decades, there has been growing interest in potential oral sunscreens. While some agents have been shown to reduce the severity of sunburn and decrease photosensitivity, these products cannot replace sunscreen. The FDA issued a statement in May 2018 warning that there are no oral sunscreens [63].

Polypodium leucotomos is a tropical fern grown in Central and South America. Polypodium leucotomos extract (PLE) is available as OTC topical or oral formulations. Studies with the oral preparation have shown that it increases the UV dose required for immediate pigment darkening and minimal erythemal dose [64]. PLE may be protective against the development of polymorphous light eruption, [65] and UVB- and psoralen plus UVA-induced toxicity [66, 67]. PLE is rich in phenolic compounds and has mainly antioxidative and anti-inflammatory effects [68].

Skin Cancer Prevention

The daily use of broad-spectrum sunscreen is recommended to prevent UV-induced skin damage. Photoprotection should also include seeking shade, wearing photoprotective clothing, including sunglasses and wide-brimmed hats, and avoiding sunbeds and tanning parlors. Protection of the eyes is extremely important as UV-induced ocular disease includes cataracts, eyelid malignancies, photokeratitis, pterygium, droplet keratopathy, macular degeneration, and potentially uveal melanoma [69–71]. Skin cancers are among the most common malignancies affecting humans, and the incidence of both melanoma and keratinocyte cancers has increased over the past decades [72, 73]. The average annual number of adults treated for skin cancer in the United States increased from 3.4 million in 2002–2006 to 4.9 million in 2007–2011 [74]. While the use of sunscreen is a key component of sun-safe behavior, epidemiological studies have yielded conflicting results about the relationship between skin cancer and sunscreen use.

Experimental studies have shown that the correct use of broad-spectrum sunscreens decreases the rate of new actinic keratoses [75] and lowers the incidence of squamous cell carcinoma. However, the literature regarding the prevention of basal cell carcinomas and cutaneous melanomas is mixed. Some studies failed to show a reduction of these cancers with the use of sunscreens, [18, 76–78] and there have even been suggestions that sunscreen use may actually increase the risk of melanoma [79]. However, this association may be related to failure to control for confounding factors [80]. Yet, others have demonstrated a reduced incidence of new melanomas in an Australian cohort of patients applying sunscreen, although the results were only marginally significant [81]. The failure of a protective effect of sunscreens on the development of basal cell carcinomas in prospective studies may be related to the significant lag time between sun exposure and the development of basal cell carcinomas [82, 83].

Sunscreen Use in Children

UV protective measures should start in infancy, as it is well known that sun exposure at a young age has been associated with an increased risk of skin cancer in later years [84, 85]. Childhood represents a period of heightened susceptibility to UVR [84]. Furthermore, children often spend prolonged periods in the sun due to outdoor activities. The AAD recommends keeping babies under 6 months of age out of direct sunlight. Parents of infants who are 6 months and older may apply a broad-spectrum, water-resistant sunscreen with an SPF of 30 or higher to their children's exposed skin. Inorganic sunscreen ingredients zinc oxide or titanium dioxide may cause less irritation to their skin.

Conclusion

It is well known that excessive UV exposure can lead to sunburns, photoaging, and skin cancers. When correctly applied in the proper amount and frequency, sunscreens will protect against the damaging effects of UVR. Sunscreen application to exposed areas is only one part of adequate photoprotection and should be practiced in combination with photoprotective clothing, wide-brimmed hats, sunglasses, avoidance of midday sun exposure, and seeking shade. People with sensitive skin, children, and those worries about potential systemic absorption of organic sunscreens may prefer to use inorganic sunscreen filters.

References

1. Emri G, Paragh G, Tósaki Á, Janka E, Kollár S, Hegedűs C, et al. Ultraviolet radiation-mediated development of cutaneous melanoma: an update. J Photochem Photobiol B. 2018;185:169–75.
2. Alkan A, Köksoy EB. Vitamin D deficiency in cancer patients and predictors for screening (D-ONC study). Curr Probl Cancer. 2019;
3. Wang SQ, Tanner PR, Lim HW, Nash JF. The evolution of sunscreen products in the United States--a 12-year cross sectional study. Photochem Photobiol

Sci Off J Eur Photochem Assoc Eur Soc Photobiol. 2013;12(1):197–202.

4. Gallagher RP, Rivers JK, Lee TK, Bajdik CD, McLean DI, Coldman AJ. Broad-spectrum sunscreen use and the development of new nevi in white children: a randomized controlled trial. JAMA. 2000;283(22):2955–60.

5. Rabe JH, Mamelak AJ, McElgunn PJS, Morison WL, Sauder DN. Photoaging: mechanisms and repair. J Am Acad Dermatol. 2006;55(1):1–19.

6. Widmark EJ, University College LLS, University College LLS. Ueber den Einfluss des Lichtes auf die Haut [electronic resource] [Internet]. [Stockholm : Samson and Wallin]; 1889 [cited 2019 Feb 15]. 78 p. Available from: http://archive.org/details/b21634336

7. Rigel DS, Weiss RA, Lim HW, Dover JS. Photoaging. 1st ed. Andover, MA: Informa Healthcare; 2004. 416 p.

8. Urbach F. The historical aspects of sunscreens. J Photochem Photobiol B. 2001;64(2–3):99–104.

9. Piz Buin [Internet]. [cited 2019 Feb 2]. Available from: https://www.pizbuin.com/en/our-heritage/

10. Schalka S, Reis VMSD. Sun protection factor: meaning and controversies. An Bras Dermatol. 2011;86(3):507–15.

11. Greiter F, Bilek P, Doskoczil S, Washüttl J, Wurst F. Methods for water resistance testing of sun protection products. Int J Cosmet Sci. 1979;1(3):147–57.

12. Bryden AM, Moseley H, Ibbotson SH, Chowdhury MMU, Beck MH, Bourke J, et al. Photopatch testing of 1155 patients: results of the U.K. multicentre photopatch study group. Br J Dermatol. 2006 Oct;155(4):737–47.

13. Norval M, Wulf HC. Does chronic sunscreen use reduce vitamin D production to insufficient levels? Br J Dermatol. 2009 Oct;161(4):732–6.

14. Kechichian E, Ezzedine K. Vitamin D and the skin: an update for dermatologists. Am J Clin Dermatol. 2018;19(2):223–35.

15. Moan J, Dahlback A, Lagunova Z, Cicarma E, Porojnicu AC. Solar radiation, vitamin D and cancer incidence and mortality in Norway. Anticancer Res. 2009;29(9):3501–9.

16. Kannan S, Lim HW. Photoprotection and vitamin D: a review. Photodermatol Photoimmunol Photomed. 2014;30(2–3):137–45.

17. Narayanan DL, Saladi RN, Fox JL. Review: ultraviolet radiation and skin cancer. Int J Dermatol. 2010;49(9):978–86.

18. Lautenschlager S, Wulf HC, Pittelkow MR. Photoprotection. Lancet Lond Engl. 2007;370(9586):528–37.

19. Petersen B, Wulf HC. Application of sunscreen-theory and reality. Photodermatol Photoimmunol Photomed. 2014;30(2–3):96–101.

20. Narbutt J, Philipsen PA, Harrison GI, Morgan KA, Lawrence KP, Baczynska KA, et al. Sunscreen applied at ≥ 2 mg cm-2 during a sunny holiday prevents erythema, a biomarker of ultraviolet radiation-induced DNA damage and suppression of acquired immunity. Br J Dermatol. 2018;

21. Azurdia RM, Pagliaro JA, Diffey BL, Rhodes LE. Sunscreen application by photosensitive patients is inadequate for protection. Br J Dermatol. 1999;140(2):255–8.

22. Wulf HC, Stender IM, Lock-Andersen J. Sunscreens used at the beach do not protect against erythema: a new definition of SPF is proposed. Photodermatol Photoimmunol Photomed. 1997;13(4):129–32.

23. Stenberg C, Larkö O. Sunscreen application and its importance for the sun protection factor. Arch Dermatol. 1985;121(11):1400–2.

24. Diffey BL. People do not apply enough sunscreen for protection. BMJ. 1996;313(7062):942.

25. Sunscreen FAQs | American Academy of Dermatology [Internet]. [cited 2018 Dec 30]. Available from: https://www.aad.org/media/stats/prevention-and-care/sunscreen-faqs

26. 14:00-17:00. ISO 24442:2011 [Internet]. ISO. [cited 2019 Feb 15]. Available from: http://www.iso.org/cms/render/live/en/sites/isoorg/contents/data/standard/04/65/46521.html

27. Wang SQ, Xu H, Stanfield JW, Osterwalder U, Herzog B. Comparison of ultraviolet A light protection standards in the United States and European Union through in vitro measurements of commercially available sunscreens. J Am Acad Dermatol. 2017;77(1):42–7.

28. Bielfeldt S, Klette E, Rohr M, Herzog B, Grumelard J, Hanay C, et al. Multicenter methodology comparison of the FDA and ISO standard for measurement of in vitro UVA protection of sunscreen products. J Photochem Photobiol B. 2018 Dec;189:185–92.

29. Scherschun L, Lim HW. Photoprotection by sunscreens. Am J Clin Dermatol. 2001;2(3):131–4.

30. Tong E, Fischer G, Smith SD. Cosmetic versus medicine: how does your country define sunscreen? J Drugs Dermatol JDD. 2018;17(8):899–904.

31. Schneider SL, Lim HW. A review of inorganic UV filters zinc oxide and titanium dioxide. Photodermatol Photoimmunol Photomed. 2018;

32. Smijs TG, Pavel S. Titanium dioxide and zinc oxide nanoparticles in sunscreens: focus on their safety and effectiveness. Nanotechnol Sci Appl. 2011;4:95–112.

33. Ruszkiewicz JA, Pinkas A, Ferrer B, Peres TV, Tsatsakis A, Aschner M. Neurotoxic effect of active ingredients in sunscreen products, a contemporary review. Toxicol Rep. 2017;4:245–59.

34. Newman MD, Stotland M, Ellis JI. The safety of nanosized particles in titanium dioxide- and zinc oxide-based sunscreens. J Am Acad Dermatol. 2009;61(4):685–92.

35. Mohammed YH, Holmes A, Haridass IN, Sanchez WY, Studier H, Grice JE, et al. Support for the safe use of zinc oxide nanoparticle sunscreens: lack of skin penetration or cellular toxicity after repeated application in volunteers. J Invest Dermatol. 2018;

36. Grande F, Tucci P. Titanium dioxide nanoparticles: a risk for human health? Mini Rev Med Chem. 2016;16(9):762–9.
37. Hanson KM, Gratton E, Bardeen CJ. Sunscreen enhancement of UV-induced reactive oxygen species in the skin. Free Radic Biol Med. 2006;41(8):1205–12.
38. Millington KR, Osmond MJ, McCall MJ. Detecting free radicals in sunscreens exposed to UVA radiation using chemiluminescence. J Photochem Photobiol B. 2014;133:27–38.
39. Nohynek GJ, Dufour EK. Nano-sized cosmetic formulations or solid nanoparticles in sunscreens: a risk to human health? Arch Toxicol. 2012;86(7):1063–75.
40. Sunscreens E. 2018. G to EWG's 2018 Guide to Safer Sunscreens [Internet]. [cited 2019 Jan 9]. Available from: https://www.ewg.org/sunscreen/report/executive-summary/
41. Antoniou C, Kosmadaki MG, Stratigos AJ, Katsambas AD. Sunscreens--what's important to know. J Eur Acad Dermatol Venereol. 2008;22(9):1110–8.
42. DiNardo JC, Downs CA. Dermatological and environmental toxicological impact of the sunscreen ingredient oxybenzone/benzophenone-3. J Cosmet Dermatol. 2018;17(1):15–9.
43. Kullavanijaya P, Lim HW. Photoprotection. J Am Acad Dermatol. 2005;52(6):937–58. quiz 959–62
44. Gonzalez H, Farbrot A, Larkö O, Wennberg A-M. Percutaneous absorption of the sunscreen benzophenone-3 after repeated whole-body applications, with and without ultraviolet irradiation. Br J Dermatol. 2006;154(2):337–40.
45. Schlumpf M, Schmid P, Durrer S, Conscience M, Maerkel K, Henseler M, et al. Endocrine activity and developmental toxicity of cosmetic UV filters--an update. Toxicology. 2004;205(1–2):113–22.
46. Calafat AM, Wong L-Y, Ye X, Reidy JA, Needham LL. Concentrations of the sunscreen agent benzophenone-3 in residents of the United States: national health and nutrition examination survey 2003–2004. Environ Health Perspect. 2008;116(7):893–7.
47. Kim S, Choi K. Occurrences, toxicities, and ecological risks of benzophenone-3, a common component of organic sunscreen products: a mini-review. Environ Int. 2014;70:143–57.
48. Huo W, Cai P, Chen M, Li H, Tang J, Xu C, et al. The relationship between prenatal exposure to BP-3 and Hirschsprung's disease. Chemosphere. 2016;144:1091–7.
49. Schneider SL, Lim HW. Review of environmental effects of oxybenzone and other sunscreen active ingredients. J Am Acad Dermatol. 2019;80(1):266–71.
50. Downs CA, Kramarsky-Winter E, Segal R, Fauth J, Knutson S, Bronstein O, et al. Toxicopathological effects of the sunscreen UV filter, Oxybenzone (Benzophenone-3), on coral planulae and cultured primary cells and its environmental contamination in Hawaii and the U.S. Virgin Islands. Arch Environ Contam Toxicol. 2016;70(2):265–88.
51. SB2571 [Internet]. [cited 2019 Jan 4]. Available from: https://www.capitol.hawaii.gov/session2018/bills/SB2571_.HTM
52. Bill Text - AB-60 Sunscreen: oxybenzone and octinoxate. [Internet]. [cited 2019 Jan 21]. Available from: https://leginfo.legislature.ca.gov/faces/billTextClient.xhtml?bill_id=201920200AB60
53. Hoegh-Guldberg O, Kennedy EV, Beyer HL, McClennen C, Possingham HP. Securing a long-term future for coral reefs. Trends Ecol Evol. 2018;33(12):936–44.
54. Bruno JF, Côté IM, Toth LT. Climate change, coral loss, and the curious case of the parrotfish paradigm: why don't marine protected areas improve reef resilience? Annu Rev Mar Sci. 2019;11:307–34.
55. Narla S, Lim HW. Sunscreen: FDA regulation, and environmental and health impact. Photochem Photobiol Sci Off J Eur Photochem Assoc Eur Soc Photobiol. 2020;19(1):66–70.
56. Afonso S, Horita K, Sousa e Silva JP, Almeida IF, Amaral MH, Lobão PA, et al. Photodegradation of avobenzone: stabilization effect of antioxidants. J Photochem Photobiol B. 2014;140:36–40.
57. Beasley DG, Meyer TA. Characterization of the UVA protection provided by avobenzone, zinc oxide, and titanium dioxide in broad-spectrum sunscreen products. Am J Clin Dermatol. 2010;11(6):413–21.
58. Nash JF. Human safety and efficacy of ultraviolet filters and sunscreen products. Dermatol Clin. 2006;24(1):35–51.
59. Matta MK, Zusterzeel R, Pilli NR, Patel V, Volpe DA, Florian J, et al. Effect of sunscreen application under maximal use conditions on plasma concentration of sunscreen active ingredients: a randomized clinical trial. JAMA. 2019;321(21):2082–91.
60. Matta MK, Florian J, Zusterzeel R, Pilli NR, Patel V, Volpe DA, et al. Effect of sunscreen application on plasma concentration of sunscreen active ingredients: a randomized clinical trial. JAMA. 2020;323(3):256–67.
61. Aldoori N, Dobson K, Holden CR, McDonagh AJ, Harries M, Messenger AG. Frontal fibrosing alopecia: possible association with leave-on facial skin care products and sunscreens; a questionnaire study. Br J Dermatol. 2016;175(4):762–7.
62. Debroy Kidambi A, Dobson K, Holmes S, Carauna D, Del Marmol V, Vujovic A, et al. Frontal fibrosing alopecia in men: an association with facial moisturizers and sunscreens. Br J Dermatol. 2017;177(1):260–1.
63. Commissioner O of the. Press Announcements - Statement from FDA Commissioner Scott Gottlieb, M.D., on new FDA actions to keep consumers safe from the harmful effects of sun exposure, and ensure the long-term safety and benefits of sunscreens [Internet]. [cited 2019 Feb 16]. Available from: https://www.fda.gov/NewsEvents/Newsroom/PressAnnouncements/ucm608499.htm
64. Kohli I, Shafi R, Isedeh P, Griffith JL, Al-Jamal MS, Silpa-Archa N, et al. The impact of oral Polypodium leucotomos extract on ultraviolet B response:

a human clinical study. J Am Acad Dermatol. 2017;77(1):33–41.e1.

65. Tanew A, Radakovic S, Gonzalez S, Venturini M, Calzavara-Pinton P. Oral administration of a hydrophilic extract of Polypodium leucotomos for the prevention of polymorphic light eruption. J Am Acad Dermatol. 2012;66(1):58–62.

66. González S, Pathak MA, Cuevas J, Villarrubia VG, Fitzpatrick TB. Topical or oral administration with an extract of Polypodium leucotomos prevents acute sunburn and psoralen-induced phototoxic reactions as well as depletion of Langerhans cells in human skin. Photodermatol Photoimmunol Photomed. 1997;13(1–2):50–60.

67. Middelkamp-Hup MA, Pathak MA, Parrado C, Garcia-Caballero T, Rius-Díaz F, Fitzpatrick TB, et al. Orally administered Polypodium leucotomos extract decreases psoralen-UVA-induced phototoxicity, pigmentation, and damage of human skin. J Am Acad Dermatol. 2004;50(1):41–9.

68. Lim HW, Arellano-Mendoza M-I, Stengel F. Current challenges in photoprotection. J Am Acad Dermatol. 2017;76(3S1):S91–9.

69. Behar-Cohen F, Baillet G, de Ayguavives T, Garcia PO, Krutmann J, Peña-García P, et al. Ultraviolet damage to the eye revisited: eye-sun protection factor (E-SPF®), a new ultraviolet protection label for eyewear. Clin Ophthalmol Auckl NZ. 2014;8:87–104.

70. Sliney DH. Photoprotection of the eye - UV radiation and sunglasses. J Photochem Photobiol B. 2001;64(2–3):166–75.

71. Kaliki S, Shields CL. Uveal melanoma: relatively rare but deadly cancer. Eye Lond Engl. 2017;31(2):241–57.

72. Lomas A, Leonardi-Bee J, Bath-Hextall F. A systematic review of worldwide incidence of nonmelanoma skin cancer. Br J Dermatol. 2012;166(5):1069–80.

73. Karimkhani C, Green AC, Nijsten T, Weinstock MA, Dellavalle RP, Naghavi M, et al. The global burden of melanoma: results from the Global Burden of Disease Study 2015. Br J Dermatol. 2017;177(1):134–40.

74. Guy GP, Machlin SR, Ekwueme DU, Yabroff KR. Prevalence and costs of skin cancer treatment in the U.S., 2002-2006 and 2007-2011. Am J Prev Med. 2015;48(2):183–7.

75. Darlington S, Williams G, Neale R, Frost C, Green A. A randomized controlled trial to assess sunscreen application and beta carotene supplementation in the prevention of solar keratoses. Arch Dermatol. 2003;139(4):451–5.

76. Gallagher RP. Sunscreens in melanoma and skin cancer prevention. Can Med Assoc J. 2005;173(3):244–5.

77. Huncharek M, Kupelnick B. Use of topical sunscreens and the risk of malignant melanoma: a meta-analysis of 9067 patients from 11 case-control studies. Am J Public Health. 2002;92(7):1173–7.

78. Vainio H, Bianchini F. IARC handbooks of cancer prevention: Volume 5: Sunscreens. New York, NY: Oxford University Press; 2001.

79. Westerdahl J, Ingvar C, Måsbäck A, Olsson H. Sunscreen use and malignant melanoma. Int J Cancer. 2000;87(1):145–50.

80. Dennis LK, Beane Freeman LE, VanBeek MJ. Sunscreen use and the risk for melanoma: a quantitative review. Ann Intern Med. 2003;139(12):966–78.

81. Green AC, Williams GM, Logan V, Strutton GM. Reduced melanoma after regular sunscreen use: randomized trial follow-up. J Clin Oncol Off J Am Soc Clin Oncol. 2011;29(3):257–63.

82. Waldman RA, Grant-Kels JM. The role of sunscreen in the prevention of cutaneous melanoma and nonmelanoma skin cancer. J Am Acad Dermatol. 2019;80(2):574–576.e1.

83. Chesnut C, Kim J. Is There Truly No Benefit with Sunscreen Use and Basal Cell Carcinoma? A Critical Review of the Literature and the Application of New Sunscreen Labeling Rules to Real-World Sunscreen Practices. J Skin Cancer [Internet]. 2012 [cited 2019 Feb 15];2012. Available from: https://www.ncbi.nlm.nih.gov/pmc/articles/PMC3357551/

84. Whiteman DC, Whiteman CA, Green AC. Childhood sun exposure as a risk factor for melanoma: a systematic review of epidemiologic studies. Cancer Causes Control. 2001;12(1):69–82.

85. Dobbinson S, Wakefield M, Hill D, Girgis A, Aitken JF, Beckmann K, et al. Children's sun exposure and sun protection: prevalence in Australia and related parental factors. J Am Acad Dermatol. 2012;66(6):938–47.

Bed Bugs

Marlous L. Grijsen and Bernard Naafs

Key Points
- Bed bug infestations are rapidly spreading throughout the world and have become a major public health concern.
- Bed bugs are wingless, flat reddish-brown arthropods that are approximately 5–6 mm long.
- Bed bugs are attracted to their hosts, which preferably are humans, by exhaled carbon dioxide and body heat.
- Cutaneous symptoms are characterized by erythematous and/or urticarial papules with a central hemorrhagic punctum.
- The diagnosis is confirmed after identification of the parasite, its excretions, and/or exoskeletons.
- Successful eradication and control can be achieved by integrated pest management, whereby non-chemical and chemical approaches are combined.

Introduction

Whether staying in a luxurious five-star hotel or an inexpensive hostel when travelling around the world, a common nuisance that travelers may encounter is bed bugs. These tiny pests can cause discomfort resulting in bites and scratch marks on the body and bed sheets covered with blood stains. Bed bugs can disrupt a peaceful night's sleep and create an unpleasant experience for travellers.

Bed bugs (Heteroptera) are wingless, flat, reddish-brown, oval-shaped ectoparasites that are approximately 5–6 mm long when unfed (Fig. 1). They are more or less comparable, in size and color, to an apple seed and can be visualized with the naked eye [1]. Bed bugs belong to the insect family *Cimicidae*. Two of the more than 90 species counting family, feed on humans: the *Cimex lectularius*, the common bed bug that is distributed globally, and *Cimex hemipterus,* the tropical bed bug that is found in tropical climates. The common bed bug is aptly named: in Latin, *Cimex* stands for bug, and *lectularius* for bed or couch [2]. Both species are fairly similar, although an experienced entomologist is able to distinguish them from one another.

M. L. Grijsen (✉)
Oxford University Clinical Research Unit Indonesia,
Faculty of Medicine Universitas Indonesia, Jakarta,
Indonesia

Centre for Tropical Medicine and Global Health,
Nuffield Department of Medicine, University of
Oxford, Oxford, UK
e-mail: mgrijsen@oucru.org

B. Naafs
Foundation Global Dermatology,
Munnekeburen, the Netherlands

Kilimanjaro Christian Medical University,
Moshi, Tanzania

W. Robles (ed.), *Skin Disease in Travelers*, Updates in Clinical Dermatology,
https://doi.org/10.1007/978-3-031-57836-6_35

335

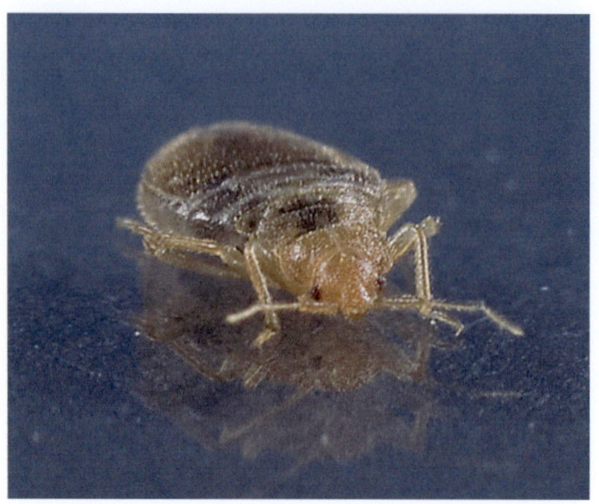

Fig. 1 The common bed bug, also called *Cimex lectularius*

Epidemiology

Bed bugs have traditionally been common in low- and middle-income countries, especially in settings of extreme poverty due to lack of hygiene and crowding. In the 1950s, bed bugs had been eradicated in many high-income countries through pesticides like DDT (dichloro-diphenyl-trichloroethane). Since the 1990s, however, there has been an unprecedented resurgence of bed bug infestations around the world, including large cities in Europe, the United States, Asia, and Australia. In Toronto, for example, single-family residences, apartments, and homeless shelters were affected by bed bugs [3]. International travel, immigration, urbanization, and resistance to insecticides have contributed to this revival [1, 4–6]. Infestations are rapidly spreading throughout the world and have become a major public health concern causing a significant socioeconomical impact [7]. In addition to hotels and households, bed bugs are also spreading to office environments and cinemas, in fact to any dwelling where people sit or sleep [8].

Bed bugs hide from daylight in cracks and crevices of beds, along the seams of matrasses, in box springs, in old furniture, or in cracks in the floor, the wall, or thatched roofs. Bed bugs travel along with people hiding in their suitcases and backpacks where they can survive for weeks to months without food. Bed bugs may also travel themselves from one room to the other through water pipes and gutters [2]. Travel agencies nowadays warn their customers and encourage them to check for their presence in hotel rooms illustrating the severity of this public health problem. Entomologists and pest control industries believe that the *C. lectularius* will be the most challenging indoor pest of our generation [1]. Healthcare workers are increasingly confronted with bedbug-related symptoms, although in most cases, these are not recognized as such, as people are not aware their house or workspace is infested by bedbugs [9, 10].

The Life Cycle of the Bed Bug

During sexual reproduction, male bed bugs, the aedeagus, pierce a hole in the abdominal wall of females and inseminate directly into the abdominal cavity (hemocoel). Female bed bugs have evolved a pair of specialized reproductive organs (paragenitalia) at the site of penetration. These organs known as the ectospermalege and mesospermalege (collectively referred to as spermalege), serve as sperm receptacles from where the sperm diffuses through the female hemolymph, to reach the ovaries resulting in fertilization. This traumatic insemination is also known as hypodermic insemination [11]. The females of the common bed bug (*C. lectularius*) lay about 5–10 eggs per day and between 200 and 500 in a lifetime; *C. hemipterus* females lay up to 50 eggs in a lifetime. *C. lectularius* has five developmental life stages, referred to as instars or nymphal stages. Eggs hatch within 9–12 days into nymphs. Each stage requires a blood meal to molt to the next stage. As bed bugs, like all insects, have their skeleton on the outside of their body (exoskeleton), they need to shed their exoskeleton before molting to the next stage. After accomplishing five nymphal stages, the bed bug becomes an adult. At room temperature (22 °C), the developmental process from egg to adult takes around 5–6 weeks [12, 13]. As bed bugs complete their life cycle, they gradually reduce their water requirements and develop a high tolerance for dehydration [14]. Bed bugs have an average life span of 6–12 months but can survive up to 1 year without a blood meal in cool conditions. They form dense aggregations or clusters, which helps them to preserve water and increase their survival [14].

Feeding

At night, bed bugs sneak out of their hiding places to attack their victims. Their preferred hosts are humans, although bed bugs may also feed on other warm-blooded animals, such as pets and poultry [15, 16]. Bed bugs hide within 1 or 2 m of the host and are attracted to them by the production of carbon dioxide and body temperature. Bed bugs move fast, approximately 90–120 cm/min [12]. Once the bed bug has located its victim, it pierces the skin with its mouthparts to find a capillary space that allows the blood to flow into its body rapidly. The parasite has a snout (proboscis) with which it penetrates through the epidermis into the dermis. Through a small duct, the snout injects anesthetics and anticoagulants. Bed bugs may puncture the skin several times before they start to feed ("mapping" of the skin). Once they have settled, they will feed for 3–5 min unless they get interrupted by the host's sudden movements. The arthropods will then look for another nearby site resulting in multiple sequential bites on the exposed areas of the host (Peres, [17] An Bras Dermatol 2018). Bed bugs stay close to each other and release aggregation pheromones to help relocate their shelters after a blood meal [13]. Once they have returned to their harborage, the bugs enter into a quiescent state to digest their meal. Bed bugs feed every 3–7 days once their metabolic reserves have been depleted.

Clinical Features

Bed bug bites generally present as small erythematous maculopapular lesions with little to no inflammatory reaction. They may have a central hemorrhagic punctum, but in many cases, this is barely visible (Fig. 2a). In atopic individuals, bites may also occur as papular urticaria caused by hypersensitivity reactions. In predisposed individuals, bites may also present as vesicles or bullae [18]. Typically, bites are arranged in a linear array or in a triangular shape of at least three to five bites (Fig. 2b), each a few centimeters apart, and referred to as "breakfast, lunch and dinner," although this is not necessary [19]. They often occur on the exposed areas of the body that are in contact with the mattress and involve the face, neck, and extremities. Bites are painless and may be noticed upon waking up or after a few days. Scratching of pruritic lesions may cause secondary bacterial infections, prurigo nodules, and/or scars. Systemic reactions like asthma or anaphylaxis are rare, although they have been reported in the past [20, 21].

Bedbugs are seldom seen by the patient, but the bed sheets, which may be covered with blood

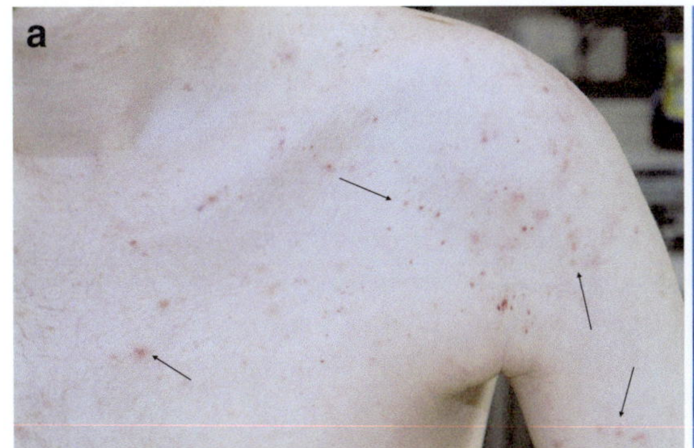
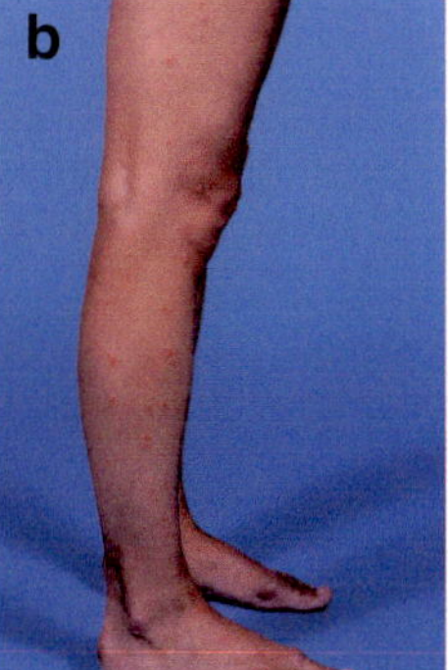

Fig. 2 (**a, b**) Bed bug bites illustrating erythematous maculopapular lesions in a linear or triangular cluster of which some, illustrated by the arrow, have a central hemorrhagic punctum

stains and fecal spotting, may give away some clues. Bed bugs may disrupt everyday life and have a social and economic impact. Patients may suffer sleep deprivation affecting the patients' emotional and psychological well-being.

Diagnosis

Bed bugs are a clinical diagnosis. In general, insect bites are challenging to identify as symptoms can vary significantly between people. Bed bugs may easily be confused with other arthropod bites (mosquitoes, fleas, or scabies) or skin rashes such as hives, prurigo nodularis, dermatitis herpetiformis, drug reactions, or chickenpox [13]. Several urticarial lesions aligned along a limb may suggest bed bugs. Signs and symptoms that may help to differentiate bed bugs from other insect bites are as follows: dog and cat fleas bite around the ankles, human fleas invade warm body spaces (armpits, the genital area, and between the buttocks), and scabies predilection sites include flexural surfaces of the wrists, between digits, axillae, umbilicus, genital area and buttocks. Scabies can also be confirmed by a skin scraping. A skin biopsy may help to differentiate bed bugs from inflammatory dermatoses. The ultimate proof of diagnosis is the identification of the parasite, its excretions (dark specks), and/or empty exoskeletons that are pale yellow and, e.g., can be found along the seams of a mattress. A thorough inspection of the house, in particular bedrooms and living areas, or work space is needed. This often requires consultation by an experienced professional as bed bugs are masters in hiding; flat as they are they can hide in all nooks and crannies and under rims of textiles. They may be found under baseboards, in cracks and crevices of beds, behind wallpaper, in electrical sockets, in chests and drawers, suitcases, bags, or even shoes. Box springs are another perfect hiding place. Some people can smell bed bugs, as they emit a characteristic musty, "sickly sweet" odor [13]. Trained sniffer dogs may also help in detecting bed bugs and are particularly useful for large facilities such as hotels, theaters, and office buildings [12].

Treatment and Prevention

Cutaneous reactions to bed bug bites are often self-limiting and genuinely resolve within 10 days. Topical corticosteroids, oral antihistamines, and anti-prurigonosa (menthol, calamine, or any other anti-pruritic) may help relieve symptoms. In case of severe pruritus, systemic glucocorticoids may be used, although this is rarely needed. Water and soap, antiseptic solutions, and/or topical or systemic antibiotics may be needed to prevent or treat secondary bacterial infections. Bed bugs may cause significant psychological distress requiring additional psychological support and treatment.

To prevent the risk of bed bug infestations, cracks and crevices must be sealed and hotel rooms and second-hand furniture must be inspected. Successful eradication and control can be achieved by integrated pest management, whereby various non-chemical and chemical approaches are combined [13]. A relatively easy and affordable technique to rapidly reduce the bed bug biomass is vacuum cleaning. This method will eliminate the eggs as well making success more likely [22]. The vacuum machines should be thoroughly cleaned after each use and contain disposable bags that can be removed and sealed. Bed linen and other textile materials covering the infestation should be washed or steamed at 60 °C or frozen at −20 °C for at least 2 h. These procedures are cumbersome but will be effective and kill the bugs and the eggs. In most cases, however, professional exterminators need to be consulted. Bed bug populations have become resistant to many of the conventional commercially available insecticides. Non-professional use of these pesticides is a public health concern and may harm the environment [23].

Transmission of Infectious Diseases

Bed bugs are suspected of potential vectors of infectious diseases, in particularly hepatitis B virus (HBV), *Trypanosoma cruzi* that causes Chagas' disease, and more recently reported methicillin-resistant *Staphylococcus aureus*

(MRSA) [2, 24, 25]. To date, however, there has been no compelling evidence that bed bugs are able to transmit infectious diseases to humans. In fact, bed bugs may contain "neutralizing factors" that attenuate the virulence of micro-organisms and decrease the ability of transmissibility [26].

Conclusion

Bed bugs are becoming a public health concern. Dermatological findings may include an erythematous rash, papular urticaria, and/or pruritus depending on the number of bites. Systemic involvement is rare. There is no evidence that bed bugs may transmit infectious diseases to humans, although they may cause significant psychological distress. Treatment includes steroid cream combined with antihistamines, and eradicating the infestation effectively by pest control.

References

1. Potter MG. The perfect storm: an extension view on bed bugs. Am Entomol. 2006;52(2):102–4.
2. Goddard J, deShazo R. Bed bugs (Cimex lectularius) and clinical consequences of their bites. JAMA. 2009;301(13):1358–66.
3. Hwang SW, Svoboda TJ, De Jong IJ, Kabasele KJ, Gogosis E. Bed bug infestations in an urban environment. Emerg Infect Dis. 2005;11(4):533–8.
4. Lee IY, Ree HI, An SJ, Linton JA, Yong TS. Reemergence of the bedbug Cimex lectularius in Seoul, Korea. Korean J Parasitol. 2008;46(4):269–71.
5. Romero A, Potter MF, Potter DA, Haynes KF. Insecticide resistance in the bed bug: a factor in the pest's sudden resurgence? J Med Entomol. 2007;44(2):175–8.
6. Paul J, Bates J. Is infestation with the common bedbug increasing? BMJ. 2000;320(7242):1141.
7. Scarpino SV, Althouse BM. Uncovering the hidden cost of bed bugs. Proc Natl Acad Sci USA. 2019;116(15):7160–2.
8. Chittoor J, Wilkison BD, McNally BW. What's eating you? Bedbugs. Cutis. 2019;103(1):31–3.
9. Reindhardt K, Harder A, Holland S, Hooper J, Leake-Lyall C. Who knows the bed bug? Knowledge of adult bed bug appearance increases with people's age in three countries of Great Britain. J Med Entomol. 2008;45(5):956–8.
10. Seidel C, Reinhardt K. Bugging forecast: unknown, disliked, ocacasionally intimate. Bed bugs in Germany meet unprepared people. PLoS One. 2013;8(1):e51083.
11. Morrow EH, Arnqvist G. Costly traumatic insemination and a female counter-adaptation in bed bugs. Proc Biol Sci. 2003;270(1531):2377–81.
12. Parola P, Izri A. Bedbugs. N Engl J Med. 2020;382(23):2230–7.
13. Doggett SL, Dwyer DE, Peñas PF, Russell RC. Bed bugs: clinical relevance and control options. Clin Microbiol Rev. 2012;25(1):164–92.
14. Benoit JB, Del Grosso NA, Yoder JA, Denlinger DL. Resistance to dehydration between bouts of blood feeding in the bed bug, Cimex Lectularius, is enhanced by water conservation, aggregation, and quiescence. Am J Trop Med Hyg. 2007;76(5):987–93.
15. Cater J, Magee D, Edwards KT. Severe infestation of bedbugs in a poultry breeder house. J Am Vet Med Assoc. 2011;239(7):919.
16. Clark S, Gilleard JS, McGoldrick J. Human bed bug infestation of a domestic cat. Vet Rec. 2002;151(11):336.
17. Peres G, Yugar LBT, Haddad JV. Breakfast, lunch, and dinner sign: a hallmark of flea and bedbug bites. An Bras Dermatol. 2018;93:759–60.
18. Thomas I, Kihiczak GG, Schwartz RA. Bedbug bites: a review. Int J Dermatol. 2004;43(6):430–3.
19. Peres G, Yugar LBT, Haddad JV. Breakfast, lunch, and dinner sign: a hallmark of flea and bedbug bites. An Bras Dermatol. 2018;93(5):759–60.
20. Bircher AJ. Systemic immediate allergic reactions to arthropod stings and bites. Dermatology. 2005;210(2):119–27.
21. Parsons DJ. Bedbug bite anaphylaxis misinterpreted as coronary occlusion. Ohio State Med J. 1955;51(7):669.
22. Doggett SL. Non-chemical methods of bed bug control: a case study. Prof Pest Manag. 2009;13:27–9.
23. Schmidt E, Levitt J. Dermatologic infestations. Int J Dermatol. 2012;51(2):131–41.
24. Lowe CF, Romney MG. Bedbugs as vectors for drug-resistant bacteria. Emerg Infect Dis. 2011;17(6):1132–4.
25. Delaunay P, Blanc V, Del Guidice P, et al. Bedbugs and infectious diseases. Clin Infect Dis. 2011;52(2):200–10.
26. Lai O, Ho D, Glick S, Jagdeo J. Bed bugs and possible transmission of human pathogens: a systematic review. Arch Dermatol Res. 2016;308(8):531–8.

Skin Diseases in Refugees

Maria Lucia Dell'Anna and Aldo Morrone

One day,
when things are going well,
you will look back and
you will feel proud
not to have given up

Hevrin Khalaf (15/11/84–12/10/19)

Key Points
- Persecution, conflicts, and human rights violations force people to flee their homes and seek safety in Europe.
- The skin is a mirror that tells the journey experience, previous experiences of the refugees, and/or the signs of torture.
- Dermatologist may be the first professional to come across and recognize lesions potentially due to torture.
- The medical intervention must be carried out in a multidisciplinary perspective, taking into account the ethical and cultural aspects of healthcare for refugees.

M. L. Dell'Anna · A. Morrone (✉)
San Gallicano Dermatological Institute IRCCS IFO, Rome, Italy
e-mail: marialucia.dellanna@ifo.it;
aldo.morrone@ifo.gov.it

Each Number Is a Person: Introduction to Demographic, Political, and Social Environment

The movement of people who look for a better, safe, and healthy life started some time ago when *homo* species gained an upright posture and they needed to move to find more animals to hunt and more land to cultivate for their social group. The type of essential goods changed during the time, but the primary need to ensure a safe and better economic and social condition for himself and for his own family is the same [1–4].

The foundation of Rome, between history and legend, is intriguingly linked to these natural human events. Rome, in its original territory, extends over seven hills. One of the seven hills of Rome is the Capitol. Two hills, the Arx and the Capitolium, originally characterized the hill, separated by a small valley, named Asylum, that the first king Romulus used to welcome the inhabitants of the nearby towns. The strategic position of the hill with very steep

W. Robles (ed.), *Skin Disease in Travelers*, Updates in Clinical Dermatology,
https://doi.org/10.1007/978-3-031-57836-6_36

sides made it a real acropolis of the city, a bulwark for the defense of the inhabitants from external attacks. Asylum, physical place and idea, was thus intrinsically part of the community concept.

In the past two centuries, Asian and European people have moved to North and South America to find jobs, to save one's life, or to be free to sing, dance, and read [5]. Within Europe, when the people from the Mediterranean area (including South Italy) went to North Europe, conditions of extreme misery were left behind, arriving in more or less large and rich cities that reserved their at least wary looks and attitudes. And some centuries before, Central and Southern Europe had been "invaded" by northern peoples attracted by better living conditions and the presence of cities [6, 7].

Persecution, conflicts, and human rights violations continue to force people to flee their homes and seek safety in Europe. Nobody loves to stay in a place where there is war, hunger, and violence. And now, Europe has become the goal for many people.

The displaced person who has been forced to cross national boundaries and who cannot return home safely has been named a refugee. According to UNHCR, refugees are people who have fled war, violence, conflict, or persecution and have crossed an international border to find safety in another country. They often have had to flee with little more than the clothes on their back, leaving behind homes, possessions, jobs, and loved ones. Refugees are protected by international law. The 1951 Refugee Convention is a key legal document and defines a refugee as "someone who is unable or unwilling to return to their country of origin owing to a well-founded fear of being persecuted for reasons of race, religion, nationality, membership of a particular social group, or political opinion."

Many risk their lives and face a treacherous journey. In the first period of 2020, 19,000 people entered Europe, including sea (16,000) and land (3200) arrivals. The main involved countries are Italy, Greece, Spain, Cyprus, and Malta. The dangerous journey probably caused the death by drowning of 160 people.

Going a little back in time, 63,311 people have risked their lives reaching Europe by sea so far in 2019 and 1028 drowned so far in 2019 (UNHCR data). In 2018, 142,000 people arrived and 2300 died during the journey to Europe.

Previously, in the first half of 2017, over 105,000 refugees and migrants entered Europe, and an estimated 362,000 refugees and migrants risked their lives crossing the Mediterranean Sea in 2016, with 181,400 people arriving in Italy and 173,450 in Greece.

The main countries of origin were Afghanistan (30%), Syria (17%), Bangladesh (6%), Congo (5%), Algeria (4%), Iraq (4%), Cote di'Ivoire (4%), Sudan (3%), and Palestine (3%).

Despite the attempts by International Organizations and some progress in increasing the number of safe pathways to Europe, these opportunities are far too few to offer a feasible alternative to risky irregular journeys for people in need of protection.

Those arriving in Europe need adequate reception and assistance, particularly those with specific needs, including unaccompanied and separated children and survivors of sexual and gender-based violence, and access to fair and efficient asylum procedures [8, 9].

On the borders between Turkey and the European Union (EU), arriving people have included Syrians, Afghans, Iranians, Sudanese, and other nationalities; they are women, children, and families, in precarious conditions.

While the situation on Turkey's western borders and Greece and the movement of several thousand people are of concern, the humanitarian disaster unfolding in northwest Syria affects some 950,000 internally displaced people.

The deteriorating situation in Syria accounts for the increased amount of refugees, whose primary destinations are countries in central and northern Europe, following the eastern Mediterranean route through Turkey and Greece. However, the closure (February 2016) of the Greek–Former Yugoslav Republic of Macedonia (FYROM) border has caused the popular "Balkan route" to shut down. In addition, the EU–Turkey agreement (March 2016) drastically limited the legal arrival of more refugees to Greece, who instead will try to reach Europe through irregular ways, risking their lives. The final result is that more than 62,000 refugees are currently blocked in Greece, without the prospect of reaching any countries. Moreover, refugee camps (or "hotspots"), originally aimed for short-term stays, had to be turned into long-term shelters, and as they were not designed to host such large amounts of refugees, they became overcrowded. Therefore, new challenges have arisen as the facilities are not adequate; thus, the living conditions are considered inappropriate. Another important issue that has come up is that these camps may host a considerable number of unaccompanied minors, especially children with an unknown vaccination status, suffering from the war and the uncertainty of the journey to a new place to resettle. Consequently, both their physical and mental health have been disturbed.

In Greece (Lesvos, Chios, and Samos), some 1200 people arrived in early March 2020 [10].

The Skin Health. General Consideration

Overall health condition of refugee people is acceptable. People approaching a long dangerous journey are generally in good health. However, the skin is a mirror that tells the previous experience starting from food/water availability and quality to hygiene, WASH quality, and dangerous environment, including chemical poisons (i.e., seawater plus gasoline mixture), long sun exposure, human violence, and self-injuring.

The current situation in Lybia, as reported by an official international source, accounts for 355,672 Libyans currently internally displaced, 447,707 returned internally displaced people, and 48,621 registered refugees and asylum seekers. The disastrous events occurring in Lybia during the last 2 years have precipitated the living conditions of people who pass through Libya to reach Europe [11].

The survivor people who reach Europe arrive with clear obvious signs on the skin of the camp's experience [12, 13].

The involvement of the skin in infectious process is in second place (22%), after the respiratory tract (64%), and is followed by the urinary tract (7%) and the gastrointestinal tract (6%). Conditions in facilities are often woefully inadequate [14–19]. Mediterranean arrivals into Europe have plummeted since the 2015 crisis, but arrivals to Greece have risen in the last year and made chronic overcrowding on the islands much worse. The risks faced by the most vulnerable individuals, pregnant women, new mothers, the elderly, and children are among the worst seen in refugee crises around the world.

Considering all the possible steps of the journey, people, including children, arriving in Europe "*may have fled conflict, lost family members, been away from home for months, even years, with some enduring horrific abuses during their journeys, but their suffering doesn't stop at the border*" (Pascale Moreau, Director of UNHCR's Europe Bureau).

In the camps, the main aspects potentially and currently affecting the health of the refugee people are water, sanitation, and health service access [20, 21].

When arriving in resettlement areas, refugees and asylum seekers face discrimination including housing, education, and healthcare access, with likely health consequences. Discrimination can range from physical violence and direct threats and insults to systemic limitations around access to resources [22].

Focus on Italy

Before 2012, most migrant people arrived in Italy from North Africa. In the following years, according to the worsening of conflicts in the North African and Middle Eastern countries, the nationalities composition changed mainly due to the increase of Syrians and Eritreans. In 2015, the Eastern Mediterranean route became predominant, mainly for people from Syria, leading to a drop in the arrivals in Italy to about 150,000.

Eritreans, Nigerians, and Somalis continue to follow the Mediterranean flow.

When migrant people arrive in Italy, the skin pathological conditions most frequently observed are scabies (58%), skin and soft tissue infections (10%), itch (9%), pediculosis (head lice) (9%), dermatitis (8%), insect bites (2%), burns (2%), and skin mycoses (1%) [19, 20].

According to the statistical data provided by the Italian Government, 4139 people were asylum seekers in Italy in October 2019 (+33% with respect to September 2019). The migrant people who arrived in Italy by sea in this current year (January to April 2020) are 2794, against 524 in the same period of 2018 [23].

When considering Europe in January 2020, 65,000 applications were registered (+9% with respect to data from December 2019). Asylum seekers are mainly from Syria, Afghanistan, Colombia, Venezuela, and Iraq [24].

The resettlement of refugees or asylum seekers in Italy is mainly based on small structures (flats, communities), where the risk of overcrowding is partially limited. Skin diseases are mainly expressions of previously acquired conditions, developed during the journey or during the stay in first reception centers.

Most Recurrent Infectious Skin Pathological Conditions

Cutaneous leishmaniasis may affect migrant people from areas of conflict and political instability, such as Afghanistan and Syria, suggesting that as mass migration of refugees continues, CL will be increasingly encountered in intake countries. The parasite is an intracellular pathogen with two forms of life cycles, one inside the vector (female sandfly) of variable species depending on geographical distribution and the other life cycle inside the host (human and animals). Some forms of leishmaniasis need a reservoir mostly an animal. The pathogenic complexes to man include the following: *Leishmania major*: mainly causes zoonotic cutaneous leishmaniasis (ZCL) and mucocutaneous leishmaniasis (MCL) in the Old World; *Leishmania aethiopica*: mainly causes ZCL and diffuse cutaneous leishmaniasis in Eastern Africa; *Leishmania tropica*: mainly

causes cutaneous leishmaniasis of the Old World; and *Leishmania donovani*: mainly causes visceral leishmaniasis, MCL, and post kala-azar dermal leishmaniasis. Over 90% of cases occur in the region Middle East and North Africa Afghanistan, Algeria, Iran, Iraq, Saudi Arabia, Syria, Ethiopia, and Sudan. The majority (76%) of cases occurred in patients <15 years of age and the disease affected the extremities more frequently than the face. Notably, 71% of patients presented with a single lesion and 27% presented with two lesions. Ulcerative cutaneous leishmaniasis was the predominant form (89%) [25–27].

Tungiasis is an ectoparasitic disease caused by skin penetration by the female *Tunga penetrans* or, less commonly, *Tunga trimamillata flea*. It is endemic in Latin America, the Caribbean, and sub-Saharan Africa (Brazil, Madagascar, Uganda, and Ethiopia). Tungiasis is usually acquired from walking barefoot or with open-toed shoes. An early-stage lesion is a 1-mm red-brown macule that evolves into a nodule with a central dark punctum. Subsequent flea engorgement from egg production leads to swelling, erythema, pruritus, and pain. Eventually, egg release and parasite death trigger severe inflammation, leading to a black-crusted papule that heals with a punched-out scar. Dermoscopy can be useful Tungiasis is self-limited because the organism typically dies within 6 weeks after penetration. Treatment aims to reduce symptom severity and prevent secondary infection. Surgical removal of the organism is crucial. This can be achieved through shave or punch biopsy procedures. Early on, sterile needles can also be used before multiple embedded fleas or extensive inflammation occur. Secondary bacterial infection requires appropriate antibiotics.

Pediculosis is an infestation of lice on the body, head, or pubic region that occurs worldwide. Lice are ectoparasites of the order Phthiraptera that feed on the blood of infected hosts. Among the risk factors for pediculosis, there is close contact with infected persons, infrequent showering, an inability to wash and heat-dry clothing, and cold weather, which decreases the frequency of showering and changing clothes [28, 29].

Head lice (*Pediculus humanus*) are a public health problem affecting all demographics. Head lice are ovoid-shaped, 2–3-mm arthropods. They are obligate human parasites that spend their entire life cycle on the scalp, feeding off blood every few hours. Female lice live 30 days and lay approximately 10 eggs daily. Nits are transparent, flask-shaped, 0.5-mm eggs found on hair shafts, typically 1–4 mm above the scalp. Transmission occurs via direct head-to-head contact, but lice can survive several days on fomites, including hairbrushes or headgear. Most cases occur in children, particularly females, likely because of cultural hair length differences. Pruritus, papular urticaria, excoriations, and cervical/occipital lymphadenopathy can occur. Diagnosis is achieved via direct observation of lice or nits on hair shafts. Dermoscopy distinguishes eggs containing nymphs from empty, translucent "pseudonymphs" (hair casts, hair product debris, or seborrheic dermatitis). Pruritus and disturbed sleep may cause school and work absences. Head lice can also carry and transmit *Staphylococcus aureus* and *Streptococcus pyogenes*.

Common lesions include excoriations and eczematous patches; papular urticaria and bullae may be seen. Prurigo nodules, lichenification, and hyperpigmentation are present in chronic infestation. Moreover, scratching predisposes to impetigo, ecthyma, and cellulitis. Diagnosis is carried out on the basis of clothing seams evaluation. When the infestation is chronic or severe, severe iron deficiency anemia and eosinophilia occur.

Body lice transmit *Bartonella quintana*, which causes *"trench" fever* (headache, dizziness, conjunctival injection, severe shin pain, lymphadenopathy, macular evanescent rash, and relapsing fevers lasting 4–8 days), recently seen in refugees after the civil war in Burundi. Diagnosis is based on culture, serology, immunohistochemical staining, or molecular tests. Treatment consists of the administration of gentamicin (3 mg/kg/day for 2 weeks) followed by doxycycline (200 mg/day for 4 weeks).

The body louse also transmits *Borrelia recurrentis*, which causes louse-borne *relapsing fever* (LBRF). Most LBRF cases originate from the Horn of Africa (Ethiopia, Eritrea, and Somalia), where *B. recurrentis* is endemic and concentrated poverty contributes to sporadic epidemics. LBRF is an emerging infectious disease in Europe, seen in refugees and asylum seekers who acquired the infection in the Horn of Africa, either during their journey through North Africa where migration routes into Europe join or in Europe through contact with new refugee arrivals. LBRF presents with an initial phase of high-grade fever, headache, dizziness, myalgias, and fatigue, followed by shorter, less severe relapses every 7–19 days. Complications include mucocutaneous hemorrhage, neurologic dysfunction, and liver or renal failure. Mortality is 40% for untreated cases and 2–5% when treated. Treatment is with a single dose of intramuscular penicillin G (400,000–800,000 units) or doxycycline 200 mg once.

P. humanus also transmits *Rickettsia prowazekii*, which causes *epidemic typhus*. While infected lice die within weeks, humans are the principal reservoir, remaining infected for life, with outbreaks associated with war, famine, crowding, refugee camps, and cold weather. Flying squirrels serve as a zoonotic reservoir in periods between outbreaks. Exanthema appears as widespread maculopapular lesions becoming petechial ones. Other features include fever, nausea, diarrhea, delirium, respiratory failure, and shock, with mortality of 60% in the absence of therapy Diagnosis is made via serology. First-line treatment is doxycycline 200 mg once [30].

The overall management of body lice must address poor hygiene and clothing infestation. Regular showering/bathing is important. Clothes should be discarded appropriately or washed and dried using high heat. Associated bacterial infections should be treated with appropriate antibiotics and eczematous lesions with topical corticosteroids. Physicians should involve social services to address underlying factors driving infestation.

Pubic lice (Phthirus Pubis) infestation can involve multiple body regions. A diagnosis warrants screening for other sexually transmitted infections and, in children, considering the pos-

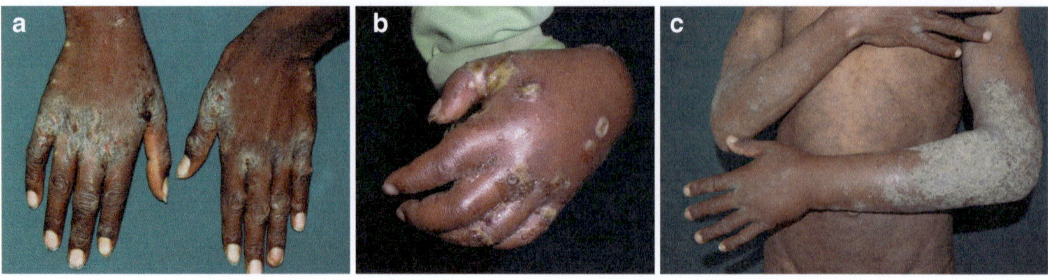

Fig. 1 Scabies. Lesions on the hands in the initial phase (**a**) and after bacterial super-infection (**b, c**)

sibility of abuse pubis infestation occurs on hairs of the scalp, axilla, chest, thighs, pubic area, and eyebrows. Pubic lice are not known to transmit other infections. A diagnosis of pubic lice warrants screening for other sexually transmitted infections. While pediatric pubic lice infestation can occur through shared sleeping arrangements with infected individuals or contact with fomites, abuse should be considered The first-line treatment of pubic lice is topical 1% permethrin. Topical 0.5% ivermectin lotion is also approved by the FDA. Petrolatum jelly is useful for treating eyelash infestation. Oral ivermectin is a second-line therapy but has not been approved by the FDA. Shaving is therapeutic and decreases the likelihood of recurrence. All clothing/linens used in the preceding 3 days should be washed and dried at temperatures.

The prolonged stay in over-crowed facilities, both during the journey (boats) and during the intermediate stops (detention camps), facilitates the high prevalence of *scabies*, in addition to pediculosis. According to these environmental conditions, it is frequent among refugees from the Middle East and Africa. Migrants (often families with numerous children) live—at least temporarily—in overcrowded facilities. However, refugees usually have no crusted scabies and no skin contact that would be sufficient for transmission to the native population. These refugees therefore are unlikely to cause major outbreaks outside these facilities, despite all the alarms. Indeed, migrants and refugees do not represent a generally increased risk of infection (parasites, measles, tuberculosis, and hepatitis) for the general population [31, 32] (Fig. 1a–c).

Most Recurrent Non-infectious Skin Pathological Conditions

In some refugee camps (Kenya), *scurvy* occurs. It is a relatively rare micronutrient deficiency disease due to inadequate access to fresh fruits and vegetables. The main observed symptoms include calf pain, chest pain, gingival swelling, lethargy, fatigue, and hyperkeratotic skin changes [33].

Refugee people from South Darfur camps with skin disorders represent 93% of the general camp population. Even if the infectious processes represent the main dermatological diseases (57% of total skin diseases), the non-communicable ones are dermatitis/eczema (10.5%), disorders of skin appendages (8.7%), atrophic skin disorders (7.4%), disorders of pigmentation (7.4%), hypertrophic skin disorders (6.4%), benign neoplasm (1.9%), dermatoses due to animal injury (0.4%), bullous dermatoses (0.1%), and malignant neoplasm (0.1%). Hypertrophic and atrophic disorders of the skin were mainly lesions of scarification (mostly atrophic) (5.7%) and keloids (5.6%). Vitiligo, probably due to a chemical stressful mechanism, was the most common depigmentary disease. The frequent triggers of this chemical vitiligo are a mix of methylated spirit, lime, and potash, applied to the face and scalp after shaving, or the black henna. The scarification is often used to identify an ethnic group membership (tribal scars): people coming from Nyala region (South Darfur) are mostly marked with horizontal straight lines on their cheeks; the Dinka, from South Sudan, exhibit serrated and fan-shaped scars and the Nuer (always from South Sudan) carry out horizontal scars; and

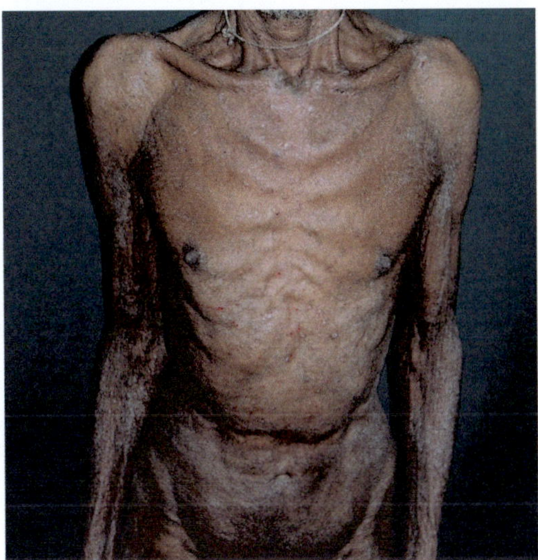

Fig. 2 Scabies. Diffuse lesions in people suffering from malnutrition

other Nilotic groups are marked with different tribal-specific scars on the foreheads rather than straight lines on their cheeks [34].

Among the Syrian refugees in Jordan, the most common diagnostic group is that of inflammatory conditions (80%), mainly represented by atopic dermatitis and eczemas (34%), followed by acne and psoriasis. The dry and arid climate, living predominantly outdoors, the lack of shade in the campsite, the ritual washings prior to prayer (wudhu) in Muslim communities, and limited access to emollients are among the leading causes of eczema. Moreover, sunburns are also frequent [35, 36] (Fig. 2).

Human-Induced Injury: Torture

Torture is usually associated with slavery and genocide and, along with them, it is condemned as a crime against humanity. There is a crucial common ground between these crimes, which explains and justifies why they are commonly abhorred.

Dermatologists may be the first and only physicians to find a lesion potentially due to torture, considering that the skin alterations may be the most evident appearance of the sign of torture.

However, dermatologist and each physician should be able to differentiate it from dermatological or systemic diseases. The signs of torture can be classified as acute and chronic lesions and for each one, the differential diagnosis must be carried out. The complete skin assessment must be a crucial step in the overall approach to the people who are survivors of torture, as dermatologist expertise is complementary to the coroner one [12, 13, 37].

However, still now there is poor access of the people victims of torture to the health system for several different reasons. The sense of shame, the fear of not being understood, the removal of what they were forced to endure, not knowing that they can receive help, and the fear of retaliation all represent a true hindrance to the complaint and thus to the "taking care." The approach to the people possibly victims of torture should be a holistic approach, where alongside the need to make a diagnosis, which anyway has, in any case, a crucial practical and legal value, the person must regain confidence in himself/herself and he/she must trust the interlocutor. This process takes time. It requires a willingness to listen and sometimes even silence. However, this process is the only way for these people to regain dignity. "Taking care" is a more complex clinical and anthropological experience than "caring."

Sometimes, both acute and chronic lesions are possibly due to repeated assaults and time spent between medical examination and violence suffered (Figs. 3a,b and 4).

Sometimes, it is not possible to immediately examine the person and the only thing possible is to deduce from the behavior, the journey, and the origin country that the person may have been tortured.

The diagnostic pathway thus starts with the observation of the person, trying to grasp even indirect requests for interview and help. Trust must also be gained by leaving aside direct questions, even on obvious skin or orthopedic injuries, if the person does not want to talk about it. Establishing a relationship of trust is therefore the first step in order to start a real diagnostic and therapeutic path. Only after this phase, it is pos-

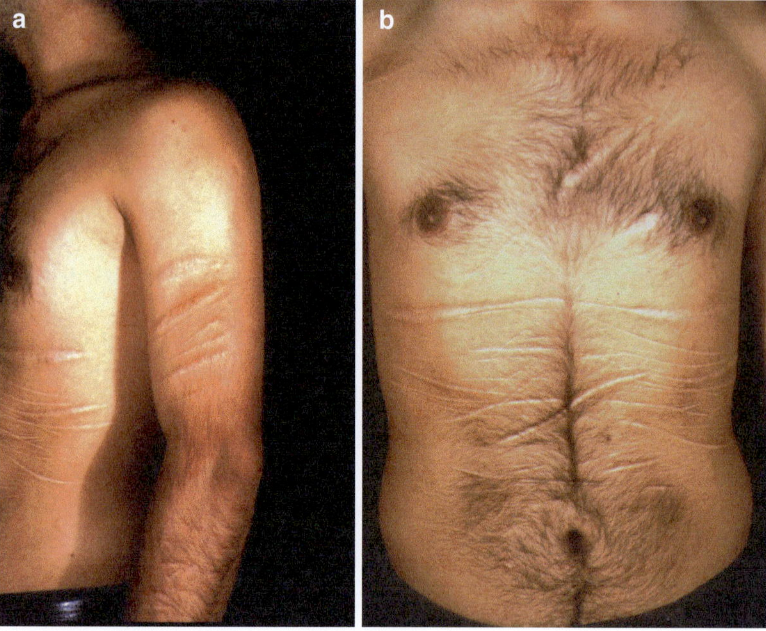

Fig. 3 Lesions on leg (**a**) and trunk (**b**) due to whip

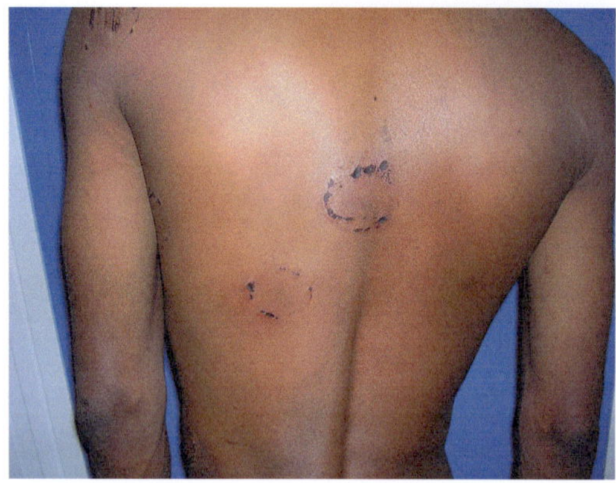

Fig. 4 Lesions due to human bite during the journey from Africa to Sicily

sible to proceed with the examination of the injuries if the person victim of possible torture wants it. Otherwise, it is necessary to strengthen the relationship of trust and possibly start a psychotherapeutic path. The acute lesions include the following:

- *Abrasions* reflecting the contours of the instrument or surface that inflicted the injury. There is a change of pigmentation (Hypo or hyperpigmentation) when repeated or deep abrasions occur.

- *Contusions* and bruises, whose extent and severity depend on applied force, structure, and vascularity of the contused tissue. Their absence, however, does not exclude violence.
- *Lacerations* on the protruding parts of the body, but if the violence is applied with sufficient force the skin can be torn on any part of the body.
- Erythema or edema, due to *burns*. However, electric burns are undetectable if water or gels are used.
- Cutting by knife, bayonet, or broken glass.
- *Petechiae*, due to asphyxiation.
- *Necrosis* due to chemicals.

The lesions carried out some time ago appear as follows:

- *Cicatricial alopecia*, linear circular zone (after prolonged application of tight ligatures).
- *Bruises*, gradually changing to violet, green, dark yellow, or pale yellow and then disappearing. It is very difficult, however, to date it accurately.
- *Scars*, resulting from whipping and representing healed lacerations; if due to cigarette

burns, appearing as circular or ovoid, macular scars with a hyper or a hypopigmented center and a hyperpigmented, relatively indistinct periphery; if due to burns applied with an electrically heated metal rod or gas lighter, they reflect the shape of the instrument and sharply demarcated with narrow hypertrophic or hyperpigmented marginal zones; if the nail matrix is burnt striped, thin, deformed nails with subsequent growth, appear; hypertrophic scars occur if pepper or other noxious substances are applied to open wounds.

The treatment requires a multidisciplinary approach, involving dermatologist, psychiatrist, orthopedist, and neurologist. The aim of the taking care includes caring for the physical lesions and taking care of the mental fractures.

However, the skin lesions due to torture must be differentiated by those due to self-injuring and those due to traditional medicine (i.e., coining or cupping).

It is relevant to know that self-injuring behavior (cutting, abrasions, and bruises) often is carried out by people already victims of torture, producing a mixed and overlapping scenario.

Independently on the etiology of abrasions/cutting, particular attention should be put on the possible subsequent infection, mainly when people live or lived in poor hygienic environments [37–41].

References

1. Schierup MH. The last pieces of a puzzling early meeting. Science. 2020;369(6511):1565–6. https://doi.org/10.1126/science.abe2766.
2. Matsu'ura S, Kondo M, Danhara T, Sakata S, Iwano H, Hirata T, Kurniawan I, Setiyabudi E, Takeshita Y, Hyodo M, Kitaba I, Sudo M, Danhara Y, Aziz F. Age control of the first appearance datum for Javanese Homo erectus in the Sangiran area. Science. 2020;367(6474):210–4. https://doi.org/10.1126/science.aau8556.
3. Carotenuto F, Tsikaridze N, Rook L, Lordkipanidze D, Longo L, Condemi S, Raia P. Venturing out safely: the biogeography of Homo erectus dispersal out of Africa. J Hum Evol. 2016;95:1–12. https://doi.org/10.1016/j.jhevol.2016.02.005.
4. Kappelman J, Alçiçek MC, Kazanci N, Schultz M, Ozkul M, Sen S. First Homo erectus from Turkey and implications for migrations into temperate Eurasia. Am J Phys Anthropol. 2008;135(1):110–6. https://doi.org/10.1002/ajpa.20739.
5. Hirschman C, et al., editors. Handbook of international migration, The: The American experience. Russell Sage Foundation, 1999. JSTOR, www.jstor.org/stable/10.7758/9781610442893. Accessed 9 Oct. 2020.
6. Simek R. "The emergence of the viking age: circumstances and conditions", "The vikings first Europeans VIII - XI century - the new discoveries of archaeology". 2005, pp. 24–25.
7. Baug I, Skre D, Heldal T, et al. The beginning of the viking age in the west. J Mari Arch. 2019;14:43–80. https://doi.org/10.1007/s11457-018-9221-3.
8. https://www.who.int/bangladesh/emergencies/rohingyacrisis/
9. www.unhcr.org/centralafrica/
10. https://www.msf.org/greece-evicts-vulnerable-refugees-leaves-them-streets
11. UNHCR Update on Lybia. 27 March 2020. www.unhcr.org
12. Morrone A. How we can approach survivors of torture. J Eur Acad Dermatol Venereol. 2019;33(7):1199–200. https://doi.org/10.1111/jdv.15724.
13. Morrone A. The skin and the catastrophes. J Eur Acad Dermatol Venereol. 2002;16(3):207–9. https://doi.org/10.1046/j.1468-3083.2002.00489.x.
14. Kloning T, Nowotny T, Alberer M, Hoelscher M, Hoffmann A, Froeschl G. Morbidity profile and sociodemographic characteristics of unaccompanied refugee minors seen by paediatric practices between October 2014 and February 2016 in Bavaria, Germany. BMC Public Health. 2018;18:983.
15. Di Meco E, Di Napoli A, Amato LM, Fortino A, Costanzo G, Rossi A, Mirisola C, Petrelli A, The INMP Team. Infectious and dermatological diseases among arriving migrants on the Italian coasts. Eur J Pub Health. 2018;28(5):910–6.
16. Pontarelli A, Marchese V, Scolari C, Capone S, El-Hamada I, Donato F, Moioli R, Girardi E, Cirillo DM, Castelli F, Matteelli A. Screening for active and latent tuberculosis among asylum seekers in Italy: a retrospective cohort analysis. Travel Med Infect Dis. 2019;27:39–45.
17. Ghosh S, Dronavalli M, Raman S. Tuberculosis infection in under-2-year-old refugees: Should we be screening? A systematic review and meta-regression analysis. J Paediatr Child Health. 2020; https://doi.org/10.1111/jpc.14701.
18. Lips P, de Jongh RT. Vitamin D deficiency in immigrants. Bone Reports. 2018;9:37–41.
19. Malik MS, Afzal M, Farid A, Khan FU, Mirza B, Waheed MT. Disease status of Afghan refugees and migrants in Pakistan. Public Health. 7:185. https://doi.org/10.3389/fpubh.2019.00185.

20. Kampouras A, Tzikos G, Partsanakis E, Roukas K, Tsiamitros S, Deligeorgakis D, Chorafa E, Schoina M, Iosifidis E. Child morbidity and disease burden in refugee camps in Mainland Greece. Children. 2019;6:46. https://doi.org/10.3390/children6030046.

21. Ozturk MK. Skin diseases in rural Nyala, Sudan (in a rural hospital, in 12 orphanages, and in two refugee camps). Int J Dermatol. 2019;58:1341–9.

22. Ziersch A, Due C, Walsh M. Discrimination: a health hazard for people from refugee and asylum-seeking backgrounds resettled in Australia. BMC Public Health. 2020;20:108. https://doi.org/10.1186/s12889-019-8068-3.

23. https://www.interno.gov.it/it/temi/immigrazione-e-asilo

24. https://ec.europa.eu/eurostat/statistics-explained/index.php/Asylum_statistics

25. Bongiorno G, Di Muccio T, Bianchi R, Gramiccia M, Gradoni L. Laboratory transmission of an Asian strain of Leishmania tropica by the bite of the southern European sand fly Phlebotomus perniciosus. Int J Parasitol. 2019;49:417–21.

26. Boggild AK, Caumes E, Grobusch MP, Schwartz E, Hynes NA, Libman M, Connor BA, Chakrabarti S, Parola P, Keystone JS, Nash T, Showler AJ, Schunk M, Asgeirsson H, Hamer DH, Kain KC, GeoSentinel Surveillance Network. Cutaneous and mucocutaneous leishmaniasis in travellers and migrants: a 20-year GeoSentinel Surveillance Network analysis. J Travel Med. 2019:1–11. https://doi.org/10.1093/jtm/taz055.

27. Abdalla NM, Abdelgani AM, Osman AA, Mohamed MN. Demographical and population dynamics impact on public health of cutaneous Leishmaniasis in Al-Madinah Almonawra, Saudi Arabia. Afr Health Sci. 2019;19(3):2421–30. https://doi.org/10.4314/ahs.v19i3.16.

28. Coates SJ, Thomas C, Chosidow O, Engelman D, Chang AY. Ectoparasites pediculosis and tungiasis. J Am Acad Dermatol. 2020;82(3):551–69. https://doi.org/10.1016/j.jaad.2019.05.110.

29. Woodruff CM, Chang AY. More than skin deep: severe iron deficiency anemia and eosinophilia associated with pediculosis capitis and corporis infestation. JAAD Case Rep. 2019;5:444–7.

30. Bouillon R, Leen A. Nutritional rickets: historic overview and plan for worldwide eradication. J Steroid Biochem Mol Biol. 2020;198:105563.

31. Sunderkötter C, Aebischer A, Neufeld M, Löser C, Kreuter A, Bialek R, Hamm H, Feldmeier H. Increase of scabies in Germany and development of resistant mites? Evidence and consequences. J German Soc Dermatol. 2018; https://doi.org/10.1111/ddg.13706.

32. Cheng TA, Mzahim B, Koenig KL, Alsugair A, Al-Wabel A, Saad Almutairi B, Maysa E, Kahn CA. Scabies: application of the novel identify-isolate-inform tool for detection and management. West J Emerg Med. 2020;21(2):191–8. https://doi.org/10.5811/westjem.2020.1.46120.

33. Ververs M, Muriithi JW, Burton A, Burton JW, Lawi AO. Scurvy outbreak among south sudanese adolescents and young men —Kakuma Refugee Camp, Kenya, 2017–2018. MMWR. 2019;68:3.

34. https://www.unhcr.org/news/briefing/2020/8/5f3248204/clashes-sudans-west-darfur-force-2500-seek-safety-chad.html

35. Saikal SL, Ge L, Mir A, Pace J, Abdulla H, Leong KF, Benelkahla M, Olabi B, Medialdea-Carrera R, Padovese V. Skin disease profile of Syrian refugees in Jordan: a field-mission assessment. JEADV. 2020;34:419–25.

36. Morrone A. A letter from a Syrian refugee camp in Lebanon: Dr. Aldo Morrone. Int J Dermatol. 2016;55(9):937–8. https://doi.org/10.1111/ijd.13424.

37. Dowd A. Uprooted minds: displacement, trauma and dissociation. J Anal Psychol. 2019;64(2):244–69.

38. Luci M. Displacement as trauma and trauma as displacement in the experience of refugees. J Anal Psychol. 2020;65(2):260–80.

39. Medical, Social, and Civic Needs of Displaced Persons. Bernard Naafs, Roderick Hay, Aldo Morrone, in Skin Disorders in Migrants. Editors: Morrone, Aldo, Hay, Roderick, Naafs, Bernard (Eds.). Skin disorders in migrants (pp. 5–7). https://doi.org/10.1007/978-3-030-37476-1_2.

40. Abuse, Self-Harm, Torture Signs, and PTSD. Aldo Morrone, Maria Lucia Dell'Anna in Skin Disorders in Migrants. Editors: Morrone, Aldo, Hay, Roderick, Naafs, Bernard (Eds.). Skin disorders in migrants (pp. 163). https://doi.org/10.1007/978-3-030-37476-1_20.

41. Essential medicines for immediate care in refugee camps. Peter Bakker in skin disorders in migrants. Editors: Morrone, Aldo, Hay, Roderick, Naafs, Bernard (Eds.). Skin disorders in migrants (pp. 233). https://doi.org/10.1007/978-3-030-37476-1_26.

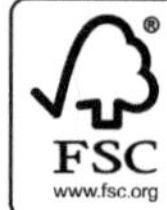

If you have any concerns about our products,
you can contact us on
ProductSafety@springernature.com

In case Publisher is established outside the EU,
the EU authorized representative is:
Springer Nature Customer Service Center GmbH
Europaplatz 3, 69115 Heidelberg, Germany

Printed by Libri Plureos GmbH
in Hamburg, Germany